Physiological and Pathological Aspects
of Eye Movements

Documenta Ophthalmologica
Proceedings Series volume 34

Editor: H.E. Henkes

Dr W. Junk Publishers   The Hague - Boston - London   1982

Physiological and Pathological Aspects of Eye Movements

Proceedings of a Workshop held at the Pont d'Oye Castle,
Habay-la-Neuve, Belgium, March 27-30, 1982
Sponsored by the Commission of the European Communities,
as advised by the Committee on Medical and Public Health Research

Edited by
A. Roucoux and M. Crommelinck

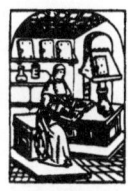

1982
Dr W. Junk Publishers
for the Commission of the European Communities

Distributors:

for the United States and Canada
Kluwer Boston, Inc.
190, Old Derby Street
Hingham, MA 02043
USA

for all other countries
Kluwer Academic Publishers Group
Distribution Center
P.O.Box 322
3300 AH Dordrecht
The Netherlands

Library of Congress Cataloging in Publication Data
Main entry under title:

Physiological and pathological aspects of eye movements.

  (Documenta ophthalmologica. Proceedings series ;
v. 34)
    1. Eye--Movements--Congresses. 2. Eye--Movement
disorders--Congresses. I. Roucoux, A.
II. Crommelinck, M. III. Commission of the European
Communities. IV. Commission of the European Communities.
Committee on Medical and Public Health Research.
V. Series. [DNLM: 1. Eye movements--Congresses.
2. Nystagmus--Congresses. W3 D0637 v.34 / WW 400 P578
1982]
QP477.5.P48 1982   612'.846   82-17986

ISBN-13: 978-94-009-8002-0   e-ISBN-13: 978-94-009-8000-6
DOI: 10.1007/978-94-009-8000-6

Publication arranged by:
Commission of the European Communities
Directorate-General Information Market and Innovation,
Luxembourg

EUR 8180

LEGAL NOTICE

Neither the Commission of the European Communities nor any person acting on behalf of the
Commission is reponsible for the use which might be made of the following information.

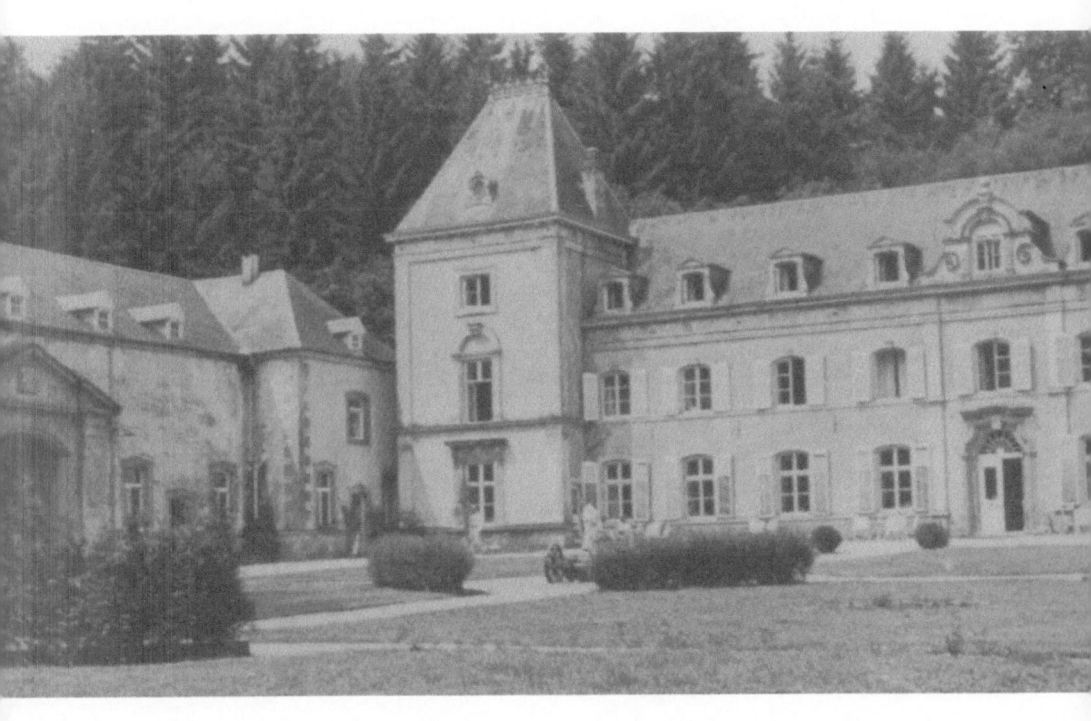

Pont d'Oye Castle, Habay-la-Neuve, Belgium.

CONTENTS

X

INTRODUCTION

This volume contains the proceedings of a workshop entitled "Physiological and Pathological Aspects of Eye Movements" held at the Pont d'Oye Castle, Habay-la-Neuve, Belgium. March 27-30 1982.

The meeting was sponsored by the European Communities. It brought together specialists of oculomotricity mainly from Europe but also from North-America. With such actions, the Communities want to encourage international and multidisciplinary contacts between researchers of a particular field. Oculomotor neuroscientists, for quite a long time, have developed such contacts. This cooperation — this is not so common in biological research — embodies various approaches, from basic mechanisms to behavioral studies, but also this applied science that medicine is or should be. Many basic discoveries about eye movement mechanisms, made with the help of human of animal subjects, have found rapid medical applications in neurology, neuro-ophthalmology or otolaryngology. This is illustrated in this book by the fact that results obtained on rats or cats are interspersed with reports of clinical investigations.

The workshop was mainly focused onto three themes: (a) eye and head movements in man, (b) visuo-vestibular interaction and (c) eye-head coordination. In each theme, one or more "review" papers were included. In addition, most of the oral presentations or posters on display mainly contained unpublished material.

It is our hope that this book will be useful to the scientific reader but will also contribute showing the intense vitality of eye movement research outside the restricted sphere of academies and universities. It is our wish that such workshop will be repeated and will further materialize the European community of neuroscientists.

We wish to thank Prof. E. Levi from the Directorate-General for Science, Research and Development who greatly helped organizing the Workshop.

Finally, we are certain that those who met in the Pont d'Oye will keep an excellent memory of this pleasant and welcoming place.

The Editors

CONTROL OF GAZE IN MAN: SYNTHESIS OF PURSUIT, OPTOKINETIC AND VESTIBULO-OCULAR SYSTEMS

H. COLLEWIJN, P. CONIJN, A.J. MARTINS[+], E.P. TAMMINGA and
G.C. VAN DIE (Rotterdam, Netherlands and [+]College Park, Md, USA)

INTRODUCTION

Human vision with maximal spatial resolution is only possible
in the narrow sector of the visual field covered by the fovea. As
a consequence we have to frequently redirect our gaze to examine
a larger part of the world in any detail. This sampling process
in space and time can be studied in a simplified form with a
stationary observer (a subject on a biteboard) looking at a stationary pattern. As shown already by Dodge (1903) and later by
many others (e.g. Yarbus, 1967) our eye movements under such
circumstances consist almost exclusively of step-displacements,
called saccades. Significantly, the afoveate rabbit makes practically no eye movements in a similar condition. Except for some slight
tremor and drift, the rabbit's eye is kept stable most of the time
when the head is fixed (see Collewijn, 1981). Also human subjects
with a stabilized head maintain a steady gaze in the intersaccadic
intervals, especially when they are instructed to fixate a small
target. A difference with the rabbit (and probably all other mammals
as well, inclusive monkeys) is that humans tend to make frequent
small saccades (microsaccades) which, however, can be suppressed
by voluntary effort. Standard deviations of about 5 min arc on both
the horizontal and vertical meridian have been reported for human
fixation (for reviews see Steinman et al., 1973; 1982). A visual
target is necessary to maintain this kind of stability. In the
dark, the eyes of rabbit (Collewijn, 1970) as well as man
(Skavenski and Steinman, 1970) drift with velocities of about 1o/s.
Thus, even with the head stabilized we need visual feedback to
maintain a steady gaze.
    The control of gaze under more natural circumstances is compli-
cated by two facts. Firstly, many visual targets are moving and,
secondly, our heads are moving. Real object motion is usually
restricted to parts of the visual surroundings which move relative
to a stationary background. We are able to pursue such moving
objects to keep their image in the fovea. For this we use not
only saccades, but also smooth, continuous eye movements. Although
several studies have analysed the dynamic performance of this
pursuit system, practically all our knowledge is based on experiments in which the head is stabilized and a single moving target
is shown without a background. A stationary background, present
under normal conditions, might considerably influence pursuit by
providing an opposite motion stimulus as soon as the target is
pursued with a smooth eye movement. Thus, pursuit in the real world
has to deal with conflicting stimuli on the central and peripheral
retina. We know that a moving background without a distinct target
induces a global form of pursuit, known as optokinetic nystagmus
(OKN). Major questions then in the understanding of pursuit and OKN
concern the interplay between target and background, the role of
the central and peripheral retina, and eventually the selective
attentional processes that determine that something is a target.
    Control of gaze becomes enormously more complex when we allow
motion of the head. In a first approximation, simple rotation of the
head can be added to rotations of the eye in the head, gaze being

Roucoux, A. and Crommelinck, M. (eds.): Physiological and Pathological Aspects of Eye Movements.
© *1982, Dr W. Junk Publishers, The Hague, Boston, London.* ISBN-13: 978-94-009-8002-0

the sum of eye and head position. Coordinated eye and head movements could then be described as the output of an expanded oculomotor system, incorporating not only the traditional extraocular muscles but also the neck muscles and most other muscles used in postural control. However, most head and body movements are not made to direct our gaze, and should not result in displacements of gaze. To filter out the non gaze related head movements the vestibulo-ocular reflex (VOR), specifically the canal-ocular reflex was developed. This provides compensatory eye rotations which are opposite and roughly equal to head rotations, in cooperation with the visually induced OKN.

These compensatory eye movements reduce the slip-velocities of the retinal images. They must be of fundamental importance in vision, independently of the development of foveal vision, as they are functioning very well in the afoveate rabbit and indeed in all species studied.

The VOR and visual pursuit systems must function together in a symbiotic way (Robinson, 1977) because neither of the two systems alone has sufficient dynamic range to cover the full spectrum of natural head motion. Visual control of eye movements is restricted by a long delay (about 100 ms) and rather low limits on velocity and acceleration (Lisberger et al., 1981), but works well for low and steady velocities. The VOR is fast and effective through all but the lowest naturally occurring frequencies, but being a feed-forward system it will by itself not maintain a correct gain under changing conditions. Only the visual system can signal whether the control of eye movements is optimal.

The requirements for adaptation of compensatory eye movements, on a short as well as long term are indeed formidable. One reason is the structure of our body: even for apparently simple rotations the rotational axes of head and body do not coincide with each other or with the nodal point of the eye's optical system. The other reason is the three-dimensional structure of the world, in which targets and backgrounds are at different optical distances. These facts alone make that a standard gain of unity for compensatory systems would be inappropriate.

However, in real life motion is even more complex. Pure rotations of the head are a rarity; normal head motions will consist of a mixture of rotatory and linear displacements. As soon as linear displacements occur, true compensation for the whole visual field by counterrotation of the eye is by definition impossible. Furthermore, parallax motion between close and distant objects will occur. All these factors make that optimal stabilization of the retinal image during unrestricted head movements can be achieved by counterrotation of the eye only for a selected, small part of the surroundings. Logically one would expect vision to be optimized for the central retina. Thus, we can argue that all compensatory movements (visual and vestibular) and their adaptation should be controlled mainly by the central part of the retina, since this part is crucial for our vision, and since motion information provided by the peripheral retina will be often uncorrelated or in conflict. This holds also for the adaptive processes necessary on a slightly longer term as a result of growth, degeneration, damage or the simple wearing of eye glasses, which magnify or reduce the visual surroundings and their apparent motion induced by head movements.

Such considerations have led us to conducting experiments which address the following questions:

-What is the contribution of the central and peripheral retina
 to OKN?
-What is the effect of a stationary, structured background on
 pursuit, and of a moving background on fixation?
-How effective is compensation by the VOR during natural head
 movements?
-How fast does the VOR change its amplitude to adapt to
 altered requirements?
-How well can we pursue continuously moving targets by
 coordinated eye and head movements?

OPTOKINETIC NYSTAGMUS
Methods
Horizontal eye position was measured with the technique of the
scleral induction coil in a rotating magnetic field (Collewijn,
1977). The scleral coil was embedded in a self-adhering silicone
annulus, mounted around the limbus (Collewijn et al., 1975). This
technique provides linear recording of gaze direction over angles
up to 360° with perfect stability, resolution better than 0.1^o and
absolute calibration (invariant for annuli and subjects). Subjects
were seated with the head on a chin rest in the center of a hemi-
cylindrical, homogeneously white screen with a radius of 0.8 m.
The optical stimulus was projected from a central rotating cylinder
and consisted of square wave gratings with different spatial
frequencies. The pattern extended 90° to both sides, 38° upwards,
67° downwards and could be rotated at velocities of 6 - 180°/s in
both directions. The projection system could be partly occluded by
cylindrical masks of different sizes, which deleted selected sectors
of the projected stripe pattern. The angular position of the mask
was coupled to the eye position by a servo-positioning system in
such a way that the exposed and masked parts of the pattern remained
projected on the same selected parts of the retina, even though the
eyes were moving. In this way the optokinetic contribution of the
different parts of the retina could be systematically investigated.
Vision was monocular; the eye without the annulus was covered.
Subjects were instructed to pay full attention to the moving stripe
pattern, wherever it was located, without attempting to deliberately
pursue a particular stripe. Trials of 16 s were digitally stored by
a computer. The average slow phase velocity was calculated after
deletion of all saccades and expressed as gain, the ratio slow
phase eye velocity / stimulus velocity. Thus the values presented
are averages, not maxima.

Results
Full field stimulation: effects of pattern and velocity.
Average gain for 5 subjects and 2 directions during unobstructed
stimulation of the whole right retina at velocities from 6 - 180°/s
is shown in the upper series of graphs (squares) in Fig. 1. The
different lines represent stimulus gratings with a period of 2°
(1° white - 1° black); 5°; 10° and 20°. These data suggest several
conclusions. The maximal gain, reached for the lower stimulus velocities (6 and 12°/s) is smaller than unity and of the order of 0.9.
(Standard deviations were about 0.15). Higher stimulus velocities
result in progressively decreasing gain, to about 0.2 at 180°/s.
These trends were not systematically influenced by the spatial
frequency of the pattern in the range used (0.05 - 0.5 cycles/deg).

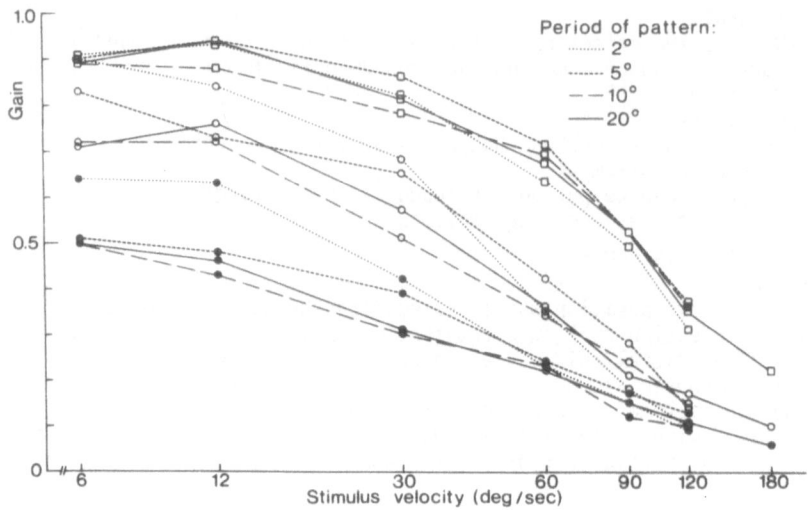

Fig. 1. Optokinetic slow phase gain as a function of velocity and wavelength of pattern. Open squares: full field stimulus (width 180°). Closed circles: central 20° of retina unstimulated. Open circles: only central 20° of retina stimulated.

Central or peripheral stimulation.
The lower set of graphs (filled circles) in Fig. 1 shows responses to the same stimuli with a central sector of 20° (10° at each side of the fixation point) deleted. Although this eliminated only 11% of the stimulus surface, the effect was dramatic. Gain decreased to 1/3-1/2 of the full field values. Once more gain was similar for the various patterns, except that at the lower velocities the pattern with the 2° period was slightly more effective.

The middle set of graphs (open circles) in Fig. 1 shows the effect of masking the whole stimulus except the central 20° centered around the fixation point. The responses were inferior to those in the full field situation, but considerably better than with peripheral stimulation. The response to the pattern with 2° period was peculiar as it was identical to the full field response at 6°/s and to the peripheral response at 120°/s.

Gain as a function of the width and location of the retinal stimulus is shown in Fig. 2 (averages and S.D. of 5 subjects), for a stimulus of 12°/s and 5° wavelength. On the left side, the effect of progressive peripheral masking is shown. At this moderate velocity, OKN gain decreased only slightly even when just a central sector of 5°° (exposing two contrast lines) was stimulated. The central retinal location of this narrow stimulus was critical for this result, as a stimulus 10° wide centered at 10° to the right or left of the fovea (columns) was a relatively poor stimulus. The right side of Fig. 2 shows the complementary situation, in which an increasing central sector was occluded. Even a central occlusion only 5° wide significantly lowered OKN gain, which declined further to about 1/3 of full field level when a zone of 30° was deleted. Once again the central retinal location of the occlusion was critical; a shift of the 10° mask from the center to 10° peripheral (columns) restored OKN gain to almost full field value.

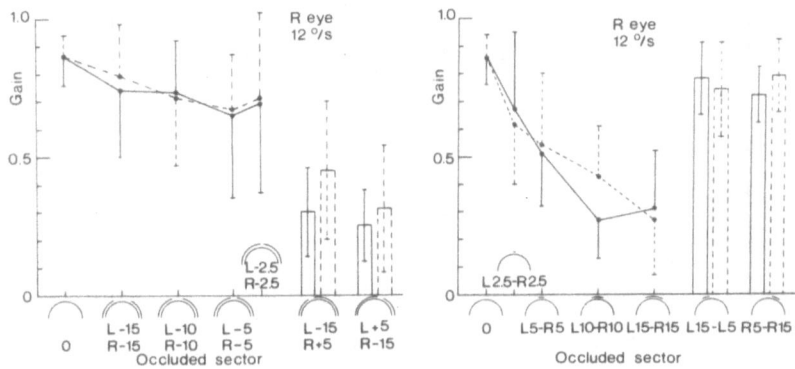

Fig. 2. Optokinetic slow phase gain as a function of stimulated retinal sector. The occluded zones are indicated on the abscissa. Continuous lines: rotation to the left; interrupted lines: rotation to the right.

Effect of central scotoma.

We had the opportunity to record OKN in a patient (female, age 60) with a circumscript, absolute central scotoma of the right eye (Fig. 3) with an extension of about 10 x 20°. The ethiology of the lesion was unknown but it had been present and stationary since childhood. Vision with the left eye was completely normal. We tested both eyes separately and monocularly (coil in the seeing eye) with full field stimulation. The results, shown in detail in Fig. 4, demonstrate a decrease in OKN gain of the scotomatous eye strikingly similar to the defect induced in normal subjects by a central occlusion.

Conclusions

These results, parts of which have been published in greater detail (Van Die, Collewijn, 1982), show conclusively that the central retina is of paramount importance in the control of OKN. Fig. 2 suggests that a central sector 5° wide is about as powerful to elicit OKN as the entire retina peripheral to this area. Similar relations were found in the patient with a central scotoma of very long standing. Our results agree with the tendencies found in several previous investigations for man (Cheng, Outerbridge, 1975; Dubois, Collewijn, 1979b), monkey (Körner, Schiller, 1972) and rabbit (Dubois, Collewijn, 1979a). They do not support the claims by Hood (1967, 1975) that OKN is predominantly controlled by the peripheral retina.

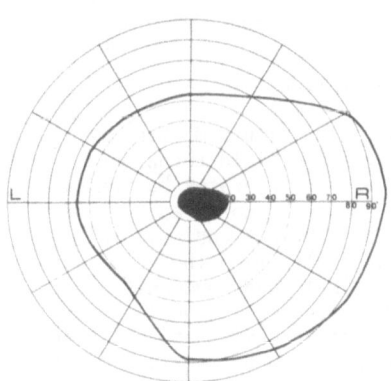

Fig. 3. Visual field of right eye of patient with central, absolute scotoma.

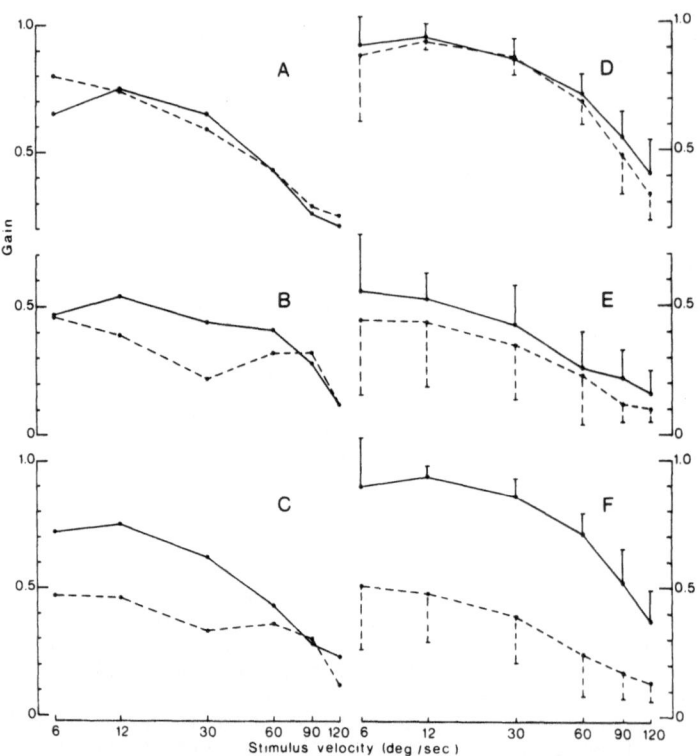

Fig. 4. OKN gain of patient with central scotoma of right eye and normal left eye (A - C) and average gain of 5 normals (D - F) with various maskings of the stimulus. A: normal eye of patient; D: full field stimulation in normals. B: scotomatous eye of patient; E: normals with central sector of 20⁰ masked. In A, B, D and E lines represent left rotation, dots right rotation. C: averages for both directions for normal (line) and scotomatous eye (dots) of patient. F: average gains for both directions for 5 normal subjects during full field stimulation (line) and stimulation with central 20⁰ deleted (dots). Pattern wavelength: 5⁰.

THE VESTIBULO-OCULAR REFLEX AND ITS ADAPTATION
Methods
These experiments were done in collaboration with R.M. Steinman, using the "Maryland version" of the revolving field technique. Implementation of digital techniques in this apparatus has resulted in a resolution better than 1 min arc. Subjects were seated on a motor-driven chair at 12.2 m distance of a bright and colorful target. They were either oscillated passively, with the head supported on a biteboard or made active sinusoidal head movements, paced by a metronome. Both types of motion were tested in the light and in complete darkness. Subjects were tested in their habitual visual conditions as well as after putting on positive or negative glasses. These changed the magnification factor of relative motion of the visual world induced by head motion. To maintain retinal stability the subjects had to recalibrate their compensatory eye movements. We measured the effects of such changed conditions upon the VOR,

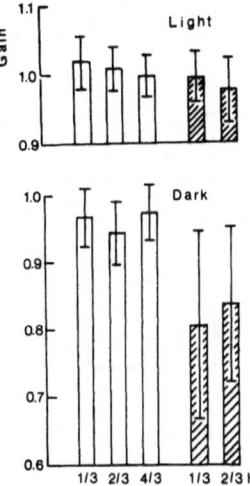

Fig. 5. Gain of compensatory
eye movements in the light and
dark for active (open columns)
and passive (hatched columns)
head motion at an amplitude of
about 17° and frequencies as
indicated. Average (and 1 S.D.)
effective values for 5 subjects
in baseline conditions.

recorded in light and darkness. The visual stimulus (inclusive a
small background) subtended 4.7°. In most cases the altered optical
conditions caused blurred vision as the spectacles' refraction was
not correct for maximal acuity.

The apparatus recorded the absolute angles in space of the eye
and head. Eye position in the head was derived as the difference.
These we shall call *nominal* angles. When spectacles are worn the
effective gaze direction is changed as a function of the magnification factor of the glasses. Thus, nominal and effective values
have to be distinguished for the direction of gaze and for the gain
of compensatory eye movements. For the derivation of the rather
complex relations between these several parameters we refer to
Collewijn et al. (in preparation). Several aspects of this work
have been already reported (Steinman, Collewijn, 1980; Collewijn et
al., 1981a, b; Steinman et al.,1982).

Results
Baseline performance.
The average effective gains (incorporating magnification factors
for subjects wearing spectacles normally) for 5 subjects in baseline condition are shown in Fig. 5. Several important trends can be
seen. During active head motion in the light gain is close to
unity, although it is rarily precisely one. The slight deviation
of gain from unity (by usually less than 5%) results in appreciable
modulation of gaze by head movements, as evident in the graphs of
gaze. As an example see the baseline performance (Fig. 6A) of a
myopic subject (AM) wearing negative glasses which make the ideal
value of his nominal gain for the right eye (recorded here) 0.86,
corresponding to a perfect effective gain of 1.0. Actually, his
right eye had a nominal gain of 0.90 and an effective gain of 1.04
in the light, with as a result slight overcompensation (motion of
effective gaze out of phase with the head). This amount of instability was commonly found. In addition to the possible causes of a
non-unity gain discussed in the Introduction we should mention that
the power of the left and right spectacle glasses of AM was unequal,
and that the left eye showed an effective undercompensation (gain
0.96). Different demands on both eyes appear to result in a compro-

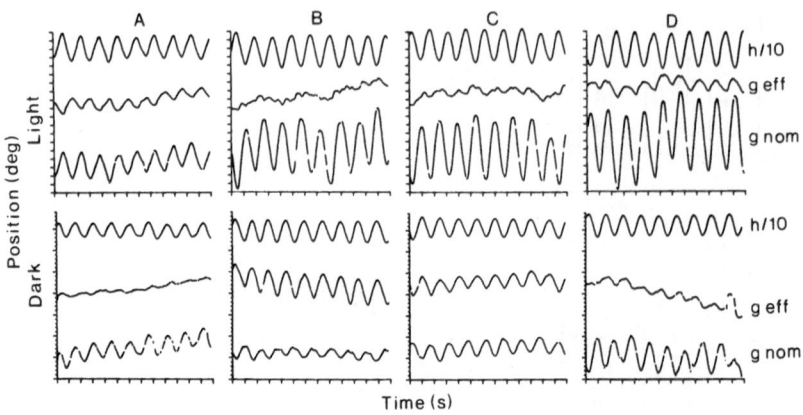

Fig. 6. Recordings of head position (divided by 10) and nominal and effective cumulative gaze with saccades deleted during active head movements at 2/3 Hz in light and dark. A: baseline condition with negative spectacles. B, C, D: 5, 10 and 40 min after change to +5 D spectacles. Subject AM.

mise as the eyes seem to be unable to change their gain individually.

For passive motion in the light, effective gain (averaged over subjects, frequencies and eyes; Fig. 5) was slightly lower (0.985 + 0.041 S.D.) than during active motion (1.014 + 0.035 for the same frequencies). This difference was significant ($\bar{p}$<0.001), but the apparent effect of frequency was not significant.

For active head motion in the dark average effective gain (3 frequencies, 2 eyes) was 0.963 + 0.044 (S.D.), which was 0.045 lower than for similar motion in the light. The difference, although surprisingly small, was highly significant (p<0.0005). The difference is visible in Fig. 6A, which instead of the slight overcompensation in the light shows almost perfect compensation in the dark.

Finally, for passive motion in the dark (at 1/3 and 2/3 Hz) gain was 0.821 + 0.127 (S.D.), compared to 0.957 + 0.046 (S.D.) for the same frequencies during active movement. The difference of 0.136 was highly significant (p<0.0005). Notice that also the variability (S.D.) was higher than in any other condition. Some other recent reports in which the VOR was tested by active head motion (Takahashi et al., 1980; Tomlinson et al., 1980) have similarly mentioned gains much closer to unity than the traditionally reported values for this frequency range, varying between 0.43 (Meiry, 1971) and 0.54 - 0.90 (Barnes, Forbat, 1979) with many other results in between these values (Benson, 1970; Gonshor, Melvill Jones, 1976a; Barr et al., 1976). Such values, measured with passive motion, are clearly not representative for the performance of the VOR during normal, active movement. Mental arithmetic activity of the subject is often used to maintain alertness, although the relation of calculation to a steady gaze is not obvious and such activity could even be distractive. Specific instructions to the subject to fixate an imagined, stationary target while being rotated passively have resulted in higher VOR gains (Barr et al., 1976). However, the simple instruction to move the head actively may be at least as effective.

At this moment we do not know whether the improvement of the VOR by active head motion is due to the specific activity of the

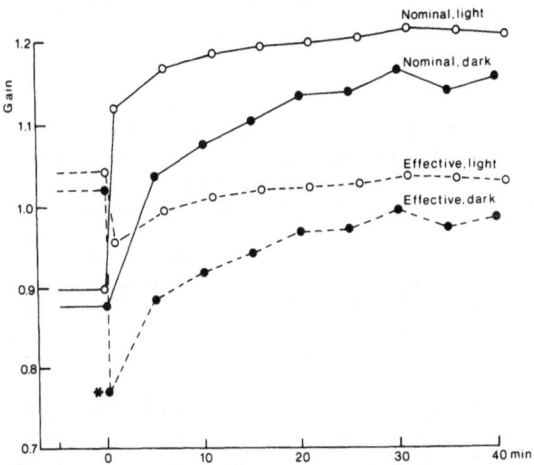

Fig. 7. Time course of nominal and effective gain for the same experiment as shown in Fig. 6. Asterisk: theoretical level to which effective gain in the dark was reduced by the positive spectacles.

subject or to additional proprioceptive signals from the neck, which may contribute to ocular stability via the cervico-ocular reflex. However, the status of this reflex in man is far from clear (Barnes, Forbat, 1979; Barlow, Freedman, 1980).

Adaptation of the VOR.
The results described above make it abundantly clear that the VOR is not a stationary system with a constant input-output relation. On the contrary, it is subject to strong modulatory influences. One of the relevant signals in this respect is systematic retinal image slip in conjunction with head motion. Such slip calls for increase or decrease in gain of the VOR, depending on the sign.

Adaptation of the VOR to modified visual motion signals has been clearly demonstrated in recent years in man (Gauthier, Robinson, 1975; Gonshor, Melvill Jones, 1976a, b), monkey (Miles, Eighmy, 1980) and several non-primates. Dissociations between head and eye movements were generally effected by inverting prisms or telescopic spectacles with a magnification factor far removed from 1 (viz. 0.5 or 2.0). The resulting adaptation was slow (taking several days or weeks) and incomplete. We contend that the demands in these experiments were high and that adaptation to smaller, more physiological changes is fast and virtually complete.

As an example, Fig. 6 shows the changes of the VOR in light and dark during a period of 40 min after AM changed his normal, negative glasses for positive glasses (+5 D). This required his compensatory eye movements to enlarge by 36%. The head was oscillated actively at 2/3 Hz during the whole period while the subject fixated the target or was briefly in darkness to measure the VOR in the dark.

The time course of the nominal and effective gain is shown in Fig. 7. The change from negative (reducing) to positive (magnifying) spectacles required the nominal eye movements to change from undercompensation to overcompensation. In the light, this change was readily achieved. In Fig. 6 B (light) the eyes move already out of phase with the head and the amplitude is growing further in the later recordings (Fig. 6 C, D). After 40 min the effective gaze movements in the light were virtually identical to those in the baseline condition. The time course of these changes in the light (Fig. 7) was very fast and effective gain reached an early asymptotic level close to the original level after about 30 min. The fact that these changes were not instantaneous illustrates that even in the light plasticity (learning) is involved in addition to mere algebraic summation of visual and vestibular responses.

The more interesting point is the immediate transfer of these changes to the VOR measured in darkness. Even after only 5 min training (Fig. 6 B, dark) the nominal gaze movements were in counterphase instead of in phase (Fig. 6 A, dark) and the amplitude was rapidly growing in the later recordings (Fig. 6 B - D, dark). After 30 min, effective gain in the dark was restored to 0.98 (Fig. 7), compared to the baseline value of 1.02.

This result was typical for our experiments on short term adaptation. We have to conclude that adaptation of compensatory eye movements (in light and darkness) is much faster than generally assumed until now and can be controlled by a small, central, blurred stimulus.

TARGET AND BACKGROUND
Methods
Eye movements were recorded with the scleral coil and phaselocked amplification. The horizontal and vertical components were separated by 90^0 phase shifts in the magnetic fields and detection systems Robinson, 1963). Subjects were seated with the head supported on a chin rest and viewed a large translucent screen (90 x 90^0), upon which stimuli were projected via servo-controlled mirrors. The targer was a bright laser spot (dia 7 min arc); the background was a fine random dot pattern (elements 15 min arc). Motion of the stimuli was numerically controlled by the computer which was also used to store and process the data. Calculations included separation of smooth and saccadic components, calculation of gain and phase in the frequency domain and of the retinal position error in the time domain. Only some aspects of these experiments are discussed here. We have briefly reported some effects of a background before (Tamminga, Collewijn, 1981). Here we shall discuss only two-dimensional pursuit of single sine waves, triangular waves and mixtures of sine waves, which were two-dimensionally composed into circular, rhomboid and pseudo-random motion.

Results
Pursuit with and without a structured background.
The most conspicuous effect of a background was a shift from smooth to saccadic pursuit, the sum of these components remaining about equal in amplitude. Examples of pursuit of a target following a circular or rhomboid trajectory are shown in Fig. 8 as a function of time and in Fig. 9 as two-dimensional plots. The circular motion without background (Fig. 8 A) was pursued quite smoothly with few saccades, as should be expected for this highly regular motion. A stationary background caused a slowdown of the smooth pursuit with the insertion of frequent corrective saccades. Fig. 9 also shows that without a background saccades were mostly made in a radial direction as course corrections, while with a background they were made mainly in a tangential direction to catch up with the target. Pursuit of rhomboid motion is much more difficult than pursuit of circular motion. Especially the corners create difficulties, although

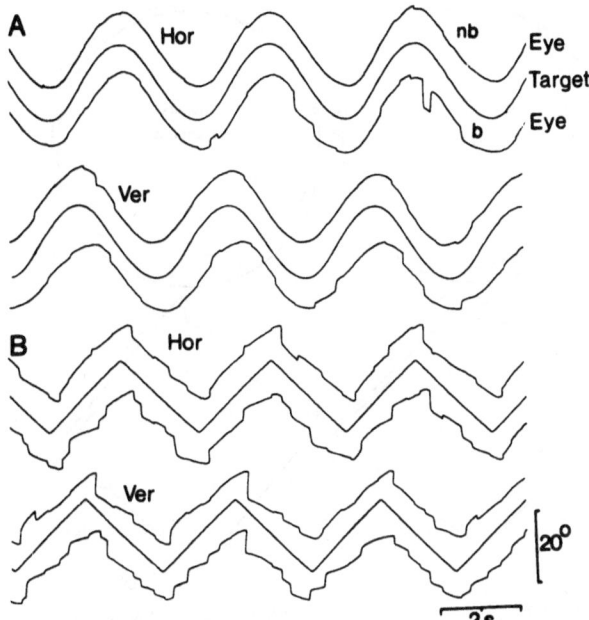

Fig. 8. Horizontal and vertical pursuit of sine waves and triangular waves (frequency 0.275 Hz; amplitude 10°) with 90° phase shift to form a circle (A) and a rhomboid (B). Of each group of three traces the middle one represents target position and the others eye position during pursuit without background (nb; upper trace) and with background (b; lower trace).

they are completely predictable. Even without a background a considerable number of saccades is made (Fig. 8 B, 9). In the presence of a background pursuit deteriorated further and the number of saccades increased.

An additional feature of the pursuit of rhomboid motion (Fig. 9) was the frequent occurrence of directional errors, independent of the presence of a background. This resulted frequently in the rotation of the figure formed by the eye motion relative to the trajectory of the target. The rotation was in the sense of the target motion and thus appears to be anticipatory in nature.

The average effect of the background on smooth pursuit gain is summarized for 5 subjects in Table 1 for two-dimensional pursuit of a rhomboid motion (frequency 0.275 Hz; amplitude 10°; horizontal and vertical velocity components 11°/s). To exclude any unspecific effect of an illuminated background all pursuit tasks were also done while the background was illuminated diffusely at the average luminance level of the structured background. The values in Table 1

Table 1. Average gain ($\pm$ S.D.) of 5 subjects for smooth pursuit of rhomboid motion.

Direction	Background		
	Dark	Light	Structured
Horizontal	0.829 + 0.052	0.838 + 0.050	0.728 + 0.106
Vertical	0.798 + 0.132	0.770 + 0.128	0.621 + 0.151

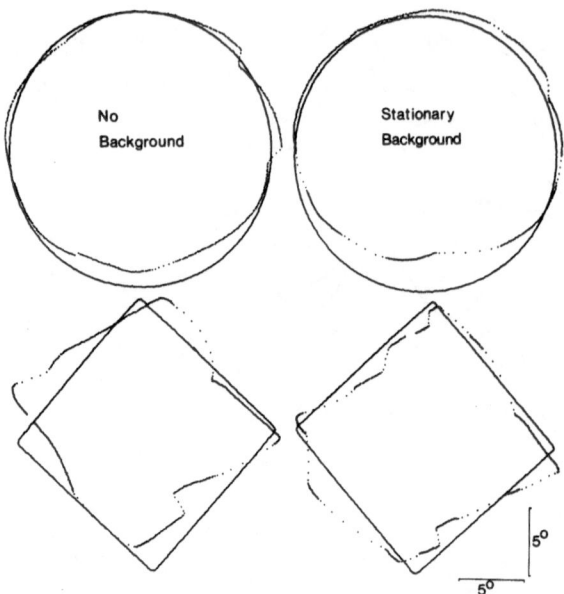

Fig. 9. X-Y plots of pursuit of a circular and rhomboid target motion with and without a stationary background. Target motion is clockwise, 1 revolution/3.64 s. Interval between two successive points in eye position plot: 8 ms.

represent average smooth pursuit gain ($\pm$ S.D.) after deletion of the saccades and of the corners. It is clear that smooth pursuit is inhibited by a structured, but not by a homogeneously lighted background. However, this does not result in a systematically larger distance of the retinal image of the target from the fovea. This error, summed for pursuit in symmetrical directions (right-left; up-down) has an average value not significantly different from zero and a pseudo-normal distribution which can be characterized by its standard deviation. Some values of this are given in Table 2 for pursuit of a circular, rhomboid and pseudo-random trajectory. It is obvious that the error is hardly increased by a background. This means that the increased number of saccades is effective in limiting the error to the same level as tolerated without a back ground. Other tendencies revealed by Table 2 are that the vertical

Table 2. Average standard deviations (in degrees) for 5 subjects of retinal error during two-dimensional pursuit of different stimulus configurations.

Configuration	Component	Background		
		Dark	Light	Structured
Circle	Horizontal	0.459	0.358	0.459
(0.275 Hz)	Vertical	0.562	0.508	0.621
Sum of sines	Horizontal	0.558	0.412	0.506
(0.15-0.78 Hz)	Vertical	0.642	0.501	0.636
Rhomboid	Horizontal	0.553	0.538	0.629
(0.275 Hz)	Vertical	0.671	0.679	0.703

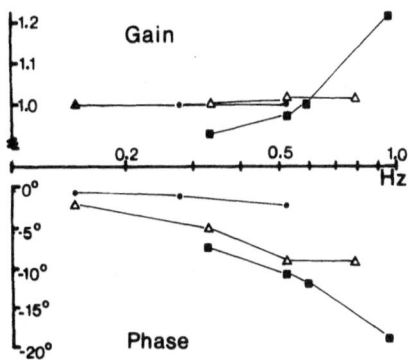

Fig. 10. Bode plots for horizontal pursuit of sine waves. Total eye movement including saccades. Dots: 3 single sine waves, measured in separate trials. Triangles: sum of 4 sine waves (0.15 - 0.78 Hz). Squares: sum of 4 sine waves (0.34 - 0.95 Hz).

error is always slightly larger than the horizontal error and that the error increases in the order pursuit of circle - two-dimensional sum of sines - rhomboid.

Analysis of the total eye movement (saccadic plus smooth) in the frequency domain shows that errors develop as a result of deviations of gain as well as phase from the ideal values of 1.0 and 0⁰. Moreover the pursuit system is not stationary but dependent on the type of stimulus. This is illustrated for horizontal pursuit in the Bode plots of Fig. 10. Single sine waves, tested individually are tracked with unity gain and a very small phase error, attributable to a delay of about 100 ms. A mixture of sines in the same frequency range (triangles) is pursued with about the same gain but considerably larger phase lag. A similar mixture of slightly higher frequency (Fig. 10, squares) is pursued with a phase lag of about 20⁰ and a gain increased to about 1.2 at 1 Hz. Several of these trends have been known for a long time (e.g. Stark et al., 1962).

Fixation with a moving background.
Typical fixation patterns for a stationary target (the same laser spot) are shown in Fig. 11, and the average standard deviations for 5 naive subjects for fixation periods of 30 s are shown in Table 3. Without a background standard deviations were equal in horizontal and vertical direction. They were larger than the values (about 5 min arc) typically mentioned in the literature. This may be due to the fact that they were obtained in completely naive subjects who participated for the very first time in an oculomotor experiment, while the recorded periods were rather long (30 s) and contained several blinks. More important than the absolute value is the effect of a background. When it was stationary, it reduced the standard deviation of fixation in both dimensions, mainly by reducing drift velocities (Fig. 11 B and C). A horizontally moving background (frequency 0.275 Hz; amplitude 1⁰) induced a marked response. The slow component followed the background with an average gain of 0.2 for this particular stimulus (but otherwise not linearly related

Table 3. Average standard deviations (in degrees) of fixation for 5 naive subjects.

Condition	Horizontal	Vertical
No background	0.197	0.192
Stationary background	0.157	0.163
Moving background	0.228	0.142

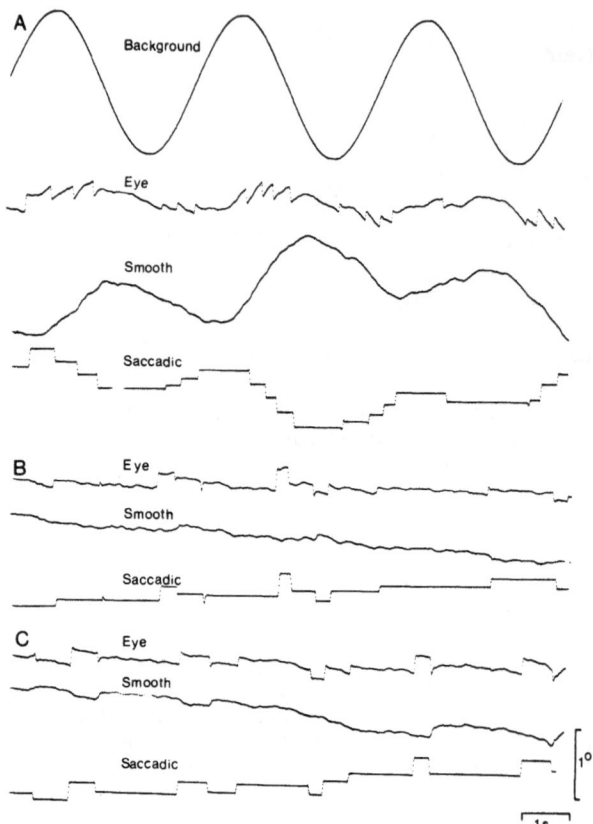

Fig. 11. Fixation in the presence of a moving background (A), a stationary background (B) and no background (C). Total horizontal eye movements are shown (Eye) as well as computer-reconstructed cumulative smooth and saccadic components.

to stimulus amplitude) and an average phase lag of 90°. Of course, pursuit of a similar frequency in a normal way shows practically no phase lag (Fig. 10). Thus, the eye is not simply dragged along with the background, nor does it follow the apparent opposite target motion which is often vividly perceived in this experiment. Rather, eye displacement is in phase with the velocity of this perceived target movement. More research will be needed to understand this phenomenon.

Remarkably, the absolute fixation error is only slightly increased by the moving background (Table 3), because the induced smooth movements are almost completely offset by saccades in the opposite direction. The vertical component of fixation was not affected by the horizontal motion of the background.

Conclusions
Pursuit and fixation are demonstrably affected by a structured background. However, this influence is limited and any deficiencies of the smooth eye movements are corrected by saccades which maintain overall accuracy of gaze.

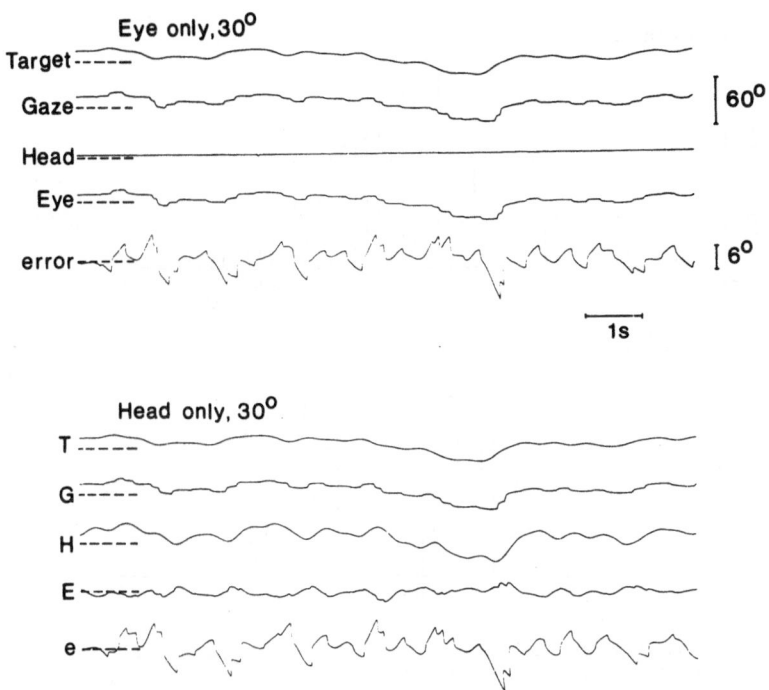

Fig. 12. Movements of target, gaze, head, eye and retinal position error (effective gaze minus target; shown at 10 x higher sensitivity). An identical episode of target motion is pursued with the eye only and with a maximal contribution by head movements. Maximal deviation of target: 30°. Interrupted lines represent zero levels.

PURSUIT WITH COORDINATED EYE AND HEAD MOVEMENTS
Methods
The same equipment was used with which OKN was investigated, except that a second sensor coil was attached to the head. The target was a similar laser spot as used in the other pursuit experiments. Its position on the cylindrical screen was linearly controlled up to eccentricities of 60°. Due to the short distance of the target (0.8 m) the sum of nominal eye and head angles is not equivalent to effective gaze. Appropriate corrections have been discussed in Collewijn et al. (1982) and can be expressed in simplified form as: *gaze = head + 0.89(eye in head)*. The target motion consisted of the sum of 15 non-harmonic sine waves in the range 0.045 - 2.2 Hz, with maximal deviations of 15, 30 or 50° from the center. Subjects were instructed to pursue the target either with eye movements alone *(eye only)* or with a maximum contribution by head movements *(head only)*. Trials lasted 66.7 s. Data processing was similar to that for the other pursuit experiments.

Results
Fig. 12 shows recordings of pursuit under the *eye only* and *head only* instructions, for identical episodes of the target motion. The instruction *eye only* was completely effective as the head did not move. The instruction *head only* elicited head pursuit movements which were often larger than the target movements but showed a

18

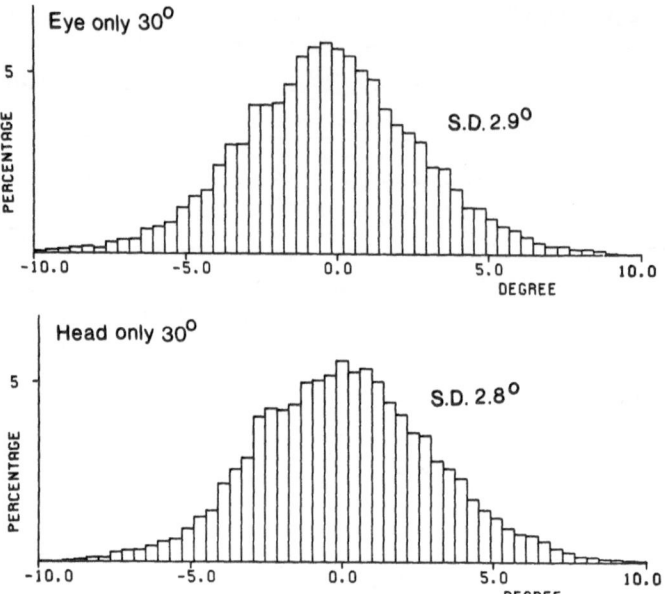

Fig. 13. Distribution of retinal position error during pursuit without and with head movements. Maximal target deviation: 30°. Average values for 4 subjects.

considerable lag. The movements of the eye in the head were very different in the two cases, but the displacements of the gaze were very similar. A real surprise is the shape of the error signal (the difference between target and gaze). The similarity between the two error traces, even in small details, is amazing. In numerous instances almost exactly the same saccades or group of saccades were made at exactly the same moments. All saccades were in the direction of the zero error level and many terminated close to it. Also the smooth components in the error signal were highly similar in the two conditions, although the movement of the eye in the head was very different. Thus, the retinal position of the target followed a virtually identical trajectory under the two conditions, although the position and motion of the eye in the head was entirely different in the two cases.

The similarity of the error under the two conditions is further corroborated by histograms (Fig. 13) of the distribution of retinal position error, computed as the average for 4 subjects. The shape and standard deviation of the distributions obtained under the two instructions are identical.

A first conclusion from these findings is that the trajectory of the retinal image of a moving target is highly stereotyped (at least within one subject and one session) and independent of the position or velocity of the eye in the head. In this respect the oculomotor responses appear to be deterministic.

Analysis in the frequency domain confirms the identity of the gaze/target relation in the two conditions, as shown in Bode plots for one subject in Fig. 14. These show gain and phase for each of the 15 components of the stimulus. They can be compared to the relations shown in Fig. 10. The main differences are that in Fig. 14

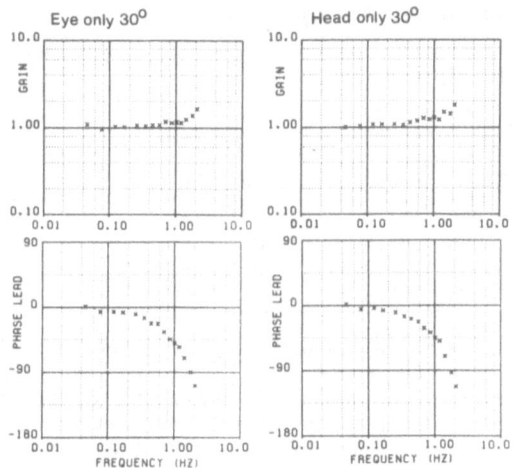

Fig. 14. Bode plots of the relation gaze/target during pursuit with and without head movements. One subject; maximal excursion of target: 30°.

the increase in gain to values above unity is even clearer for frequencies above 1 Hz and that the phase lag is much larger (45° at 1 Hz, compared to 20° for the stimulus with the highest frequency components in Fig. 10). These differences may be due to the increased complexity of the stimulus (15 instead of 4 components), the increased bandwidth or the larger amplitude. However, the presence or absence of head movements does not have the slightest effect.

Table 4 shows average values for the standard deviation of the retinal error (the mean error being zero) during pursuit with and without head movements for three different ranges of target deviation. These three stimuli contained the same 15 components but had a different power spectrum in order to keep overall velocities roughly similar. The error increased with the maximal deviation, but was unaffected by head movements.(For a target deviation of 50° pursuit with the eye only was impossible and for 40° it was very difficult).The errors are considerably larger than for pursuit of a 4-component motion with a bandwidth of 0.78 Hz and a maximal excursion of 10° (Table 2). They are also larger than the values we reported recently (Collewijn et al., 1982) for head and eye pursuit of a 6-component stimulus in the frequency

Table 4. Average standard deviations of retinal error for four subjects during eye and head pursuit.

Target motion	Target excursion range	Eye only	Head only
Sum of 15 sines 0.045-2.2 Hz	15°	2.18	2.20
	30°	2.89	2.80
	50°	-	3.46
Sum of 6 sines 0.045-0.9 Hz	15°	1.18	1.20
	30°	1.57	1.55
	40°	2.65	1.61
	50°	-	1.79

Table 5. Gain and phase of compensatory eye movements during active, irregular head movements. Average values of 3 emmetropic subjects.

Frequency range (Hz)	Light, fixation of stationary spot (0.89 eye/head)		Dark, no specific instruction (eye/head)		Dark, fixation of imaginary stationary spot (eye/head)	
	Gain	Phase	Gain	Phase	Gain	Phase
0.34-1.17	0.989	181.0	1.011	182.7	1.080	179.9
1.17-1.95	0.995	182.6	1.039	185.0	1.090	182.2
1.95-2.72	0.987	184.3	1.048	186.9	1.079	184.6
2.72-3.50	0.983	185.9	1.054	188.5	1.087	185.6

range of 0.045 - 0.9 Hz, which are also mentioned in Table 4 for comparison. The error and phase lag clearly increase with amplitude, bandwidth and possibly the number of components of the stimulus.

A second conclusion from these experiments is that head movements add to the spatial range of pursuit, but do not appreciably affect the retinal trajectory of the target's image in any other way.Thus, the effective sum of eye and head movements - gaze - remains constant in relation to the target. This means by definition that the added head movements are subtracted (with the appropriate magnification factor) from the eye movements or, in other words, that head movements during pursuit are virtually completely compensated by opposite eye movements. This extends the conclusions reached from the experiments with fixation during head movements: compensation is excellent during active head movements, whether the fixated target is stationary or moving.

To confirm the findings in Maryland for a stationary target independently, we also determined the gain of compensatory eye movements without a moving target with the apparatus in Rotterdam. The results are summarized in Table 5. Three emmetropic subjects made, at the end of the pursuit session, voluntary head movements somewhat similar to the pseudo-random target motion they had pursued before. Gain and phase were calculated for four frequency ranges. With the fixation spot present the effective gain (corrected for non-coincidence of eye and head rotational axes) was within 1 or 2% of unity. The remaining gaze instabilities were of the same order of magnitude as found in the Maryland experiments. The phase lags deviated by maximally 6^{0} from the ideal value of 180^{0} at the highest frequencies, which corresponds to a delay of about 5 ms.

Due to the vicinity of the target (0.8 m) such good compensation required the eye movements to be larger than the head movements. This is reflected in the gain of the subsequently measured VOR in the dark (inclusive any contribution by the cervico-ocular reflex). As shown in Table 5, all nominal VOR gain values were in excess of unity, possibly due to adaptation to the close target in the previous trials. The additional instruction to fixate an imagined stationary target caused a slight further elevation of the gain (Table 5).

GENERAL CONCLUSIONS

The present results suggest the following answers to the questions formulated at the end of the Introduction:

-OKN is largely controlled by the central retina. Stimulation of a central sector of 20^{0} produces almost normal OKN whereas a complementary peripheral stimulus excluding the central retina

results in a strongly decreased OKN. A similar decrease was
found in a patient with a central scotoma.
-A stationary structured background slows smooth pursuit down
by 20 - 30%. The deficit is supplemented by saccades and the
overall accuracy of pursuit is unaffected.
-Compensation by the VOR during active head movements is excellent in the light and almost as good in the dark. Deviation
from unity gain in the light does not exceed a few percent.
-Adaptation of the VOR in the light and in the dark to changes
in visual magnification factor up to 36% is very fast. The
changes have a time constant of 10 min or less and are virtually complete within 30 min.
-The quality of pursuit and even the details of the retinal
trajectory of the image of the target are identical in the
absence and presence of active head movements. The latter only
extend the useful pursuit range.

REFERENCES
Barlow D and Freedman W (1980) Cervico-ocular reflex in the normal
adult, Acta otolaryngol. 89, 487-496.
Barnes GR and Forbat LN (1979) Cervical and vestibular afferent
control of oculomotor response in man, Acta otolaryngol. 88, 79-87.
Barr CC, Schultheis LW and Robinson DA (1976) Voluntary, non-visual
control of the human vestibulo-ocular reflex, Acta otolaryngol.
81, 365-375.
Benson AJ (1970) Interactions between semicircular canals and gravi-
ceptors. In Busby DE, ed. Recent advances in aerospace medicine,
pp. 249-261. Dordrecht (Holland), Reidel.
Cheng M and Outerbridge JS (1975) Optokinetic nystagmus during
selective retinal stimulation, Expl. Brain Res. 23, 129-139.
Collewijn H (1970) The normal range of horizontal eye movements in
the rabbit, Expl. Neurol. 28, 132-143.
Collewijn H (1977) Eye- and head movements in freely moving
rabbits, J. Physiol. (London) 266, 471-498.
Collewijn H (1981) The oculomotor system of the rabbit and its
plasticity. Studies of brain function, Vol. 5. Berlin, Springer.
Collewijn H, Van der Mark F and Jansen TC (1975) Precise recording
of human eye movements, Vision Res. 15, 447-450.
Collewijn H, Martins AJ and Steinman RM (1981a) Natural retinal
image motion: origin and change, Ann. NY Acad. Sci. 374, 312-329.
Collewijn H, Martins AJ and Steinman RM (1981b) The time course of
adaptation of human compensatory eye movements, Doc. Ophthal. Proc.
(Den Haag) 30, 123-133.
Collewijn H, Conijn P and Tamminga EP (1982) Eye-head coordination
in man during the pursuit of moving targets. In Lennerstrand G,
Zee DS and Keller EL, eds. Functional basis of ocular motility
disorders. Oxford, Pergamon, in the press.
Dodge R (1903) Five types of eye movement in the horizontal
meridian plane of the field of regard, Am. J. Physiol. 8, 307-329.
Dubois MFW and Collewijn H (1979a) The optokinetic reactions of the
rabbit: relation to the visual streak, Vision Res. 19, 9-17.
Dubois MFW and Collewijn H (1979b) Optokinetic reactions in man
elicited by localized retinal motion stimuli, Vision Res. 19,
1105-1115.
Gauthier GM and Robinson DA (1975) Adaptation of the human vestibulo-
ocular reflex to magnifying lenses, Brain Res. 92, 331-335.

Gonshor A and Melvill Jones G (1976a) Short-term adaptive changes in the human vestibulo-ocular reflex arc, J. Physiol. (London) 256, 361-379.

Gonshor A and Melvill Jones G (1976b) Extreme vestibulo-ocular adaptation induced by prolonged optical reversal of vision, J. Physiol. (London) 256, 381-414.

Hood JD (1967) Observations upon the neurological mechanism of optokinetic nystagmus with especial reference to the contribution of peripheral vision, Acta otolaryngol. 63, 208-215.

Hood JD (1975) Observations upon the role of the peripheral retina in the execution of eye movements, J. Oto-Rhino-Lar. Borderlands 37, 65-73.

Körner F and Schiller PH (1972) The optokinetic response under open and closed loop conditions in the monkey, Expl. Brain Res. 14, 318-330.

Lisberger SG, Evinger C, Johanson GW and Fuchs AF (1981) Relationship between eye acceleration and retinal image velocity during foveal smooth pursuit in man and monkey, J. Neurophysiol. 44,229-249.

Meiry JL (1971) Vestibular and proprioceptive stabilization of eye movements. In Bach-y-Rita P, Collins CC and Hyde JE, eds. The control of eye movements, pp.483-496. New York, Academic Press.

Miles FA and Eighmy BB (1980) Long-term adaptive changes in primate vestibuloocular reflex. I. Behavioral observations, J. Neurophysiol. 43, 1406-1425.

Robinson DA (1963) A method of measuring eye movement using a scleral search coil in a magnetic field, IEEE Trans. Biomed. Electron. BME-10, 137-145.

Robinson DA (1977) Vestibular and optokinetic symbiosis: an example of explaining by modelling. In Baker R and Berthoz A, eds. Control of gaze by brain stem neurons, pp. 49-58. Amsterdam, Elsevier.

Skavenski AA and Steinman RM (1970) Control of eye position in the dark, Vision Res. 10, 193-203.

Stark L, Vossius G and Young LR (1962) Predictive control of eye tracking movements, IRE Trans. Human Factors Electron. HFE 3, 52-57.

Steinman RM, Haddad GM, Skavenski AA and Wyman D (1973) Miniature eye movement, Science 181, 810-819.

Steinman RM and Collewijn H (1980) Binocular retinal image motion during active head rotation, Vision Res. 20, 415-429.

Steinman RM, Cushman WB and Martins AJ (1982) The precision of gaze, Human Neurobiol. in the press.

Takahashi M, Uemura T and Fujishiro T (1980) Studies of the vestibulo-ocular reflex and visual-vestibular interactions during active head movements, Acta otolaryngol. 90, 115-124.

Tamminga EP and Collewijn H (1981) The effect of a structured background on human oculomotor pursuit of visual targets, Doc. Ophthal. Proc. (Den Haag) 30, 134-143.

Tomlinson RD, Saunders GE and Schwarz DWF (1980) Analysis of human vestibulo-ocular reflex during active head movements, Acta otolaryngol. 90, 184-190.

Van Die G and Collewijn H (1982) Optokinetic nystagmus in man: role of central and peripheral retina and occurrence of asymmetries, Human Neurobiol. in the press.

Yarbus AL (1967) Eye movements and vision. New York, Plenum Press.

ACKNOWLEDGEMENTS
This research was supported in part by the Foundation for Medical Research FUNGO (grant nr. 13-46-27) and the National Science Foundation (grants BNS 77-16474 and BNS 80-13508).

GAZE FIXATION AND PURSUIT IN HEAD FREE HUMAN INFANTS

A. ROUCOUX, C. CULEE and M. ROUCOUX (Laboratoire de Neurophysiologie, University of Louvain, Brussels, Belgium)

1. INTRODUCTION

Vision plays a major role in the organization of the human
newborn behavior. Many observations show that soon after
birth, the infant manifests interest for his visual surroundings (Bower, 1966; Brazelton et al, 1966; Barten et al,
1971; Fantz et al, 1975, Haith et al, 1977; Miranda et al,
1977; Dubowitz et al, 1980; Banks and Salapatek, 1981).
In some studies visual target fixation saccades have simply
been counted (Kessen et al, 1972; Aslin and Salapatek, 1975;
Salapatek et al, 1980).
Other authors more quantitatively analyzed eye movements
with D.C. E.O.G. recording. The observations were done with
head fixed (Dayton et al, 1964;Kremenitzer et al, 1979) or
head free with a monitoring of head movements (Trevarthen
and Tursky, 1969; Tronick and Clanton, 1971).It is shown in
the head fixed situation (Dayton et al, 1964) that no smooth
pursuit exists before two months of age for a target moving
at 16°/sec. Kremenitzer (1979),in a similar experimental
situation demonstrates that three days old babies display
smooth pursuit of targets moving slower than 14°/sec. The
periods of smooth pursuit however do not exceed 15% of the
total time during which infants pay attention to the target.
Trevarthen and Tursky (1969) and Tronick and Clanton (1971)
also recorded head movements but give few quantitative data
about eye-head coordination mechanisms in smooth pursuit or
saccadic movements and their evolution with age.
The present study is a first attempt to quantify eye and
head movements during pursuit or rapid shifts of gaze in infants and analyze their evolution with age.

2. METHODS

Data obtained in four infants (three boys and one girl) are
reported here. The subjects were full-term babies free of any
perinatal problem and judged normal by routine neurological
examination. Recording sessions were conducted while the infants were alert in state 3 or 4 according to Prechtls's scale
of alertness (Prechtl and Benteima, 1964): subjects are awake,
eyes open, moving spontaneously. Sessions were stopped if
fussing or crying occured. Horizontal eye movements were recorded by electrooculography. Two Beckman miniature electrodes were placed each at an outer canthus. Signals were sent
to D.C. coupled amplifiers. A small coil was also affixed

Roucoux, A. and Crommelinck, M. (eds.): Physiological and Pathological Aspects of Eye Movements.
© *1982, Dr W. Junk Publishers, The Hague, Boston, London.* ISBN-13: 978-94-009-8002-0

to the mid-forehead in order to record head movements by the
magnetic field technique (Roucoux et al, 1980). The subject
sat with his (her) head at the center of the field coils, on
his (her) mother's lap, head and trunk resting against the
mother's body, inclined backward at about 30° from the vertical (Casaer and Akiyama, 1973). The baby's trunk was slightly
restrained by the mother, leaving arms and legs free. The mother herself sat on a chair supporting the coils. Targets consisting of black and white "Mickey's" heads subtending angle of
ten to two degrees were rear-projected onto a tangent translucent screen placed at a distance of 80cm from the infant's
eyes. Targets could be moved horizontally by means of a gal-
vanometer-mounted mirror. Eye, head and target positions were
stored on magnetic tape. Eye movement signal was calibrated
by presenting the target respectively at 0, 15 and 30° to the
left or to the right, visually observing the subject's saccades, and noting on the tape, the moments at which he (she)
appeared to fixate. A mean of the voltages corresponding to
a serie of successful fixations was taken as calibration.
Head movement calibration was done with a dummy coil. Gaze
position in space was obtained by summing suitably calibrated
eye and head position signals.

3. RESULTS
3.1. Fixation saccades
Contrary to the adult, infants fixate peripheral targets by
means of several successive hypometric saccades. The number
of saccades increases with the eccentricity of the target and
progressively decreases with age. The acquisition of targets
by one saccade is realized at eight weeks for targets situated at 15°, at twelve weeks for eccentricities of 30° and
still later for 45 degrees. The latency of eye saccades is
much larger than in the adult until one year of age (400ms
versus 200 ms).
Fig. 1 illustrates fixation saccades aimed at a 15 degrees
target. At five weeks two or even three successive saccades
are made. At eight and twelve weeks, two saccades are still
sometimes present. At twelve months, the pattern becomes
adult-like. For this eccentricity, head movements are almost
absent.
Fig. 2 shows the different fixation patterns for 30 degrees
targets. At five weeks, three to four saccades are made,
one or two at eight and twelve weeks and only one at twelve
months. For this eccentricity, head moves slightly and an
adequate compensating movement is seen on the eye's trace
for all ages.
On fig. 3 are shown the patterns for 45° fixations. At five
weeks, this target is apparently not perceived and not fixated. At eight weeks, two or three saccades are made. At twelve weeks, subject J.B. grossly undershoots the target by making only two small saccades. At twelve months, the whole
pattern is close to that exhibited by the adult as illustrated (C.C.) for comparison. The coordinated head movement is

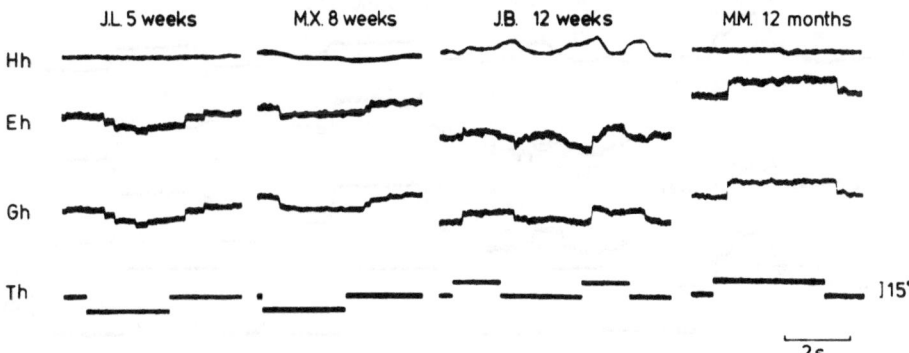

Fig. 1. *Eye and head fixation movements made by infants at different ages for a target eccentricity of 15 degrees. Hh: horizontal head movement; Eh: horizontal eye movement; Gh: horizontal gaze (Eh + Hh); Th: horizontal displacement of the target. The amplitude calibration is valid for all traces.*

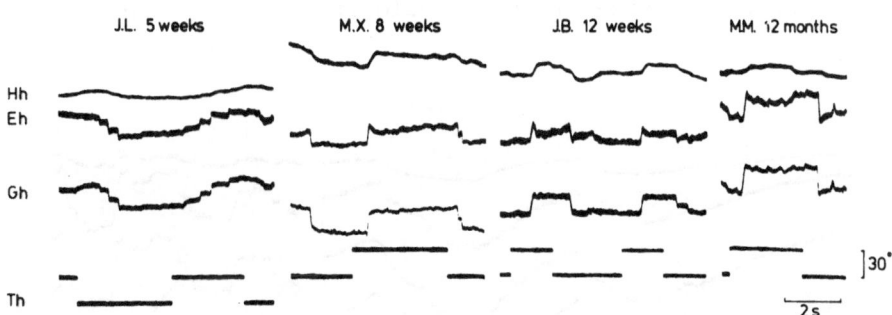

Fig. 2. *Eye and head fixation movements made by infants at different ages for a target eccentricity of 30 degrees.*

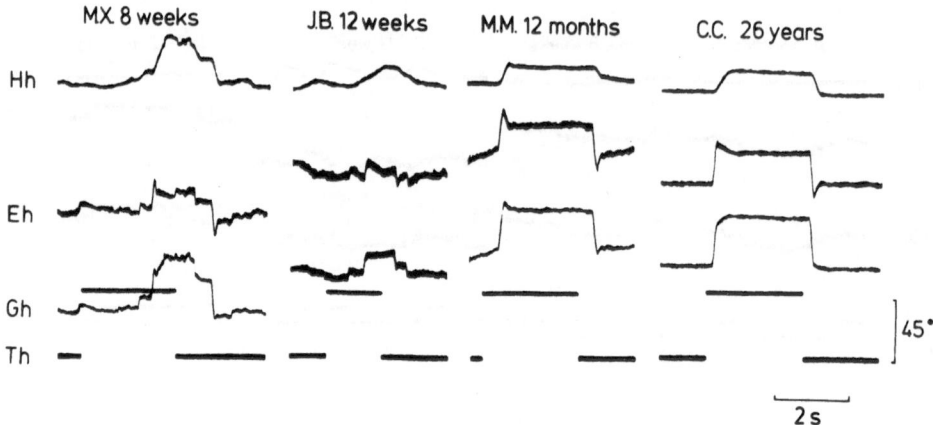

Fig. 3. *Eye and head fixation movements made by infants of different ages for a target eccentricity of 45 degrees. The adult pattern (C.C.) is shown for comparison.*

is noticeably larger for this eccentricity and the adequate compensatory eye movement present in all cases except at eight weeks in some cases.

3.2. Smooth pursuit

From five weeks on, babies are able to smoothly pursue a visual target, provided that its velocity is low enough.

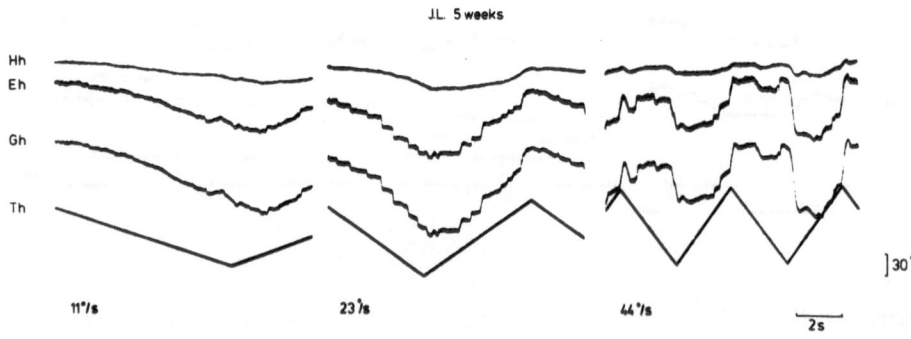

Fig. 4. *Eye and head pursuit movements made by an infant of five weeks at different velocities.*

With age, the maximum velocity of smooth pursuit increases. At one year, pursuit capacities are still lower than in the adult. In the youngest subjects we have tested so far (five weeks) almost 100% of the time the baby pays attention to the target, is occupied by smooth tracking with both head and eye for an 11°/sec. velocity. Corrective eye saccades are small and rare. When target velocity increases up to 23°/sec., eye saccades appear more frequently. Their amplitude also increases . They are interspersed with smooth pursuit, the velocity of which is most of the time too small. Head movement is smooth. At 44°/sec., smooth head-eye movements have almost disappeared. Instead fixations can be observed interrupted by visually very large saccades (up to 60 degrees). These large saccades are always synchronous with rapid head movements. At this velocity, head pursuit is virtually absent.

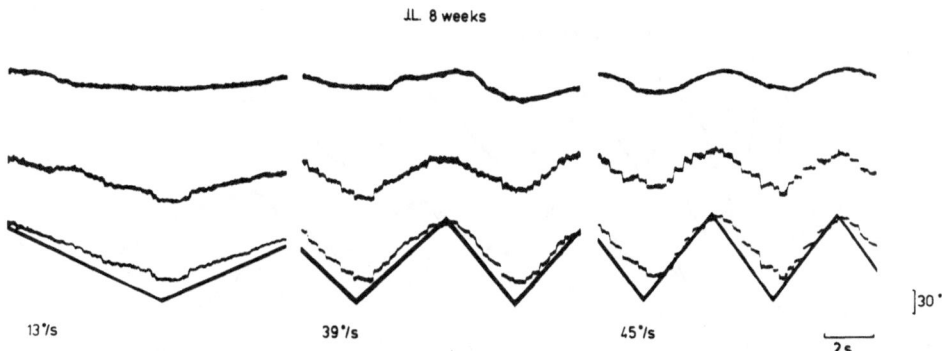

Fig.5. *Eye and head pursuit movements made by an infant of eight weeks at different velocities.*

At eight weeks (fig.5) pursuit capacities improve: at 39 and 45°/sec. smooth pursuit eyes movements very rarely match target velocity and thus corrective saccades are frequent. Head movements are smooth.
At one year (fig.6) smooth pursuit becomes almost adequate at 45°/sec. At 55°/sec., adequate smooth pursuit is still present for short periods of time, though quite large saccades appear. Head movement is most of the time smooth but its velocity adapts slowly to target velocity changes. By comparison, the adult performance is illustrated on fig. 7.

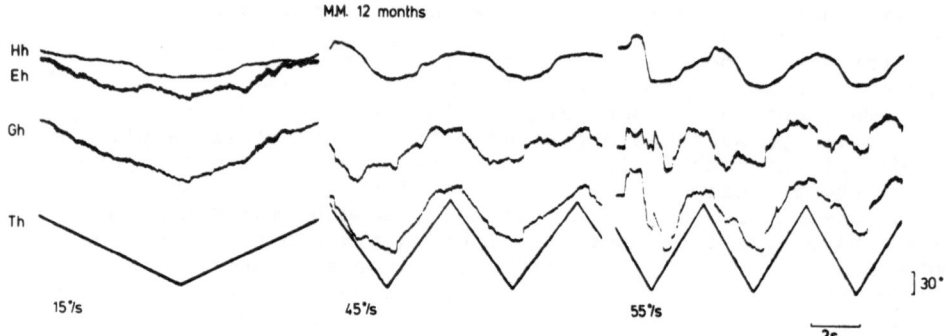

Fig. 6. *Eye and head pursuit movements made by an infant of twelve months at different velocities.*

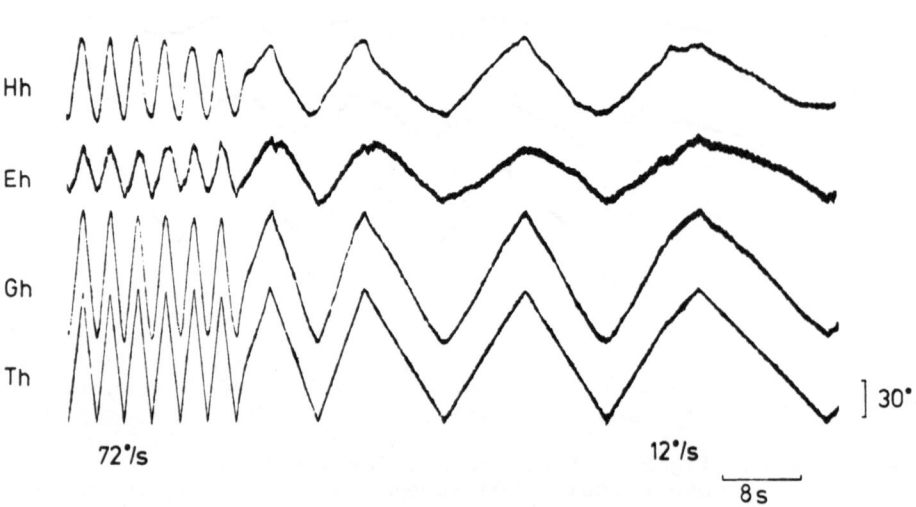

Fig. 7. *Eye and head pursuit movements made by an adult at different velocities.*

Note that half the amplitude of the movement is accomplished by the head, the other half by the eye in the orbit.

4. DISCUSSION

This preliminary study of eye and head movements in infants
has been focused on two types of gaze movements: fixation
saccades and pursuit.

4.1. Fixation saccades

Though it has previously been shown that infants already
very early display saccadic eye motility, few quantifications
have been done. Moreover the contribution of the head in this
behavior has never been investigated.

Our main conclusion is that in young infants (five weeks),
visual fixation can be elicited in a range of about 30 degrees from the midline. This fixation is accomplished by several small and hypometric saccades. With age, both the extent of the visuo-motor field and the amplitude of the individual saccade increase. Aslin and Salapatek (1975) have
shown a limitation of the visuomotor field to about 30 degrees for ages of one to two months. Macfarlane et al. (1976)
measure a field of 25 degrees for their neonatal group and
35 degrees for seven weeks old subjects. Also in accordance
with our findings is the observation (Aslin and Salapatek,
1975) of multiple saccades, the number of which increases
with the eccentricity of the target. The appearance of these multiple saccades is thus not caused by a restriction of
head movements as hypothesized by Macfarlane et al (1976).
The longer than adult latency of fixations has also been described by Aslin and Salapatek (1975). We did not however
made a detailed analysis of this value nor of its variation
with target eccentricity or age. Our data reveal that, from
a few weeks on, the eye-head coordination during orienting
or fixation movements seem basically similar to that of the
adult (Bartz, 1966): almost all fixations are executed by a
combined eye-head rotation, the head movement is slower than
the eye saccade and gaze is stabilized at the end of the saccade by a compensating movement most probably of vestibular
origin (Dichgans et al, 1974).

4.2. Pursuit

Our results show that infants, from the age of five weeks
are able to smoothly pursue a moving visual target of a size
of a few degrees with a combined eye-head pattern similar
to that of the adult. What characterizes the improvement of
performance with age is an increase of the highest gaze velocity attainable. These results are in disagreement with
studies taking the functional immaturity of the fovea during
the first month as the cause of an inability to pursue
smoothly (Dayton et al, 1964; Bronson, 1974). Kremenitzer
et al (1979) however, demonstrated the presence of smooth
pursuit in newborns aged of three to five days. These movements are rare (15% of the total time) and slow ($<15°/S$).
Our data show that, in older infants (one month), pursuit
is present 100% of the time the baby pays attention to the
target, for similar velocities. The improvement of pursuing
ability, however is slow and progressive with age. At one

year, performance is still lower than in the adult. In the
first weeks of life however, the infant capabilities improve
rather rapidly. Our data would favor the hypothesis according
to which the central retina, soon after birth, already pos-
sesses some functional specialization (Lewis and Maurer,
1980). They also suggest that the physiological development
of the foveal zone is progressive. Moreover, it appears from
our records, that the eye-head coordination pattern during
smooth pursuit does not change qualitatively with age. At a
few weeks already, infants are able to "suppress" their
vestibulo-ocular reflex in order to realize combined eye and
head smooth pursuit movements. Only when velocity passes
beyond a certain value does an "afoveate" pattern appear
(smooth head movement accompanied by a serie of eye saccades,
Collewijn, 1977). Another interesting phenomenon is that,
although unable to make large fixation saccades, the young
infant can exhibit very large saccades during high velocity
pursuit attempts, always synchronous with rather fast head
movements. The tight linkage between eye and head, also,
is a characteristic of afoveate animals.

5. REFERENCES

Aslin RN and Salapatek P (1975) Saccadic localization of
  visual targets by the very young human infant, Perception
  and Psychophysics, 17(3), 293-302.
Banks MS and Salapatek P (1981) Infant pattern vision: a
  new approach based on the contrast sensitivity function,
  Journal of Experimental Child Psychology , 31(1), 1-45.
Bartens S, Birns B and Ronch J (1971) Individual differen-
  ces in the visual pursuit behavior of neonates, Child
  Development, 42, 313-319.
Bartz AE (1966) Eye and head movements in peripheral vision:
  nature of compensatory eye movements, Science ,152,
  1644-1645.
Bower TG (1966) The visual world of infants, Scient. Am.,
  215, 80-92.
Brazelton TB, Scholl ML and Robey JS (1966) Visual respon-
  ses in the newborn, Pediatrics, 37, 284-290.
Bronson G (1974) The postnatal growth of visual capacity,
  Child Development, 45, 873-890.
Casaer P and Akiyama Y (1973) Is body posture relevant for
  neonatal studies ? Acta Paediatrica Belgica, 27, 418-423.
Collewijn H (1977) Eye and head movements in freely moving
  rabbits, J. Physiol. (London), 266, 471-498.
Dichgans J, Bizzi E, Morasso P and Tagliasco V (1974)
  The role of vestibular and neck afferents during eye-head
  coordination in the monkey, Brain Research, 71, 225-232.
Dayton GO, Jones MH, Steele B and Rose M (1964) Developmen-
  tal study of coordinated eye movements in the human infant,
  Archives of Ophtalmology, 71, 871-875, 1964.
Dubowitz LMS, Dubowitz V, Morante A and Verghote M (1980)
  Visual function in the preterm and full term newborn in-
  fant, Develop. Med. Child. Neurol., 22, 465-475.

Fantz R, Fagan JF and Miranda SB (1975) Early visual selectivity. In Infant Perception- from Sensation to Cognition,
ed. by LB Cohen and P Salapatek, pp. 249-345, Academic
Press, New York, San Francisco, London.
Haith MM, Bergman T and Moore MJ (1977) Eye contact and face scanning in early infancy, Science, 198, 853-855.
Harris P and Macfarlane A (1974) The growth of the effective
visual field from birth to seven weeks, Journal of Experi-
mental Child Psychology, 18, 340-348.
Kessen W, Salapatek P and Haith M (1972) The visual respon-
se of the human newborn to linear contour, Journal of Ex-
perimental Child Psychology, 13, 9-20.
Kremenitzer JP, Vaughan HG, Kurtzberg D and Dowling K (1979)
Smooth-pursuit eye movements in the newborn infant, Child
Development, 50, 442-448.
Lewis TL and Maurer D (1980) Central vision in the newborn,
Journal of Experimental Child Psychology, 29, 475-480.
Macfarlane A, Harris P and Barnes I (1976)Central and peri-
pheral vision in early infancy, Journal of Experimental
Child Psychology, 21, 532-538.
Miranda SB, Hack M, Fantz RL, Fanaroff AA and Klaus MH
(1977) Neonatal pattern vision: a predictor of future men-
tal performances ? , 91, 642-647.
Prechtl H and Beintema D (1964) The neurological examination
of the full-term newborn infant. Little Club Clinics in
Developmental Medicine n°12. London, The spastics Society
Medical Education, William Heinemann, Med. Books.
Roucoux A, Guitton D and Crommelinck M (1980) Stimulation
of the superior colliculus in the alert cat. II. Eye and
head movements evoked when the head is unrestrained.
Exp. Brain Res., 39, 75-85.
Salapatek P, Aslin RN, Simonson J and Pulos E (1980) Infant
saccadic eye movements to visible and previously visible
targets, Child Development, 51, 1090-1094.
Trevarthen C and Tursky B (1969) Recording horizontal ro-
tations of head and eyes in spontaneous shifts of gaze,
Behav. Res. Meth. & Instru., 1(8), 291-293.
Tronick E and Clanton C (1971) Infant looking patterns,
Vision Res., 11, 1479-1486.

PREDICTIVE MECHANISMS IN HUMAN SMOOTH PURSUIT MOVEMENT

Wolfgang Becker and Albert F.Fuchs
Universität Ulm, Sektion Neurophysiologie
D-7900 Ulm
and
Regional Primate Research Center
University of Washington
Seattle,Washington 98195,USA

1. Introduction

If a human observer is presented with a target moving at constant speed he can, almost within a single reaction time period, "lock" onto this target and start to track with virtually no retinal slip. This ability is difficult to explain if one considers the pursuit system merely as a simple servo mechanism responding to velocity and position errors (Young,1971). Therefore a variety of alternative mechanisms have been invoked, among them many which involve some form of "prediction". Vossius and Werner (1969) for example have proposed an extrapolating prediction, based on a Taylor expansion of current target movement into future. They and others (e.g. Eckmiller,1978) had observed that the smooth pursuit response can "bridge" short gaps of target presentation. Before the idea of predictive extrapolation can be pursued however, it needs a quantitative experimental basis. As a step toward such a basis the present report considers the smooth pursuit component that remains when a moving target is suddenly removed from sight.

2. Methods

In a first series of experiments a highly predictable pattern of target movement was used. The target consisted of a light spot (diameter 1/4 deg), rear projected onto a translucent tangent screen. At regular intervals it moved from right to left and vice versa with constant velocity over an angular distance of 40 deg .The velocity (5,10, or 20 deg/sec) remained the same throughout an experimental session. Between moves there was a pause of constant length during which the target made two small up-and-down movements which helped the observer to synchronize his response with the next horizontal movement. During about 40 % of all moves the target was blanked for various time periods leaving the observer in complete darkness. The blanking periods were random with regard to their occurrence, their length, and their position along the target track. In some experiments they could start right at the beginning of the target movement. Observers were instructed to "track the horizontal target movement as accurately as possible" and to "continue tracking, if the target disappears, so as to be right on target when it reappears". Four observers participated in this series,among them the two authors.

The observers' eye movements were recorded by means of a suction lens with embedded induction coil (Collewijn et al, 1975) and stored on computer tape, together with tar-

Roucoux, A. and Crommelinck, M. (eds.): Physiological and Pathological Aspects of Eye Movements.
© *1982, Dr W. Junk Publishers, The Hague, Boston, London.* ISBN-13: 978-94-009-8002-0

get position and blanking signals. Using interactive
computer software all saccadic components were then
removed and replaced by a linear interpolation of the
smooth movement before and after the saccade. After
removal of the saccades the eye position curves were
averaged, separately for each blanking condition. By
digitally differentiating these averages, average smooth
velocity curves were obtained.

3.Results

3.1 Survey
The observers who all were familiar with the basic
aspects of smooth and saccadic eye movements felt quite
uncertain about their tracking performance during
blanking periods. They noticed the increased number and
size of saccadic eye movements occurring in the dark, but
were generally surprised to see, at the conclusion of a
recording session, the considerable amount of smooth
velocity they had continued to produce between saccades.
This continued smooth velocity component was obvious
already in the very first trials of an experimental
session.

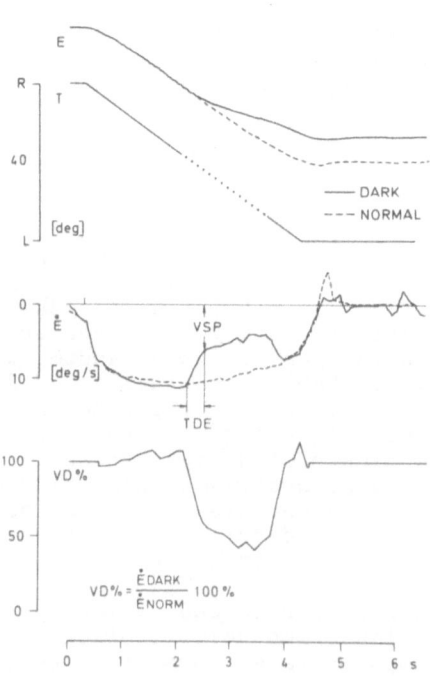

Figure 1. Example of
smooth pursuit res-
ponse to a target mo-
vement of 10 deg/sec.
Dashed curves, average
(n=20) of trials
without blanking of
target ("NORMAL").
Continuous curves,
trials (n=8) with
blanking ("DARK"). E,
desaccadized eye po-
sition ("smooth eye
position"). Ė, smooth
velocity. T, target
position; dotted seg-
ment indicates blan-
king period. VD%, ve-
locity in trials with
blanking normalized
to velocity without
blanking. TDE, du-
ration of fast ini-
tial decay of velo-
city ("decay time").
VSP, residual velo-
city at beginning of
"plateau period".

A typical profile of averaged smooth velocity is shown in Fig.1. After blanking the smooth velocity initially undergoes a sudden and steep decay. The velocity does not reduce to zero however, but stabilizes at a new level. This level represents what we call the "residual velocity". The residual velocity either remains almost constant while the blanking period continues, or declines slowly as in the example shown in Fig.1. The near constancy of the residual velocity becomes particularly clear if it is normalized to the velocity in trials without blanking (trace VD% in Fig. 1). Velocity profiles of the type shown in Fig.1 which are characterized by an initial fast deceleration and a subsequent "plateau" of slow or no velocity changes were by far the most frequent to occur (62%). In other cases the velocity showed no well defined transition between fast decay and subsequent plateau (12%) or declined along an exponential curve (9%). However, all observed velocity patterns appear to be variants of a same basic scheme and do not constitue truely different entities. Target velocity and blanking conditions (period of visible target movement preceding blanking) had no obvious effect upon their frequency of occurrence. The only exception are trials where the target was blanked right at the beginning of its movement; they will be considered separately.

3.2 Initial decay of velocity
The decay time, TDE (cf.Fig.1), of each observer had a constant value which was independent of the velocity decrement associated with the initial period of fast deceleration. It had mean values (standard deviations) of 191 (70), 258 (32), and 280 (91) msec in three of our observers. (No reliable value can be given for the 4th observer who had participated in only one experiment and tended to have an exponential decay). The decay time being constant, the magnitude of deceleration was proportional to the velocity decrement. The decelerations resulting from blanking were larger in magnitude than the initial accelerations in response to the start of the target movement. The average (across observers) acceleration during velocity increments from 0 to 8.6 deg/sec, for example, was 18.5 deg/sec , while the average deceleration associated with a 8.6 deg/sec drop of the velocity after blanking, was 34.5 deg/sec . A comparison to the pursuit decelerations that result if an always visible target suddenly slows down is not available, at present. We feel however that these decelerations would not be faster than those observed in responses to blanking. This would imply that, after blanking, the smooth velocity behaves as if the observer had actually seen the target slow down to the residual velocity.

36

3.3 Residual velocity

The direction of the residual velocity was identical to that of the target movement. This was true also for small target velocities (5 deg/sec). Therefore drift phenomena, such as spontaneous vestibular nystagmus, are not at the origin of the residual smooth movement; they would result in an unidirectional movement. Furthermore, the magnitude of the residual velocity clearly is a function of target velocity. This was established by measuring "VD%0.7", the normalized residual velocity occurring 700 msec after the beginning of the fast velocity decay (or approximately 450 msec after its end). VD%0.7 was considered to be representative of the initial part of the plateau period. Examined as a function of target velocity, VD%0.7 was approximately constant in all three observers who had partipated in experiments with different velocities. Thus, the normalized residual velocity appears to be independent of target velocity, at least in the velocity range explored in the present experiments (5-20 deg/sec).

The normalized residual velocities obtained at different target velocities were pooled, therefore, and used to construct an average time course of the velocity during blanking for each of the observers (Fig.2). The leftmost point of each of the individual curves shown in Fig.2 represents the instant at which the velocity begins to deviate from its normal profile. The second point marks the end of the fast decay period, and the following points give the velocity measured at constant intervals from the beginning of the deviation. The curves confirm the qualitative impression that the residual velocity following the fast decay period is only slowly declining. Averaged across observers the normalized residual velocity approximately had a value of 60% at the outset of the plateau period.

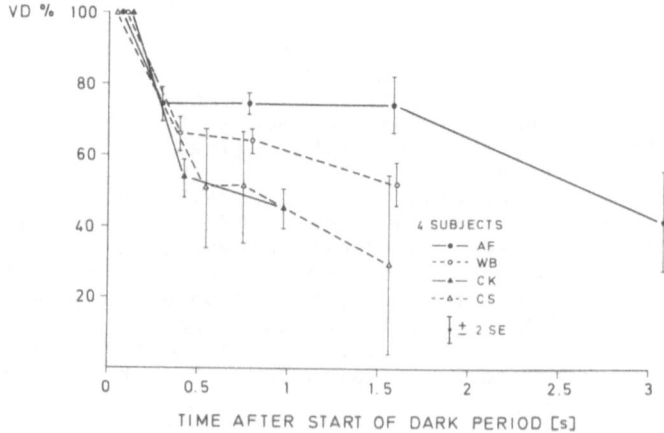

Fig.2 Time course of the normalized residual velocity.

3.4 Blanking at beginning of target movement

A closer inspection of the velocity profiles from all experiments revealed that, quite regularly, the smooth movement had started prior to the actual target movement despite the fact that the target still was seen to be stationary in the horizontal direction (cf.Figs.1&3).The lead time of the smooth movement ranged from 50 to 200 msec. In order to investigate for how long a time period this truely predictive generation of smooth "pursuit" can be maintained, we had the target disappear in synchrony with the onset of its horizontal movement in some experiments. Although no target movement could be perceived in this situation, the observers continued to accelerate their smooth movement along the same velocity profile as when responding to the start of an always visible target movement (Fig.3). Only 200 to 300 msec after the - invisible - start of the target movement began the velocity to deviate from its normal profile and to decelerate for a short period of time. Thereafter there was even another, albeit slower, period of acceleration with still no target movement being visible. Thus the predictive generation of a known velocity profile can be sustained for up to 500 msec (= 200 msec lead time + 300 msec period of continuing acceleration).

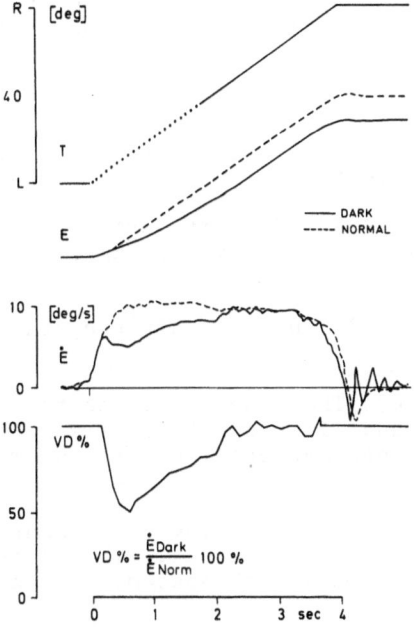

Figure 3. Example of predictive smooth pursuit movement in trials whith blanking synchronous to start of target movement. Same presentation as in Fig. 1.

4. Conclusions

The residual velocity occurring after blanking is suggestive of nystagmus aftereffects. Besides the well known optokinetic afternystagmus, also a pursuit afternystagmus (PAN) has been reported (Muratore and Zee, 1979). The time course and the normalized velocity ("gain") of PAN are compatible with those of the residual velocity. However, in order to induce PAN, long periods (2 min) of unidirectional smooth pursuit have been used while the residual velocity is seen after very brief periods of tracking already. This does not preclude a link between the two phenomena. If one interpretes PAN as the output of a storage mechanism which is slowly charged by a prolonged pursuit movement, then the residual velocity could well result from a rapid charging of the storage mechanism by a predictor of target movement. The smooth acceleration observed in the absence of a visible target movement demonstrates that prediction exists indeed and that it can be translated into appropriate motor commands. Among its benefits is certainly the possibility to synchronize the pursuit movement with known regularities of the target movement.

We consider our results compatible with the idea that the structure controlling the smooth pursuit response contains an integrating component which can be charged by a predictor of future target movement, to a value equivalent to at least 60% of the predicted velocity. In case of slow target movements this may indeed help to reduce retinal slip and yet to operate the system at low open loop gain without danger of uncontrolled oscillations.

5. References

Collewijn H, van der Mark F, and Jansen TC (1975) Precise recording of human eye movement. Vision Res. 15,447-450

Eckmiller R and Mackeben M (1978) Pursuit eye movements and their neural control in the monkey. Pflügers Arch. 377, 15-23

Muratore R and Zee DS (1978) Pursuit after-nystagmus. Vision Res.19, 1057-1059.

Vossius G and Werner J (1969) The functional control of the eye-tracking-system and its digital simulation. Congress of the International Federation of Automatic control (IFAC), Warsaw

Young LR (1971) Pursuit eye tracking movements.In Bach-y-Rita P, Collins CC, and Hyde JE eds. The control of eye movements, pp 429-423, New York,Academic Press

----
Supported by DFG Be 783/1 and 783/2-1, and NIH RR 00166 and EY 00745

BIPHASIC AFTEREFFECTS OF VESTIBULAR STIMULI, OPTOKINETIC NYSTAGMUS AND PURSUIT - COMMON INTEGRATORS ?

J. Dichgans and E. Koenig
(Neurological Clinic, University of Tübingen, W.-Germany)

SUMMARY
Primary (phase I) and secondary (phase II - opposite in direction) afternystagmus after vestibular, optokinetic and pursuit stimuli of different duration and velocity were quantitatively studied in humans to determine the charge and discharge characteristics of the underlying central storage mechanisms. Three different storage mechanisms were identified: 1. A common integrator for the vestibular and the retinal periphery dependent optokinetic system gives rise to optokinetic afternystagmus I and prolongs the decay of vestibular afternystagmus I. Its vestibular charge is fast and the OKN charge slower (30 s). It discharges within 1 min and is related to storage of ego motion sensation. 2. An integrating mechanism for pursuit with a rapid charge (2 s) and a fast discharge (10 s) stores a velocity signal concerning object motion possibly playing a role in prediction of pursuit. 3. Secondary afternystagmus is a common feature of vestibular stimuli and prolonged optokinetic and pursuit stimulation. It shows rapid charge for vestibular and slower charge for OKN and pursuit stimuli, but slow discharge after vestibular and visual stimuli. Its gain is lower than the one of primary vestibular, optokinetic and pursuit afternystagmus. The secondary nystagmus integrator is independent of whether or not nystagmus occurs during stimulation. Its inputs seem to bypass the phase I integrator.

INTRODUCTION
Whereas secondary vestibular (VAN II) and secondary optokinetic afternystagmus (OKAN II) are well known for a long time, the underlying mechanisms are still not completely understood. In recent years efforts in the analysis of the optokinetic and vestibular systems have centered on primary vestibular (VAN I-per- and postrotatory) and primary optokinetic afternystagmus (OKAN I). Similar characteristics of the two phenomena led to the assumption of a common storage mechanism (Cohen et al., 1977; Raphan et al., 1979). There is good evidence that this common integration is achieved in the brainstem involving the vestibular nuclei (Dichgans and Brandt, 1972; Waespe and Henn, 1977). The vestibular nuclei receive inputs from the vestibular endorgans as well as from the retina. Optokinetic input is effective whenever large field motion is seen. Since secondary nystagmus of reversed direction is also observed after both kinds of stimulation when applied in isolation and shows similar characteristics, it is tempting to assume a common integrator also for secondary nystagmus (Waespe et al., 1978). The latter may represent an adaptational process to counteract primary vestibular and optokinetic

Roucoux, A. and Crommelinck, M. (eds.): Physiological and Pathological Aspects of Eye Movements.
© 1982, Dr W. Junk Publishers, The Hague, Boston, London. ISBN-13: 978-94-009-8002-0

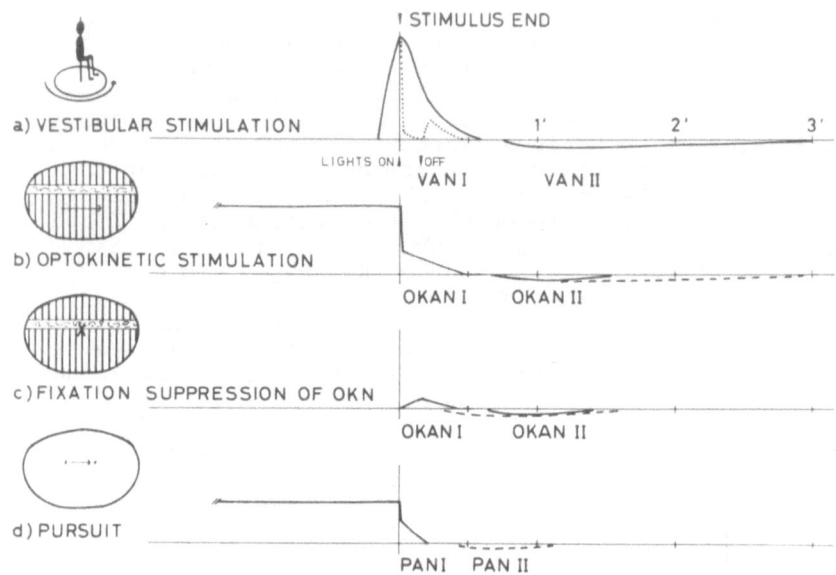

FIGURE 1. Stimuli applied and typical characteristics of
afternystagmus observed (continuous lines), reduction of
vestibular afternystagmus I by intermittent fixation of
a stationary horizon (dotted line), long lasting secondary
optokinetic and pursuit afternystagmus (dashed lines) after prolonged optokinetic and pursuit stimulation.

afternystagmus. Previous studies (Mackensen, Rudolf,
1962; Brandt et al., 1974; Koenig, Dichgans, 1981) however
indicated that secondary nystagmus (VAN II and OKAN II)
are not dependent on the actual occurrence of nystagmus,
but are a response to the stimulus itself. In this paper
we compare primary and secondary nystagmus after vestibular, optokinetic and pursuit stimulation, and the effects of fixation during these stimuli to determine the
characteristics of primary and secondary nystagmus and
their possible interdependence.

METHODS
4 subjects were seated on a rotatory chair with their
heads in a headrest. The chair was surrounded by a cylindrical drum which could be rotated about the same axis.
Both chair and drum could be rotated independently or
coupled at servo controlled velocities up to 180 °/s and
accelerations up to 18 °/s². Eye movements were recorded
by electrooculography using d-c coupling. They were

calibrated using voluntary saccades between each trial. Horizontal and vertical eye movements as well as drum and chair acceleration and signals monitoring on and off of both drum illumination and the fixation target were recorded on paper charts.

Vestibular stimuli (Fig. 1a) consisted of chair accelerations of 18 °/s² for 10 s in the dark. Deceleration of the chair was initiated after 4-5 min, when VAN II had definitely ceased.

To test the influence of fixation-suppression on vestibular nystagmus (Fig. 1a, dotted line) chair and drum were coupled and accelerated simultaneously. At the end of the acceleration the drum was illuminated for intervals of 2, 5, 10, 20, 30 s and 1, 2, 3 min presenting the "stationary" inner wall of the drum to the subject. The inner wall of the drum was covered with 48 alternating black and white stripes (7.5° wide) and a small band at eye level covered with coloured comic strip figures as an additional foveal stimulus.

To study the influence of full field optokinetic stimulation (stimulating both the pursuit and the large field dependent OKN-system simultaneously, Fig. 1b) only the drum was rotated at velocities of 30, 90 and 180 °/s and illuminated for intervals of 2, 10, 30 s and 1, 3 and 15 min.

To test the pursuit system in isolation (Fig. 1d) single target stimulation was achieved by means of 8 LEDs mounted on the inner wall of the drum at eye level at equal distances of 45°. LEDs in the peripheral visual field were masked, leaving an aperture of 60° width in front of the subject, so that only 1 faintly lit spot was visible for 3/4 of the stimulus duration (45/60) and 2 light spots for the remaining time to elicit a refixation saccade. Subjects were asked to attentively pursue both the full field and single target stimulus.

To test fixation-suppression of OKN (Fig.1c) and of pursuit (not shown) subjects were asked to fixate a stationary light spot mounted immediately in front of the wall of the drum.

Eye movements were analyzed manually. All data mentioned in the result section refer to average values of the 4 subjects tested.

RESULTS

Pure vestibular stimulation (Fig. 1a) by a body acceleration of 18 °/s² elicited a maximum slow phase velocity (SPV) of primary vestibular nystagmus (VAN I) of approximately 90 °/s (gain 0.5) which decayed on the average within 37 s (cumulative amplitude 1150°). After a pause of about 10 s, secondary vestibular afternystagmus (VAN II) started and slowly increased in velocity reaching a maximum of approximately 7 °/s 1 min after the end of the vestibular stimulus. Then VAN II slowly decayed and ceased on the average 175 s after the termination of the body acceleration. Cumulative amplitude of VAN II averaged 635°.

Fixation after the end of the vestibular stimulus (Fig.

DURATION OF OKAN I AND II

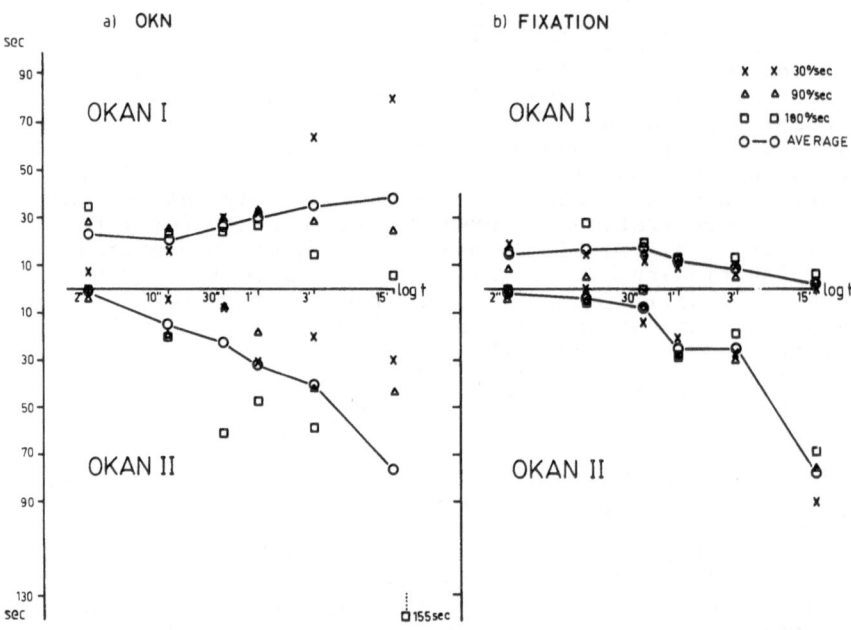

FIGURE 2. Duration of optokinetic afternystagmus I and II after different durations of (a) OKN or (b) fixation-suppression of OKN with three different stimulus velocities (30, 90, 180 °/s).

1a, dotted line) leads to a rapid decrease of SPV of VAN I. After an intermittent fixation of the stationary scene VAN I reappears (after fixation periods of up to 20 s), but does not reach the SPV of VAN I without prior fixation at the corresponding time. VAN I ceases somewhat earlier after fixation (29 s after stimulus termination). The duration and cumulative amplitude of VAN II was not reduced by prior fixation, but instead was somewhat larger with the shorter fixation intervals (up to 30 s). Pilot experiments showed that even the presence of the stationary horizon throughout the acceleration phase did not affect VAN II.

Full field optokinetic stimulation leads to afternystagmus (OKAN I) even after short stimulus durations of 2 s (average initial SPV just after lights off about 20 °/s). OKAN I increases with stimulus durations up to 1 min (average cumulative amplitude 170°, maximally 250° with the 90 °/s stimulus, Fig. 2a). And so does the initial SPV of OKAN I (average 28 °/s after 30 s of stimulation). OKAN I duration increases with low stimulus velocities (30 °/s) up to 15 min of stimulus duration (average 70 s),

DURATION OF PAN I AND II

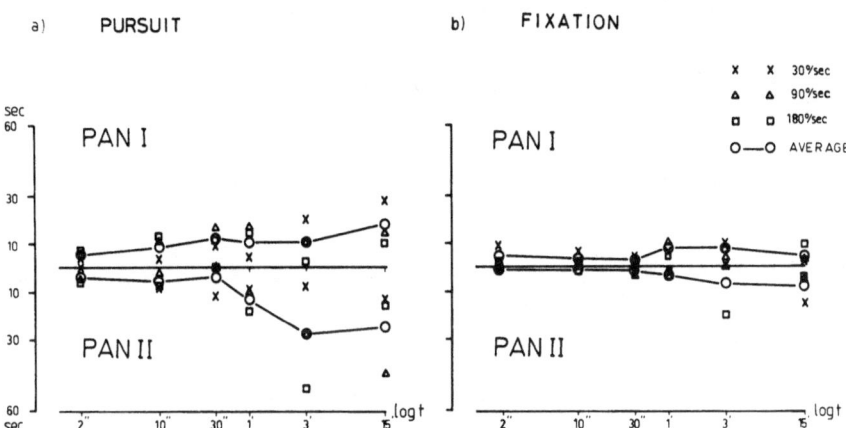

FIGURE 3. Duration of pursuit afternystagmus I and II after different durations of (a) pursuit or (b) fixation-suppression of pursuit with three different stimulus velocities (30, 90, 180 °/s).

but decreases with high stimulus velocities lasting only 5 s after a 15 min stimulation at 180 °/s. The average duration of OKAN I with all stimulus velocities and durations was about 30 s. OKAN II may be observed if stimuli last for more than 10 s. Its duration (up to 155 s after the 180 °/s stimulus) and cumulative amplitude (up to 724°) increase with stimulus speed and duration up to the longest stimulus tested (15 min, Fig. 2 a). Suppression of OKN throughout full field stimulation reduces OKAN I, but does not abolish it (Fig. 2b). The maximum of SPV of OKAN I no longer occurs immediately after lights off. Instead, SPV increases slowly over several seconds indicating an outlasting effect of the prior fixation. After optokinetic stimulation of 3 and 15 min OKAN I may be missing. Again OKAN II does not start immediately after switching the lights off, but rises slowly over about 10 s and lasts up to 80 s. Pursuit stimulation by only one (and intermittently two) small moving targets elicits PAN I (pursuit afternystagmus I) and after prolonged stimulation PAN II (Fig. 1d). Even though, according to most of the literature, one would not easily assume a convergence to the visual-vestibular

44

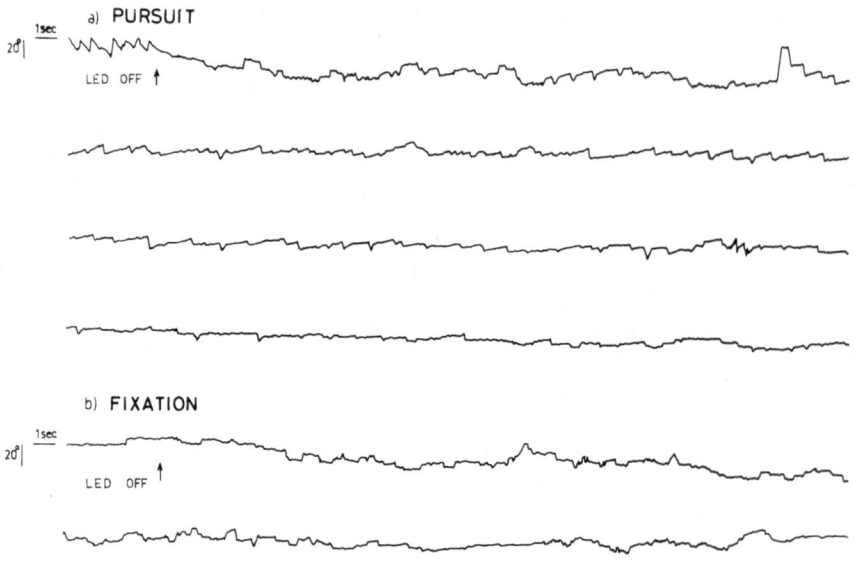

PAN I AND II AFTER STIMULATION FOR 3min (90°/s)

a) PURSUIT

1sec

20°|

LED OFF ↑

b) FIXATION

1sec

20°|

LED OFF ↑

FIGURE 4. a) Original recording of primary and secondary pursuit afternystagmus after 3 min of pursuit with 90 °/s stimulus velocity, b) original recording of eye movements after the same stimulus as in a), but with fixation suppression of pursuit.

integrator, storage is indicated by a short lasting PAN I (average cumulative amplitude 45° after the 1 min stimulus, up to 65° after 1 min of stimulation with 180 °/s, Fig. 3a). The initial SPV of PAN I reaches about 30 °/s after 2 s stimuli and a maximum of about 39 °/s after 30 s of stimulation. PAN II reaches an average cumulative amplitude of 45° after 3 min of stimulation (original recording in Fig. 4a). Pursuit afternystagmus seems to be elicited by the repetitive tracking and not by the visual stimulus, e.g. it is probably an oculomotor aftereffect. The latter statement was suggested by the results of presenting the identical pursuit stimulus and suppressing pursuit by fixation of a stationary target. In this case almost invariably neither primary nor secondary afternystagmus were observed (Fig. 4b). Rarely, however, the 1 or 2 light spots moving across the retina during fixation were able to elicit a slight selfmotion sensation, then a very weak afternystagmus was occasionally seen (Fig. 3b).

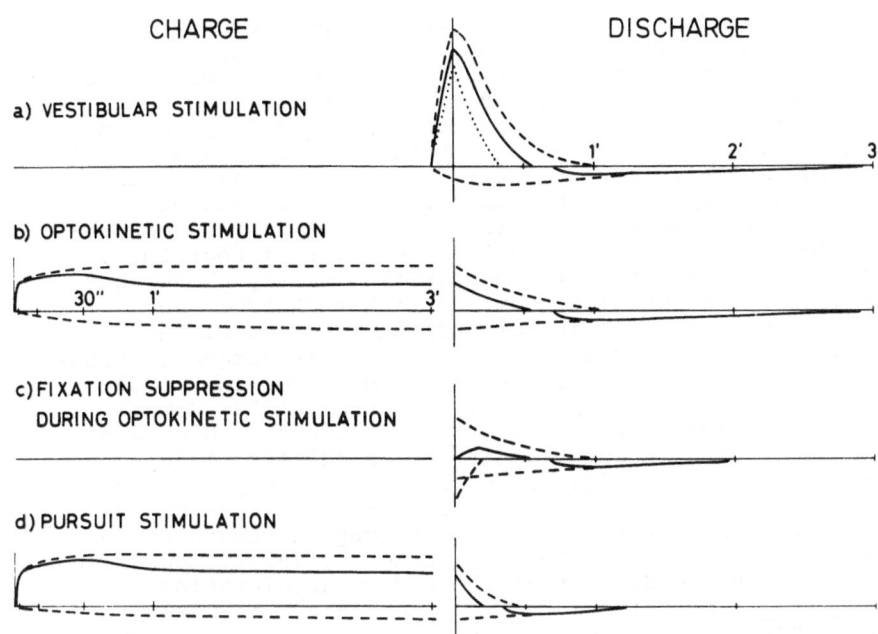

CHARGE   DISCHARGE

a) VESTIBULAR STIMULATION

b) OPTOKINETIC STIMULATION

c) FIXATION SUPPRESSION
   DURING OPTOKINETIC STIMULATION

d) PURSUIT STIMULATION

FIGURE 5. Charge and discharge of afternystagmus (continuous lines) as well as the suggested charge and discharge properties of the underlying central integrating
mechanisms (interrupted lines) and the cupula (dotted
lines in a).

DISCUSSION
The results of aftereffects of vestibular, optokinetic
and pursuit stimulation, as well as fixation suppression,
may help to understand some of the basic characteristics
of the underlying storage mechanisms. The results and
some of the interpretations suggested are graphically
presented in Fig. 5. This figure schematically depicts
data on the temporal summation (charge) within the neural mechanisms responsible for afternystagmus (on the
left) as well as on their discharge characteristics (on
the right).
Vestibular stimulation (Fig. 5a) leads to a cupula deflection which slowly decays after the termination of
acceleration. During the decay three mechanisms contribute to vestibular nystagmus: 1. The slowly decaying
cupula deflection modulates the discharge rate for about
20 s throughout its return phase (time constant 7 s,
Fernandez, Goldberg, 1971; Büttner, Waespe, 1981).
2. A storage mechanism in the vestibular nuclei storing
activity of the peripheral nerve (throughout the acceleration and the cupula return phase) prolongs primary

vestibular afternystagmus beyond the termination of cupula return (Buettner, Büttner, 1979; Raphan et al., 1979). 3. The activity of the storage mechanism forming the basis of primary afternystagmus, however, outlasts VAN I. The slow rise of VAN II (the result of a second integrator with an opposite effect) seems to be due to the vanishing counteraction of this storage. It must be noted that the observed nystagmus up to this point invariably results from the probably linear interaction of two mutually counteractive storage mechanisms, the VAN I and OKAN I storage in the vestibular nuclei (vestibular nucleus integrator) and the storage responsible for secondary nystagmus (secondary integrator). The latter is active throughout the primary phase, but initially,is outweighed by the higher charged, but faster decaying vestibular nucleus integrator. The vestibular nucleus integrator may be discharged by fixation of a stationary target or scene (Collins, 1968; Raphan et al., 1979; Buettner, Büttner, 1979; Koenig, Dichgans, 1981). Primary vestibular neurons which are not modulated by optokinetic inputs (Keller, 1976; Büttner, Waespe, 1981) however are obviously not affected by fixation, as they seem to recharge the vestibular nucleus integrator throughout the cupula return phase (Cohen et al., 1981; Koenig, Dichgans, 1981). Recharging was seen up to 20 s after the end of acceleration.

Full field optokinetic stimulation (Fig. 5b) leads to a rather rapid charge of a storage mechanism. The amount of charge after different stimulus durations can be inferred from the initial SPV of afternystagmus and is schematically shown in Fig. 5b. Most of the charge is accumulated within the first 2 s (in contrast to Cohen et al., 1981) who used an optokinetic stimulus without our features to improve foveal pursuit. The maximum, however, was reached also in our experiments after 30 s of stimulation. The slight drop of the initial SPV of OKAN with long stimulus durations is interpreted as the consequence of the slow build up of charge in the counteractive secondary integrator. The decay of OKAN I shows similar properties to that of VAN I, if one takes into account that the input from the semicircular canals throughout the cupula return phase is missing (Raphan et al., 1979). OKAN I lasts about 30 s, the discharge of the underlying storage mechanism again is supposed to last until OKAN II has reached its maximum (about 1 min after stimulus termination). So the data conform with the hypothesis of a common storage mechanism for OKAN I and VAN I (Raphan et al., 1979).

Pursuit afternystagmus I (PAN I, Fig. 5d) first demonstrated by Muratore and Zee (1979) and as an oculomotor aftereffect in a different optokinetic paradigm by Brandt et al. (1974) shows about the same initial SPV as OKAN I (similar charge characteristics), but a much more rapid decay thereafter. The initial SPV reaches about the same high level after 2 s of stimulation and then still increases somewhat to a maximum after 30 s. The initial fast rise may be the correlate of a prediction mechanism

for pursuit, the latter segment suggests a slow build up
of charge independent of prediction. The fact that duration and cumulative amplitude of PAN I amount to only
30 % of that of OKAN I is inconclusive with respect to
the question whether PAN I and OKAN I are driven by the
same integrator. The same initial SPV, but the much
shorter duration of PAN I however suggest two different
discharge time constants and therefore two mechanisms.
The experiment of Brandt et al. (1974) proves that both
the retinal periphery dependent OKAN (vestibular nucleus)
integrator and the pursuit integrator may be charged independently. During full field optokinetic stimulation
both integrating mechanisms are charged simultaneously.
The pursuit integrator stores activity related to slow
eye movements (slow phase of nystagmus or pursuit) when
those are repetitively elicited into one direction, the
vestibular nucleus integrator stores motion information
either from the vestibular or the visual system (predominantly from the retinal periphery).
The independent existence of a subsystem for velocity
storage in the pursuit system may also be demonstrated
by the characteristics of OKAN I after fixation suppression of OKN (Fig. 5c). The slow rise of OKAN I after
stimulus end may be an outlasting effect of the fixation
impetus. It may be speculated that the intention to
fixate generates an internal pursuit signal opposite to
the direction of the optokinetic stimulus. This pursuit
signal may charge the PAN I integrator. Thus in the case
of the afternystagmus after fixation-suppression of OKN
we might have studied the discharge of the oppositely
charged PAN I and vestibular nucleus integrating mechanisms.
The storage mechanism for secondary nystagmus is probably
common to the vestibular, to the retinal periphery dependent optokinetic and to the pursuit system. Vestibular
and full field optokinetic stimulation charge it strongly
whereas pursuit leads to less secondary nystagmus. The
amount of charge accumulated in the storage mechanism is
about the same after an 18 °/s² body-acceleration for
10 s (final velocity 180 °/s) and a prolonged 180 °/s optokinetic stimulus (OKAN II cumulative amplitude 724°,
duration 170 s, VAN II: 635°, 175 s). OKAN II is missing
with stimuli shorter than 10 s and increases up to the
longest stimulus tested (15 min). Thus the discharge properties of the secondary integrators seem to be very similar, the charge characteristics, however, are different.
Secondary nystagmus is directly elicited by the stimulus
and does not depend on the execution of primary after-
nystagmus. Fixation-suppression during primary vestibular afternystagmus (Collins, 1968; Cohen et al., 1981;
Koenig, Dichgans, 1981) as well as during OKAN I (Waespe
et al., 1978) reduces the primary afternystagmus, but not
the secondary one; instead secondary nystagmus is frequently stronger.
We thus suggest that there are 3 central integrating
mechanisms besides the mechanical integration properties
of the cupula: The integrator in the vestibular nucleus

responsible for OKAN I and the prolongation of the time
constant of VAN I, a storage mechanism for pursuit,
probably used for prediction and a secondary integrator
with a low gain and a long discharge time constant
counteracting all kinds of primary afternystagmus (VAN I,
OKAN I, and PAN I).

REFERENCES
Brandt T, Dichgans J and Büchele W (1974) Motion habituation: Inverted self-motion perception and optokinetic
after-nystagmus, Exp. Brain Res. 21,337-352.
Buettner W, Waespe W and Henn V (1976) Duration and direction of optokinetic after-nystagmus as a function of
stimulus exposure time in the monkey, Arch. Psychiat.
Nervenkr. 222, 281-191.
Buettner UW and Büttner U (1979) Vestibular nuclei activity in the alert monkey during suppression of vestibular
and optokinetic nystagmus, Exp. Brain Res. 37,581-593.
Büttner U and Waespe W (1981) Vestibular nerve activity
during vestibular and optokinetic nystagmus, Exp. Brain
Res. 41,310-315.
Cohen B, Matsuo V and Raphan T (1977) Quantitative analysis of the velocity characteristics of optokinetic
nystagmus and optokinetic after-nystagmus, J. Physiol
(London) 270,321-344.
Cohen B, Henn V, Raphan T and Dennett D (1981) Velocity
storage, nystagmus and visual vestibular interactions in
humans, Ann. N.Y. Acad. Sci. 374,421-433.
Collins WE (1968) Special effects of brief periods of
visual fixation on nystagmus and sensations of turning,
Aerospace Med. 39,257-266.
Dichgans J and Brandt T (1972) Visual vestibular interaction and motion perception. In Dichgans J and Bizzi E,
eds. Cerebral control of eye movements and motion perception, pp. 327-338 (Vol. 82) Bibliotheca Ophthalmologica,
Basel, Karger.
Fernandez C and Goldberg JM (1971) Physiology of peripheral neurons innervating semicircular canals of the
squirrel monkey. II Response to sinusoidal stimulation
and the dynamics of the peripheral vestibular system,
J. Neurophysiol. 34,661-675.
Keller EL (1976) Behaviour of horizontal semicircular
canal afferents in alert monkey during vestibular and
optokinetic stimulation, Exp. Brain Res. 24,459-471.
Koenig E and Dichgans J (1981) Aftereffects of vestibu-
lar and optokinetic stimulation and their interaction,
Ann. N.Y. Acad. Sci. 374,434-445.
Mackensen G and Rudolf U (1962) Untersuchungen zur
Physiologie des optokinetischen Nachnystagmus. III.
Mitteilung. Ein Beitrag zur Entstehung des optokine-
tischen Nachnystagmus, Albrecht v. Graefes Arch.
Ophth. 165,60-70.
Muratore R and Zee DS (1979) Pursuit after-nystagmus,
Vision Research 19,1057-1059.
Raphan T, Matsuo V and Cohen B (1979) Velocity storage
in the vestibulo-ocular reflex arc, Exp. Brain Res.
35,229-248.

Waespe W and Henn V (1977) Vestibular nuclei activity
during optokinetic afternystagmus in the alert monkey,
Exp. Brain Res. 30,323-330.
Waespe W, Huber T and Henn V (1978) Dynamic changes of
optokinetic after-nystagmus caused by brief visual
fixation periods in monkey and man, Arch. Psychiat.
Nervenkr. 226,1-10.

THE COORDINATION OF PURSUIT AND SACCADIC EYE MOVEMENTS IN THE
SCANNING OF A MOVING SCENE.

Paolo Viviani

Laboratoire de Physiologie Neurosensorielle

C.N.R.S. - Paris

1-ABSTRACT

The visual exploration of a scene in relative motion with respect to
the observer requires the joint action of the two main oculomotor modes:
the smooth pursuit mode to stabilize the scene with respect to the head,
and the saccadic mode to capture the visual targets.The coordination of
these two modes is studied in the case of reading eye movements. We
provide a quantitative description of the changes that displacements of
different amplitude, direction and velocity induce in the parameters of
the saccadic sequences. The possible strategies for planning a saccade
to a moving visual target are discussed and compared with the results.
It appears that such planning has access to, and is contingent upon, information on the smooth pursuit components, and therefore that the coordi
nation of pursuit and saccadic movements entails more than the simple
vectorial summation of the two components.

2-INTRODUCTION

One of the most remarkable aspects of the oculomotor system is the
sharp difference, both qualitative and functional, between its two main
modes of operation: saccadic scan and smooth pursuit. It is indeed quite
unique in the whole motor system that one and the same neuromuscular
complex has evolved specific control modes to satisfy specific needs.
Nothing of the kind has for instance happened in the case of the tongue
movements which eventually took up the all important task of speaking
withouth evolving a task-specific mode of operation.

Even more intriguing are the instances when these two sharply different
types of eye movements are called upon simultaneously (Feinstein and
Williams,1972).This happens more frequently than we may perhaps realize:
whenever the visual scene and the observer are in relative motion, the

Roucoux, A. and Crommelinck, M. (eds.): Physiological and Pathological Aspects of Eye Movements.
© *1982, Dr W. Junk Publishers, The Hague, Boston, London.* ISBN-13: 978-94-009-8002-0

exploratory scanning of the scene requires in fact the coordinated action
of both the pursuit and saccadic systems.Ideally, the smooth pursuit
should stabilize the visual scene with respect to the retina in order to
provide a workable frame of reference for the planning of the saccades.
In actual facts, however, perfect stabilisation is seldomly,if ever,achie
ved (Stark et al.,1962), expecially when the relative displacement between the scene and the observer is unpredictable (Michel and Melvill Jones,
1966; St Cyr and Fender,1969 a,b). Thus the planning of the saccades also
requires the availability of proprio- and exteroceptive information on
the intervenig smooth pursuit.

The following research in an attempt to clarify the nature of this
coordination in the particular case of reading eye movements. This task
is ideally suited to our purposes because reading is certainly one of the
most familiar and stereotyped forms of oculomotor performances, and becau
se the normal (i.e. static) scanning pattern during reading has been
extensively studied (Levi-Schoen and O'Reagan,1979; Monty and Senders,1976).
An effort is made to render in a quantitative fashion some aspects of the
motor performance. However, the main concern of this preliminary work is
with the qualitative description of the oculomotor strategies. The study
includes three experiments. The first two were designed to provide a mea
sure of the difficulty that different types of displacements introduce in
the reading task, both in the case of litterary texts (Experiment I) and
random digits (Experiment II). Experiment III studies more specifically
the organisation of the eye movements.

3-APPARATUS AND GENERAL PROCEDURE

Subjects sat at 57 cm. from a translucent projection screen. At this
distance 1 cm. subtends approximately 1°. During the recording of eye
movements (Experiment III) the head of the subject was immobilized with
the help of a front rest and of an individually molded biteboard. When
only reading time was being measured (Experiments I and II),the distance
of the eyes from the screen was kept constant by the front rest,but the
head was otherwise unconstrained. The texts to be read were retroprojected
on the screen by a Leitz Pradovit 2500 slide projector. Each text was
contained in the white rectangular frame provided by the slide mounting
(angular dimension 24°x 36°). The average luminance of the frame was
100 cd/m^2 and the contrast with the dimly illuminated sorrounds was

about 10. With the help of two orthogonally mounted galvanometric mirrors
(Scanner,300-GPX) the images on the screen were displaced sinusoidally
along the three main directions: horizontal, vertical and oblique(along
the 45°/225° meridian). The maximum angular displacement in both the
horizontal and vertical direction could take one of the three values $\pm$ 5°,
$\pm$ 7.5°, $\pm$ 10°. The frame displacement in the case of oblique movements
was $\sqrt{2}$ larger than each of these values, respectively. The range of fre
quencies of the sinusoidal oscillations varied according to the values of
their amplitude (see later). In Experiments I and II the voice of the
subjects during overt reading was taped to measure reading times and to
analyze the inflectional and prosodic patterns. In Experiment III the
horizontal and vertical components of the eye movements were measured
with the search-coil technique (Robinson,1963; Collewijn et al.,1975)
which affords a dynamic accuracy of a few minutes of arc. An accurate
calibration procedure (Viviani and Swensson, 1981) was followed to obtain
a static accuracy of the same order of magnitude. Both the eye movements
and the displacements of the texts were filtered (400 Hz. cut-off),sampled
(1 KHz. sampling rate) and stored for subsequent processing.

4-EXPERIMENT I

Our first concern shall be to define the range of parameters within
which it is meaningful to explore the coordination of pursuit and saccades
in the case of dynamic reading. Experiment I provides an estimate of this
range using a global measure of performance. Quite expectedly, as the
size and frequency of the relative displacement increases, all aspects
of overt reading are progressively affected. Preliminary measurements
have however demonstrated the existence of three qualitatively different
types of behavior. For any combination of direction and amplitude of the
displacements, at the lower frequencies the presence of movement does
not modify appreciably the reading pattern. In the middle frequency range
only the rythm of reading slows down, but the inflectional and prosodic
patterns are not affected. Finally, a further increase in frequency
results, quite abruptly, into the appearance of localised slowndowns or
pauses which make the rythm very irregular and affect heavily the supra
segmental features of the voice. Moreover, subjects make many errors,
also because their understanding of the text becomes poor. This last type

of behavior can no longer be construed as normal reading. It appears thus
that reading time provides,for any combination of amplitude and direction
of the movement, an upper frequency bound within which the oculomotor
coordination subserves a qualitatively homogeneous performance. Furthermore, in the middle frequency range, it provides an appropriate behavioral
measure of the extent to which movement affects the performance.

4.1-METHOD

Texts

The texts used for the experiments consisted of 9 short excerpts of
standard french prose taken from the newspaper "Le Monde". The criterion
of selection, and some minor editing ensured that the texts could be read
with a smooth, regular prosodic rythm. All numbers and unpronounceable
acronyms were eliminated. Some particularly elaborated syntactic forms
were resolved into simpler expressions. Each text consisted of 10 lines
containing between 70 and 75 characters (including spaces). Words were
never split. The texts were typeset in Newton 55/20 font with right-end
justification, and transformed in standard 24 x 36 slides. The angular
size of the projected text was 12°x 32°.

Subjects

Ten native french-speaking subjects participated to the experiments
and were paid for their services.

Procedure

The experiments were run in three successive sessions, one for each
value of the displacement amplitude. The order of the sessions was rando
mized and counterbalanced across subjects, and they were spaced by at
least one week to prevent excessive practice with the texts. In each
session a subject read four times the entire sequence of 9 texts. The
first three times the texts were animated by an horizontal, vertical and
oblique movement respectively. The fourth time no movement was imposed.
Text no.1 was always presented at the lowest frequency,which varied as a
function of the amplitude (1.0 Hz. for $\pm$ 5°;.8 Hz. for $\pm$ 7.5°;.6 Hz. for $\pm$
10°).   For text no.2 the frequency was increased by 0.1 Hz. and so on
until text no.9 which was always read at the highest frequency (1.8 Hz.
for $\pm$ 5°; 1.6 Hz.for $\pm$ 7.5° ; 1.4 Hz. for 10°). In the case of vertical

and oblique displacements of large amplitude (7.5° and 10°),some subjects
have not been able to complete all the projected sequences because their
performance entered in third type of behavior described above(deciphering)
before reaching the highest frequency.

4.2-RESULTS

   Table I reports the means and standard deviations of the reading times
T_s (averaged over the three sessions) for all subjects and all texts in
the static condition. A two-way analysis of variance shows that the

Table I: Static Reading Times(sec.)

Text	1	2	3	4	5	6	7	8	9	
Av	33.7	34.3	36.5	37.4	35.8	37.2	37.1	37.2	38.9	
Sd	3.25	3.46	3.82	3.65	3.84	4.10	3.36	3.40	4.46	
Subject	S_1	S_2	S_3	S_4	S_5	S_6	S_7	S_8	S_9	S_{10}
Av	35.5	37.5	43.6	34.5	35.5	33.4	38.8	40.7	33.3	31.6
Sd	2.09	1.41	2.22	1.79	2.96	1.15	2.09	2.10	2.18	1.70

"subject" factor is highly significant ($F(9,80)= 26.95$, $P \ll .001$) whereas
reading times are not sognificantly different across texts ($F(8,81)= 1.67$,
$P= .118$). A significant interaction effect can be demonstrated, which
however need not to concern us in this context. For our purposes, we can
admit that texts and subjects are two independent factors of the experiments, and that the static reading times define a baseline performance
for each combination of these factors.
   Each panel in Figure I shows the results in the dynamic condition for
the indicated directions. The data points in this figure are the average
across all subjects of the ratio T_d/T_s between the individual dynamic
(T_d) and static (T_s) times. If more that 5 subjects were unable to read
the text for a given combination of amplitude, direction and frequency
of the displacements, the corresponding data point is omitted. The results
demonstrate the following points:
1) Below .7 Hz a displacement of the image has no apparent effect,under
   any condition, on the reading performance.
2) Above this value, reading times progressively increase as a function
   of frequency for all combinations of amplitude and direction.However,

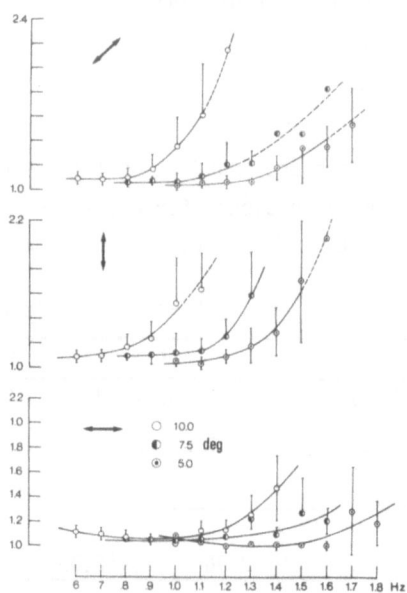

Figure 1: Reading times as a function of frequency for
all combinations of amplitude and direction of the
displacement.Average data for all subjects normalized to
the individual static times.

horizontal displacements affect the performance far less than either the
vertical   or oblique ones
3) Since oblique and vertical displacements have roughly comparable effects,
   and considering also that the former are $\sqrt{2}$ larger than the latter ,
   it is likely that the presence of a vertical component is the discrimi_
   nating factor vis à vis the horizontal case.
4) The higest frequency at which normal reading is possible for all combi_
   nations of amplitude and direction, is about 1.2 Hz.
5) The amplitude A and the frequency ω of the displacement have independent effects on reading times. If the performance were only dependent
   on the average linear velocity of the images(which is proportional to

the product $A\omega$ then reading times should be expressible by a relation of the type $T_d = f(A\omega)$. In fact, the results are in a much better agreement with the general expression $T_d = f(\omega + g(A))$, where g is some function of the amplitude and the function f only depends on the frequency. Thus, to a first approximation, increasing the movement amplitude simply results into a rightword shift of the Time/Frequency curves.

5-EXPERIMENT II

Experiment I has shown that the effects of vertical and oblique displacements on the reading performance are considerably larger than those of horizontal movements. Moreover, the analysis of the voice recordings shows that the rythm of reading during horizontal movements is fairly constant across the lines of the text. Instead, when a vertical movement component is present, the rythm slows down in the middle of the text, where the spatial references provided by the text frame are less visible. One possi ble reason for these differences may be the fact that only in the first case smooth pursuit and saccadic eye movements have the same direction. Experiment II was designed specifically to test this hypothesis by using numerical texts which can be scanned both vertically and horizontally.

5.1-METHOD

Texts

Only one text was used which consisted of a square matrix containing 100 arabic numbers arranged in 10 rows and 10 columns. Each row and each column contained a different random permutation of the first ten numerals (0 to 9). The font type, the vertical angular size and the spacing between rows was the same as in the litterary texts.

Procedure

The general experimental procedure was similar to that of Experiment I. However, only one frequency (ω = 1. Hz.) and one amplitude (A= $\pm$ 10°) was tested. These values produce a substantial reduction of the reading rate, but are still compatible with what was considered normal behavior. The displacement of the text could be either horizontal (M_h) or vertical (M_v), and the matrix could be read either row-wise (R_h) or column-wise(R_v). Four conditions are then possible:

(M_h,R_h), (M_h,R_v),(M_v,R_h),(M_v,R_v). In a single session each subject executed five times the following sequence:

1: (M_h,R_h); 2: (M_h,R_v); 3: static reading,row wise; 4: (M_v,R_h); 5: (M_v,R_v);
6: static reading, column-wise.

Subject

Four subjects, native french speakers, participated in the experiments
and were paid for their services.

5.2-RESULTS

In static conditions, reading by columns does not take significantly
longer than reading by rows. Thus, at least in the case of digits, the
performance seems to be independent of the absolute direction of the
saccades. Table II reports, for each subject and each experimental condition, the average over the five repetitions of the ratio T_d/T_s between
dynamic and static reading times.

Table II: Dynamic Reading Times for Digits(Normalized)

	S_1	S_2	S_3	S_4	Av.
(M_h,R_h)	1.09	1.27	1.09	0.86	1.08
(M_h,R_v)	1.32	2.16	2.19	1.40	1.77
(M_v,R_h)	1.09	1.15	1.36	1.29	1.22
(M_v,R_v)	1.37	1.31	1.48	1.33	1.37

On the average, the ratio T_d/T_s is higher when the direction of the
displacement is different from the direction of the saccades than in the
case when the two movements have the same direction. However, the pattern
of the results also suggests that, in contrast with the static case, the
dynamic performance also depends on the absolute direction of the saccades.
A simple linear model is used to quantify the relative weight of these
two factors. Let us suppose that the ratio T_d/T_s is equal to 1 plus the
sum of two terms. The first term takes the values k_h or k_v according to
the absolute direction of the saccades. The second term takes the value
k_d if saccades and pursuit have different directions, and 0 otherwise.
Thus, from Table II we get the following set of relations:

Condition	T_d/T_s	Exp
(M_h, R_h)	$K_h + 1$	= 1.08
(M_h, R_v)	$k_v + k_d + 1$	= 1.77
(M_v, R_h)	$k_n + k_d + 1$	= 1.22
(M_v, R_v)	$k_v + 1$	= 1.37

Solving this overdeterminated system in the least square sense, we get an estimate of the parameters k_h, k_v and k_d:

$$k_h = .015 \qquad k_v = .435 \qquad k_d = .270$$

This simple model predicts quite accurately the experimental values of the ratio T_d / T_s:

Observed	1.08	1.77	1.22	1.37
Predicted	1.015	1.705	1.285	1.435

The total lenghtning $T_d - T_s$ of the reading time can then be decomposed into three parts which correspond to the factors k_h, k_v and k_d :

	$T_d - T_s$	$k_h T_s$	$k_v T_s$	$k_v T_s$
(M_h, R_h)	0.60	0.60	0.00	0.00
(M_h, R_v)	28.25	0.00	17.43	10.82
(M_v, R_h)	11.06	0.58	0.00	10.48
(M_v, R_v)	16.89	0.00	16.89	0.00

This analysis confirms the presence of two additive factors: the mutual direction of the pursuit and of the saccades accounts for approximately one third of the total lenghtning. The absolute direction of the saccades is almost irrelevant in the case of horizontal displacements (as in static reading) but it is the dominant factor in the case of vertical displacements.

6-EXPERIMENT III.

Figure 2 illustrates a typical pattern of reading eye movements under normal (i.e. static) conditions. The lines of the text are scanned by a

very regular sequence of horizontal saccades of small amplitude (4°- 5°).
One large backward saccade with a small vertical component is generally
used to skip from one line to the next. Because reading eye movements
are so highly directional, their coordination with a pursuit component
must depend critically on the direction of the displacement.

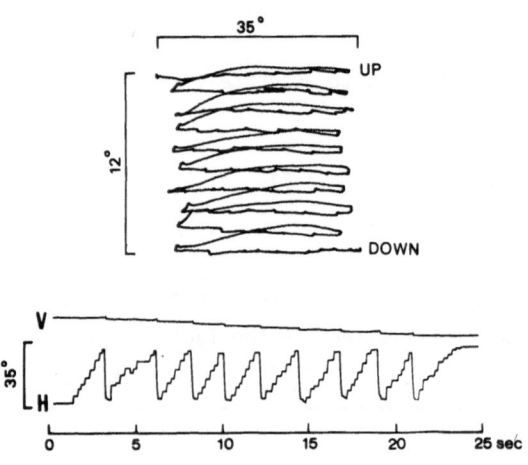

Figure 2: Typical recording of the horizontal(H) and
vertical (V) components of the eye movements during
normal (static) reading of a text used in the experiments. In the upper panel, the resulting X-Y displacement of the gaze.

In the case of horizontal displacements, the problem to be solved by
the oculomotor system is basically that of composing algebraically the
movements of the eye in space with the perceived motion of the text with
respect to the same stable external reference. When the text is displaced
vertically the problem is more complex for it involves vectorial composi-

tion of the eye and text movements. In both instances, however, the oculo
motor system must estimate the total displacement of the text after the
completion of a saccade. As we shall argue later, this seems a rather
formidable task which requires both proprio- and extero-ceptive information on the ongoing movements, as well as accurate knowledge of the in-
trinsic properties of the saccadic system itself.

In Experiment III reading eye movements both in space and with respect
to the moving frame were recorded to provide:

a) A qualitative description of the modes of coordination between smooth
   pursuit and saccadic eye movements.
b) A quantitative measure of the effects of relative motion upon the para
   meters of the saccadic sequences (Amplitude, duration and latencies).
c) The groundwork for a discussion on the possible mechanisms which permit
   the reaching of visual targets under dynamic conditions.

6.1-METHODS

Procedure

The general procedure was that of Experiment I. However, reading was
done silently because of the biteboard used to fixate the head position.
All the three directions of frame displacement were tested, but the ampli
tude was kept constant ($\pm 10°$). On the basis of the results of Experiment
I, the effects of frequency was tested only at three selected values :
.2, .6 and 1.0 Hz. which cover most of the dynamic range of interest.
Each subject participated to three identical sessions organised as
follows:

Text no.	1	2	3	3	4	5	6	6	7	8	8	9
Frequency	.2	.6	1.	static	.2	.6	1.	static	.2	.6	1.	static
Direction	→	→	→		↑	↑	↑		↗	↗	↗	

Each session begun and ended with a calibration. Sessions were spaced by
at least two weeks.

Subjects

Two payed subjects participated in the experiments. They both had a
long experience with the corneal lens used to measure eye movements.

6.2-RESULTS

The summation of pursuit and saccadic components.

Figures 3,4 and 5 show representative examples of eye movement recordings for the horizontal, vertical and oblique displacements respectively. Each of the three parts of these figures is relative to a frequency value (A: 1. Hz.; B: .6 Hz.; C: .2 Hz) and contains two sets of recordings. Those labelled "Space" represent the horizontal (H) and vertical (V) components of the eye movements with respect to the head (which is fixed in space). Those labelled "Page" represent the position of the gaze with respect to the moving frame, and have been obtained by vectorial subtraction of the frame displacement from the eye movements.

During horizontal displacements (Figure 3) the vertical eye movements are unaffected by the dynamic conditions. The horizontal eye components in space are, in all cases,the algebraic composition of the smooth and saccadic mode. However, the morphology of the resulting tracings depends on the frequency of the oscillations. At .2 Hz.(C) the subject is able to read two, or even three lines within one 5 sec. period. When the text moves to the right, the eye runs after it; when it moves to the left,the line of sight remains roughly in the straight-ahead position and scans the lines by taking advantage of the frame displacement(Bouma and de Voogd, 1974). At this frequency, the most frequently observed strategy consists of initiating the scanning of a line in coincidence with one of the two extreme positions of the frame (zero velocity). At .6 Hz. (B) it becomes difficult to apply this strategy because the time to read a line almost coincides with the period of the oscillations. As a consequence,the movements of the eyes in space become very erratic. Finally, at the highest frequency(A) several cycles of oscillation are necessary to read a line and the large backward saccades are once again synchronized frequently with the extremes of the cycles.

The most relevant aspect of these results is the striking linearity of the neuromuscular mechanisms which integrate the pursuit and saccadic components of the motor commands. In fact, even when the total displacement of the line of sight in space is very irregular (as for instance in panel B), it nevertheless contains a stair-case saccadic component quite similar to the one present in normal reading. This is demonstrated by the tracings labelled "Page" which represent the best approximation to the

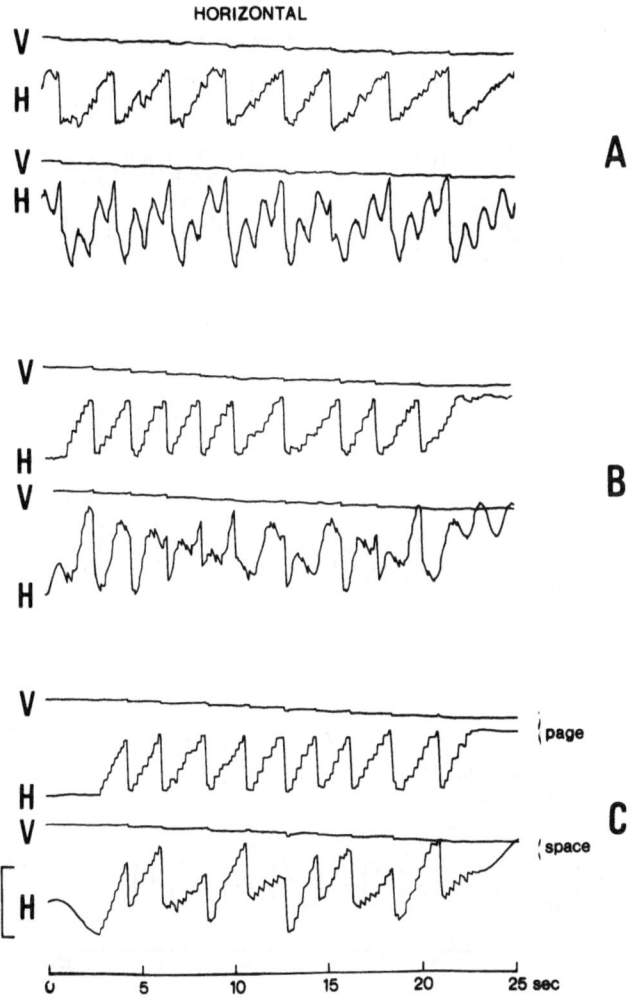

Figure 3: Reading eye movements during horizontal
sinusoidal displacements of the text. A : 1 Hz.,
B : .6Hz., C : .2 Hz. The traces noted "Page" show
the movements of the gaze with respect to the moving
frame of reference.

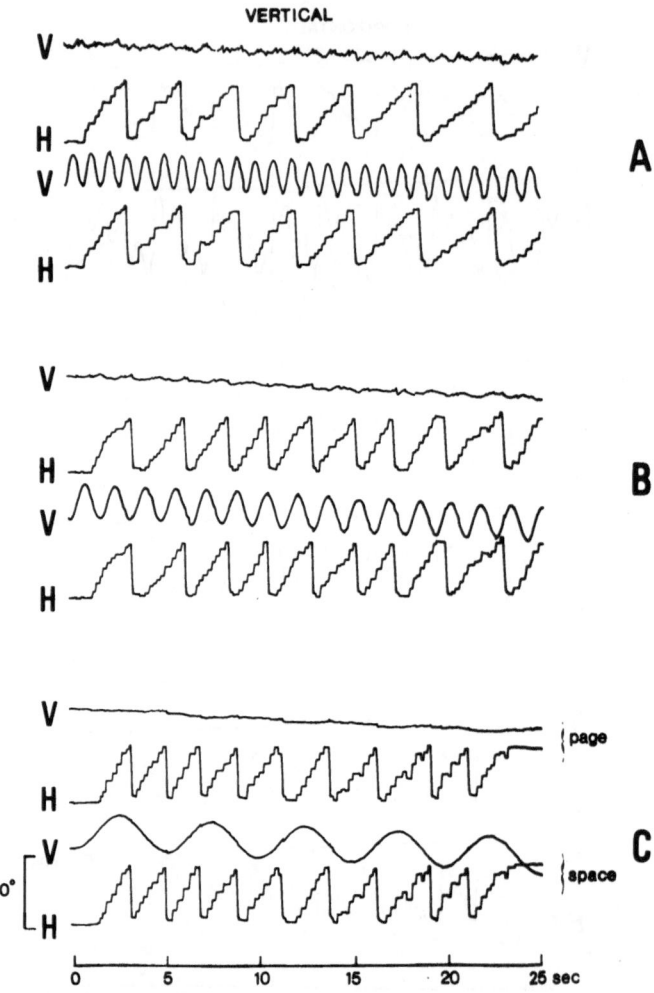

Figure 4: Reading eye movements during vertical sinusoidal displacements of the text. See Fig. 3.

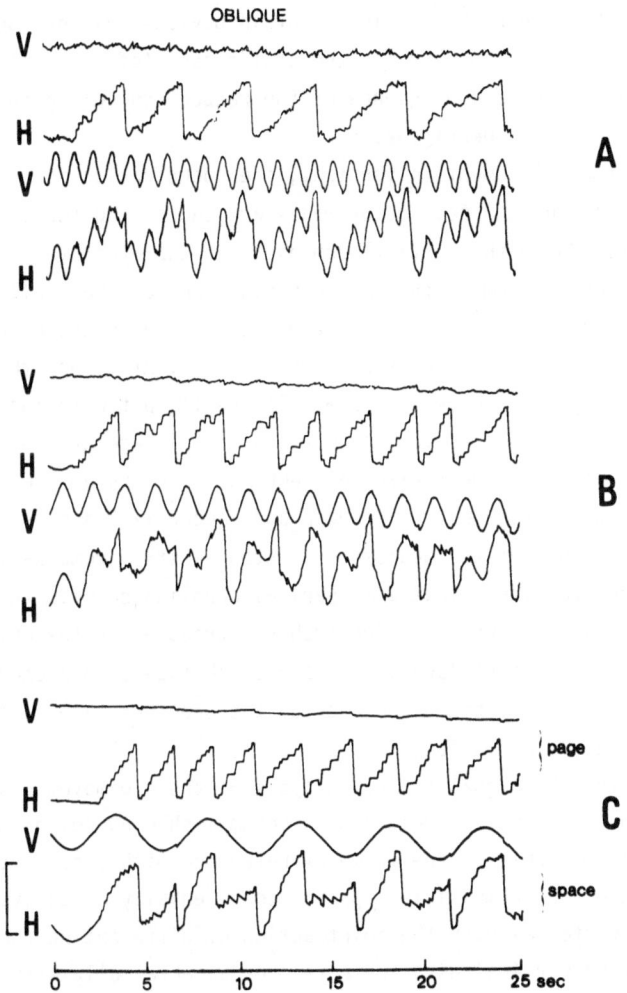

OBLIQUE

A

B

page

space

40°

0   5   10   15   20   25 sec

Figure 5: Reading eye movements during oblique
sinusoidal displacements of the text. See Fig. 3.

normal reading sequence that the observer can obtain with the help of the
pursuit system. Even when the tracings contain obvious distorsions with
respect to the analogous results for the static case (cf.Figure 11) these
distorsion appear to be a consequence of the reduced pursuit gain rather
than the effect of non-linearities.

When the text displacement is vertical, the coordination is entirely
different, because the two oculomotor modes are addressing two independent
muscular systems. While the vertical component of the eye movements in
space is the algebraic sum of the smooth pursuit and of the small line-to-
line vertical saccades, the horizontal component -both in space and accross
the text - show a pure sequence of reading saccades. At .2 Hz. this sequence is virtually undisturbed (cf.again Figure 1), but with increasing
frequency it becomes progressively slower and more irregular. This sug-
stests that the vertical and horizontal neuromuscular system are not completely independent (cf.,however, Goodwin and Fender,1973 a,b).Nevertheless,
the global performance of the oculomotor system is still remarkable,
expecially if one considers that a mechanical coupling between the horizontal and vertical components is inevitably introduced by the oblique
extraocular muscles (Jampel,1966). The case of oblique displacements
(Figure 5) presents the combined features of the previous cases and does
not require further elaboration.

In summary, the above qualitative analysis of the eye movements shows
that reading under dynamic conditions is accomplished by composing a
pursuit command to stabilize the frame of reference,with a conventional
saccadic sequence. The composition appears to be equally effective whether
is is obtained vectorially,by the joint action of different neuromuscular
sustems (as during vertical displacements), or algebraically within the
same system. However, the progressive increase in reading time with the
frequency, and the differences among directions are reflected in the
timing of the saccadic sequences.

Quantitative analysis of the saccadic sequences.

The saccadic components of the eye movements with respect to the text
were analysed as described in detail elsewhere (Viviani and Monot,1981).
Figure 6 resur..es the average results for the two subjects who participated in the experiments. Each panel represents the effect of frequency
on the indicated parameters. Once again the dynamic values of these

parameters are normalized to the corresponding static averages calculated during normal reading.

Both the number (N) and duration (T) of the fixations increase at 1 Hz.[note].The product of these two factors is approximately equivalent

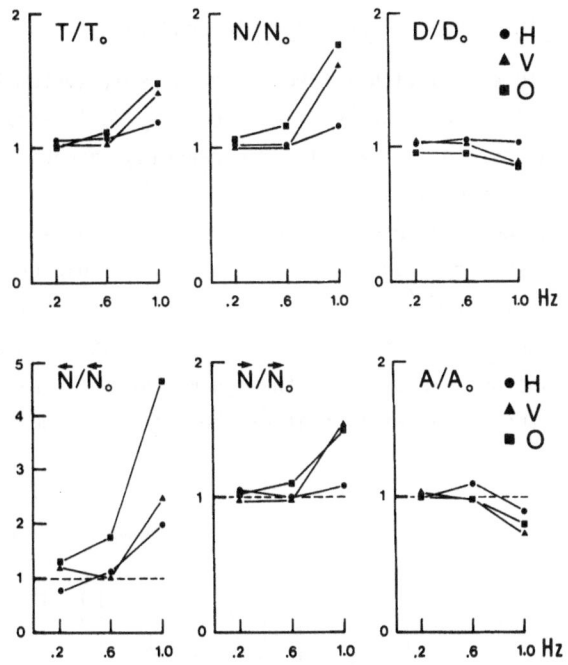

Figure 6: Parameters of the saccadic sequences as a function of the frequency(normalized values). T:fixation duration; N:number of fixations; D:saccade duration;N:number of regressive saccades; N: number of forward saccades; A: amplitude of the saccades.

Note: The slow drifts of the gaze due to the reduced gain of the pursuit were classed as fixations by the analysis as long as their velocity did not exceed 40°/sec.

to the reduction in reading rythm demonstrated in Figures 3 to 5, but is somewhat higher than the corresponding values in the case of overt reading. Although the absolute number of regressive saccades remains small, the ratio N̄/N̄o increases dramatically at the higher frequencies, expecially in the case of oblique displacements. Amplitude (A) and duration (D) of the saccades decrease pari passu, but their variations are modest.

The planning of the saccades under dynamic conditions.

After the capture of a visual target, the pursuit system keeps it in the foveal field for the amount of time necessary to 1)extract the information contained therein, and 2) plan the reaching saccade to the next target. In general, the displacement of the scene is not in the same direction of the vector connecting two successive targets. Thus,whatever its amplitude, a saccade planned along this vector would certainly miss the target by an amount which depends on the velocity of displacement of the scene. In order to obtain an accurate capture, it is instead necessary that the amplitude and direction of the eye movements be planned to reach the point where the target will be after the saccade. Figure 7 demonstra-

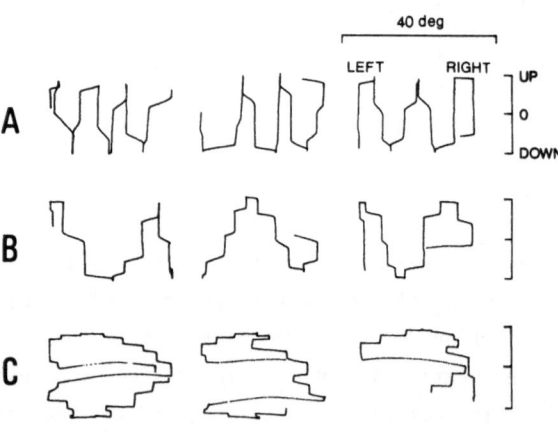

Figure 7: X-Y trajectories of the eye in space during vertical displacements. A : 1 Hz. , B : .6Hz., C : .2Hz.

te this point by showing for each frequency (A: 1 Hz.; B: .6 Hz.; C: .2 Hz.) three representative X-Y recordings of actual eye movements during verti- cal displacements of the text. As hypothesized, forward saccades are bent in the direction of the movement; their inclination is maximal in the midpoint of the displacement -where the velocity is maximum- and virtually zero at both extremes of the oscillations (zero velocity). Notice that the planning of the reaching saccade is quite accurate, for corrective saccades are almost never seen.

Figure 8 illustrate schematically the two pure strategies that may be used for the accurate planning of the movements. According to diagram A, a saccadic motor command is issued which produce a velocity vector V_s directed toward the target position <u>before</u> the movement. However, the pursuit command that made possible the previous fixation continues to act during the saccade and produces a velocity vector V_p in the direction T'-T" of the text displacement. As long as the gain of pursuit is 1, the vectorial summation of the velocities V_s and V_p automatically ensures that the target position T" after the saccade will be correctly reached. From simple geometrical considerations it results that such a scheme would predict the relation $V_p = V_s \, tg \, \varphi$ between the velocities and the

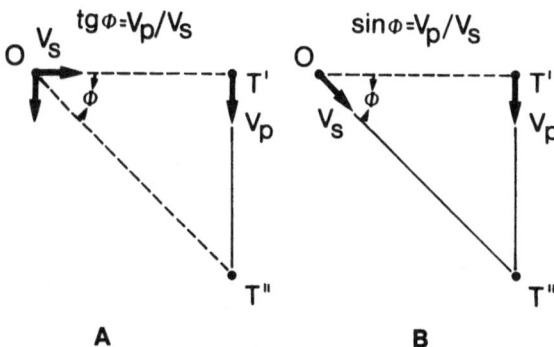

<u>Figure 8</u>: Schematic representation of the two possible pure strategies for capturing a moving visual target with a saccade.

direction of the saccades. This simple and elegant hypothesis is the generalization to the case of two-dimensional movements of the notion that saccade and pursuit velocities summate when they are in the same direction (Jürgens and Becker,1975). According to diagram B,the saccadic motor command is directly programmed to produce a velocity vector V_s pointing to the final target position T". In this case the pursuit command must be shut off during the saccade and the appropriate relation among V_s, V_p and φ is: $V_p = V_s \sin\varphi$.

In order to test these two hypotheses it is sufficient to calculate independently the velocities of the horizontal and vertical components of the total eye movement in space. In fact, if scheme A holds true, the high velocity component corresponding to the saccadic commands should only be present in the horizontal traces. Figure 9 shows an example

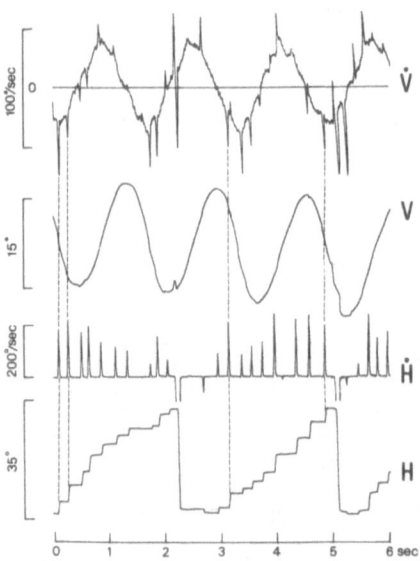

Figure 9: Reading eye movements during vertical displacements at .6Hz.Horizontal and vertical compo- nents of the position and velocity of the eye in space. Notice the presence of saccades also in the vertical component.

of displacement (H and V) and velocity ($\dot{H}$ and $\dot{V}$) traces always
in the case of vertical displacements at .6 Hz. (cf.Figure 7), and demon
strates unambiguously that both the vertical and horizontal traces contains typical saccadic components. We must therefore conclude that the
hypothesis outlined in diagram B of Figure 8 provides a more realistic
description of the saccadic planning than that of diagram A, even though
it prefigures a more complex perceptuomotor coordination (see Discussion).

As a final point,we consider again the question of the accuracy of
the motor plan. The absence of corrective saccades can be taken to suggest that the upper bound on the accuracy is of the order of magnitude
of the "Dead Zone"(approximately .5° under static conditions) which is
defined as the smallest error from the target that still elicits a corrective saccade (Rashbass,1961; Young, 1966; Viviani and Swensson,1981).
It is however interesting to verify directly that indeed amplitude and
direction of the saccadic velocity are planned,as a function of the
instantaneous pursuit velocity, according to the relation $V_p = V_s \sin\varphi$
suggested by the diagram B of Figure 8. The results of Figure 10 provide
such a verification in one subject for a vertical displacement at .6 Hz.
In this Figure, each data point represent the direction of a saccade as
a function of the smooth pursuit velocity V_p at the time of its onset.
Since the spread of saccadic velocities is small (m=160°deg./sec. ;
σ/m =.17), we have only distinguished between the saccades with $V_s < 160°$
(data points ●) and those with $V_s > 160°$ (data points o). The continuous
line is the linear regressions corresponding to $V_s = 115$ deg./sec.
Despite the fact that different values of V_s have been pooled together,
the data indicate a very precise correlation ($r = .89$) between V_p and
the inclination of the saccade $\sin\varphi$. This provides additional evidence
that saccades are planned to aim directly at the final target position.

7-DISCUSSION

Reading a moving text is possible, with normal prosodic and stress
patterns, up to a displacement velocity of about 30°/sec. Under dynamic
conditions the movements of the eyes are quite complex, but can still be
decomposed into a pursuit component, and a sequence of saccades similar
to those occurring during normal reading. However, all the parameters of
the saccadic component (number and duration of the fixations, number of

72

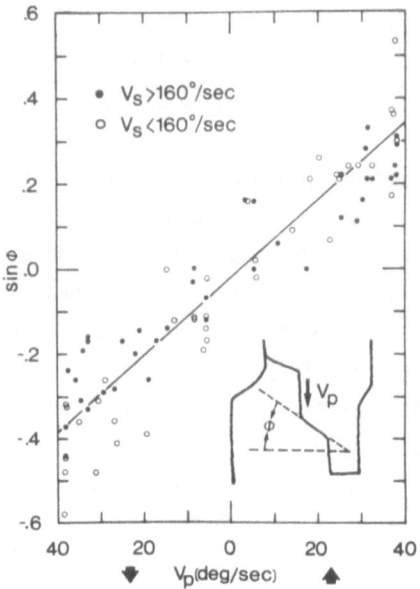

Figure 10: Relation between the velocity of the
smooth pursuit V_p and the direction of the saccades.
Vertical displacements at .6Hz. Notice that at this
frequency the gain of the pursuit is close to 1 and
the pursuit velocity almost coincides with the displacement velocity V_d (see Discussion).

regressive saccades etc.) depart progressively from their normal values.
Moreover, the fixations are increasingly affected by slow drifts due to
the reduced pursuit gain. The decrease in reading rythm with velocity appears to be a specific consequence of the reduced effectiveness with which
the two main oculomotor modes cooperate to capture and stabilize the
intended visual targets. More specifically, if we admit that the local
frame of reference is set up by the vector that is pursued by the eye
(Stoper, 1973; Stern and Emelity, 1978; Pernier et al., 1969), we may
then suppose that the progressive faltering of the pursuit system at the
higher velocities makes the establishment of such a frame more and more
problematic. In its turn, this would affect the correct planning of the

saccades, if indeed they are programmed with respect to a retino-centric
reference.

The analysis of the eye movements has suggested that the coordination
of the two oculomotor modes entails more than the simple summation (algebraic or vectorial) of the respective motor commands. The tentative scheme
given in Diagram B of Figure 8 can then be used to outline the problem
that the visuo-motor control mechanisms must solve to ensure en effective
performance. Assuming that the velocity of the displacement is constant,
the quantities relevant to the planning of a saccade in a dynamic condition are indicated in the schematic diagram of Figure 11. In this scheme
ΔX is the angular distance between the point being fixated (0) and the
initial position of the target (T'), A and ΔT are the amplitude and
duration of the saccade to the final target position T", V_d is the displacement velocity and ψ is the angle between the direction of the movement

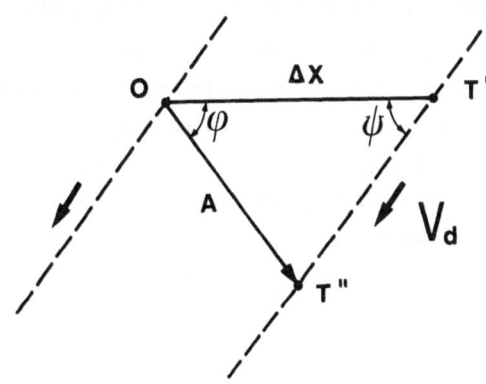

Figure 11: Schematic representation of the
planning of a saccade.

and the vector OT'. Planning the saccade amounts formally to dermining
its intended amplitude and direction φ . However, the amplitude of a saccade is related to its duration by the Main Sequence Law (Yarbus, 1957;
Robinson, 1964; Stark, 1968) which, in the range of values relevant in this
context can be expressed as a power law : $\Delta T = k A^b$. Combining this
expression with simple trigonometric considerations, leads to the following

non-linear system:

$$A^2 = \Delta X^2 + k^2 \, V_p^2 \, A^{2b} - 2k \Delta X \, V_p \, A^b \cos \psi$$

$$\cos \varphi = (\Delta X - k \, V_p \, A^b \cos \psi)/A$$

The first equation contains quantities which can be measured by the visual system (ΔX, ψ, V_p), as well as parameters which are characteristic of the saccadic system (k,b) and may be supposed to be available. Solving for the unknown term A and substituing in the second equation one can calculate the other unknown φ.

In conclusion, we must admit the possibility for the visual system to provide simultaneously a distance and a velocity estimate (Barmack, 1970). In particular, it should be noted that estimating the amplitude and direction of the velocity vector V_p poses an interestingly complex problem. In fact, when the gain of the pusuit loop is close to 1 (small values of V_p), only the motor command itself can provide such an estimate. However, as soon as the gain decreases, this efferent information must be complemented with an afferent sensory information on the retinal slip.

The above-going discussion was only meant to indicate the logical necessity of integrating both proprio- and extero-ceptive informations to the motor plan for capturing a moving target with a saccade. It should be obvious how unlikely it is that the perceptuo-motor system perform the specific calculations outlined above, or, for that matter, any computation at all. However, our analysis suggests the level of sophistication that the intervening processes, whatever they are, must display to afford the observed performances.

Aknowledgements
This research was partly supported by CCETT/CNRS RA-7689 Research Grant. We wish to thank Ms. Annie Monot for her precious assistence.

REFERENCES

Barmack, N.H. (1970)
Modification of eye movements by instantaneous changes in the velocity of visual targets. Vision Res., 10, 1431-1441

Bouma, H. and de Voogd, H.D. (1974)
On the control of eye saccades in reading. Vision Res., 14, 273-284

Collewijn, H., Mark, F. van der, and Jansen, T.C. (1975)
Precise recording of human eye movements. Vision Res., 15, 447-450

Feinstein, R. and Williams, W.J. (1972)
Interaction of the horizontal and vertical human oculomotor systems : the vertical smooth pursuit and horizontal saccadic systems. Vision Res. 12, 45-52

Goodwin, A.W. and Fender, D.H. (1973a)
The interaction between horizontal and vertical eye-rotation in traking tasks. Vision Res., 13, 1701-1712

Goodwin, A.W. and Fender, D.H. (1973b)
Recognition of component differences in two-dimensional oculomotor tracking tasks. Vision Res., 13, 1905-1913

Jampel, R.S. (1966)
The action of the superior oblique muscle. Arch. Opthalmol., 75, 535-544

Jürgens, R. and Becker, W. (1975)
Is there a linear addition of saccades and pursuit movements? in : G. Lennerstrand and P. Bach-y-rita (Eds.) Basic Mechanisms of Ocular Motility. Oxford: Pergamon Press

Levi-Schoen, A. and O'Reagan, K. (1979)
The control of eye movements in reading (A Tutorial). in : P.A. Kolers, M.E. Wrolstad and H. Bouma (Eds.) Processing of Visible Language, I. New-York: Plenum.

Michel, J.A. and Melvill Jones G. (1966)
Dependence of visual tracking capability upon stimulus predictability. Vision Res., 9, 1149-1165

Monty, R.A. and Senders, J.W. (Eds.) (1976)
Eye Movements and Psychological Processes, I. Hillsdale, N.J.: Erlbaum.

Pernier, J., Jeannerod, M. and Gerin, P. (1969)
Elaboration et décision des saccades : adaptation à la trace du stimulus. Vision Res., 6, 707-716

Rashbass, C. (1961)
The relatioship between saccadic and smooth eye tracking movements. J. Physiol.(London), 159, 326-338

Robinson, D.A. (1963)
A method for measuring eye movements using a search coil in a magnetic field. IEEE Trans. Bio. Med. Electron., 10, 137-145

Robinson, D.A. (1964)
The mechanics of human saccadic eye movemnts. J. Physiol.(London), 174, 245-264

Stark, L., Vossius, G. and Young, L.R. (1962)
Predictive control of eye tracking movements. IRE Trans. Human Factors
Electron., HEF-3, 52-57

Stark, L. (1968)
Neurological Control Systems. New-York: Plenum

St Cyr, G.J. and Fender, D.H. (1969a)
Non linearities of the human oculomotor system : gain. Vision Res., 9,
1235-1246

St Cyr, G.J. and Fender, D.H. (1969b)
Non linearities of the human oculomotor system : time delays. Vision Res.,
9, 1491-1503

Stern, L.D. and Emelity, D. (1978)
Evidence for frames of reference based on pursuit eye movements.Percept.
Psychophys., 24, 521-528

Stoper, A.E. (1973)
Apparent motion of stimuli presented stroboscopically during pursuit
movements of the eye. Percept. Psychophys., 13, 201-211

Viviani, P. and Monot, F. (1981)
L'exploration visuelle de textes alpha-numériques en mouvement. Internal
Report: Laboratoire de Physiologie Neurosensorielle: Paris

Viviani, P. and Swensson, R. (1982)
Saccadic eye movements to peripherally discriminated visual targets.
J. Exp. Psychol.:HPP, 8, 113-126

Yarbus, A.L. (1957)
Eye Movements and Vision. New-York: Plenum

Young, L.R. (1966)
The dead zone to saccadic eye movements. Proc. Symp. Biomed. Eng.
(Milwaukee),1,360-362

DEPENDENCE OF SACCADIC PREDICTION ON ASYMMETRICAL PERIODIC STIMULUS

S. RON (Occupational Health and Rehabilitation Institute at
Loewenstein Hospital, Raanana, Israel)

1. INTRODUCTION

In man, the saccadic response to a visual random unpredictable
target is known to have a delay of about 250 msec. When the target
motion is a periodic square move in the horizontal plane, this
delay gradually decreases as the tracking proceeds, until the eye
actually overtakes the target. Thereafter, the eyes continue to
move accurately with the target with little or no time lag (Stark
et al., 1962; Dallos, Jones, 1963; Fuchs, 1967). This prediction
is not an "either-or" property of the prediction system (Michael,
Melvill Jones, 1966; Stark, 1968). When a subject is presented
with a periodic square wave target, after about 10 cycles a rapid
buildup of prediction occurs, changing the periodicity and changing
the (mean) prediction depending on the cycle duration.
When the subject is presented with a periodic target displacement
for eye movements prediction, coordination between the two hemispheres has to take place. It might be presumed that some timing
control takes place in certain neural networks; the timing of the
periodic movements is due to an oscillator in the neural networks.
Once the period of the oscillator has been learnt, the visual
target displacement might not become of prime importance for the
repetitive movement but rather of a correcting function since the
eyes will continue to move at about the learned cycle rate. Correction will be in both cycle duration and amplitude accuracy.
Presenting the subject with an asymmetrical target, the eye movement response will be different; the subject must learn the two
phase period duration. In this paradigm, the eye movement response
was dependent on the asymmetry and cycle time. Furthermore, under
certain conditions, seeing the target had only limited effect in
repeating cycle duration or cycle asymmetry.

2. CHANGING CYCLE DURATION, FIXED SYMMETRY

Eye movement time response (T) and phase duration response (R) were
measured for each phase of the cycles (Fig. 1,A). We define the
term "prediction" as any time ranging from 150 msec delay to an
anticipation response shorter than half the cycle time but not exceeding 500 msec. Under this definition, anticipation may be so
great that the eye has a chance to see itself in error (termed
"overprediction" if greater than 100 msec, by Stark, 1968). The
eye may still not correct itself, but rather await the expected
change of target position.
When a symmetrical square wave was presented, the eye movement
response was dependent on the cycle duration. In the majority of
subjects, although the target presentation was a symmetrical square
wave, it had a different (mean) prediction when the eyes moved in
one direction or the other. The difference (15 to 80 msec), however, was almost independent on cycle duration. When the subject
was asked to follow an imaginary target at the same pacing, the
eye movements response was surprisingly accurate for long cycles.

Roucoux, A. and Crommelinck, M. (eds.): Physiological and Pathological Aspects of Eye Movements.
© *1982, Dr W. Junk Publishers, The Hague, Boston, London.* ISBN-13: 978-94-009-8002-0

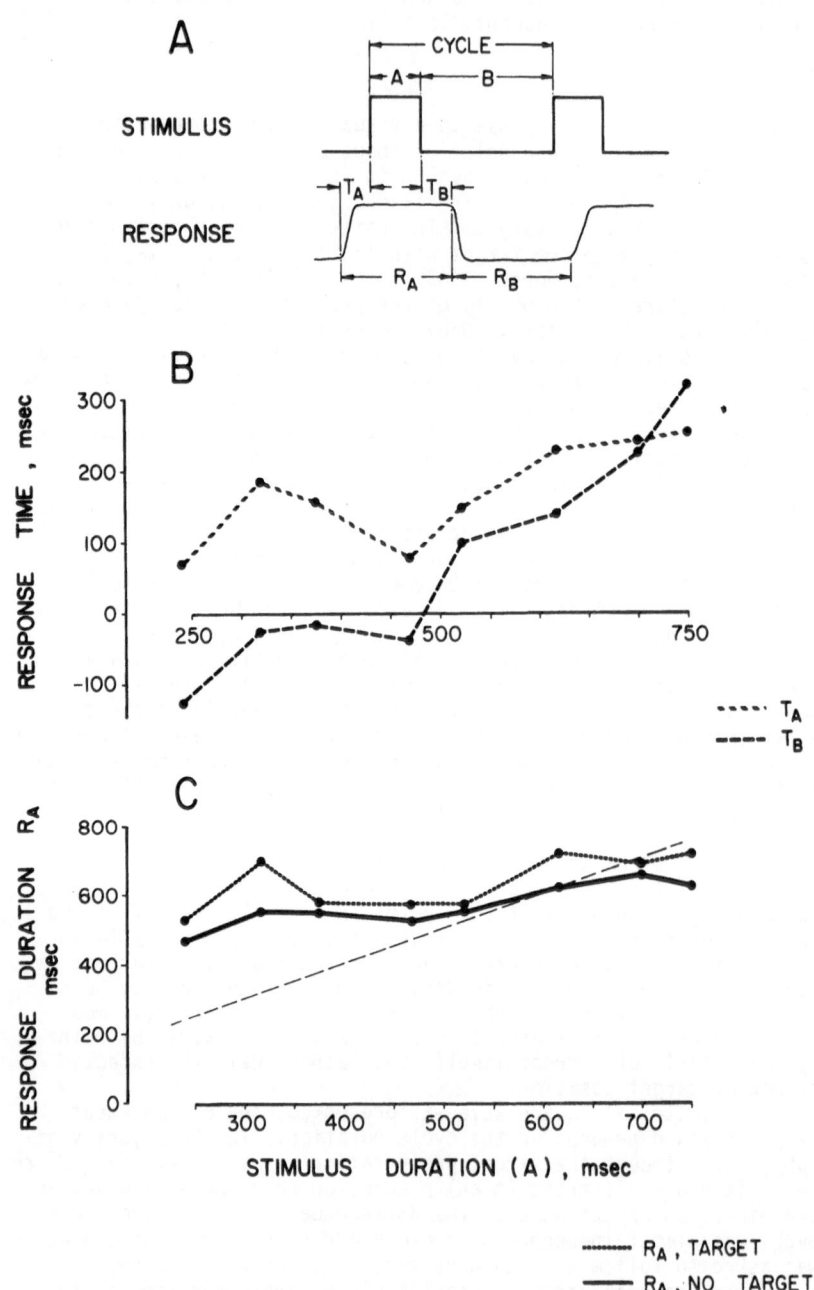

FIGURE 1. A) A diagram presenting the symbols related to stimulus and response. The response time (T_A and T_B) and response duration (R_A and R_B) for each phase of the cycle (A and B). Response time B), and response duration C) dependency on stimulus duration when cycle was fixed at 1.5 sec. Each dot is the mean of 50 measurements.

3. CHANGING TARGET ASYMMETRY, FIXED CYCLE

For a fixed cycle of 1.5 sec only the long phase (T_B) response time was strongly dependent on the asymmetry (A/B) (Fig. 1,B). Looking at a target that moves at a fixed cycle duration but with asymmetrical phases, concentrates our attention on the short phase, trying to predict it and paying less attention to the long phase, presumed by the subject to be the "steady state". Occasionally, a subject might concentrate on the long phase for short periods and then the two response times (T_A and T_B) will interchange. As the asymmetry ratio decreases and approaches one, the prediction of the two phases was about the same but not equal.

The correlation between the response time of the two phases (T_A and T_B) was high (> 0.35) in all subjects studied, which indicates that there is an interhemispheral response time relationship. Possibly, this results from coupling information which is trans-fered between the predictor mechanisms of the two hemispheres. The response durations to each phase (R_A and R_B) were only weakly correlated (< 0.40) to the asymmetry, i.e. the eyes tended to make a symmetrical response for each phase of the asymmetrical target displacement. One example of response duration of the short phase is illustrated in Fig. 1,C. If during the experiment the target is switched off and the subject is asked to continue at the same pace as before, the response was an eye movement with a higher tendency to reproduce the target phase duration. Apparently, reproducing an asymmetrical cycle is easier when there is no target and the subject concentrated his attention on the difference in the phase duration rather than on predicting the target. These results are consistent in all subjects but one, where the response was un-correlated to the asymmetry and was the same with or without target presentation.

4. CHANGING CYCLE DURATION, FIXED ASYMMETRY

Presenting a periodic square wave target with fixed asymmetry and changing cycle duration, the response time (T_A and T_B) for both short and long phases depended on cycle duration; after the cycle reached about 4 sec duration, both responses approached a delay of 150-200 msec (Fig. 2,A). The eye movement responses predicted both phases of the cycle but with a different prediction time; the responses always predicted the short phase better than the long phase with the subject paying probably less attention to the long phase and considering it as the "steady state". As the cycle dur-ation became larger than 4-8 sec (depending on the subject) both responses were delayed approaching the delay of an unpredictable target. The different prediction response to the asymmetrical target suggests that there are probably two predictors, each having access to one saccadic generator.

The response time of the two phases (T_A and T_B) were correlated (> 0.3) with a decreasing correlation when the cycle duration increased above 3 sec, indicating some interhemispheral relation-ship between the two predictors. The duration response of each phase (R_A and R_B) was also correlated with cycle duration (> 0.4) and decreased for cycles above 4 sec. One example of response duration dependency on cycle time is illustrated in Fig. 2,B. When the subject was asked to follow at the same pacing after the target was switched off the response duration for each phase was less correlated to cycle duration than when the target was present.

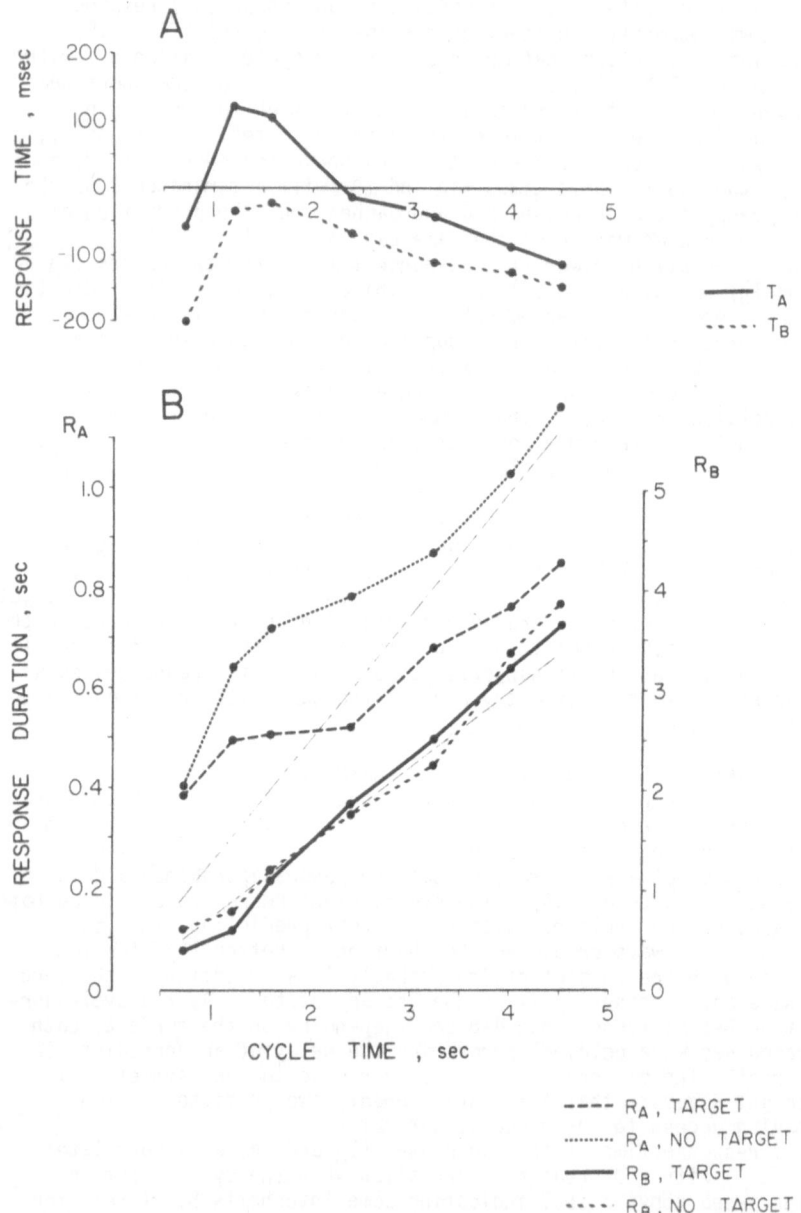

FIGURE 2. A) Response time and, B) response duration dependency on cycle time when the asymmetry was fixed at A/B = ¼. Symbols are the same as in Fig. 1.

5. DISCUSSION

Eye movement response to an asymmetrical periodic square wave target, within a certain cycle range, predicted the target on both cycle phases (T_A and T_B). The response to each phase duration (R_A and R_B) were well estimated by the subjects both when the experiment was done with target and without. The asymmetrical response can be presumed to be the result of an oscillator and a predictor in each hemisphere within the saccadic system. If the two oscillators are set at the periodic cycle time but are phase shifted, the combined response will be an asymmetrical periodic saccadic response. The output of each oscillator is advanced or delayed by the variation of a predictor or delay mechanism and accordingly the saccadic response. The predictor learns the phase duration during the first 6-12 cycles and is able to trigger the saccadic pulse generator, thus, predicting the oscillator output. It might be argued that the two predictors that learned the pace duration are enough to generate a periodical saccadic response that is both asymmetrical and predictive to the two phases of the cycle. This is difficult to assume since under certain experimental conditions subjects tended to respond with an equal phase duration to the asymmetrical cycle but still maintained the cycle duration. Furthermore, experiments in our laboratory on brain injured indicate that as a result of the injury some patients might lose the saccadic prediction ability on the injured side but still maintain the cycle duration time. The assumption of only two predictors is also weakened by the experimental results showing subject's ability to make an asymmetrical saccadic response when no target was present. The predictor and oscillator in each hemisphere interact and are inter-dependent and intra-dependent between the hemispheres. The degree of functional interaction was highly dependent on the subject's attitude, concentration and training. During the experiment each subject chose his own strategy for the task (e.g. counting to mark time). Still, the response time and phase duration (T_A and R_A) for the short phase presentation were highly correlated but not for the long phase (T_B and R_B). Concentrating on one phase of the cycle pre-occupied the subject's attention choosing the most noticeable one, which is the short phase.

The current saccadic system mathematical models lack some basic components of the prediction mechanism. The ability of the system in predicting an asymmetrical square target with changing cycle duration might provide some of the necessary data.

REFERENCES

Dallos PJ and Jones RW (1963) Learning behavior of the eye fixation control system. IEEE Trans. Autom. Control. AC-8,218-227.

Fuchs AF (1967) Periodic eye tracking in the monkey. J. Physiol. 193,161-171.

Michael JA and Melvill Jones G (1966) Dependence of visual tracking capability upon stimulus predictability. Vision Res. 6,707-716.

Stark L (1968) Predictive control. In Stark L, Neurological control systems, studies in bioengineering, pp.236-249. New York, Plenum Press.

Stark L, Vossius G and Young LR (1962) Predictive control of eye tracking movements. IRE Trans. Hum. Factors Electron. HEE-3,52-57.

Sugie N (1971) A model of predictive control in visual target tracking. IEEE Trans. Sys. Man Cybern. SMC-1,2-7.

CAN TRAINING BE TRANSFERED FROM ONE OCULOMOTOR SYSTEM TO ANOTHER?

S. RON (Occupational Health and Rehabilitation Institute at
Loewenstein Hospital, Raanana, Israel)

1. INTRODUCTION

"Transfer of training" refers to the effects of prior training on
subsequent performance of a task, the latter differing in some way
from the task utilized during the original training. Transfer of
training in the intact CNS has long been studied by psychologists,
yielding findings that were ambivalent to later investigators:
that it is possible to produce positive (increased) as well as
negative (decreased) transfer effects in motor-learning situations.
Later studies formulated the conditions of transfer where subjects
under the more complex input conditions were able to learn most or
all of the skill components required under less complex input
conditions, while the reverse was not true.
The above common definitions are of little help when we ask
whether training can be transfered from one oculomotor system to
another. It refers to transfer of one skill to another in the
same type of modality (e.g. same 'type' of motor act) or, similar
tasks. Furthermore, previous studies (Sage, 1971) indicate that
there is no transfer where training of a motor task was transfered
to another such task when the basic movement pattern is not shared
in both tasks.

2. IMPROVING OCULOMOTOR OUTCOME THROUGH TRAINING

The oculomotor activity is believed to be the most precise of all
skeletal muscle movements and is therefore probably the most sus-
ceptible to damage or insult of the CNS. When the CNS has sustained an insult, the impaired system has to exploit its plastic
capacity to improve the outcome of the system. The natural recovery that takes place has two time constants: immediately
following the insult, and a second one which takes weeks or months.
In the intact oculomotor system, plastic changes were demonstrated
(Balliet, Nakayama, 1978) in tortional eye movements where gain
improvement was shown in subjects receiving training. In another
study, subjects with extraocular paresis were trained and saccadic
gain improvement was achieved (Ciuffreda et al., 1979). In brain
injured patients, to facilitate improvement of the second time
constant, each oculomotor system underwent training (Ron, Hackett,
1979; Ron, 1981) with the result of shortening the recovery time
constant. Among a group of 22 patients studied, the minimal time
constant of the saccadic gain in patients not receiving training
was 7 months whereas in those receiving training it was 1.5 months.
Similar shortening of the time constant was found for the OKN
smooth phase velocity gain (3 versus one months) and for the smooth
pursuit gain (4 versus 1.5 months). One example of the saccadic
gain temporal change in a patient receiving training is shown in
Fig. 1 and of smooth pursuit in Fig. 2. In the limited sample
studied, patients receiving training reached a higher gain at the
end of the training compared with non-trained patients.
When the CNS has sustained an insult, the transfer function which
relates the input sensory signal to the output command might change
in consequence. The impaired system has to exploit its plastic

Roucoux, A. and Crommelinck, M. (eds.): Physiological and Pathological Aspects of Eye Movements.
© *1982, Dr W. Junk Publishers, The Hague, Boston, London.* ISBN-13: 978-94-009-8002-0

84

capacity for modifying internal signals so that the efferent signal remains unchanged. Some of these changes take place during the recovery period, as has long been known, to yield an improved outcome (Daroff, Hoyt, 1971; Ron, 1979). In motor function, to restore motor action, physiotherapy is commonly employed to change the level at which a function takes place and involves the patient's residual capacity in the performance of habitual activity. The purpose of training is to achieve a higher functional capacity of the machinery (higher gain) more quickly (shorter time constants). Mechanisms that are involved in this task are probably adaptation, modification, gain control, to mention only a few. Admittedly, in spite of the recent advances in the study of neuronal plasticity (Tsukaharu, 1981), we still lack some of the basic experimental results to explain the behavioral changes in terms of the cellular or neuronal plasticity in the central nervous system.

3. TRANSFER OF TRAINING IN THE OCULOMOTOR SYSTEM
Transfer of OKN training to the vestibular system has been demonstrated, i.e. a transfer of training across sensory modalities. The results indicate an enhanced (Young, Henn, 1974) decline or unchanged response in the vestibular system as a result of unidirectional OKN training (Pfaltz, Kato, 1974; Pfaltz, Novak, 1977). In the impaired oculomotor system, the majority of the patients' natural improvement occurs at a different rate dependent on site and extent of injury. Training a system improves the outcome to reach a higher gain faster. Training, however, might facilitate the activities of other oculomotor systems. Fig. 3 illustrates the results obtained and compares the improvement rate of patients receiving OKN training (bidirectional), with those not receiving training. The gain change through the follow-up period is represented with a straight line. In Fig. 3,A OKN results are compared

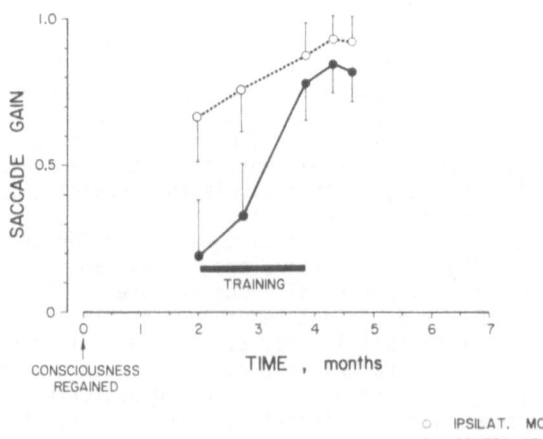

FIGURE 1. Temporal changes of saccadic gain in one patient receiving training. The subtending angle was 30 degrees; each dot represents 15 measurements and bars are one standard deviation.

with smooth pursuit and in Fig. 3B with saccades. While there
was no change in the saccadic trend there was a marked improvement
in the OKN smooth phase gain change.
Similar transfer of training was found when patients were trained
to make smooth pursuit movements. In the two populations, smooth
pursuit and OKN smooth phase had a marked improvement, compared
with saccade gain which had only a small improvement. When subjects underwent saccade training there was no marked change in
gain trend in either smooth pursuit or OKN smooth phase (Fig. 4).
Thus, there was no transfer of training to either system.

4. DISCUSSION

No condition is of greater importance to the acquisition of motor
skills than practice. It may be argued that the 'natural practice'
is the required process that the patients need. Improper practice,
however, may actually perpetuate errors. The schedule of practice
and the use of a bio-feedback system during practice were probably
of paramount importance in the success of training outcome. Training twice daily for 15-30 minutes, 5 days a week for several weeks
proved in most cases to be adequate although no attempts were made
to find the 'optimal' schedule for training.
The two most obvious effects of practice are first, increasing the
speed of performance, and second, increasing accuracy, or decreasing errors. Training the patients proved to achieve both goals,
although the amount of success obviously depended also on the site
and extent of brain lesion that the patient sustained. The

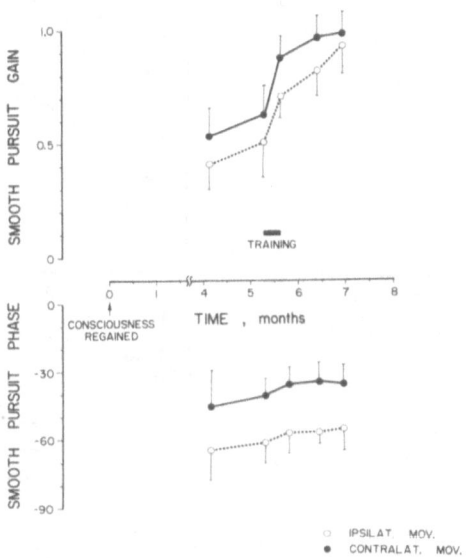

FIGURE 2. Temporal changes of smooth pursuit gain (top) and phase
(bottom) in one patient receiving training. The subtending angle
was 30 degrees, stimulus cycle was 0.5 Hz ; each dot represents
15 measurements and bars are one standard deviation.

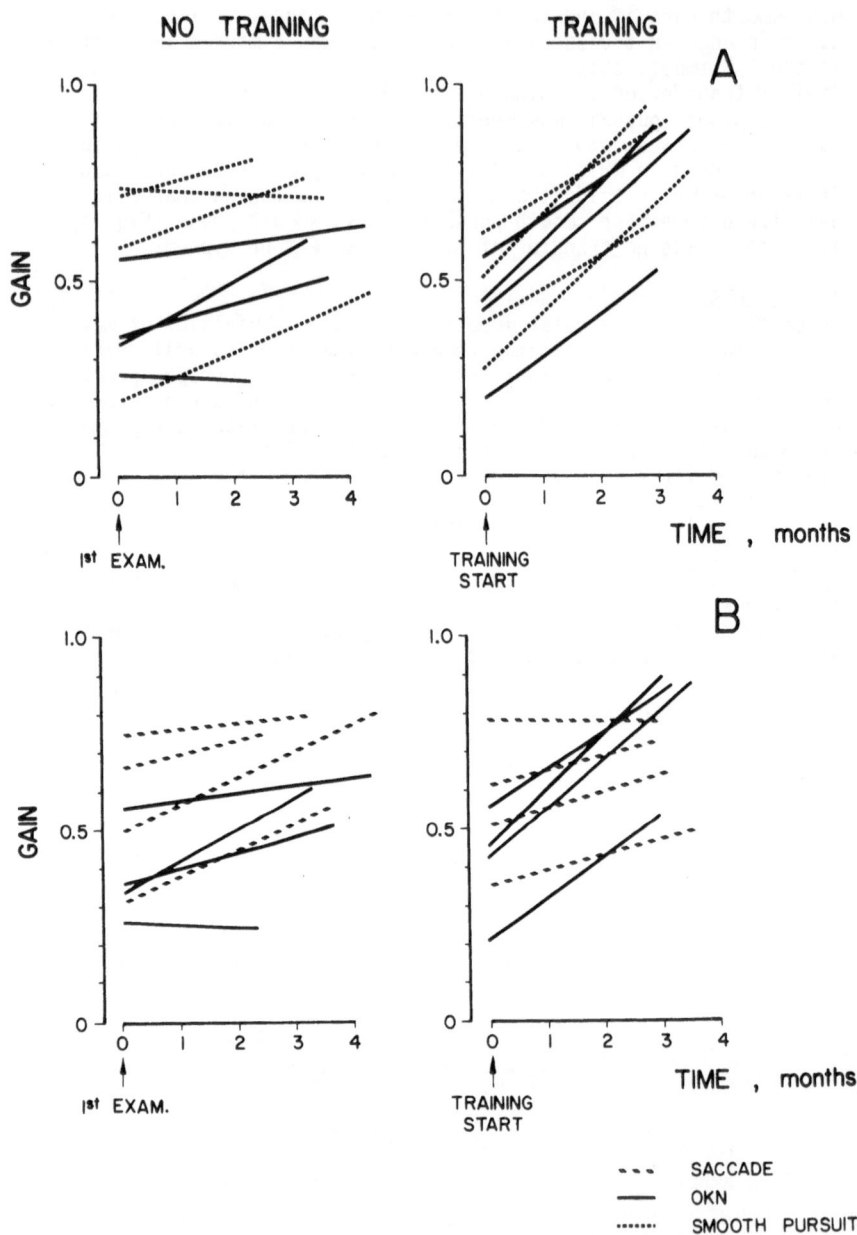

FIGURE 3. The gain change of contralateral saccades, ipsilateral OKN smooth phase and smooth pursuit when the subjects were trained in optokinetic movements. Each straight line represents one patient through the follow-up period. Comparison of gain trend in the various patients between A) saccades and OKN smooth phase and, B) saccades and smooth pursuit.

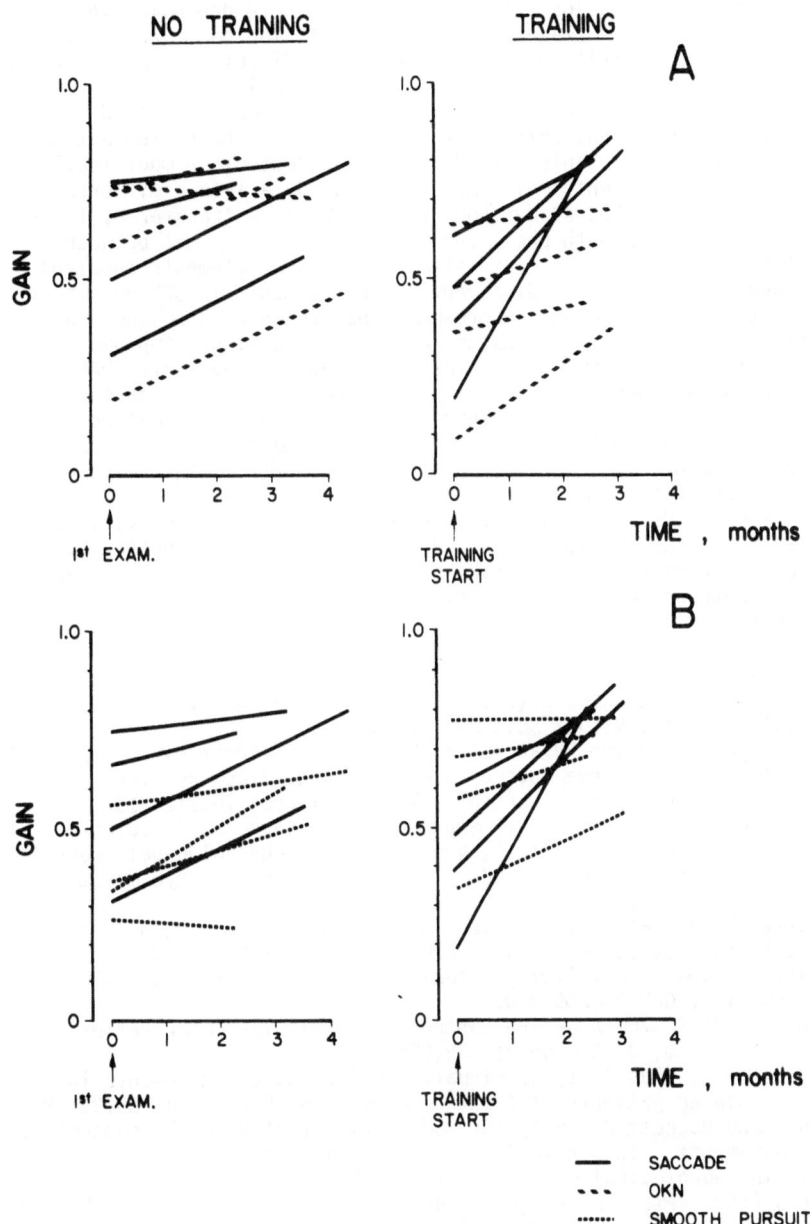

FIGURE 4. The gain change of contralateral saccades, ipsilateral OKN smooth phase and smooth pursuit when the subjects were trained in saccadic movements. Each straight line represents one patient through the follow-up period. Comparison of gain trend in various patients between A) OKN smooth phase and smooth pursuit and, B) OKN smooth phase and saccades.

restoration of function follows a different path depending on
whether the brain sustained concussion or lesion not directly related to the specific motor performance, or directly related. We
presume that in our patient population even patients who underwent
surgery still belonged to the first class. It was suggested
(Robinson, 1976; Ron, 1979) that improvement of the system outcome
is through some mechanism of adaptive gain control or modification
of the neural elements which map the input data into a different
output action. This study shows that there is a transfer of training between OKN smooth phase and smooth pursuit but not between
either one and the saccadic system. The neural elements involved
in saccade response are different to the elements in OKN or smooth
pursuit. Thus, it might be presumed that training a subject to
make saccades without 'transfer' of learning will not improve con-
comitantly the outcome of the latter systems. Conversely, OKN or
smooth pursuit does not involve neural machinery of the saccadic
system. Whether the improvement of OKN and smooth pursuit response
when one of the systems is trained is the result of some shared
neural elements or the result of some components of the learned
task transfered to the other system (Sage, 1971) is not clear from
this study. We are clearly lacking more experiments to distinguish
between the two possibilities. We would then be in a better position to provide the model makers with the elements of the interaction between neural substrates of the different oculomotor
systems.

REFERENCES
Balliet R and Nakayama K (1978) Training of voluntary tortion,
Invest. Ophthal. Visual Science, 17,304-314.
Ciuffreda JK, Kenyon RV and Stark L (1979) Different rates of functional recovery of eye movements during orthoptics treatment in an
adult amblyope, Invest. Ophthal. Visual Science, 18,213-219.
Daroff RB and Hoyt WF (1971) Supranuclear disorders of ocular control systems in man: clinical, anatomical and physiological correlation. In Collins CC and Hyde JE ed. The control of eye movements,
pp.175-235, New York, Academic Press.
Pfaltz CR and Kato I (1974) Vestibular habituation. Interaction of
visual and vestibular stimuli, Archs. Otolar, 100,400-448.
Pfaltz CR and Kato I (1977) Optokinetic training and vestibular
habituation, ORL 39,309-320.
Robinson DA (1976) Adaptive control of vestibulo-ocular reflex by
the cerebellum, J. Neurophys. 39,954-959.
Ron S (1979) Plasticity of visually controlled eye movements in
brain injured patients, XII Inter. Conf. Med. Biol. Eng. 55.2,1-2.
Ron S and Hackett P (1979) The modifiability of visually controlled
eye movements. In Schmid R and Zambarbiri D, ed. Eye movement analysis in neurological diagnosis, Italy, Nat. Res. Council, pp.176-198.
Ron S (1981) Plastic changes in eye movements of patients with trau-
matic brain injury. In Fuchs AF and Becker W, ed. Progress in oculomotor research, pp.233-240. New York, Amsterdam, Oxford, Elsevier/
North-Holland.
Sage GH (1971) Introduction to motor behavior, a neuropsychological
approach. Reading, Mass., Addison-Wesley Pub. Comp.
Tsukahara N (1981) Synaptic plasticity in the mammalian central nervous system, Ann. Rev. Neurosci. 4,351-379.
Young LR and Henn VS (1974) Selective habituation of vestibular
nystagmus by visual stimulation, Acta oto-lar. 77,159-166.

ACQUIRED PENDULAR NYSTAGMUS: Characteristics, pathophysiology and pharmacological modification

J.J. ELL, M.A. GRESTY, B.R. CHAMBERS, L.J. FINDLEY
Medical Research Council, Neuro-otology Unit,
Institute of Neurology, National Hospital, Queen Square,
London, WC1N 3BG, England.

INTRODUCTION
Pendular nystagmus is an oscillatory movement of the eye which
has a sinusoidal rather than a "saw-tooth" wave form (Figure 1).
It may be congenital, acquired in association with neurological
diseases, or voluntary (trick nystagmus). This report discusses
the manifestations of acquired pendular nystagmus in 20 of our
own patients together with a further 32 cases from the literature.
Complete clinical details of these patients have been published
elsewhere (Gresty et al, 1982). Albeit a rare disorder, pendular
nystagmus is important because of its implications for the
organisation of the oculomotor system, the pathophysiology of
tremor and for the severe visual handicap it may produce. For
the latter reason emphasis has been laid on the pharmacological
modification of the nystagmus with a view to treatment.

CHARACTERISTICS OF ACQUIRED PENDULAR NYSTAGMUS
Acquired pendular nystagmus may take the form of uni-ocular
or binocular sinusoidal oscillations about any or all of the axes
of rotation of the globe. The movements of the two eyes may
be conjugate, disconjugate or dissociated and tend to be
unaffected by eye position in the orbit. All the different
combinations of pendular nystagmus encountered in our patients
are illustrated in Figure 2. An example of conjugate nystagmus
would be a horizontal (bilateral) pendular nystagmus. An example
of disconjugate movement is pendular convergence nystagmus.
Dissociated pendular nystagmus may consist of any combination
of movements. Thus one eye may be moving about the principal
axis whilst the other rotates under the combined influence of
vertical and horizontal pendular movements. Alternatively,
one eye may be stationary whereas the other has a nystagmus.
Figure 2 does not show all horizontal combinations of movement
yet our observations so far suggest that any combination is
possible.

Acquired pendular nystagmus has a typical amplitude up to a
limit of approximately 5°. It is sinusoidal in wave form, usually
with little harmonic distortion (Figure 1). The nystagmus has a
set frequency which ranges from 2 Hz to 5 Hz with a modal
frequency of 3 Hz. The fact that all forms of acquired pendular
nystagmus have wave forms of similar amplitudes which fall on
a unimodal frequency distribution suggests that they have similar
pathophysiology and can be considered as a single clinical entity.

Roucoux, A. and Crommelinck, M. (eds.): Physiological and Pathological Aspects of Eye Movements.
© 1982, Dr W. Junk Publishers, The Hague, Boston, London. ISBN-13: 978-94-009-8002-0

PENDULAR NYSTAGMUS: right eye horizontal, left eye rotatory. M.S.

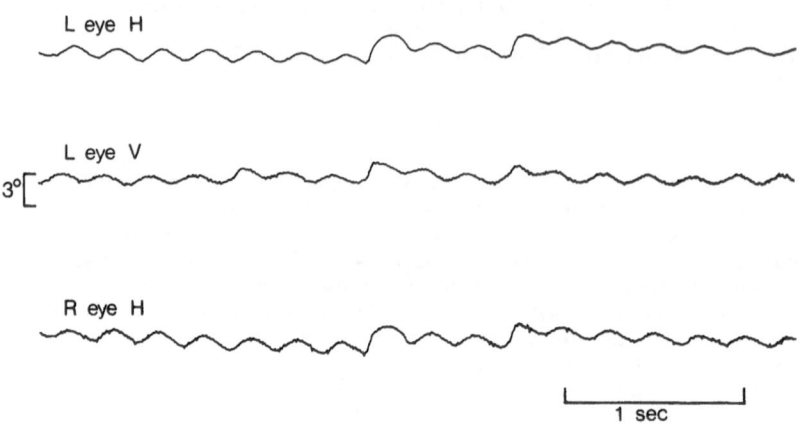

L eye H

L eye V

3°[

R eye H

1 sec

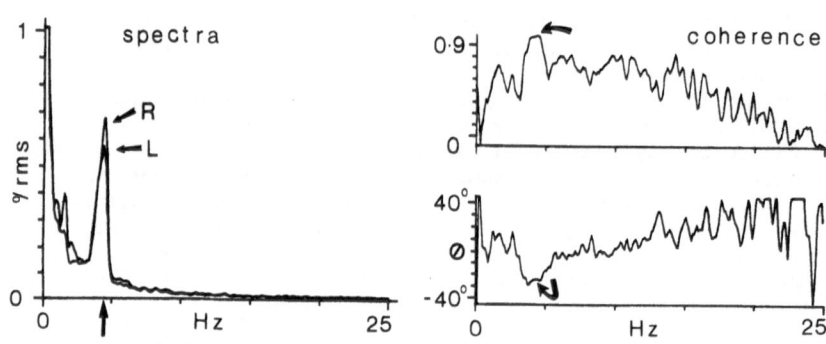

spectra

1

⁹rms

R

L

0

0   Hz   25

coherence

0·9

0

40°

∅

-40°

0   Hz   25

Figure 1 - Examples of raw records of pendular nystagmus in a patient with Multiple Sclerosis (M.S.) H. horizontal; V. vertical; L. left; R. right. Below, examples of the spectra calculated on recordings of the horizontal movements of the eyes averaged over 50, 10.24 second overlapping samples. The coherence indicates a high degree of relationship between the movements. The phase ∅ indicates that the movements are to a slight degree convergent (30°).

A feature of pendular nystagmus which has important implications for pathophysiology is that movements of one or both eyes about different rotational axes are (with the exception of only two of our patients) highly synchronised. Evidence for this comes from two sources. Firstly, in cases of rotatory pendular nystagmus, one can observe minimal variation in the trajectory of movement of the globe indicating that the vector components of horizontal and vertical movement maintain a constant frequency and phase relationship. Secondly, in cases of binocular pendular nystagmus,

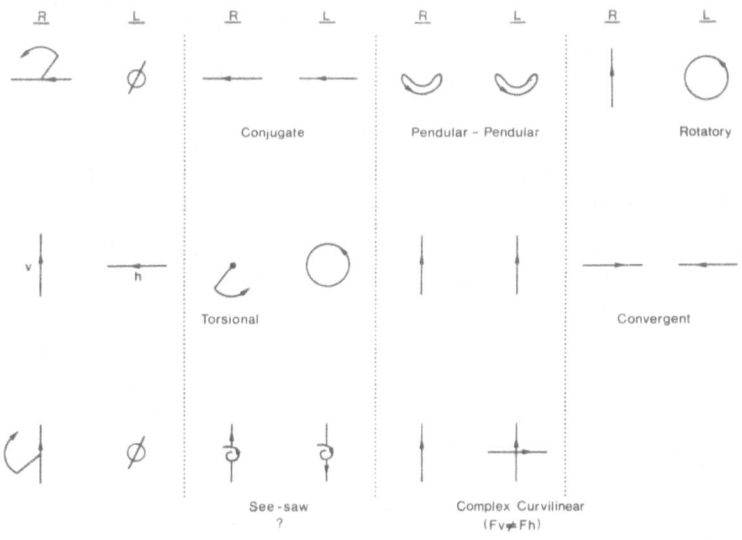

COMBINATIONS OF TRAJECTORIES OF THE POLE OBSERVED IN
ACQUIRED PENDULAR NYSTAGMUS

Conjugate   Pendular – Pendular   Rotatory

Torsional   Convergent

See-saw ?   Complex Curvilinear (Fv≠Fh)

Figure   2

recordings of the movements of the two eyes demonstrate that the
wave forms of both maintain the same phase relationship with each
other, sometimes with such precision that they may be generated
by one and the same underlying mechanism.   The properties of
constant phase relationship and co-varying amplitude are termed
Coherence* and may be assessed using a spectrum analyser.   With
the exceptions of the unusual varieties of nystagmus described
below, coherence measurements made on binocular movements in our
group of patients demonstrated that the movements were always
highly synchronised (eg, Figures 1, 4).

In rare cases (and so far only monocular nystagmus) we have found
different frequencies of movement in the horizontal and vertical
planes producing a nystagmus which is irregular in trajectory.   In
the table of Figure 2 this is termed "complex curvilinear".
----

*Coherence is a measurement of the degree to which the various
frequency components of two signals co-vary in amplitude and
maintain constant phase relationships.   Coherence is expressed
on a scale of 0 - 1.   0 indicates that the signals are unrelated
and 1 indicates that they are completely inter-dependent.
Appropriately, levels of statistical significance can be attributed
to a coherence measurement depending upon the number of averages
taken to derive the measurement.

Coherence =
$$\text{Coherence} = \frac{\text{Average of (magnitude of cross spectrum)}^2}{\text{Average (power spectrum 1st signal)} * \text{Average (power spectrum 2nd)}}$$

A rare form of nystagmus termed "see-saw" in which the eyes
execute alternating pendular movements in the vertical plane
and also retract, the upwards movement being synchronised with
the retraction, has frequency characteristics similar to those
of the other acquired pendular nystagmus. For this reason
we have tentatively classified see-saw nystagmus with pendular
nystagmus.

There are numerous behavioural characteristics of pendular
nystagmus which seem quite arbitrary and defy classification. For
example although most are continuous through waking life, some
appear only on vergence movements. We have observed a pendular
nystagmus which comprised crescendo-decrescendo transients
reminiscent of rhythmical myoclonus. Another monocular form was
provoked only when the subject fixated intently with the one eye.

ASSOCIATION WITH NERVOUS DISEASE AND OTHER CLINICAL SIGNS

More than 50% of our patients with acquired pendular nystagmus
had multiple sclerosis. One third or more had brain stem vascular
disease or angioma. It is occasionally seen in association with
ambylopia and optic atrophy in which case it has been assumed
to represent some form of sensory defect nystagmus. However, in
our experience, with monocular pendular nystagmus in an
amblyopic eye, there has been evidence of concurrent neurological
illness such as migraine.

The most common clinical signs associated with pendular nystagmus
in our patients were skew deviation - 15%, squint - 5%,
internuclear ophthalmoplegia - 66%, convergence failure - 90%
and supranuclear palsy. All the major oculomotor functions
(saccades, pursuit, vestibulo-ocular reflex and optokinetic
responses) could be intact in the presence of pendular nystagmus
and disorders of these functions did not correlate with any
manifestation of the nystagmus.

Acquired pendular nystagmus has interesting relationships with
concurrent somatic tremor. Two distinct forms of tremor of the
upper limbs occur in patients with posterior fossa lesions (Findley,
Gresty, 1981). Tremor at 4 - 5 Hz which frequently occurs
during intentional movement and is attributed to lesions of the
dentato-thalamic projection pathway and tremor at about 3 Hz
which is of larger amplitude, occurs only during posture and tends
to have an irregular wave form. Tremor at this lower frequency
can sometimes involve the palate, pharynx and larynx and
diaphragm in which case associated pendular nystagmus is referred
to as "ocular myoclonus". In up to one quarter of our patients
pendular nystagmus occurred in association with 3 Hz somatic tremor
and in all cases was closely related in frequency.

In one patient with a brain stem infarction who subsequently
developed oculo-palatal myoclonus the coherences between eye,
pharynx and index finger movements were found to be 0.9 or
higher over 100 spectral averages (Figure 3) indicating a very
high degree of synchronisation at a probability level of less than
1%. Such an extraordinary degree of inter-relationship is not a
characteristic of similar movements in multiple sclerosis.

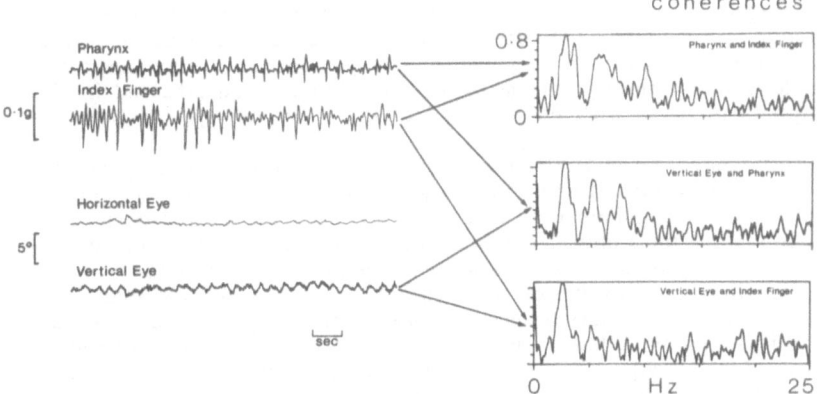

Figure 3 - Recordings of movements of the eyes, pharynx and finger in a stroke patient with oculo-palatal myoclonus. Coherences indicating a very high degree of synchronisation were calculated on 100, 10.24 sec. overlapping samples.

Pendular eye movements seen in multiple sclerosis and in some vascular diseases may appear identical to the nystagmus of oculo-palatal myoclonus. However, the high degree of synchronisation between the nystagmus and the body movements in the latter, may indicate a different neuro-physiological mechanism. We suggest that the term ocular myoclonus be restricted to examples in which there is such synchronisation with somatic movement.

MECHANISM OF PENDULAR NYSTAGMUS

Aschoff et al (1974) maintained that pendular nystagmus was a sign of cerebellar disease and resulted from a failure on the part of the roof nuclei to maintain stable eye position. The evidence for this came from two sources. One was that in the patients reviewed by Aschoff and his colleagues there was a high incidence of other neurological signs of cerebellar disease. Secondly in patients with the syndrome of "oculo-palatal-laryngeal-pharyngeal-diaphragmatic myoclonus" previous pathological studies had revealed lesions of the dentate nuclei of the cerebellum and hypertrophy of the inferior olive (Van Bogaert, Bertrand, 1928: Guillain et al, 1933).

The view that pendular nystagmus is attributable to dysfunction of the cerebellar nuclei cannot be maintained in all cases, for stimulation studies of the role of the cerebellum in oculomotor function have revealed binocular projections (Nashold et al, 1969; Ron, Robinson, 1973). The occurrence of purely monocular pendular nystagmus, therefore, cannot be explained in terms of cerebellar disease (Castaigne, 1979). In addition our own study.

unlike that of Aschoff et al, did not confirm the evidence of a high prevalence of cerebellar signs amongst patients with pendular nystagmus. On the contrary, only one third of our patients had unequivocal signs of cerebellar disease. Exact localisation of the lesion was possible in only two of our patients. In each case the lesions were angiomatous malformations which were situated in the high brain stem with no evidence of extension to the cerebellum.

The observation that the most common oculomotor neurological signs associated with pendular nystagmus are internuclear and juxta-nuclear lesions would suggest that the structural damage responsible for pendular nystagmus is near the oculomotor nuclei. It is almost certain that the mechanism(s) responsible for generating the rhythm of the nystagmus is at a similar level proximal to the final common oculomotor pathways. The reasons for this are as follows. Firstly the nystagmus is almost purely sinusoidal in wave form and, therefore, produced by reciprocal activity in agonist muscles. For this to occur the generating mechanism must have access to the motor-neurones of both muscles and, therefore, be at a supranuclear level. Secondly, because the major oculomotor systems may be intact in the presence of pendular nystagmus, and in particular the velocity of saccadic eye movements may be normal, it is unlikely that the abnormality responsible for the nystagmus is in the final common pathway. Because the nystagmus is an active motor phenomenon we presume that the immediate cause of the rhythmical activity is deafferentation of a nervous structure which is capable of going into oscillation. Concerning the nature of the rhythm generator in pendular nystagmus several features indicate that it may consist of instabilities in individual neurones rather than oscillatory processes in neuronal circuits. Firstly the frequency of the nystagmus is low in comparison with estimates of timing one may attribute to any oculomotor feedback system. This means that if a loop were involved then its processing time would have a heavy pharmaco-logical weighting. Secondly the frequency and pharmacological properties of pendular nystagmus are similar to those of some associated somatic tremor indicating that they may share a common rhythm generating mechanism. If there is a common mechanism then it is unlikely to involve processing around neuronal circuits because nervous structures involved in somatic and ocular movements are so dissimilar. On the other hand one can readily envisage that both oculomotor and somatomotor neuronal mechanisms utilise individual types of neurones with similar membrane properties.

In overview the mechanism responsible for pendular nystagmus is likely to be at a level proximal to the oculomotor neurones, not on the final common pathway nor involving the major oculomotor systems and is probably a form of instability in a mechanism with similar characteristics to those responsible for associated somatic tremor.

Speculation arises as to the normal function of this mechanism which, when disordered, gives rise to pendular nystagmus. The principal clue as to its normal function lies in the fact that one eye, and in particular one set of muscles alone, may be affected. Bender (1980) has stressed that in any ocular movement all extra-ocular muscles are involved, albeit their relative contributions may be small. The net result is that the eye is aligned on target

with all asymmetries of muscle action and secondary actions
compensated. In the case of binocular movements the signals fed to
the two sets of ocular muscles must be subtly different to take into
account the right/left mirror imaging of orbital muscle as well
as the secondary corrections required for each eye. Therefore, it
is reasonable to propose a "secondary corrective" mechanism which
makes the final small corrections due to orbital asymmetries and
secondary actions of muscles which are necessary for binocular
alignment and orthophoria. Such a mechanism under different
conditions of movement would require restricted access to the
individual muscle pairs in each eye and thereby produce
synchronised monocular effects or synchronised binocular effects
in restricted muscle groups. It is possible that this mechanism
could give rise to pendular nystagmus. If this is correct then
pendular nystagmus becomes a further example of a disorder of
conjugate gaze along with its most common associated clinical
signs of skew, squint and internuclear ophthalmoplegia.

The visual handicap produced by pendular nystagmus can be
considerable with almost all patients experiencing loss of acuity
because of oscillopsia.. A comparison of visual acuity before and
after treatment of the nystagmus indicates that up to 4 lines of
the Snellen chart may be gained by its suppression. Scanning
patterns necessary for reading may be impaired more than a
simple measurement of acuity would suggest. We have seen
patients in whom acuity was near normal but who were severely
handicapped in general locomotor activities, reading and viewing
motion pictures. Accordingly it would be desirable to develop
a suppressant drug regime.

PHARMACOLOGICAL MODIFICATION OF PENDULAR NYSTAGMUS
To date we have attempted to modify pendular nystagmus with a
variety of pharmacological agents including: L-Dopa;
Baclofen; Clonazepam; Prochlorperazine; Carbamazepine and
Tetrabenazine. Modification of the amplitude of pendular nystagmus
has been achieved with three drugs, viz Ouabaine,which had an
exacerbating effect, and Hyoscine and Lignocaine, which temporarily
abolished the nystagmus.

The rationale for assessing the effects of intravenous Ouabaine on
pendular nystagmus comes from the hypothesis that the nystagmus
arises from instability at the neuronal membrane level. We,
therefore, chose a drug having a generalised action on cell
membranes. Its specific action on neurones is one of alteration of
the trans-membrane potential through inhibition of the sodium pump.

The results of a 250 ugm intravenous injection of Ouabaine in a
double blind placebo controlled study on a patient with multiple
sclerosis are shown in Figure 4.

Measurements were taken of the amplitude of his horizontal monocular
nystagmus. After administration, nystagmus amplitude rose from
a peak level of about 2.5° to a magnitude of 5° over an interval of
5 minutes. Amplitude then decreased until baseline level was attained
13 minutes after administration. This pharmacodynamic response
profile corresponds closely to the known pharmacokinetic properties
of Ouabaine. In comparison, normal saline had no effect on nystagmus
amplitude.

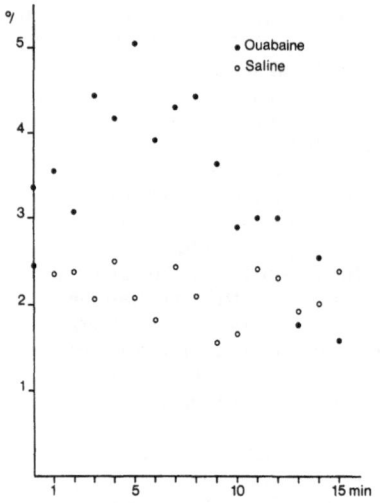

Figure 4 – Pharmacodynamic effects of Ouabàine on the amplitude (in degrees peak °/) of pendular nystagmus in a controlled study against normal Saline.

Since Charcot's original observations (ref 8) Hyoscine has been known to possess a suppressive effect on involuntary movements in neurological disease and trials on many of our patients have shown that this action extends to pendular nystagmus. Unfortunately the side effects of Hyoscine prevent its long term application.

The rationale for using Lignocaine stems from its membrane stabilising properties (although its modes of action have not yet been fully elucidated). Dramatic and encouraging results were found in the three multiple sclerosis patients with pendular nystagmus who have so far been assessed on acute intravenous doses of 100 mg. Lignocaine in double blind placebo controlled trials. The results of one such trial are illustrated in Figure 5 which shows the effects of intravenous Lignocaine followed some ten minutes later by 200 ugm of Hyoscine on a monocular rotatory nystagmus. We found that although Lignocaine effectively abolished the nystagmus without producing untoward side effects, its effects were short lived. Hyoscine 200 ugm administered after Lignocaine prolonged the period of suppression up to one hour, without causing unacceptable side effects. The serendipitous finding that somatic tremor could also be suppressed by intravenous Lignocaine is illustrated in Figure 6. The figure presents raw data records of postural tremor of the upper limbs and binocular pendular nystagmus in a patient with multiple sclerosis. The tremor was measured with the arms in posture and flexed with the index fingers pointing towards the nose as if the patient were executing the familiar "finger to nose test". The dramatic reduction in nystagmus 10 minutes after intravenous administration of Lignocaine is also evident in the postural tremor.

PRE DRUG SPECTRA

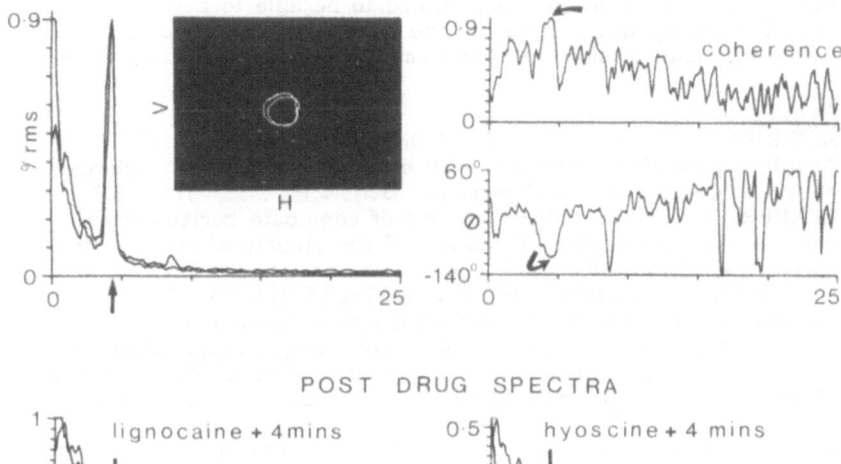

POST DRUG SPECTRA

Figure 5 – Modification of rotatory nystagmus with intravenous Lignocaine and Hyoscine. Spectral calculations were averaged over 50, 10.24 sec overlapping samples.

EFFECT OF LIGNOCAINE ON PENDULAR NYSTAGMUS AND POSTURAL TREMOR (MULTIPLE SCLEROSIS)

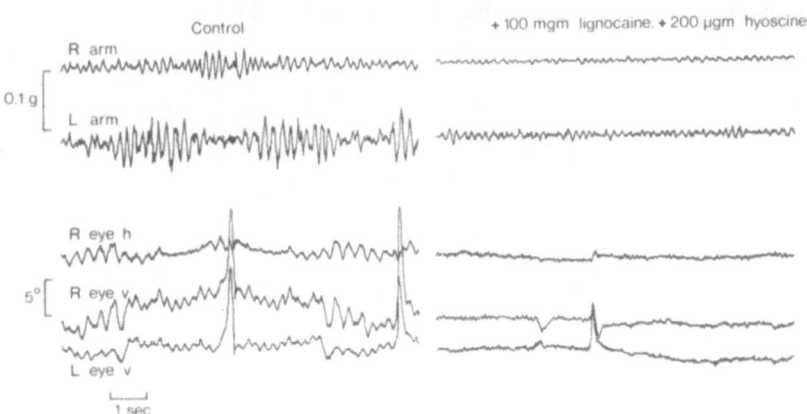

Figure 6

The finding that Lignocaine administered intravenously is capable of suppressing pendular nystagmus gives new hope for the development of a therapeutic drug regime. Lignocaine derivatives now exist for oral administration. With trials of oral preaparations underway we hope in the near future to be able to develop an effective therapeutic regime for the suppression of pendular nystagmus and possibly certain forms of associated somatic tremor.

REFERENCES:

ASCHOFF, J.C., CONRAD, B., KORNHUBER, H.H. (1974) Acquired pendular nystagmus with oscillopsia in multiple sclerosis: a sign of cerebellar nuclei disease. J.N.N.P. 37 : 570 - 577

BENDER, M.B. (1980) Brain control of conjugate horizontal and vertical eye movements. A survey of the structural and functional correlates. Brain 103 : 23 - 69

CASTAIGNE, P., CHAIN, F., PIERROT-DESEILIGNY, C., LARMANDE, P. (1979) Le nystagmus de circumduction monoculaire. Étude clinique, oculographique et électro-myographique d'un cas dans la sclérose en plaques. Rev. Neurol. (Paris) 135 : 51 - 57

FINDLEY, L.J., GRESTY, M.A. (1981) Tremor. Br. J. Hosp. Med. 26 : 16 - 32

GRESTY, M.A., ELL, J.J., FINDLEY, L.J. (1982) Acquired pendular nystagmus. J.N.N.P. (in press)

GUILLAIN, G., THUREL, R., BERTRAND, I. (1933) Examen anatomo-pathologique d'un cas de myoclonies vélo-pharyngo-oculo-diaphragmatiques associées à des myoclonies squelettiques synchrones. Rev. Neurol. (Paris) 2 : 801 - 812

NASHOLD, B.S., SLAUGHTER, D.G., GILLS, J.P. (1969) Ocular reactions in man from deep cerebellar stimulation and lesions. Arch. Ophthal. 81 : 538 - 543

ORDENSTEIN, L. (1868) Sur la paralysie agitante et la sclérose en plaques generalisée. Delahaye (Paris) Ref. to M. Charcot.

RON, S., ROBINSON, D.A. (1973) Eye movements evoked by cerebellar stimulation in the alert monkey. J. Neurophysiol. 36 : 1004 - 1022

VAN BOGAERT, L., BERTRAND, I. (1928) Sur les myoclonies associées synchrones et rythmiques par lésions en foyer du tronc cérébral. Rev. Neurol. (Paris) 1 : 203 - 214

EYE MOVEMENT DISORDERS IN MULTIPLE SCLEROSIS AND OPTIC NEURITIS

J.P.H. REULEN, E.A.C.M. SANDERS[1] and L.A.H. HOGENHUIS[2]
(Department of Medical Physics, Vrije Universiteit,
Amsterdam)

[1] Department of Neurology
    Military Hospital "Dr. A. Mathijsen", Utrecht

[2] Department of Neurology
    Hospital "De Goddelijke Voorzienigheid", Sittard

POSTER SUMMARY
Horizontal saccadic and smooth pursuit eye movements
were studied in 84 patients with multiple sclerosis
(MS) and 21 patients with optic neuritis (ON).
The MS patients, clinically classified in subgroups,
showed subclinical eye movement disorder in 80 % of the
the definite, 74 % of the probable and 60 % of the
possible category. Five of the ON patients (25 %) showed a subclinical eye movement deficit. They all were
young patients with a recent history of ON. In a group
of 27 MS patients with symptoms of spinal cord involvement only, 14 established subclinical oculomotor
discorder indicating the involvement of cerebral structures in the demyelination process.
A study of correlation between specific eye movement
parameters and results of visual evoked response (V.E.R.)
tests revealed that saccadic latency or smooth pursuit
abnormalities are not correlated with prolonged VER latencies (P-100 peak latency). This indicates that lesions
beyond the primary visual pathway substantially contribute to both parameters of oculomotor dysfunction.
A significant correlation between prolonged saccadic
latency and smooth pursuit deficit is found. The occu-
rence of internuclear ophthalmoplegia (INO) is significantly related with saccadic latency increase. This
finding indicates that demyelination in patients with
an established INO may not be restricted exclusively
to one or both medial longitudinal fasciculi (MLF)
but extends to other brainstem structures which are
functionally related to the programming of saccades.
The findings substantiate the value of standardised,
objective examination of eye movements in the detection and clarification of subclinical lesions in the
central nervous system of patients with an early diagnosis of MS or ON.

Details are embodied in a paper submitted for publication

Roucoux, A. and Crommelinck, M. (eds.): Physiological and Pathological Aspects of Eye Movements.
© *1982, Dr W. Junk Publishers, The Hague, Boston, London.* ISBN-13: 978-94-009-8002-0

THE MEASUREMENT OF EYE MOVEMENT USING DOUBLE MAGNETIC INDUCTION

J.P.H. REULEN, L. BAKKER (Department of Medical Physics, Vrije Universiteit, Amsterdam)

POSTER SUMMARY
The poster describes a new method for the accurate measurement of human eye movements. This eye-contact method is based on double magnetic induction and allows for a lead-free eye coil. The major characteristics of the method are a resolution of 8 minutes of arc, a linearity up to 15 degrees and a frequency bandwidth of 3 kHz. Further improvement of resolution is possible based on theory and experiment. Results of measurements on human eye movements are presented. The new technique considerably improves eye movement measurement with eye-contact methods, based on magnetic induction. The method is applicable to man and animal.

Accepted for publication in:
"IEEE Transactions on Biomedical Engineering"

Roucoux, A. and Crommelinck, M. (eds.): Physiological and Pathological Aspects of Eye Movements.
© *1982, Dr W. Junk Publishers, The Hague, Boston, London.* ISBN-13: 978-94-009-8002-0

THE VERTICAL VESTIBULO-OCULAR REFLEX

R. Baker, W. Graf* and R. F. Spencer**
Dept. of Physiology & Biophysics, NYU Medical Center
New York, NY 10016 *Rockefeller Univ. New York, NY 10021
**Dept. Anatomy, Medical Col Virginia, Richmond, VA 23298

If causal and teleological reasoning were clearly diametrically opposed attitudes, then tackling the central organization of vertical eye movements would indeed be a formidable task. This opening, and light, assertion is partially explained by the subsequent lengthy introduction to some of the problems posed by the descriptive, but unfortunately misnamed, "vertical" vestibulo-ocular reflex (VOR). Many in the oculomotor field believe the key to understanding vertical eye movements depends to a large extent on first understanding the vertical VOR reflex pathways. Experiments carried out to date ranging from the sensory to motor periphery suggest that the excellent performance of the vertical VOR is achieved at the level of the second order vestibular neurons. Accordingly these cells must be the center of focus in the upcoming years. At the outset it should also be appreciated that many eye movement related signals, even vestibular, appearing at target sites of second order vestibular neurons could be obtained either directly or indirectly via more than one pathway. Therefore, critical experiments will always require correlation between physiology and morphology. With the above view in mind, experiments initiated nearly a decade ago in lateral-eyed (rabbit) and frontal-eyed animals (cats) have recently been brought to a level that can now form a concrete basis for providing a better understanding of central vertical VOR organization (Baker, Berthoz, 1974; Baker et al. 1972; Baker et al. 1973; Baker, Spencer, 1981; Baker et al., 1981; Baker et al. 1982; Cohen, Suzuki, 1982; Gacek, 1971; Ghelarducci et al. 1977; Graf et al. 1981; Highstein, 1973; Ito et al. 1973; Ito et al. 1976a,b,c; McCrea et al. 1981; Precht, Baker, 1972; Uchino et al. 1978; Uchino et al. 1980a,b; Uchino et al. 1981; Yamamoto et al. 1978; Yoshida et al. 1981). The brief summary below begins by elaborating on the behavioral basis of vertical VOR organization in mammals and extends up to the questions now being asked including some comment on their implications. More focus is placed on VOR organization in the cat and the readers indulgence is requested until the ensuing papers (in preparation) appear with the detail concerning points ever so sparsely presented now. Admitting that we are not convinced that any of the questions posed or answers suggested are as straightforward as outlined is not difficult at this point.

As one moves presumably higher in the vertebrate phylum the eyes have shifted from a lateral to frontal position to allow stereoscopic vision to replace panoramic sight. Although many principles of retinal processing of light stimuli remain common to all animals, there is, nevertheless, considerable development of retinal receptors and optic nerve fibers to increase retinal capacity for detecting contrast change and movement. Accordingly, evolution has greatly expanded the cen-

Roucoux, A. and Crommelinck, M. (eds.): Physiological and Pathological Aspects of Eye Movements.
© 1982, Dr W. Junk Publishers, The Hague, Boston, London. ISBN-13: 978-94-009-8002-0

Spatial relationship between semicircular canals, optic axis and extraocular muscles

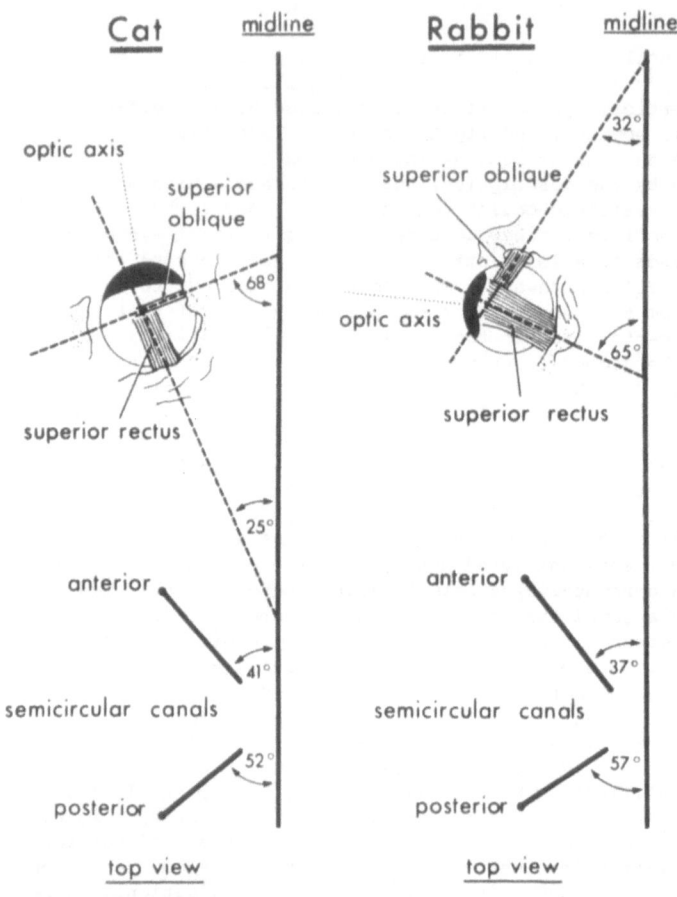

Figure 1. Spatial relationships in the cat and rabbit were selected from Figure 1 of Simpson, Graf (1981). The lines of action for the superior rectus and superior oblique muscles remain nearly parallel to the ipsilateral anterior and posterior canals. A similar canal arrangement is likely for the inferior rectus and inferior oblique muscles.

tral organization of visual centers to, on one hand, carry out visual processing, and the other, to implement an extensive array of motor performances. Compensatory eye movements are intimately linked to the successful performance of the visual system. Indeed associated with the above mentioned phylogenetic improvements in visual capacity are the basic compensatory movements initiated by vestibular and optokinetic stimuli which are augmented in many higher order species by the ability to di-

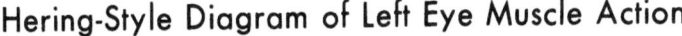

Hering-Style Diagram of Left Eye Muscle Action

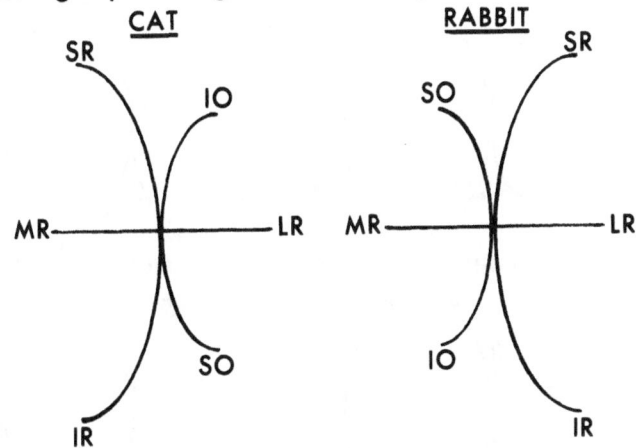

Figure 2. Comparison of the actions of extraocular muscles in cat and rabbit presented in the form of a Hering-style diagram. Note that the primary muscle actions do not change as the recti produce elevation-depression and the obliques-torsion. Secondary roles are reversed as extensively discussed by Graf, Simpson (1981) and Simpson, Graf (1981).

rect the attention of the eye voluntarily to discrete targets in space (e.g. saccades and smooth pursuit). Understanding how these newly acquired motor activities are superimposed on the oculomotor nuclei requires that the central structure-function organization of the vestibular and optokinetic reflexes be firmly elucidated. The mandate for this approach is clear. There are ample data to argue that the CNS augments encephalization of function by adding to existing circuitry rather than re-structuring from sensory to motor periphery. As it turns out the vertical VOR is one of the best places to examine the above propostion in detail. The problem posed seems to be simple and straightforward. It begins with the observation that the orientation of the semicircular canals in most lateral and frontal-eyed species are nearly congruent although the optic axes differ by nearly 90° (Fig. 1; Graf, Simpson, 1981; Simpson, Graf, 1981). Recently it has been clearly demonstrated that one mechanism utilized, and likely a major one, is peripheral rearrangement of the insertion of vertical extraocular muscles so as to produce, mechanically, the appropriate axes for globe rotation (Fig. 2; Graf, Simpson, 1981; Simpson, Graf, 1981). For example, in the cat, torsion of both eyes is produced by rotation around the x-axis (roll) whereas in the rabbit such movements are produced by rotations around the y-axis (pitch; Fig. 3). Two points are important. In the above case, both species utilize the same primary eye muscles. Compensation can be accomplished because the pulling action of the muscles are all nearly aligned with the appropriate semicircular canal. This argument is true for either torsion or up-down movement as illustrated in 3A and B. A good example of the contribution by an individual muscle is the superior rectus

104

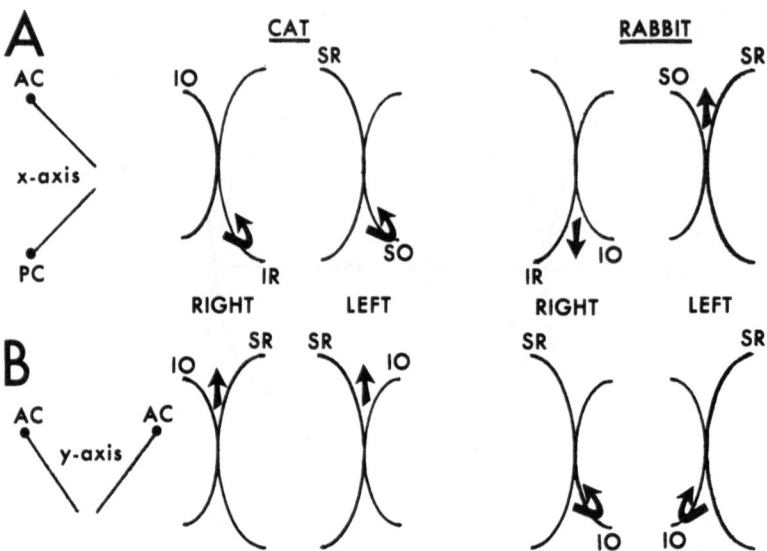

<u>Figure 3.</u> Direction of compensatory eye movements produced in
cat and rabbit following rotation around the x-and y-axes. In
A and B only the direct excitatory pair of 3-neuron VOR arcs
activated from the canals are labeled for the two eyes (see
text). In each case (A and B) the type of compensatory eye
movement is shown to differ between species yet in both they
are symmetric and parallel.

whose pulling directions lie on opposite sides of the anterior
canals in the rabbit and cat. The large change, however, only
modifies the secondary action of the muscle (i.e, extorsion vs.
intorsion). The Hering-style diagrams depict the trajectory of
optic axis in both species (Fig. 2) and illustrate a second
point whose historical origin is so lengthy it's hardly worth
documentation any longer, namely that each semicircular canal
is specifically related to the reciprocal excitatory-inhibitory
control of the motoneurons of one muscle pair in each eye
(Figs. 2-4). The above concept has been evident from the time
of the first papers in the field and, it of course, forms the
basis for 'multiple sets' of 3-neuron arcs (Szentagothai,
1943). There has been much ado about nothing in respect to the
significance of co-planar (i.e., ipsi-anterior canal and con-
tra-posterior canal) role in the vertical VOR. This intuitive
fact has always been implicitly appreciated in the literature
on compensatory movement, (Cohen, Suzuki, 1963) but only recently, has it nicely been re-emphasized in the work showing
the visual system interface to the oculomotor system is likely
via the same co-ordinate plan, in fact, probably via the same
neurons involved in the vertical VOR (Simpson et al. 1981).
Thus, it may be appreciated that the visual and vestibular system organization is not centered around a Cartesian coordinate
system, but the aforementioned non-orthogonal pairs of semicircular canals (Graf, Simpson, 1981; Simpson, Graf, 1981). Tele-
ologically there may be considerable significance to the above

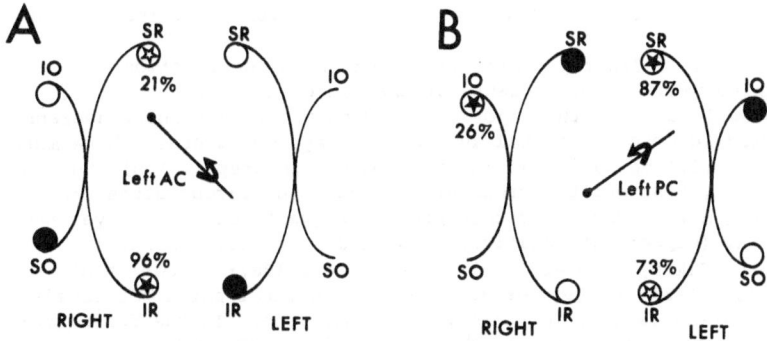

Figure 4. All excitatory and inhibitory anterior and posterior canal 3-neuron VOR pathways in the cat are presented in the form of a Hering-style diagram. In A, the left anterior canal is shown to disynaptically contact all motoneurons to the ipsilateral superior rectus and contralateral inferior oblique muscles (open circles). In addition, another 3-neuron arc contacts motoneurons to the contralateral superior rectus (open star). Two separate inhibitory VOR pathwys are illustrated. The 3-neuron arc to motoneurons innervating the oblique and ipsilateral inferior rectus form the first type (filled circles) and the second includes the contralateral inferior rectus (filled star). The percentages next to the circles indicate the approximate number of motoneurons synaptically contacted based on data from Table I of Uchino et al. 1980b. In B, connections from the posterior canal are shown as in A.

design. First it is the co-planar organization of the vertical semicircular canals that undoubtly is the singular most important design feature adhered to throughout lateral to frontal-eyed species. It doesn't change, but many other aspects of CNS organization must. Years ago, Simpson (in unpublished cogitations) expressed the view that in order to achieve bilateral canal symmetry and also maintain a balanced, maximally sensitive push-pull system, a 45 deg angle with the midsaggital plane would be desirable. In view of the consistency in peripheral semicircular canal orientation and the peripheral rearrangements between frontal and lateral eye animals at the level of the globe, one can entertain the question of how central pathways might be best organized to achieve the optimum vertical VOR. As expressed earlier this is not a simple problem. There isn't any way it will be adequately addressed by a non-experimental approach. In recent years several morphophysiological studies have demonstrated differences in extraocular motoneuron properties and motor nuclei organization between species. The presence of axon collaterals in many cat, but not rabbit oculomotor neurons is one clear example (Evinger et al. 1982). In fact, the issue of contra vs. ipsilateral localization of some vertical motoneurons has remained without good explanation, but it also is likely to be related to the above described vertical canal orientation. Nonetheless, the major focus in the upcoming years will be on second-order vertical vestibular neurons. The ensuing comments focus on vertical VOR

organization in the cat and rabbit. The morphological illus-
trations point to the extent of the circuitry, not its complexity, which needs to be considered.

Since Szentagothai's (1943) classical description of the
three neuron arc, students of the oculomotor system have frequently ignored the major role second order vestibular neurons
play in both horizontal and vertical eye movements. These mat-
ters will be addressed in time (papers in preparation), but in
short, vestibular neurons exhibit numerous target sites other
than motoneurons, and they exhibit signals related to eye movement (especially position) as well as vestibular sensiti-
vity(Baker, Spencer, 1981; Baker et al. 1982; McCrea et al.
1980, 1981; Yoshida et al. 1981). The first point for consideration is their contact with motoneurons. In the horizontal
VOR, there are separate populations of second order excitatory
neurons to the abducens and medial rectus (McCrea et al.
1980). All evidence to date, in both cat and rabbit vertical
VOR pathways, states explicitly that one canal is connected in
an excitatory fashion to, minimally, two subpopulations of motoneurons (Ito et al. 1976a, Graf et al. 1981; Uchino et al.
1980a,b). In fact, Szentagothai (1943) designated as "primary
connections" the individual canal relationship with motoneurons
for two eye muscles in the VOR. This clearly forms the basis
for the anterior and posterior canal regulation of one muscle
pair in each eye in agonist-antagonist fashion (Figs. 3,4).
However, there is no way a simple three neuron reflex arc by
itself could even begin to be adequate to produce symmetric eye
movements in either the rabbit or cat - especially in the vertical system. One can appreciate the problem rather easily by
employing the measurements of pulling axes from Fig. 1
(Simpson, Graf, 1981) and using them to approximate those of
the inferior oblique and inferior rectus muscles. Assuming in
the cat that the left posterior canal innervates the contralateral inferior rectus and trochlear nucleus one can see that
the pulling axis (i.e., force) is more closely aligned with the
optic axis (i.e., the axis of rotation is shifted by 13° from
that of the canal). The posterior canal would be better oriented at 25° from the midline to optimally favor the contralateral inferior rectus or 68° to favor the ipsilateral superior
oblique muscle. Yet, if the same VOR neuron contacts motoneuronal populations on both sides of the brain then the difference
must be averaged. Congruency between semicircular canal or-
ientations and kinematic features of muscles are important issues to be enlarged on before the adequacy of three neuron arcs
is established (Simpson, Graf in preparation).

On the other hand, the long-standing hypothesis of an individual second order neuron contacting two populations of motoneurons has recently been demonstrated to have been a correct, but substantially incomplete surmise (Graf et al. 1981;
Uchino et al. 1978,1980b). In many ways this is fortunate.
Employing the finer technical expertise available in recent
years frequently raised more physiological and morphological
problems in both the rabbit and cat than the above limited version of the three-neuron arc could explain. Several long stor-
ies are shortened by combining diverse data to support the
postulate of two distinct types of second order vestibular
neurons in the cat. The newest three neuron-arc (both discov-

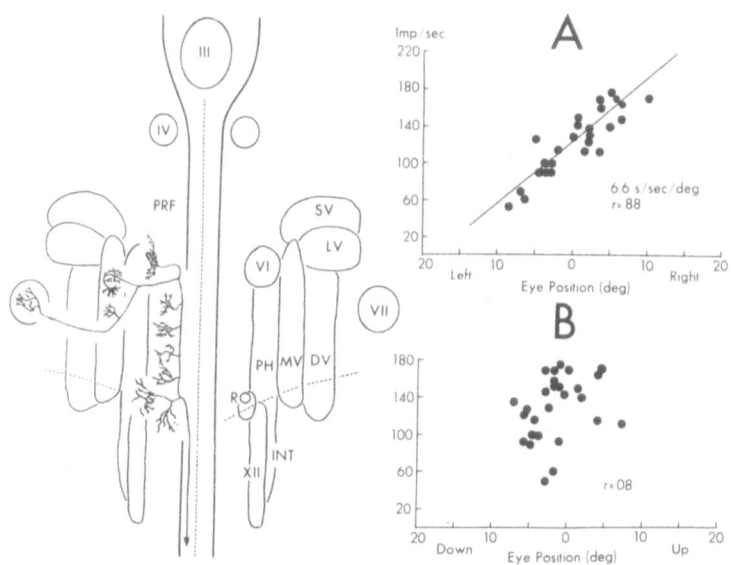

Figure 5. Morphology and eye movement related signals of an identified second order vestibular neuron recorded in the abducens nucleus. Intracellular application of HRP following recording of the activity of the vestibular neuron in the alert cat shows the diversity of termination sites in addition to the abducens nucleus. Rate-position plots for the horizontal (A) and vertical (B) directions were constructed in a conventional fashion.

ery and evolution) connects, <u>minimally</u>, three populations of motoneurons with one common signal (Graf et al. in preparation). Thus, each anterior and posterior canal is connected in an excitatory and inhibitory fashion with three pairs of eye muscles (Fig. 4). This morphology fits perfectly with the electrophysiology demonstrating bilateral excitation and inhibition between pairs of vertical eye muscles (Uchino et al. 1980b). In addition, the crossing of vestibular axons in the oculomotor nucleus (Gacek, 1971) can now be interpreted as originating solely from the collaterals of the above class of second order vestibular neurons. All semicircular canal excitatory pathways in the cat (and likely in the rabbit) reach the oculomotor complex via the contralateral MLF and all inhibitory pathways via the ipsilateral MLF (Maciewicz et al. in preparation). The percentages shown next to the bilateral VOR connections were calculated from Uchino, etal (1980b) and indicate that not all motoneurons in any subgroup receive synaptic effects from these vestibuar neurons. In fact, it seems that the inhibitory connections are more extensively distributed. The convergence between the bilateral AC-PC canal pairs is now being studied, especially as it relates to motoneuron axon collateralization in vertical motoneurons (Graf et al. 1981).

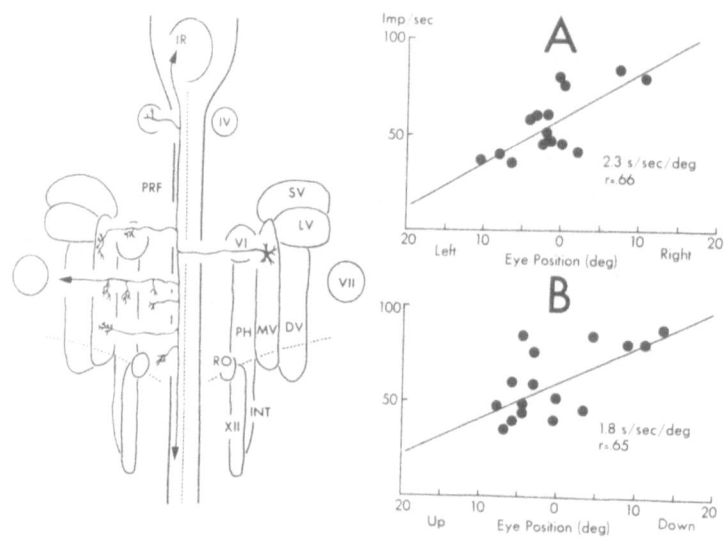

Figure 6. Morphology and eye movement-related signals of an excitatory second order vestibular neuron activated from posterior canal and terminating in the trochlear nucleus and presumably the ipsilateral inferior rectus subdivision of the oculomotor nucleus. Mulitple target sites are illustrated in the posterior brain stem. Rate-position plots for horizontal (A) and vertical (B) directions were obtained with the same procedure as in Fig. 5.

Nonetheless, the pattern of vestibular input just described already suggests different roles for certain motoneurons in compensatory VOR than in other eye movements. This leads to the questions - "What role do the additional posterior and anterior canal pathways provide in respect to the VOR and what is the relationship to other eye movement related signals in the system?"

Certainly, the additional anterior canal pathways are primarily directed toward movement of the contralateral eye and specifically are associated with the vertical recti (Fig. 4). Even in the simple vector diagrams illustrated in Fig. 1 it can be seen that the additional forces exerted would effectively place the axis of rotation more vertical as well as closer to the plane of canal rotation. In the case of the posterior canal, the pathways are directed toward the ipsilateral eye and also largely to the vertical recti. This implies that the axis of rotation for the ipsilateral eye becomes more congruent with the rotation plane of the posterior canal.

When the AC-PC connections to the oculomotor complex are viewed from the vestibular nucleus looking towards the oculomotor nuclei they seem to be associated with 'real' vertical compensatory eye movement. This observation appears to be consistent with their appearance in the cat and not in the rabbit

(Graf et al. 1981). Eye movement related signals on the two
sets of 3 neuron VOR arcs have not yet been conclusively identified; however, a reasonable prediction can be offered from
the data available in one well studied pathway, the excitatory
posterior canal to contrateral trochlear and inferior recuts
motoneurons (2 targets) and a second pathway that includes the
contralateral inferior rectus (3 targets). Combining the unpublished data in the alert cat (Graf et al. in preparation)
and prior work on vestibular input to the trochlear nucleus
(Blanks etal. 1978), suggests two distinct types of second order vestibular neuron response distinguished by the extent of
the vertical eye position signal. The latter is undoubtedly
significant for vertical plant stiffness. Two types of vertical vestibular MLF fibers are found in the alert cat; namely,
one with high position sensitivity (aprox 10 sp/sec/ deg) and
the other with a moderate gain (aprox 2 sp/sec/deg; Yoshida et
al. 1981; Graf et al. in preparation). The above numbers were
selected in order to illustrate another point found by comparing the horizontal and vertical rate position plots for identified second order vestibular neurons to the abducens (Fig. 5)
'.nd trochlear (Fig. 6) nuclei. For the neuron shown in Fig. 6,
the horizontal rate position sensitivity was actually higher
than the vertical. Exactly the opposite might be expected
from the vestibular neuron that terminates bilaterally in the
inferior rectus. Secondly the horizontal vestibular neuron
clearly does not exhibit vertical sensitivity at all (Fig.
5B). Comparison of the two examples leads to the conclusion
that horizontal position information must reach the level of
the vertical vestibular neurons in the vestibular nuclei but
that vertical position must be added to abducens motoneurons by
pathways other than horizontal second order vestibular neurons.
Recent evidence suggests other solutions and in some cases it
is via other vestibular neurons (Graf et al. 1981 and in preparation). However, for the moment the main message is that
much work remains to be carried out on second order vestibular
neurons in both the rabbit and cat vestibular nuclei. The final part of this paper comments photographically on that
subject.

     Recent studies re-evaluating pathways and distributions of
neurons in the vestibular complex indicate three points worth
emphasis now. First, the number of second order vestibular

Figure 7. Anterograde and retrograde labeling in the cat vestibular nuclei following HRP injection in the oculomotor nucleus. A-H, the vestibular afferent input to the oculomotor nucleus and the latter's afferent pathway to the vestibular complex were simultaneously studied employing HRP transport and
subsequent sensitive histochemistry. Four representative
transverse sections through the vestibular nuclei are shown
with bright field and polarized light optics to highlight the
significant connections. Vestibular nuclei topography is after
Brodal, Pompeiano (1957). Abbreviations: SV, MV, LV AND DV are
superior, medial, lateral and descending vestibular nuclei, respectively; Y, Y-group; d and v, dorsal and ventral subdivision
of Y-group; PH, prepositus nucleus; RB, restiform body; and
MLF, medial longitudinal fasciculus. All calibrations are 1mm.

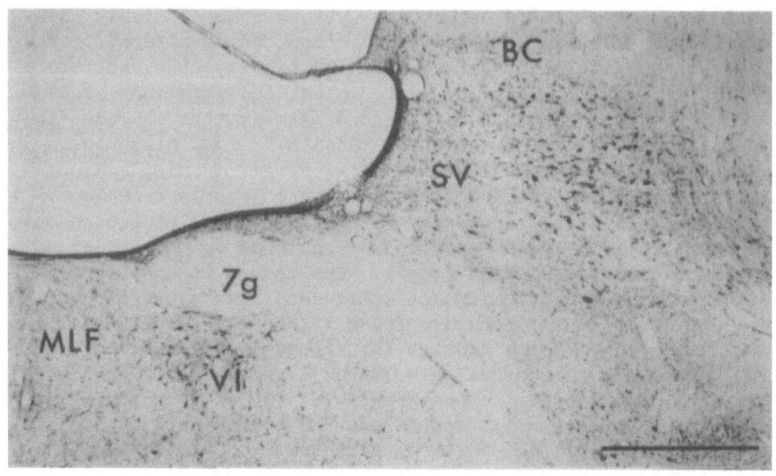

A. Transverse section near the caudal end of the superior
vestibular nucleus. Several of the large ventral vestibular
cells may lie in the rostral tip of the lateral vestibular
nucleus.

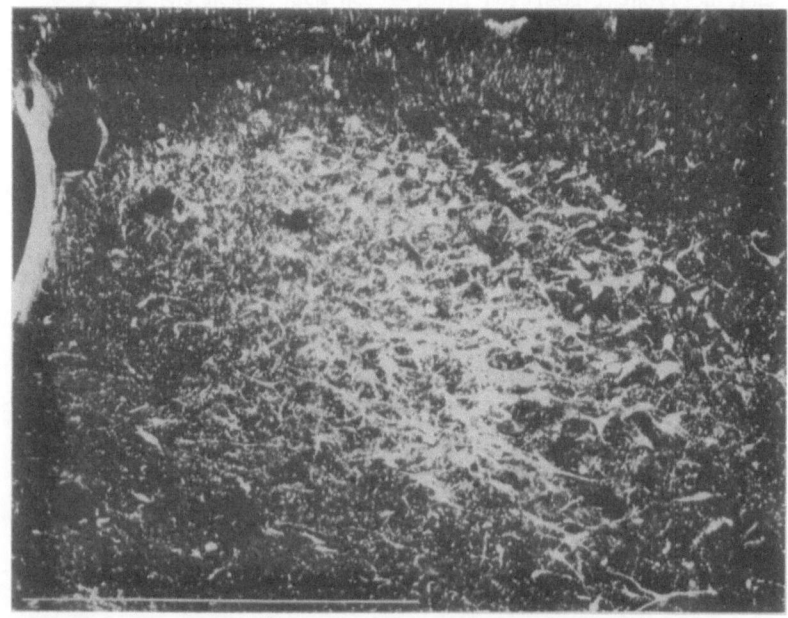

B. Enlargement of the superior vestibular nucleus shown in A.
Polarized light microscopy illustrates the density of synaptic
input to SV as well as the extensive vestibular cells with
rostral projections.

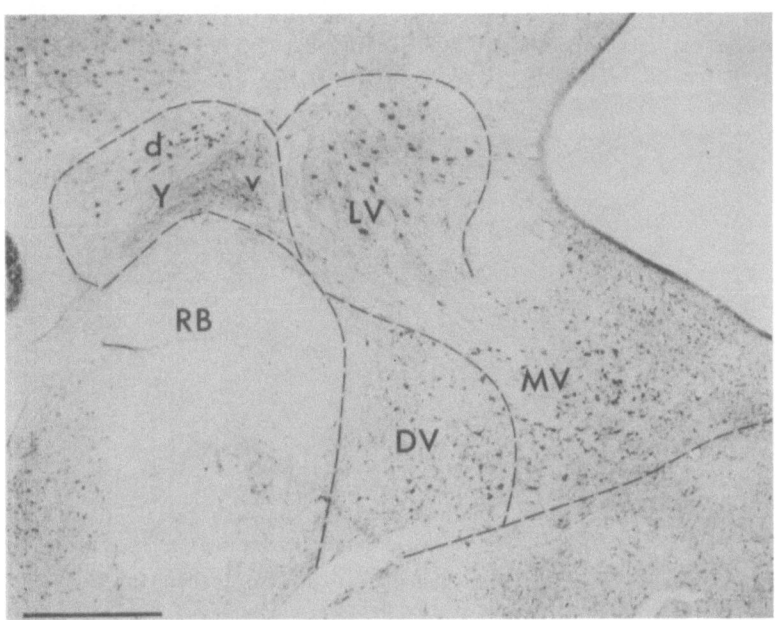

C.Transverse section through the caudal tip of the lateral vestibular nucleus and rostral part of the descending vestibular
nucleus. The dorsal and ventral parts of the Y-groups are
shown situated between the dentate nucleus and restiform body.

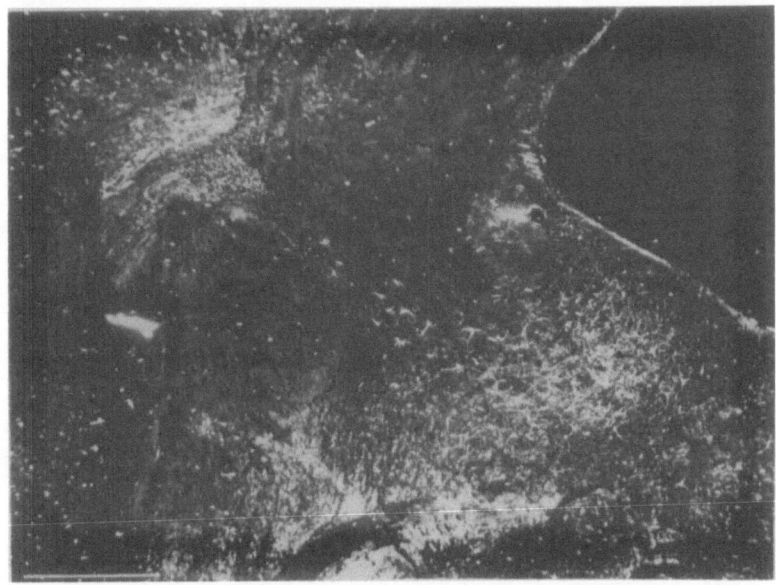

D. Same in C, but with polarized illumination. The large labeled cells in the descending nucleus are labeled in contrast

to those in the lateral vestibular nucleus. Also the retrograde (d) and anterograde (V) clearly subdivides the Y-group.

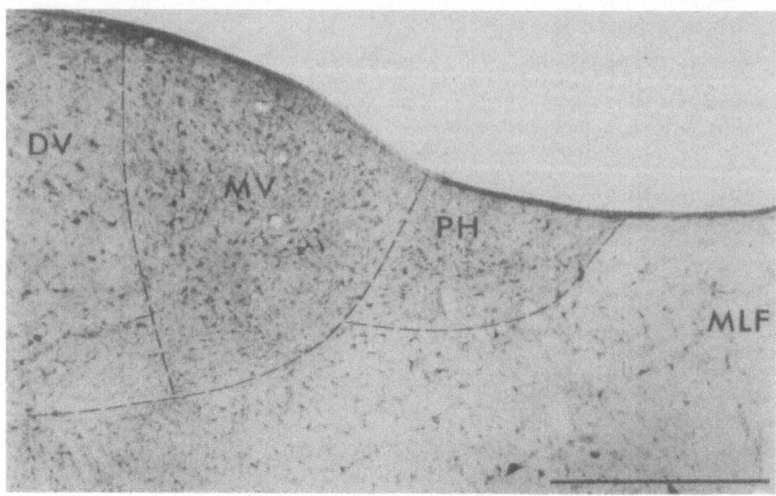

**E. Transverse section near the middle of the descending and
medial vestibular nucleus. The prepositus nucleus is also
clearly recognized.**

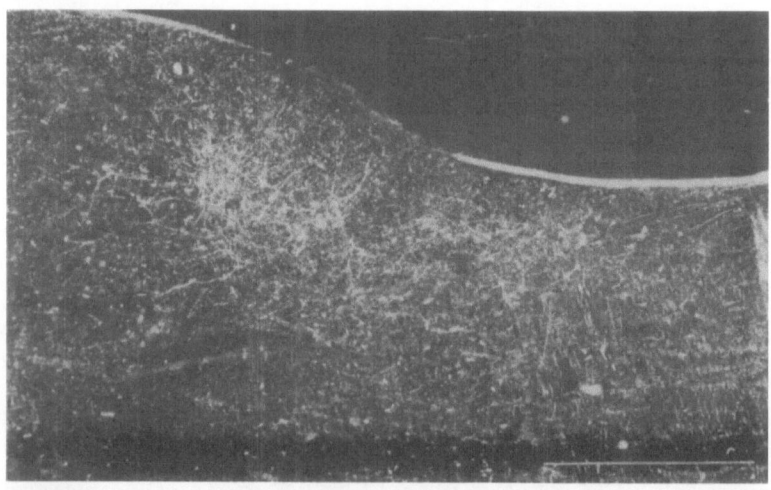

F. Same section as in E. In addition to the medial vestibular
nucleus a large number of cells are labeled in descending vestibular and prepositus nucleus. At this level, numerous cells
are found in, and around, the MLF.

neurons projecting to the oculomotor nuclei is more extensive
than previously envisioned (see Fig. 7B,D,F,H). Secondly, vertical semicircular canal pathways are comprised of neurons that
can be selectively localized in the medial, superior and descending vestibular nuclei and whose axonal pathways are in the
MLF (Uchino et al. 1981; Spencer et al. in preparation).
Thirdly, in addition to neurons distributed extensively

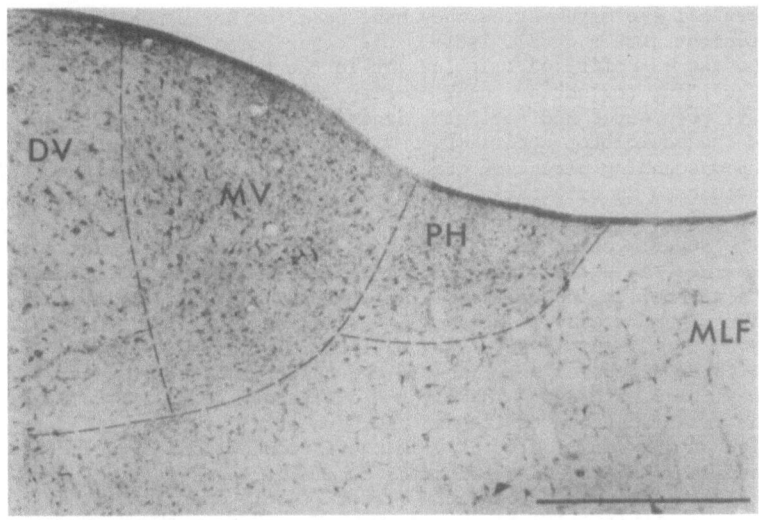

G. Transverse section near the caudal end of medial and **descending** vestibular nucleus.

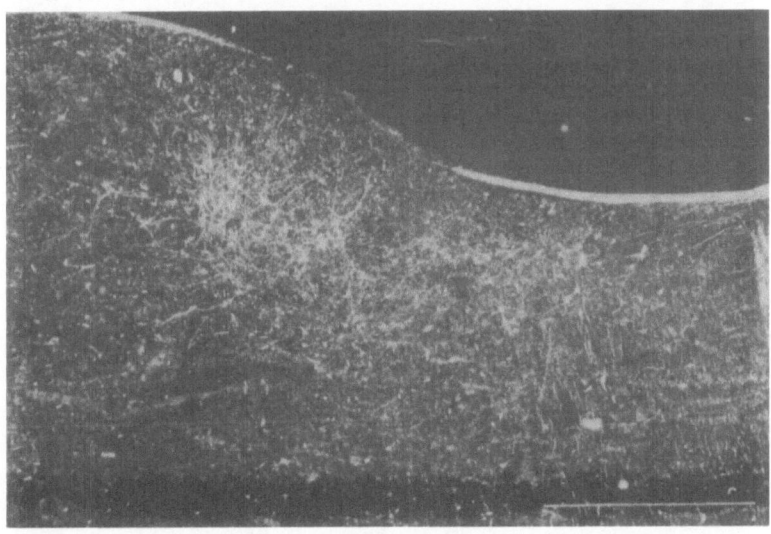

H. Same as in G. Note the continuation of a high density of cells in the caudal medial vestibular nucleus and prepositus nucleus. Anterograde labeling is still largely overlapping the same areas containing the above cells.

throughout the vestibular nucleus considerable numbers of cells are found in the prepositus nucleus proper as well as distributed in and surrounding the MLF (Fig. 7E-H). In the latter areas, irrespective of the directness of their involvement with the VOR, these neurons must be considered as significant for

vertical eye movement as they have been for horizontal eye
movement (Baker et al. 1981). One other point shown well by
the use of polarized illumination is the tremendous size of the
descending oculomotor input overlapping directly the vestibular, prepositus and reticular areas that in turn send afferents
to the oculomotor nuclei (Fig. 7). The extent of the ascending
and descending circuitry argues that the vertical VOR cannot be
envisioned as originating solely in an ascending direction from
the semicircular canals to the oculomotor nucleus.

Superimposed upon the VOR circuitry in the vestibular complex are the equally important classical relationships between
the cerebellum and bilateral vestibular nuclei, directly, and
also via commissural interaction (Baker et al. 1972; Ito et al.
1973; Ito et al. 1980c). We continue to find that Purkinje
cells in flocculus only inhibit two selected pairs of vertical
vestibular pathways - (namely the excitatory AC to iSR, cIO and
the inhibitory one to iIR and cSO; Ito et al. 1973). Thus, in
view of the reciprocity of commissural connections between the
co-planar anterior and posterior canals it seems that the cerebellum has chosen to contact, directly, only one canal path.
As a result it controls one of the reciprocal excitatory-inhibitory canal pathways in each eye. Whether the cerebellum also
influences the sets of three neuron arcs with bilateral oculomotor termination described in the cat is not important because
in any case, one must assume that the interaction between AC-
PC pairs must be sufficient to regulate all the compensatory
vertical eye movements originating from the posterior canal.
Therefore, the only structural difference is direct vs. indirect modulation in cerebellar regulation of the anterior and
posterior canal excitatory-inhibitory pathways. In a well-
tuned, balanced, push-pull system, this control might not pose
a formidable problem; however, not all vertical eye movements
are symmetrical (Anderson, 1981; King, Leigh, 1982).

In summary, the number, location, distribution, termination and eye movement related activity of second order vestibular neurons in the cat and rabbit are being pursued with emphasis on simultaneously providing information concerning both
morphological and physiological features. As was found for the
horizontal VOR, the vertical VOR will offer some special sur-
prises underlying its operation, however, it will not be any
more difficult to understand. Continued advances in circuit
description will lead to comparably good models concerning the
neuronal basis of how vertical and torsional eye movements are
synthesized centrally.

Supported by U.S. Public Health Service Research Grants,
EY02007, EY02191, and NS13742.

References:

Anderson JH (1981) Behavior of the vertical canal VOR in normal
and INC-lesioned cats. In Fuchs AF and Becker W eds Progress
in Oculomotor Research , Elsevier/North Holland: Amsterdam
397-402.
Baker R and Berthoz A (1974) Organization of vestibular nystagmus in oblique oculomotor system, J. Neurophysiol. 37, 195-217.

Baker R and Spencer RF (1981) Synthesis of horizontal eye movement in the abducens nucleus, Jap. J. EEG & EMG Suppl. 31, 49-59.

Baker R , Precht W and Llinas R (1972) Cerebellar modulatory action on the vestibulo-trochlear pathway in the cat, Exp. Brain Res. 15, 364-385.

Baker R, Precht W and Berthoz A (1973) Synaptic connections to trochlear motoneurons determined by individual vestibular nerve branch stimulation in the cat, Brain Res. 64, 402-406.

Baker R, Evinger C and McCrea RA (1981) Some thoughts about the three neurons in the vestibulo-ocular reflex. In Cohen B, ed. Ann. New York Acad. Sci. 374, 171-188.

Baker R, Spencer R and Evinger C (in press 1982) Structure-function study in the oculomotor system. In Lennerstrand G, Zee DS and Keller E eds. In Functional Basis of Ocular Motility Disorders, Oxford: Pergamon Press.

Blanks RHI, Anderson JH and Precht W (1978) Response characteristics of semicircular canal and otolith systems in cat. II. Responses of trochlear motoneurons, Exp Brain Res. 32, 509-528.

Brodal A and Pompeiano O (1957) The vestibular nuclei in the cat. J. Anat. (Lond) 91, 438-454.

Cohen B and Suzuki JI (1963) Eye movements induced by ampullary nerve stimulation, Am. J. Physiol. 204, 347-351.

Evinger C, Spencer RF and Baker R (in press 1982) Comparison of oculomotor motoneuron axon collaterals in mammals. In Lennerstrand G, Zee DS and Keller E eds. Functional Basis of Ocular Motility Disorders, Pergamon Press: Oxford

Gacek RR (1971) Anatomical demonstration of the vestibulo-ocular projections in the cat, The Laryngoscope, 81, 1559-1595.

Ghelarducci B, Highstein SM and Ito M (1977) Origin of the pre-oculomotor projections through the brachium conjunctivum and their functional roles in the vestibulo-ocular reflex. In Baker R and Berthoz A eds. The Control of Gaze, Elsevier/North Holland: Amsterdam, 167-176.

Graf W and Simpson JI (1981) The relations between the semicircular canals, the optic axis and the extraocular muscles in lateral-eyed and frontal-eyed animals. In Fuchs AF and Becker W eds. Progress in Oculomotor Research, Elsevier/North Holland: Amsterdam, 411-420.

Graf W, McCrea RA and Baker RG (1981) Morphology of secondary vestibular neurons linked to the posterior canal in rabbit and cat, Neurosci. Abst. 7, 40.

Highstein SM (1973) The organization of the vestibulo-oculomotor and trochlear reflex pathways in the rabbit, Exp. Brain Res. 17, 285-300.

Ito M, Nisimaru N and Yamamoto M (1973) Specific neural connections for the cerebellar control of vestibular-ocular reflexes. Brain Res. 60, 238-243.

Ito M, Nisimaru N and Yamamoto M (1976a) Pathways for the vestibulo-ocular reflex excitation arising from semicircular canals of rabbits, Exp. Brain Res. 24, 257-271.

Ito M, Nisimaru N and Yamamoto M (1976b) Postsynaptic inhibition of oculomotor neurons involved in vestibulo-ocular reflexes arising from semicircular canals of rabbits, Exp. Brain Res. 24, 272-283.

Ito M, Nisimaru N and Yamamoto M (1976c) Inhibitory interaction between the vestibulo-ocular reflexes arising from semicircular canals of rabbits, Exp. Brain Res. 26, 89-103.

King WM and Leigh RJ (in press 1982) Physiology of vertical gaze. In Lennerstrand G, Zee DS and Keller E eds. Functional Basis of Ocular Motility Disorders, Pergamon Press: Oxford

Lorente de No R (1933) Vestibulo-ocular reflex arc, Arch. Neurol. Psychiat. 30, 245-291.

McCrea RA, Yoshida K, Berthoz A and Baker R (1980) Eye movement related activity and morphology of second order vestibular neurons terminating in the cat abducens nucleus, Exp. Brain Res. 40, 468-473.

McCrea RA, Yoshida K, Evinger C and Berthoz A (1981) The location, axonal arborization and termination sites of eye-movement-related secondary vestibular neurons demonstrated by intra-axonal HRP injection in the alert cat. In Fuchs AF and Becker W eds. Progress in Oculomotor Research, Elsevier/North Holland: Amsterdam, 379-386.

Precht W and Baker R (1977) Synaptic organization of the vestibular-trochlear pathway. Exp. Brain Res. 14, 158-184.

Simpson JI and Graf W (1981) Eye muscle geometry and compensatory eye movements in lateral-eyed and frontal-eyed animals, Ann. N.Y. Acad. Sci. 374, 20-30.

Simpson JI, Graf W and Leonard C (1981) The coordinate system of visual climbing fibers to the flocculus. In Fuchs AF and Becker W eds. Progress in Oculomotor Research, Elsevier/North Holland: Amsterdam, 475-484.

Szentagothai J (1943) Die zentrale innervation der augenbewegungen, Arch Psychiat. Nervenkr. 116, 721-760.

Tarlov E (1970) Organization of vestibulo-oculo-motor projections in the cat, Brain Res. 20, 159-179.

Uchino Y, Hirai N and Watanabe S (1978) Vestibulo-ocular reflex from the posterior canal nerve to extraocular motoneurons in the cat, Exp. Brain Res. 32, 337-388.

Uchino Y, Hirai N, Suzuki S and Watanabe S (1980a) Axonal branching in the trochlear and oculomotor nuclei of single vestibular neurons activated from the posterior semicircular nerve in the cat, Neurosci. Letters 18, 283-288.

Uchino Y, Suzuki S and Watanabe S (1980b) Vertical semicircular inputs to cat extraocular motoneurons, Exp. Brain Res. 41, 45-53.

Uchino Y, Hirai N, Suzuki S and Watanabe S (1981) Properties of secondary vestibular neurons fired by stimulation of ampullary nerves of the vertical, anterior or posterior semicircular canals in the cat. Brain Res. 223, 273-286.

Yamamoto M, Shimoyama I and Highstein SM (1978) Vestibular nucleus neurons relaying excitation from the anterior canal to the oculomotor nucleus, Brain Res 148, 31-42.

Yoshida K, McCrea, R, Berthoz A and Vidal P.P. Eye-movement-related activity of identified second order vestibular neurons in the cat. In Fuchs AF and Becker W eds Progress in Oculomotor Research. Elsevier/North Holland: Amsterdam, 371-378.

SINGLE UNIT RECORDINGS IN THE VESTIBULAR NUCLEI OF THE ALERT MONKEY RELATED TO THE VERTICAL VESTIBULO-OCULAR REFLEX (VVOR)

H. Reisine and V. Henn (Dept. of Neurology, University Hospital, Zürich, Switzerland)

1. INTRODUCTION

Study of the vestibular system's role in oculomotor function has con-centrated on motion in horizontal planes parallel to earth to simplify experimental paradigms. Thus, the logic is that passive and active head rotations involving only events in the horizontal semicircular canals (SCC), exclusive of those for example in the vertical SCC and the otolith organs, need be correlated with the actions of only two of six extraocular muscles for one eye, i.e. the medial and lateral recti. As productive as this re-search has been in defining vestibulo-ocular relations, it is evident that head and eye movements in the horizontal plane are but a fraction of the overall eye and head motion. Involved here is the general problem of how head movement information, detected in the three dimensions of the SCC, is projec-ted onto the oculomotor system, having only two dimensions of movement--if torsions are neglected. Analysis of premotor neurons has already revealed complex iso-frequency curves in two dimensional space (Henn, Hepp, 1981). To be more specific, then, it is necessary to determine how the vestibular system interfaces with such premotor neurons, and subsequently with oculo-motoneurons.

Another notable aspect of vestibulo-ocular interfacing is that asymme-tries in vertical nystagmus have been reported in regard to gain, time constant, and visual-vestibular interaction (Matsuo, et al., 1979). As peripheral input seems to be symmetrical in all three canal planes, the question arises; at what stage are these functional asymmetries introduced. In this regard we have begun to examine the VVOR in the alert monkey, and to correlate single unit recordings in the vestibular nuclei with these reflex patterns as well as those of the horizontal vestibulo-ocular reflex. This preliminary report expresses our approach and initial findings.

2. METHODS

Experiments were performed on juvenile monkeys (Macaca mulatta). Head bolts for head fixation, silver-silver chloride DC EOG electrodes for moni-toring eye position, and a stainless steel cylinder for a micropositioner were implanted. Single units were recorded with etched, varnished tungsten microelectrodes having impedences between 1-7 MegOhm. During recording sessions the animal sat with head fixed, ventroflexed 25° to the horizon-tal plane, in a primate chair, which was fastened into a gimbal. The gimbal, in turn, was attached to a turntable. Both gimbal and turntable could be driven independently by seperate servo-controlled motors. This arrangement permitted independent horizontal and vertical axis rotations relative to the animal's head; in addition, the animal could be statically tilted in the gimbal for otolith testing. Also, a device at the bottom of the primate chair

Roucoux, A. and Crommelinck, M. (eds.): Physiological and Pathological Aspects of Eye Movements.
© 1982, Dr W. Junk Publishers, The Hague, Boston, London. ISBN-13: 978-94-009-8002-0

permitted the animal's saggital plane to be oriented at any angle relative to the gimbal plane. Thus, the device allows sinusoidal rotation in any desired vertical plane through the animal's head, e.g. face forward, 45° left ear forward (LEF), or 90° right ear forward (REF) which is now the roll axis.

The range of vestibular stimulation consisted of sinusoidal rotations of 0.1 or 0.2 Hz.; peak amplitudes were ± 25 to 30 deg and peak velocities ± 25 to 30 deg/s. Eye position traces were calibrated during sessions of combined vestibular and optokinetic stimulation (light on, optokinetic drum stationary) at 30 deg/s constant velocity rotation. For vertical eye position calibration, the animal was placed right ear down and rotated about a vertical axis.

EOG, turntable and gimbal velocity and position signals as well as single unit records were stored on magnetic tape for off-line analysis. Data was played back and written out on chart paper for hand analysis. Unit data was written out as either instantaneous frequency or averaged for 250 ms and updated every 100 ms.

3. RESULTS

As a first step, it was found essential to define the individual animal's nystagmus response.

Sinusoidally rotating the animal in the gimbal, i.e. about an earth horizontal axis, in the dark produces both upward and downward nystagmus (direction of nystagmus refers to the direction of the fast phase). Fig. 1 illustrates the results from such an experiment (0.2 Hz, ±25°).

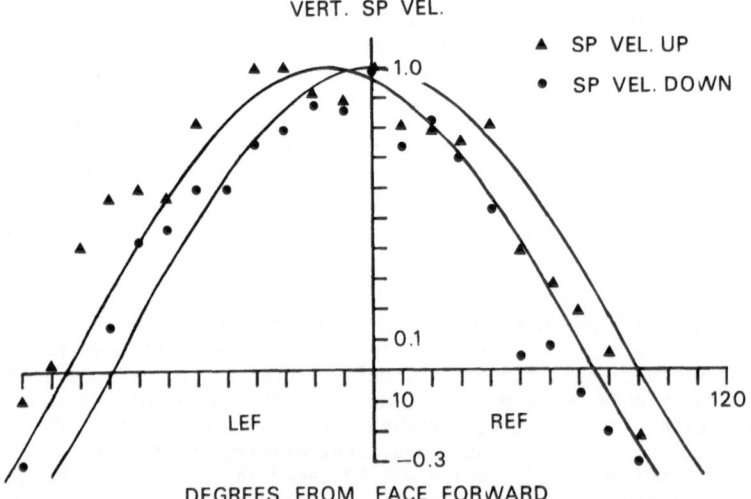

Figure 1. Relation of amplitude of slow phase velocity in the vertical plane to angle that saggital plane makes with the gimbal plane of rotation. Note that negative values of the slow phase velocity indicate a reversal of the direction of the eye movements, e.g. triangles with negative values represent downward slow phase velocity.

The ordinates represent a ratio of slow phase velocity compared to the maximal slow phase velocity obtained in the paradigm. Abscissa values indicate each 10° change in the orientation of the vertical plane through which the animal was rotated. Each ordinate value represents the average of the peak slow phase velocity for five successive cycles. The cosine curve with a peak value at the Y-axis is the predicted relation of the slow phase as a function of the angle of rotation obtained from a previous study (Blanks, et al., 1975). The second cosine curve with the peak at -15° is an approximation of a regression analysis for the combined upward and downward slow phase velocities. Our interpretation is that the 15° shift in the peak of the curve is related to individual variation and/or error in head orientation in the holding appratus. The point is that such an examination is required for each monkey before proceeding to the unit analysis. In this case the 15° LEF was thereafter defined as the face forward position. Notably, the data in Fig. 1 also demonstrate almost consistantly that upward is greater than downward slow phase velocity under the same conditions, i.e. an asymmetry exists. The cause for this is unknown.

Following the initial observation of eye movements, single units were recorded extracellularly in the vestibular nuclei. One example will be presented in detail. Data in Fig. 2 depict the experimental paradigm (A) and identification and analysis of a Type I anterior canal unit (B) recorded in the left brain stem. Records in Fig. 2A reflect the experimental conditions present when record 45° LEF in 2B was obtained. Important is that the peak discharge (approx. 50 spikes/s) occurs at a 90° phase lead relative

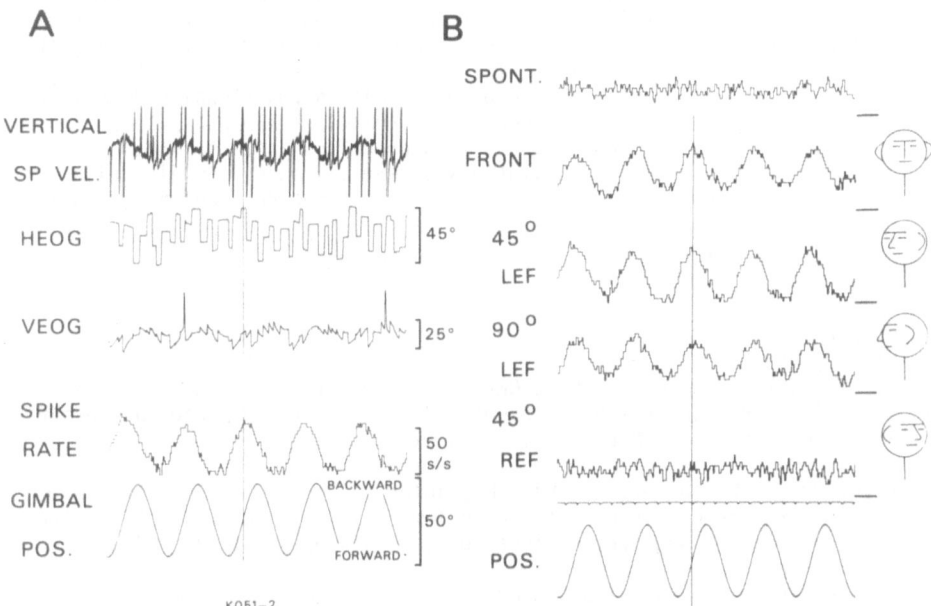

Figure 2. Experimental protocol (A) and identification of a Type I anterior canal unit (B). Note in (B), bars in bottom right of averaged rate traces indicate zero spikes/s.The records have the same calibration as in (A). Time trace in (B) indicates 1 s/division.

to gimbal position (or in phase with peak upward slow phase velocity). The sensitivity of the response is 0.9 spikes/s per deg/s. With the gimbal traveling forwards to backwards, activation of the unit correlates with that of the ipsilateral anterior canal. In B, although no eye positon records have been included, the spontaneous rate in the light is constant while the animal makes eye movements, suggesting a lack of oculomotor input. Spontaneous rate is 20 spikes/s. The ratio of the modulation at face forward and 90° LEF to the 45° LEF is 0.7 (mean= 0.7, range 0.55-0.82, n=7 units), while unit activity is nulled during rotation in the orthogonal plane, i.e. 45° REF. The ampliude changes in the unit response related to the plane of rotation, suggest that they follow a cosine curve with the peak in a plane almost parallel to the left anterior canal.

Other units were invariably tested. In analogy to the classification of units with horizontal canal input they were found to be characteristic of Type I or II, anterior or posterior canal units, with or without rapid eye movement modulation. Some units responded to static tilt suggesting an otolith input.

4. DISCUSSION

The data presented in this preliminary report point to interesting trends in analyzing the VVOR in the alert monkey. First, each animal must be fully assessed for its unique pattern of eye movement responses to the experimental paradigm; only then can the unit activity recorded from central vestibular neurons be properly correlated. Second, the VVOR in the alert monkey is asymmetric and this cannot be related to differences between the spontaneous, nor the dynamic, activity in primary vestibular afferents from the posterior vs the anterior canals (Goldberg, Fernandez, 1971; Blanks, et al., 1975). Finally, although the multiplicity of possible inputs to central vestibular neurons is great, we were usually able to functionally determine the respective canal input for a neuron, and null its response out during animal motion in the orthogonal plane. If a unit, sensitive to motion in one canal plane, was additionally modulated with eye movements, on-direction for the eye movements coincided with the direction of the vestibular activation.

ACKNOWLEDGEMENTS
Supported by a grant from the Swiss National Foundation for Scientific Research 3.718.80.

5. REFERENCES

Blanks, HI, Estes, MS and Markham, CH (1975) Physiologic characteristics of vestibular first order canal neurons in the cat. II. Response to constant angular acceleration, J. Neurophysiol. 38, 1250-1268.

Goldberg, JM and Fernandez, C (1971) Physiology of peripheral neurons innervating semicircular canals of the squirrel monkey. I. Resting discharge and response to constant angular accelerations, J. Neurophysiol. 34, 635-660.

Henn, V and Hepp, K (1981) Two-dimensional analysis of eye movements in oculomotor and premotor structures. In Fuchs, A and Becker, W eds. Progress in oculomotor research, pp 81-88. Amsterdam, Elsevier/North-Holland.

Matsuo, V, Cohen, B, Raphan, T, De Jong, V and Henn, V (1979) Asymmetric velocity storage for upward and downward nystagmus, Brain Res. 176, 159-164.

THE BRAIN-STEM MATRIX OF THE VESTIBULO-OCULAR REFLEX

L.W. SCHULTHEIS, DAVID A. ROBINSON (Departments of
Ophthalmology and Biomedical Engineering, The Johns
Hopkins University, Baltimore, Maryland U.S.A.)*

1. INTRODUCTION

This report shows how one may calculate the functional
strengths of the anatomical connections between second-
order neurons in the vestibular nuclei and the motoneurons of the extra-ocular muscles that subserve the
vestibulo-ocular reflex in all three dimensions. To
transform neural signals in the spatial coordinates
of the canals to motor commands in the coordinates of
the muscles, every canal pair must project to every
muscle pair. The strengths of these projections may
be calculated by geometrical considerations alone. In
addition, the changes in the strengths of these connections may be calculated when the reflex plastically
adapts to the chronic wearing of optical devices that
dissociate head movement and the relative movement of
the visual environment. These calculations do not say
how these modifications are made but they at least
tell numerically what must be done and a few interesting
features of these modifications emerge.

2. DERIVATION OF THE BRAIN-STEM MATRIX
2.1. Overview

The appropriate method for dealing with the vestibulo-
ocular reflex in three dimensions is to consider the
head rotation as a velocity vector $\dot{H}$ with components
$\dot{H}_z$, $\dot{H}_x$, $\dot{H}_y$ in a coordinate system such as that shown
in Fig. 1. The response is an eye rotation vector $\dot{E}$
with similar z, x, y components. Any transformation
that converts one vector to another, such as the vestibulo-ocular reflex, can be described by a matrix
[VOR],

$$\vec{E} = \begin{vmatrix} \dot{E}_z \\ \dot{E}_x \\ \dot{E}_y \end{vmatrix} = [VOR] \; \vec{H} = \begin{vmatrix} -1 & 0 & 0 \\ 0 & -1 & 0 \\ 0 & 0 & -1 \end{vmatrix} \begin{vmatrix} \dot{H}_z \\ \dot{H}_x \\ \dot{H}_y \end{vmatrix} = [-I]\vec{H}. \quad (1)$$

For an ideal reflex, the matrix [VOR] is, as shown on
the right, minus the identity matrix [-I] so that the
gain of the reflex is -1.0 in yaw ($\dot{H}_z$), pitch ($\dot{H}_x$),
and roll ($\dot{H}_y$); cross-coupling terms are all zero. The
matrix [VOR] is made up of three parts: the canals,
brain-stem, and eye muscles, (Fig. 1). The canals may be
thought of as transforming $\dot{H}$ into a vector $\vec{C}$ the components of which represent the change in neural

* This research was supported by grants EY00598 and
EY01765 from the NEI of the NIH, the U.S. Public
Health Service.

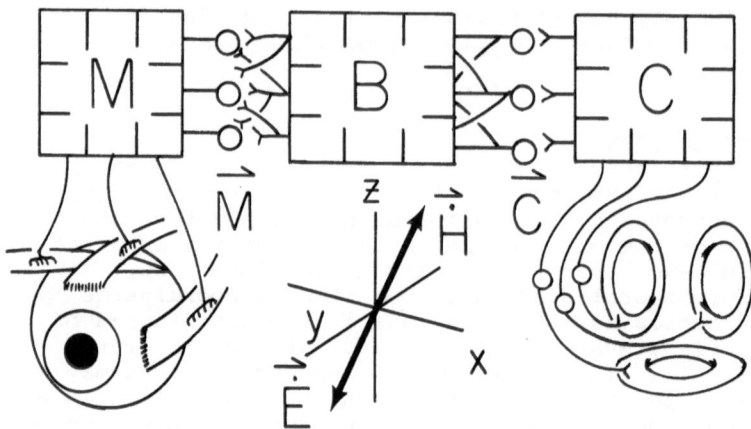

FIGURE 1.   The matrices of the vestibulo-ocular reflex.

discharge rate of the canal afferents. The canal transformation is a matrix, [C].   The brain-stem transforms
$\vec{C}$ into a vector $\vec{M}$ with components representing the
change in firing rate of motoneurons; that matrix is
called [B].   Finally, the eye muscles transform, by a
matrix [M], the neural command $\vec{M}$ into the physical
eye movement $\vec{E}$.   Thus,

$$\vec{E} = [M]\vec{M} = [M][B]\vec{C} = [M][B][C]\dot{\vec{H}}. \qquad (2)$$

From equs. (1) and (2),

$$[VOR] = [M][B][C], \qquad (3)$$

so that,

$$[B] = [M^{-1}][VOR][C^{-1}]. \qquad (4)$$

Thus, given the matrices [M], [VOR], and [C] one can
find from [B] how much each canal pair projects to
each muscle pair.

2.2. The canal matrix
The amount by which a canal is excited by $\vec{H}$ is proportional to the projection of $\vec{H}$ onto an axis perpendicular
to the plane of that canal. The six canals may be
grouped into three pairs not so much for convenience
but because the central nervous system actually per-
forms this pairing through the vestibular commissural
system.   Since a second-order, vestibular neuron is
driven both by ipsilateral excitation and disinhibition
from the contralateral side, it behaves as though it
were driven by a pair of canals perfectly aligned in a
plane midway between those of the individual canals.
Using the data of Blanks, Curthoys and Markham (1975)
for human canals, one can construct three planes, one
for each canal pair; perpendiculars to these planes are
the axes of the coordinate system of the canals. It is
then a simple matter to show (Schultheis, 1982) that,

$$\vec{C} = \begin{vmatrix} C_{lrh} \\ C_{rpla} \\ C_{ralp} \end{vmatrix} = [C] \; \vec{H} = \begin{vmatrix} 0.927 & 0 & -0.374 \\ 0.156 & -0.673 & 0.723 \\ 0.156 & 0.673 & 0.723 \end{vmatrix} \begin{vmatrix} \dot{H}_z \\ \dot{H}_x \\ \dot{H}_y \end{vmatrix} \quad (5)$$

where the canal-pair subscripts are combinations of left (l), right (r), horizontal (h), anterior (a), and posterior (p).

It can be noted that $\vec{C}$ consists of the projections, not the components of $\vec{H}$ in the canal system. Thus, [C] combines two steps: a coordinate transformation of the contravariant vector $\vec{H}$ into the skewed, canal coordinates and then a transformation within that system from components to projections. The matrix of the latter transformation is called the metric tensor of the canal space and $\vec{C}$ is a covariant vector (Pellionisz and Llinás, 1980).

2.3. The muscle matrix

Each pair of muscles rotates the eye about an axis. The three axes so defined form the coordinate system of the muscles. Pairing the axes of individual muscles for the left eye from the data of Robinson (1975), one can show (Schultheis, 1982) that,

$$\vec{E} = \begin{vmatrix} \dot{E}_z \\ \dot{E}_x \\ \dot{E}_y \end{vmatrix} = [M] \; \vec{M} = \begin{vmatrix} 1.0 & 0.016 & 0.14 \\ -0.005 & -0.906 & 0.6 \\ 0.015 & 0.424 & 0.788 \end{vmatrix} \begin{vmatrix} M_{lmr} \\ M_{sir} \\ M_{sio} \end{vmatrix} \quad (6)$$

The muscle subscripts are formed from lateral (l), medial (m), superior (s), inferior (i), recti (r), and obliques (o).

2.4. The brain-stem matrix

Assuming that the reflex is perfect ([VOR] equal to [-I]), equs. (5) and (6) may be inverted and from (4),

$$\vec{M} = \begin{vmatrix} M_{lmr} \\ M_{sir} \\ M_{sio} \end{vmatrix} = [B]\vec{C} = \begin{vmatrix} -1.024 & -0.203 & -0.131 \\ 0.146 & -0.997 & 0.212 \\ 0.212 & -0.267 & -0.919 \end{vmatrix} \begin{vmatrix} C_{lrh} \\ C_{rpla} \\ C_{ralp} \end{vmatrix} \quad (7)$$

The terms on the main diagonal reflect the principal excitatory connections: horizontal canal → contralateral (contra) lr, ipsilateral (ipsi) mr; anterior canal → ipsi sr, contra io; posterior canal → contra ir, ispi so. The other two terms in the first column are due to a small sensitivity of the vertical canals to yaw which must be suppressed by a projection from the h canals to the cyclovertical muscles. The other two terms in the first row are due to a backward tilt of the h canals making them sensitive to roll. To suppress this, the vertical canals must project to the horizontal muscles. The remaining four terms at the lower right correct for the misalignments of the vertical canals and cyclo-vertical muscles.

3. PLASTICITY

3.1. Twisting the vestibulo-ocular reflex

We (1980) showed that by associating horizontal retinal
slip with pitch head movements for several hours in
the cat, horizontal eye movement could be created
reflexively by pitch head movements in the dark. The
former were about 25% of the latter. The gains of the
reflexes in other directions were unchanged. The
matrix for this modified reflex is shown on the left
in equ. (8). This matrix may be put into (4), assuming
a similar result in humans, to find [B] shown on the
right in equ. (8). Only the last two elements in the

$$[VOR] = \begin{vmatrix} -1 & -0.25 & 0 \\ 0 & -1 & 0 \\ 0 & 0 & -1 \end{vmatrix} ; [B] = \begin{vmatrix} -1.024 & -0.017 & -0.317 \\ 0.146 & -0.999 & 0.215 \\ 0.212 & -0.27 & -0.917 \end{vmatrix} \quad (8)$$

first row have changed from equ. (7) to reflect the
altered connections from the vertical canals to the
horizontal recti. The elements changed by equal and
opposite amounts because in pitch C_{rpla} equals $-C_{ralp}$.
This matrix thus allows only pitch to induce horizontal
eye movements without affecting the gains in any other
direction. This example shows that the matrix technique
can reveal just which connections had to change and by
how much during plastic adaptation.

3.2. Gain changes in two dimensions by vision reversal

Berthoz et al. (1981) noted that wearing Dove prisms
not only reverses visual motion seen in yaw, but also
in roll, while leaving vision normal in pitch. They
also found that the gain of the torsion reflex was
half that of the others in a normal subject. Consequently, the normal reflex in humans may be closer to
that on the left in equ. (9) than the [-I] used in
equ. (1). The values in [B] associated with this [VOR],
shown at the right in equ. (9), have changed significantly from those in equ. (7); note that the second

$$[VOR] = \begin{vmatrix} -1 & 0 & 0 \\ 0 & -1 & 0 \\ 0 & 0 & -0.5 \end{vmatrix} ; [B] = \begin{vmatrix} -1.01 & -0.248 & -0.176 \\ 0.08 & -0.799 & 0.41 \\ 0.112 & 0.031 & -0.621 \end{vmatrix} \quad (9)$$

number in the last row has even changed sign. The
reasons are similar to those involved with plasticity
to be considered next. When the subject wore reversing
prisms for 19 days, the gains of the horizontal and
torsional reflex had dropped by 60%. For a subject
trying to attend to a visual task in the dark, the
adapted, vestibulo-ocular reflex would be described by
the matrix on the left in equ. (10). The corresponding
brain-stem matrix is shown on the right.

$$[VOR] = \begin{vmatrix} -0.4 & 0 & 0 \\ 0 & -1 & 0 \\ 0 & 0 & -0.2 \end{vmatrix} ; [B] = \begin{vmatrix} -0.404 & -0.121 & -0.049 \\ 0.032 & -0.682 & 0.527 \\ 0.045 & 0.208 & -0.444 \end{vmatrix} \quad (10)$$

The decrease in the upper, left term reflects the drop in the horizontal gain. The decreases in the other terms in the first row and column are due to the smaller need to eliminate cross-coupling between horizontal and cyclovertical reflexes when gains are lower. The four terms in the lower right are of most interest because they allowed the gain in roll to decrease without changing the gain in pitch. This is accomplished by decreasing the magnitudes of both main-diagonal terms by the same amount (0.117) while increasing the off-diagonal terms by the same amount. As Berthoz et al. (1981) pointed out, one cannot change the gain of one of the cyclovertical reflexes without the other unless secondary (off-diagonal) connections are altered. This is true but one can add that, although the gain of the vertical reflex did not change, comparison of equs. (9) and (10) show that all nine elements of the matrix underwent a considerable change.

These examples illustrate the use of matrices in studying plasticity of the reflex. It may be extended to an analysis of the comparative physiology of the reflex and to the prediction of the results of lesions as well, whenever one is concerned with the operation of the vestibulo-ocular reflex in all its degrees of freedom.

REFERENCES

Berthoz A Melvill Jones G and Béqué AE (1981) Differential visual adaptation of vertical canal-dependent vestibulo-ocular reflexes, Exp. Brain Res. 44, 19-26

Blanks RHI Curthoys IS and Markham CH (1975) Planar relationships of the semicircular canals in man, Acta Otolaryngol. 80, 185-196.

Pellionisz A and Llinás R (1980) Tensorial approach to the geometry of brain function: cerebellar coordination via a metric tensor, Neurosci. 5, 1125-1136.

Robison DA (1975) A quantitative analysis of extra-ocular muscle cooperation and squint, Invest. Ophthal. 14, 801-825.

Schultheis LW (1982) Cross-axis plasticity of the vestibulo-ocular reflex in the cat, Doctoral dissertation, TheJohns Hopkins University, Baltimore

Schultheis LW and Robinson DA (1981) Directional plasticity of the vestibulo-ocular reflex in thecat. In Cohen B, ed. Vestibular and oculomotor physiology; International Meeting of the Bárány Society, pp. 504-512. New York, New York Academy of Sciences.

COMPENSATORY EYE MOVEMENTS IN THE MONKEY DURING HIGH FREQUENCY SINUSOIDAL
ROTATIONS

A.BÖHMER, V.HENN, (Zürich, Switzerland) and
J.-I.SUZUKI (Tokyo, Japan)

INTRODUCTION
Vestibulo-ocular reflex (VOR) transfer characteristics are well documented
in various species for frequencies up to 1 Hz. Natural active and passive
head movements, however, have frequency components well above 1 Hz (Donaghy
1980)and accelerations exceeding several thousand deg/sec^2. Stimulation in
this range requires special apparatus which have become available only
recently at reasonable costs and therefore only few published data exist. In
this frequency range the peripheral vestibular organ is probably the exclusive
sensory organ which contributes to compensatory eye movements; data on a
possible contribution of neck afferents (cervico-ocular reflex COR), however,
are still controversial.
    Two series of experiments investigating compensatory eye movements elicited
by high frequency (up to 6 Hz) sinusoidal stimulation are presented here. VOR
and COR measurements were made in 1)normal monkeys and 2)a monkey after
selective plugging of both horizontal semicircular canals.

METHODS
Data were obtained from five alert monkeys (Macaca mulatta and M.fasci-
cularis), chronically implanted with silver-silverchloride EOG electrodes to
monitor eye position. In an additional monkey both horizontal canals were
plugged by drilling through the bony canal and filling the hole with bone
chips (fecit J.-I.S.). The monkeys were attached in a ligthweight primate
chair with the head firmly fixed by implanted bolts. A device driven by a
powerfull servo-controlled torque motor rotated sinusoidally either the
whole monkey about a vertical axis (VOR) or the trunk only while the head
stayed earth-fixed (COR). Three different peak-to-peak amplitudes (6, 12, and
24 deg) and frequencies between 0.5 and 6 Hz were tested. Phase and gain data
were measured by hand from eye and body position curves (gain = peak-to-peak
eye position divided by peak-to-peak body position; phase = eye position
relative to body position, negative values = phase lag).

RESULTS
1. Normal monkeys
A Bode plot of the horizontal VOR and VOR+OKN (stimulation in the light) is
given in fig.1. Each point represents the mean of the responses elicited by
all stimulus amplitudes (cross-subject average of five monkeys). The gain is
slightly below unity over the whole frequency range tested here and there is
a slight increase of phase lag at 6 Hz. No obvious differences were found
between stimulation in the light and in darkness. In normal monkeys cervico-
ocular reflexes were virtually absent in this frequency range.

Roucoux, A. and Crommelinck, M. (eds.): Physiological and Pathological Aspects of Eye Movements.
© *1982, Dr W. Junk Publishers, The Hague, Boston, London.* ISBN-13: 978-94-009-8002-0

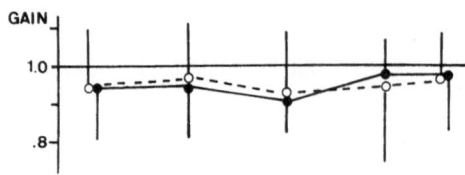

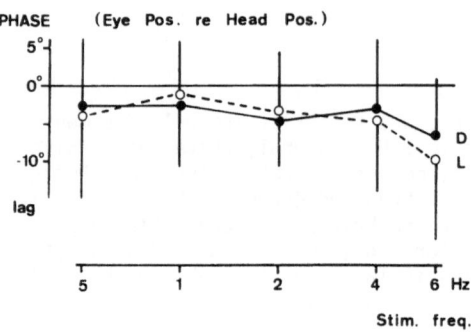

FIGURE 1. Horizontal VOR (rotation in the dark, full circles) and horizontal VOR + OKN (rotation in the light, open circles) in normal monkeys. Vertical bars = 1 S.D.)

2. Horizontal semicircular canals plugged

At first the head of the monkey was precisely ventro-flexed relative to earth horizon untill no compensatory eye movements could be induced in darkness by applied angular velocity steps about a vertical axis (100 deg/sec^2 to 100 deg/sec). In this position (nose down 33 deg) the vertical semicircular canals seemed to be orientated exactly in the vertical plane. Further forward pitching reversed vestibular nystagmus (i.e. clockwise acceleration elicited left beating nystagmus).

All further experiments were performed with the head 33 deg nose down. During the first weeks after the canal plugging sinusoidal rotation in the dark also induced no nystagmus; responses elicited in the light therefore might be considered as pure optokinetic responses, they showed a large decrease of the gain and increase of phase lag with higher stimulus frequencies (gain at 2 Hz = 0.4); with frequencies above 2 Hz no measurable compensatory eye movements could be induced.

In the following months velocity steps in the dark still failed to induce nystagmus, while compensatory eye movements developped in response to vertical axis sinusoidal rotations in the dark. A Bode plot of such responses 7 months after the canal plugging is given in fig. 2, showing a gain increase with higher stimulus frequencies and a phase lead up to 50 deg which decreased with higher frequencies.

Fig. 3 shows that the gain of these responses was more closely related to stimulus velocity than to stimulus frequency with a threshold at about 45 deg/sec, 1 month after the canal plugging. This threshold decreased to about 15 deg/sec, 7 months post-operative.

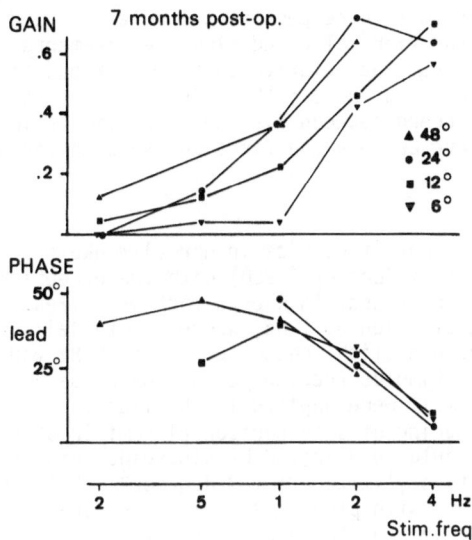

FIGURE 2. Compensatory eye movements in response to sinusoidal rotation of the whole monkey with both horizontal semicircular canals plugged. Bode plot for 4 different stimulus amplitudes 7 months after the canal plugging.

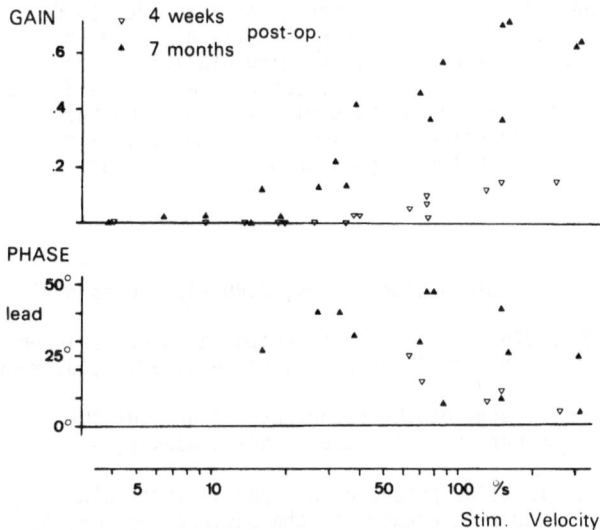

FIGURE 3. The same data as in fig. 2 (solid symbols) and data obtained 4 weeks after the canal plugging (open triangles) plotted versus stimulus velocity.

In this monkey eye movements could also be elicited by trunk rotation (COR).
The slow phases were always compensatory in respect to the relative head
movement (i.e. trunk rotations to the right elicited slow eye movements to
the right). These responses had a phase lag relative to the trunk position
which increased with higher stimulus frequencies; the gain varied between
0.05 and 0.45 without a systematic trend between 0.2 and 4 Hz stimulation
frequency and did not further improve between the first and seventh month
after the operation.

DISCUSSION
Our data on high frequency transfer characteristics in normal monkeys agree
well with those described in the cat by Donaghy (1980) with the exception of
a slight phase lead below 2 Hz that he found. In Rhesus monkeys, Miles and
Eighmy (1980) reported a phase lag of 2 deg at 1 Hz, whereas both Keller
(1978) and Furman et al. (1982) found a slight phase lead up to 6 Hz and a
1.2 peak of the gain curve at 4 Hz stimulus frequency. This peak was absent
in Keller's study when the same stimuli were applied in the light.
    Several weeks after surgical plugging of both horizontal semicircular
canals compensatory eye movements could be elicited by sinusoidal rotations
but not by steps of angular velocities (limited to 100 deg/sec^2). B.Peterson
observed the same phaenomenon in cats with plugged semicircular canals
(pers.comm. at this meeting). The origin of these responses is not clear. The
absence of nystamgus elicited by steps of angular velocity seems to exclude
input from the vertical canals. Preliminary findings in a labyrinthectomized
monkey which shows no compensatory eye movements, neither to velocity steps
nor to sinusoidal rotations, also exclude a somatic origin. The most probable
candidates for this response thus are the otolith organs, although it is
claimed that they do not respond to (low) angular acceleration as long as the
animal is centered over the rotation axis (Goldberg and Fernandez 1975). In
response to sinusoidal force variations (excentric rotation), however,
responses can be obtained from irregularly discharging otolith neurons
(Fernandez and Goldberg 1976). A Bode plot constructed from such data (l.c.,
p.1001) shows striking similarities to our Bode plot in fig.2. Further
experiments using excentrical sinusoidal rotations may lead to a better
understanding of the role of the otolith organs as possible generators of
compensatory eye movements.

REFERENCES
Donaghy M (1980) The cat's vestibulo-ocular reflex, J.Physiol (London)
    300, 337-351.
Fernandez C and Goldberg JM (1976) Physiology of peripheral neurons inner-
    vating otolith organs of the Squirrel monkey, response dynamics, J. Neuro-
    physiol 39, 996-1008.
Furman JM et al (1982) Dynamic range of the frequency response of the
    horizontal vestibulo-ocular reflex of the alert Rhesus monkey, Acta
    otolaryngol 93, 81-91.
Goldberg JM and Fernandez C (1975) Responses of peripheral vestibular
    neurons to angular and linear acceleration in the Squirrel monkey, Acta
    otolaryngol 80, 101-110.
Miles FA and Eighmy BB (1980) Long term adaptive changes in the primate
    vestibulo-ocular reflex, J.Neurophysiol 43, 1406-1425.
Keller EL (1978) Gain of the vestibulo-ocular reflex in the monkey at high
    rotational frequencies, Vision Res 18, 311-315.

CONCERNING THE LINEAR ACCELERATION INPUT TO THE NEURAL OCULOMOTOR CONTROL SYSTEM IN PRIMATES

R. Eckmiller (Div.of Biocybernetics,Dept.of Biophysics, University of Düsseldorf, West Germany)

INTRODUCTION

There is a growing body of evidence that the utricular otolith organs influence the oculomotor system as part of the otolith-ocular reflex(Barnes,1980; Blanks et al.,1978; Buizza et al.,1980; Schwindt et al.,1973). However, no quantitative descriptions of this utriculo-oculomotor pathway in primates so far exist.

This paper for the first time presents neurophysiological data from direct measurements of the dynamic responses of oculomotor motoneurons to sinusoidal linear acceleration in the alert and the anesthetized monkey. The first study(A) in alert trained monkeys compares the different neural control contributions of individual oculomotor motoneurons to a given foveal pursuit eye movement depending on whether it is caused by purely visual or by mixed visual-vestibular stimulation. The second study(B) describes the directional characteristic of motoneurons(during anesthesia) with respect to the direction of the horizontal linear acceleration vector and provides evidence that the direct utriculo-abducens pathway involves only the medial region of the ipsilateral utricle. In the third study(C) the frequency response(Bode plot) of the utriculo-abducens pathway which demonstrates a phase gap between otolith afferents and motoneurons is presented.

METHODS

Single unit activity in the III. and VI.nerve nuclei, as well as horizontal eye movements(implanted EOG electrodes) were recorded in three monkeys(Macaca fascicularis). The animals had been trained to perform foveal pursuit eye movements. Further details concerning training, surgery, and recording have been described elsewhere(Eckmiller, Mackeben,1978). For the application of sinusoidal linear accelerations in the horizontal plane a slide track with a special primate chair was designed. The upper portion of the chair can be rotated around the vertical axis and can be moved along the slide track over a total distance of 1.6 meters by means of a feedback control system having a position sensor with a resolution of 200 microns. In most experiments described in this paper the sinusoidal linear movements of the chair had an amplitude of 26.4 cm which is equivalent to 10 degrees of eye movements for pursuit of a stationary target on a screen 1.5 m away. For one set of experiments the chair was locked at various angles δ. The angle δ is defined as that between the monkey's X-axis(anterior-posterior axis) and the slide track axis, such that $\delta=90^\circ$ refers to a pure right-left movement of the chair on the track.

Roucoux, A. and Crommelinck, M. (eds.): Physiological and Pathological Aspects of Eye Movements.
© *1982, Dr W. Junk Publishers, The Hague, Boston, London.* ISBN-13: 978-94-009-8002-0

132

RESULTS

A. <u>Visual-vestibular rivalry in the neural control of
primate foveal pursuit during linear acceleration</u>

The question of whether or not the contribution of
individual oculomotor motoneurons to a given eye movement
depends on the specific sensory input is still open.
The first hint of such a dependency came from a recent
study in alert monkeys(Skavenski, Robinson,1973).
To tackle this question, foveal pursuit eye movements
which are virtually identical(with an amplitude of 10
degrees at 0.3 Hz) were elicited by two quite different
conditions of sensory stimulation:
1)Light spot(4 min. of arc in diameter) moves horizontally
on a screen 1.5 m away; monkey head stationary.
Stimulation is purely visual.

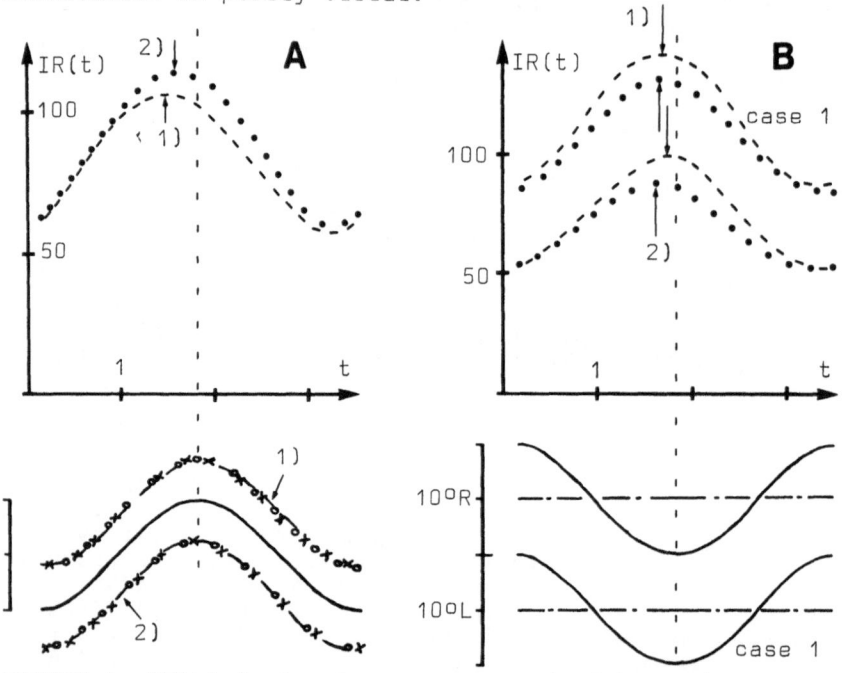

FIGURE 1. IR(t) in impulses per second of two motoneurons
during foveal pursuit with an amplitude of 10 degrees at
0.3 Hz under condition 1)(purely visual) and 2)(visual
plus otolith organ stim.). <u>Fig. 1A</u>. Top half: IR(t) of
abducens motoneuron(D7-1320); IR maximum is larger under
condition 2). Bottom half: stimulus time course(middle
trace) with vertical scale(upwards,10°R;downwards,10°L);
three superimposed(-,x,o) eye movement cycles under
condition 1)(upper trace) and condition 2)(lower trace).
Upper and lower trace were shifted on this graph relative
to middle trace. <u>Fig. 1B</u>. IR(t) of neuron(D5-1044) in
III.nerve nucleus in case 1(stim.movement centered around
10°L) and case 2(stim. movement centered around 10°R);
in both cases IR maximum is larger under condition 1).
Bottom half: common time course for stimulus and eye
movement in cases 1 and 2.

2) Light spot stationary, primate chair moves at $\delta=90^{\circ}$
on the slide track parallel to the screen. This condition
yields visual plus vestibular stimulation.
Since either visual or otolith input alone can lead to
eye movements, the oculomotor system must be able to
alter the neural weighting factor of these different
inputs if the stimulus condition changes from 1) which is
purely visual to 2) which is a superposition of visual
and otolith organ stimulation.
   Two trained monkeys were subjected to such stimuli
during single unit recordings. Fig. 1A and 1B compiles
data from two oculomotor motoneurons which demonstrate
two opposite kinds of significant dynamic differences in
the impulse rate IR(t) time course. The bottom half of
Fig. 1A gives the sinusoidal movement time course of the
stimulus(middle trace) at 0.3 Hz with the range of $\pm$ 10
degrees as indicated by the vertical scale. This stimulus
movement refers to both conditions:1)light spot movement
on the screen and 2)chair movement on the slide track.
Three superimposed full cycles of the corresponding
foveal pursuit eye movement of the right eye are drawn
above the stimulus trace for condition 1) and below for 2.
The eye movements(vertically shifted on this graph for
better visibility) are virtually identical. This is not
the case for the IR time courses of the abducens moto-
neuron(D7-1320) which are shown in the upper diagram.
The vertical dotted line marks the extreme right position
of the eye(10 deg.right) in order to study its phase lag
(Eckmiller,Mackeben,1978) relative to the IR maximum.
IR maximum and the difference between IR maximum and
minimum were significantly larger whereas the phase lead
was smaller under condition 2)(filled circles) than under
condition 1)(dashed line).
   Since identical eye movements were generated under
both conditions, one can expect the existence of other
motoneurons controlling other muscle fibers in the same
extraocular muscles, which change their neural control
contribution in the opposite manner. An example of such
a motoneuron is given in Fig. 1B. Since the movement time
courses of stimulus and eye were found to be identical
at 0.3 Hz(see:bottom half of Fig. 1A) only one common
time course is plotted in the bottom half. Another
parameter was added instead, namely the range of operation. In case 1, stimulus and eye were moving with an
amplitude of 10 degrees around the center position of
10 degrees left,and in case 2 around 10 degrees right.
The diagram above gives IR(t) of another motoneuron
(D5-1044) under both conditions for cases 1 and 2. This
neuron was recorded in the III.nerve nucleus and
presumably participated in the control of the right
medial rectus muscle. IR maximum and the difference
between IR maximum and minimum were always larger and the
phase lead was smaller under condition 1) than 2).
The occurrence of IR maximum is marked by arrows. It is
noteworthy that these significant dynamic differences
could be reproduced by repeatedly switching between
condition 1) and 2).

134

B. <u>Dependence of oculomotor neural activity on direction</u>
   <u>of acceleration</u>
In this study single unit activity was recorded in three
monkeys at levels of barbiturate anesthesia at which the
afferent visual system was functionally detached from the
oculomotor system and eye movements could only be
elicited by stepwise left and right turns of the chair.
The monkeys were subjected to sinusoidal linear
acceleration with an amplitude of 26.4 cm at 0.4 Hz. The
angle δ (see:Methods) was varied stepwise. The neurons
described here are assumed to represent oculomotor
motoneurons for several reasons.   While the monkey was
still awake, the recording site had been identified as
one of the oculomotor nuclei on the basis of neurophysiological and stereotaxic evidence.   When the monkey
performed slowly drifting eye movements under anesthesia,
these neurons increased their tonic IR with horizontal
eye movements of the expected eye(movements were recorded
for both eyes independently because they are often
decoupled during anesthesia) in the expected direction.
The following results were found: 1.The phase relationship between linear acceleration and IR(t) of abducens
motoneurons was similar to an α -otolith response
(Duensing, Schaefer,1959). Accordingly, motoneurons
recorded in the III.nerve nucleus always showed a phase
relationship similar to a β-otolith response. 2. The IR
modulation due to linear acceleration was maximal for
pure right-left movement(δ =90° or 270°) and minimal for
forward-backward movement(δ =0° or 180°).For different
neurons the optimal direction of the acceleration vector
(maximal IR modulation) varied slightly, ranging $\pm$20°
relative to pure right-left movement.

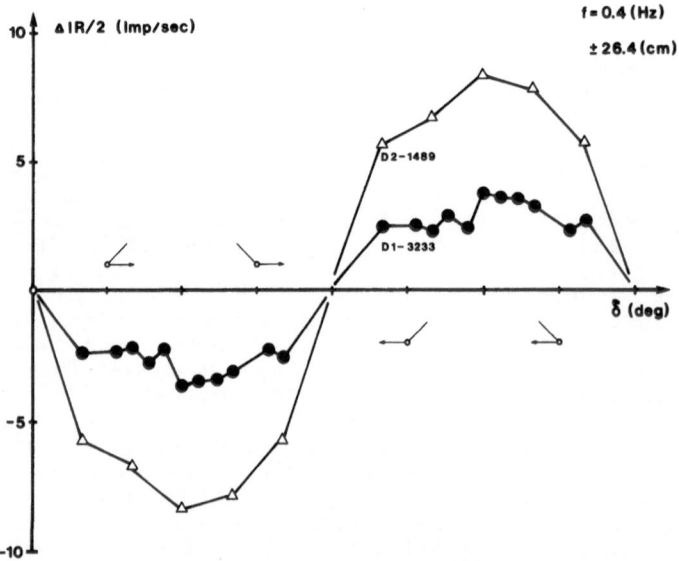

FIGURE 2. Directional characteristic of two motoneurons
during sinusoidal linear acceleration.

Typical examples of the directional characteristics are
shown in Fig. 2. Both motoneurons were located in the
right VI.nerve nucleus. The abscissa gives the angle δ
(direction of chair movement)which is also indicated by
four symbols(arrows:movement direction; circle and line:
chair center and monkey's X-axis). The ordinate(ΔIR/2
in impulses per second) represents the modulation
amplitude or maximal IR deviation(averaged over five
values from different cycles) from the tonic unmodulated
IR level(depending on eye position and level of anesthesia). This modulation amplitude did not appear to depend
on the tonic IR level for a given neuron, but was quite
different for different neurons as is demonstrated here.
Both motoneurons showed the largest IR increase for
δ=270°, which corresponds to a pure left movement.
Gradual changes of angle δ led to reductions of the
modulation amplitude. The phase lag of IR maximum
relative to acceleration(about -60 deg. for neuron D2-
1489; about -75 deg. for neuron D1-3233) did not change
significantly with angle δ.

C. Dependence of impulse rate on acceleration frequency

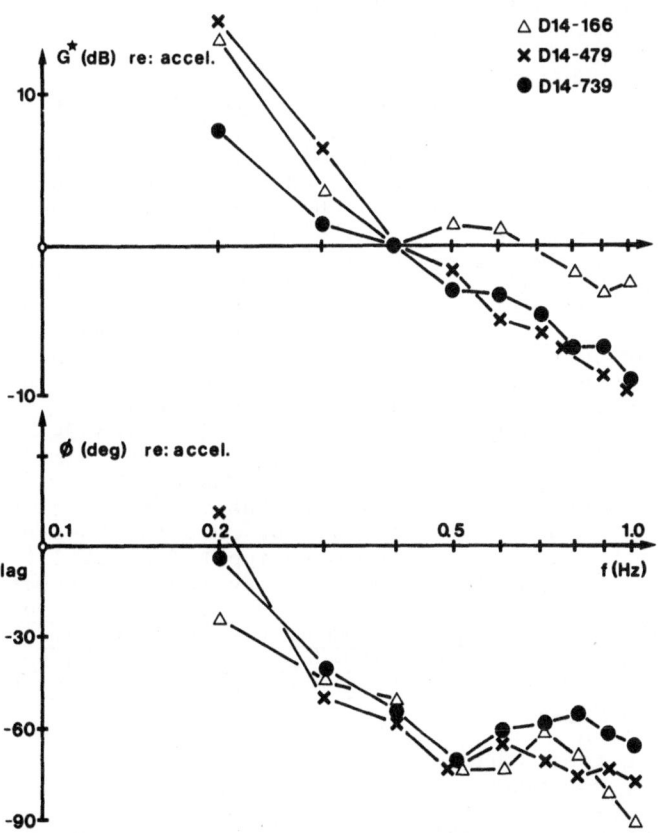

FIGURE 3. Bode plot for three motoneurons in the left
VI.nerve nucleus during sinusoidal linear acceleration.

Under the same conditions as in part B., the monkeys
were subjected to sinusoidal right-left movements(δ=90⁰).
The dynamic properties of the otolith-oculomotor pathway
were evaluated and analyzed as Bode plots in a frequency
range between 0.1 and 1.0 Hz. The movement amplitude was
maintained at a constant value of 26.4 cm for frequencies
up to 0.5 Hz, but had to be reduced at higher frequencies
because of power limitation of the slide track drive.
This should not influence the Bode plot of an approximately linear system. Fig. 3 gives such a Bode plot on a
common logarithmic frequency scale for three motoneurons
which were located in the left VI.nerve nucleus. The
gain G* in decibels was calculated on the basis of the
quotient of modulation amplitude(averaged over five
values from different cycles) and maximum stimulus
acceleration, and was arbitrarily set to 0 dB at 0.4 Hz.
The corresponding phase lag(averaged over five values)
between IR maximum and maximal linear acceleration to the
right is shown in the lower diagram. It is noteworthy
that the IR time course was about in phase with
acceleration for frequencies at or below 0.2 Hz, whereas
a phase lag of almost -90 degrees had developed at 1.0 Hz.
This clearly differs from the corresponding phase
spectrum of otolith afferents.

DISCUSSION AND CONCLUSIONS
These results demonstrate a significant modulation of
oculomotor motoneurons by linear acceleration in primates.
Although the otolith-ocular reflex in humans(and also in
monkeys) can easily be suppressed and shows a poor and
unreliable frequency response in the alert state(Barnes,
1980; Buizza et al.,1980), the data in chapter A. indicate an impact during visual-vestibular rivalry.
If the(phylogenetically youngest) foveal pursuit system
'wanted to be' dominant - after all, only the visual and
not the vestibular system can detect when the stimulus
is properly projected onto the fovea - it could inhibit
all the dynamic vestibular inputs to the motoneurons in
order to avoid difficulties(alteration of neural
weighting factors) with superimposed velocity signals
during joint stimulation of both visual and vestibular
receptors. In that case one would expect no dynamic
change in oculomotor neural activity when the stimulation
is changed from condition 1) to 2). Our results, however,
suggest that the older subsystem with input from otolith
organs is at least partly dominant during foveal pursuit.
Thus it is likely that the final 'common' pathway is, in
fact, subdivided into parts predominantly under visual
control and parts predominantly under vestibular control
and that the ultimate integration takes place only in the
extraocular muscles.
     The directional characteristic(Results, B.) shows for
the first time that oculomotor motoneurons controlling
horizontal eye movements receive maximal otolith input
during right-left acceleration and minimal input during
forward-backward acceleration. Assuming that a direct
utricular input to ipsilateral abducens motoneurons

(Schwindt et al.,1973) also exists in the monkey, <u>our</u>
<u>results can be taken as neurophysiological evidence for</u>
<u>the existence of a projection exclusively from the medial</u>
<u>region of the utricle to the ipsilateral VI.nerve nucleus</u>
(and to the contralateral medial rectus motoneurons).

The surprising feature of the frequency response
(Results, C.) which resembles data from the cat(Blanks et
al.,1978) very well, is the big increase in phase lag
with increasing frequency. Since otolith organs respond
closely in phase with acceleration in this frequency
range, this phase gap is puzzling(see also:Blanks et al.,
1978). <u>It is tempting to speculate that the increasing</u>
<u>phase lag is caused by the same neural mechanism in the</u>
<u>brain stem which transforms all neural control signals</u>
<u>for eye velocity into eye position.</u>

ACKNOWLEDGEMENTS
This research was supported by Grants Ec 43/5 and
SFB 200/A1 from the Deutsche Forschungsgemeinschaft.

REFERENCES
Barnes GR (1980) Vestibular control of oculomotor and
postural mechanisms, Clin.Physiol.Meas. 1, 3-40.

Blanks RHI, Anderson JH, and Precht W (1978) Response
characteristics of semicircular canal and otolith systems
in cat. II.Responses of trochlear motoneurons,
Exp. Brain Res. 32, 509-528.

Buizza A, Léger A, Droulez J, Berthoz A, and Schmid R
(1980) Influence of otolithic stimulation by horizontal
linear acceleration on optokinetic nystagmus and visual
motion perception, Exp. Brain Res. 39, 165-176.

Duensing F und Schaefer KP (1959) Über die Konvergenz
verschiedener labyrinthärer Afferenzen auf einzelne
Neurone des Vestibulariskerngebietes, Arch. Psychiat.
Nervenkr. 199, 345-371.

Eckmiller R and Mackeben M (1978) Pursuit eye movements
and their neural control in the monkey, Pflügers Arch.
377, 15-23.

Schwindt PC, Richter A, and Precht W (1973) Short latency
utricular and canal input to ipsilateral abducens
motoneurons, Brain Res. 60, 259-262.

Skavenski AA and Robinson DA (1973) Role of abducens
neurons in vestibuloocular reflex, J. Neurophysiol. 36,
724-738.

AN INTRACELLULAR HRP STUDY OF ABDUCENS MOTOR AND INTERNUCLEAR NEURONS IN THE ALERT SQUIRREL MONKEY

R.A. McCrea, A. Strassman and S.M. Highstein (Albert Einstein College of Medicine, Bronx, New York)

INTRODUCTION

Although the abducens nucleus has been extensively studied in the alert monkey (King et al., '76; Pola, Robinson, '78) and cat (Delgado-Garcia et al., '77, '83 in preparation) with extracellular recording, further investigation with techniques that allow single cell structure-function correlation (McCrea et al., '80) is of interest. We have chosen the squirrel monkey, Saimiri sciurius, as our experimental animal because it offers several distinct advantages over the cat or rhesus. It is a foveate, frontal-eyed primate with eye movements similar in several respects to man (Paige, '82). More importantly, squirrel monkeys are small in size and have a small brain stem (in comparison to the cat) which allows horseradish peroxidase intracellularly injected at one point to diffuse more completely throughout a given neuron. Experiments were performed in alert squirrel monkeys utilizing intra-axonal recording and staining with glass microelectrodes filled with horseradish peroxidase. The following is a report on the morphology and physiology of two broad classes of cells within the abducens nucleus, namely abducens motoneurons and internuclear neurons (Baker, Highstein, '75; Graybiel, Hartweig, '74).

METHODS

Twelve male squirrel monkeys, 600-800 gm, were implanted with a bolt on the occiput for head stabilization (Paige, '82) and a scleral search coil to measure eye movements (Robinson, '63). A plug of parietal cortex was removed to expose the cerebellar tentorium, and a small, cone-shaped chamber implanted. When the animals recovered from surgery they were trained to sit in a primate chair. Glass microelectrodes were backfilled with a 10% solution of horseradish peroxidase in 0.5M KCL, 0.05M tris buffer ph 7.2 (Highstein et al., '82); and advanced through the cerebellum to the brain stem. When an axon was penetrated, its discharge rate in relation to eye movements was recorded and horseradish peroxidase injected with depolarizing pulses of 10-20nA (total currents 1200-2400nA min). Animals survived for 24-30 hours when they were deeply anesthetized with pentabarbital and perfused through the heart with heparinized saline followed by fixative (Graham, Karnovsky, '66). Frozen sections were cut and reacted with diaminobenzidine to visualize the peroxidase reaction product (Cullheim, Kellereth, '76; Jankowska et al., '76). Neuronal morphology was analyzed, and axons reconstructed with the aid of a light microscope and a drawing tube (Zeiss).

RESULTS

Twelve internuclear neurons and four abducens motoneurons have been injected. Figure 1 shows the activity of an

Roucoux, A. and Crommelinck, M. (eds.): Physiological and Pathological Aspects of Eye Movements.
© 1982, Dr W. Junk Publishers, The Hague, Boston, London. ISBN-13: 978-94-009-8002-0

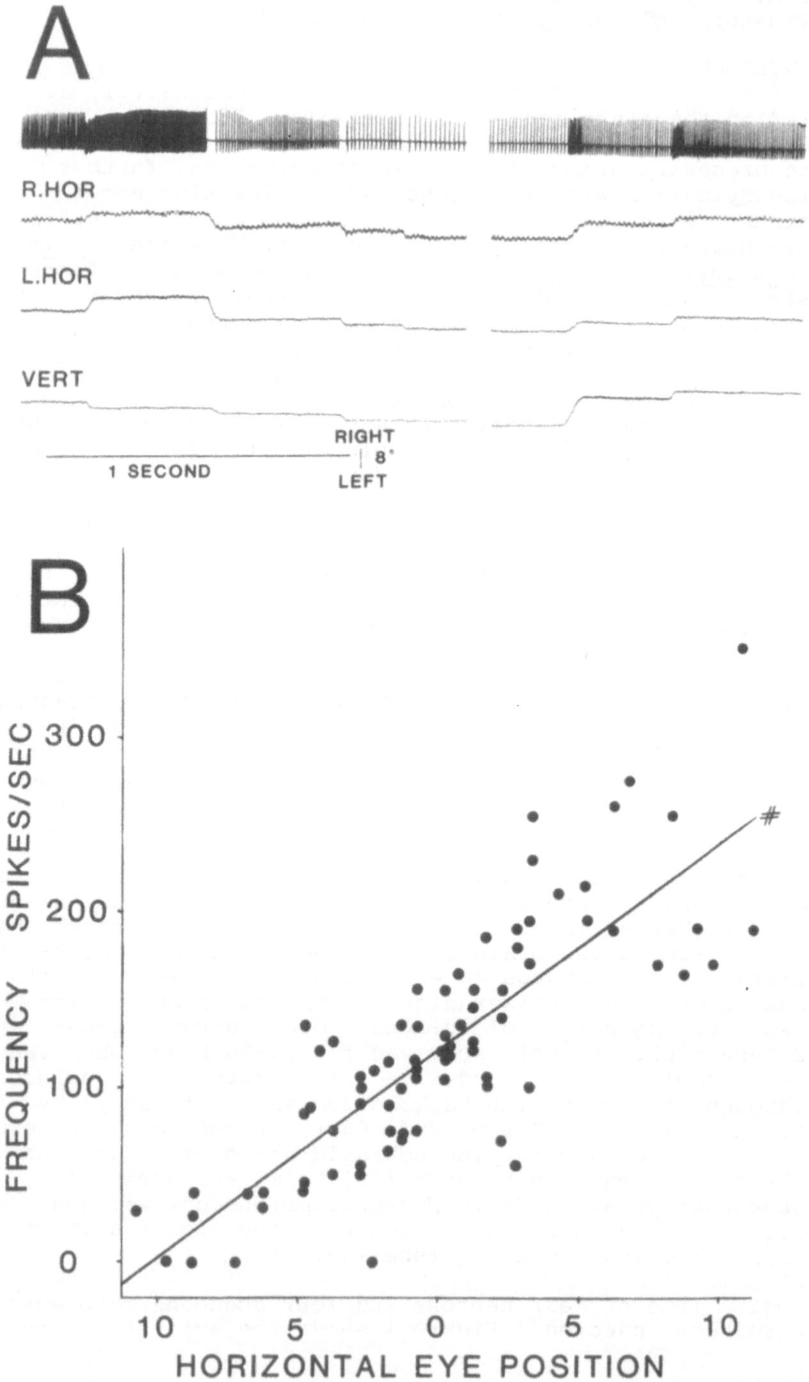

140

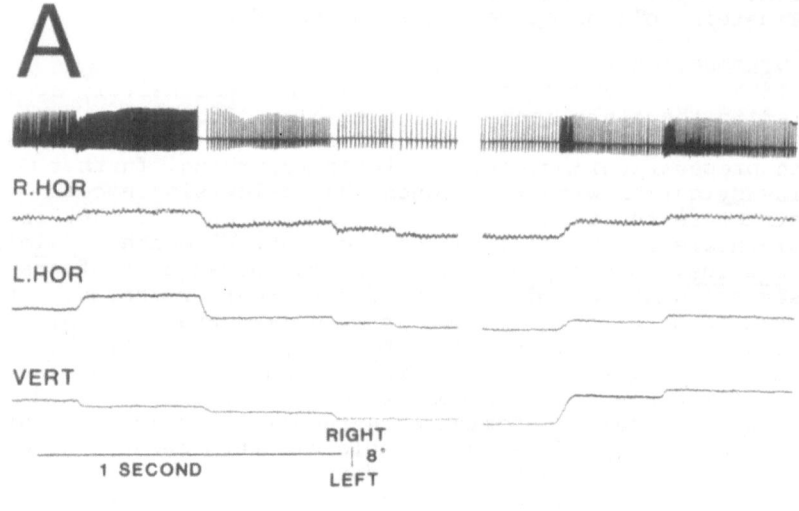

A

R.HOR

L.HOR

VERT

1 SECOND   RIGHT
                8°
                LEFT

B

FREQUENCY SPIKES/SEC

300

200

100

0

10   5   0   5   10

HORIZONTAL EYE POSITION

FIGURE 1. A) Activity of an abducens motoneuron recorded in the alert squirrel monkey. B) Rate-position plot for another abducens motoneuron. The (#) upper right indicates that right-left eye movements have been transposed.

identified motoneuron. As previously reported (Robinson, '70) the activity is burst tonic with an ipsilateral on-direction (defined by horizontal eye movements to the ipsilateral side). During periods of steady fixation, the firing frequency of motoneurons was linearly related to eye position. Figure 1 shows the spike frequency-eye position relationship for one motoneuron. The K value or slope of the plot is 11.8 and the correlation coefficient for the line is 0.84. K values of motoneurons ranged from 10-14.5. Internuclear neurons also have burst-tonic discharges as previously reported (Delgado-Garcia et al., '77), with on-directions identical to ipsilateral abducens motoneurons but defined by the pulling direction of the contralateral medial rectus extra-ocular muscle. An analysis similar to motoneurons indicated higher K values on average than the motoneurons ranging from 7-24. Both classes of cells fired a burst of action potentials before and during on-direction rapid eye movements and paused or decreased their activity for off-direction saccades or quick phases of nystagmus. Quantitative analysis in this report will be limited to rate-position data, but during a given saccade or quick phase the intrasaccadic burst frequency appeared to be slightly higher in internuclear neurons than that in motoneurons.

Motoneuron and internuclear neuron somas were distributed throughout the squirrel monkey abducens nucleus, similar to other species studied (Steiger, Buttner-Ennever, '75; Glicksman, '80), and overlapped in size. In many cases intra-axonal injection of HRP within several mm of a neuronal soma resulted in a diffusely filled motor or internuclear soma and dendritic tree. This allowed comparison of the soma-dendritic morphology of both types of cell, as well as allowing comparisons with the previously analyzed data on cat abducens motor and internuclear neurons. In the cat, roughly 5% of the motoneuron and internuclear neuron dendrites ramified outside the cellular borders of the abducens nucleus (Highstein et al., '82). However, the dendrites of both abducens motor and internuclear neurons are completely contained within the cellular borders of the squirrel monkey abducens nucleus. Similar to the cat, the dendritic territories of both classes of cells are completely overlapping within the nucleus. Figures 2A and B are reconstructions of a squirrel monkey abducens motoneuron and internuclear neuron, respectively, and figures 3A and B show examples of a feline motoneuron and internuclear neuron. In both species, abducens motoneuron primary dendrites typically branched soon after their origin from the soma and continued to branch as they

142

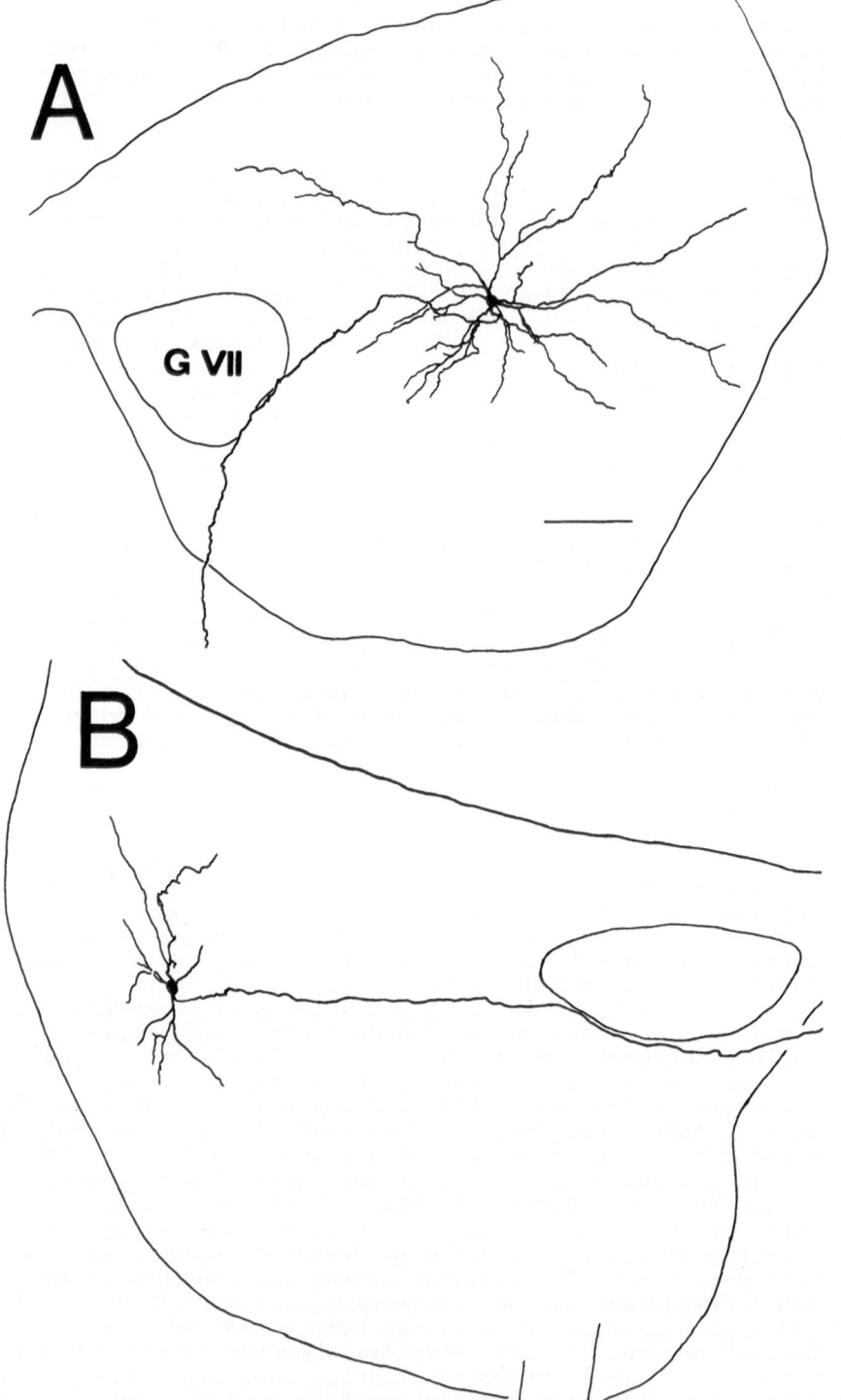

143

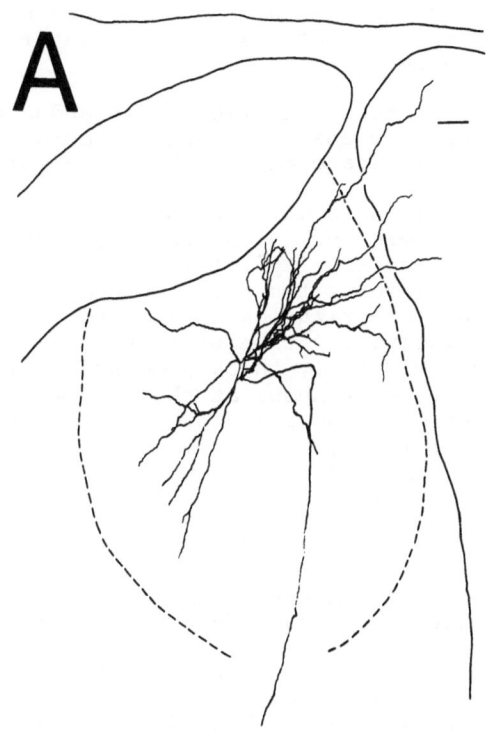

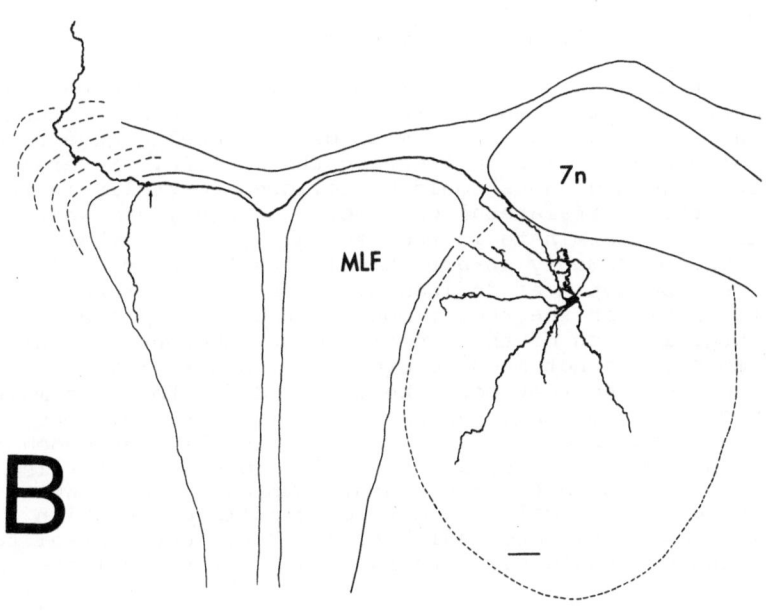

FIGURE 2. Coronal reconstruction of a squirrel monkey abducens motoneuron A) and an abducens internuclear neuron B) that were injected with HRP. 7n, facial nerve. Calibration: 100μm.

FIGURE 3. Coronal reconstruction of an abducens moto- neuron A) and an abducens internuclear neuron B) from the cat. Arrows indicate axons. GVII, facial nerve.

traveled away from the soma. In contrast, internuclear neuron dendrites were typically sparsely branched and traveled long distances with little tapering or branch- ing. Motoneuronal dendrites usually become rather fine in their terminal arborization while internuclear den- drites being relatively untapered continue to their terminations as relatively thick processes. The photo- micrographs in figure 4 show, at the same magnification, a large cat motoneuron soma and proximal dendrites (4A), and a typical cat internuclear soma and proximal den- drites (4B). Examples of dorsal motoneuron dendrites and ventral internuclear dendrites are shown in 4C and 4D. Although the motoneuron dendrites are processes of a large cell (soma diameter 77μm x 18μm), the distal dendrites of the internuclear cell (soma diameter 60μm x 9μm) shown in 4D are comparable in thickness to some of the more proximal motoneuron dendrites illustrated in 4A.

Axons of abducens motoneurons originated from axon hil- locks directed toward all parts of the nucleus, and coursed ventrally within a few hundred microns of their origin to form the abducens nerve. There were no collat- erals of abducens motoneuron axons within the nucleus in either squirrel monkey or cat. One of the four injected squirrel monkey motoneurons had an axon collateral with a small terminal field confined to the territory of the abducens nerve 1.5mm below the nucleus.

All of the injected squirrel monkey internuclear neurons gave rise to axons which crossed the midline and ascended in the contralateral MLF. None of these cells gave rise to collaterals prior to crossing the midline. Several of the injected axons could be followed rostrally in the MLF to the contralateral oculomotor nucleus, and were observed to terminate in the ventral aspect of that nucleus; presumably an area homologous to the medial rectus subgroup A as defined by Buttner-Ennever and Akert (1981) in the rhesus monkey (the precise location and organization of the medial rectus subgroup in squir- rel monkey has not been determined). Squirrel monkey internuclear neurons could be subdivided into three main groups, based on their axonal branching pattern. One group of internuclear neurons had axons which ascended in the contralateral MLF, and gave rise to no collaterals prior to reaching the oculomotor complex. The axons of a second groups of cells gave rise to collaterals which terminated within and medial to the MLF, just rostral to the abducens nucleus. A third group of internuclear

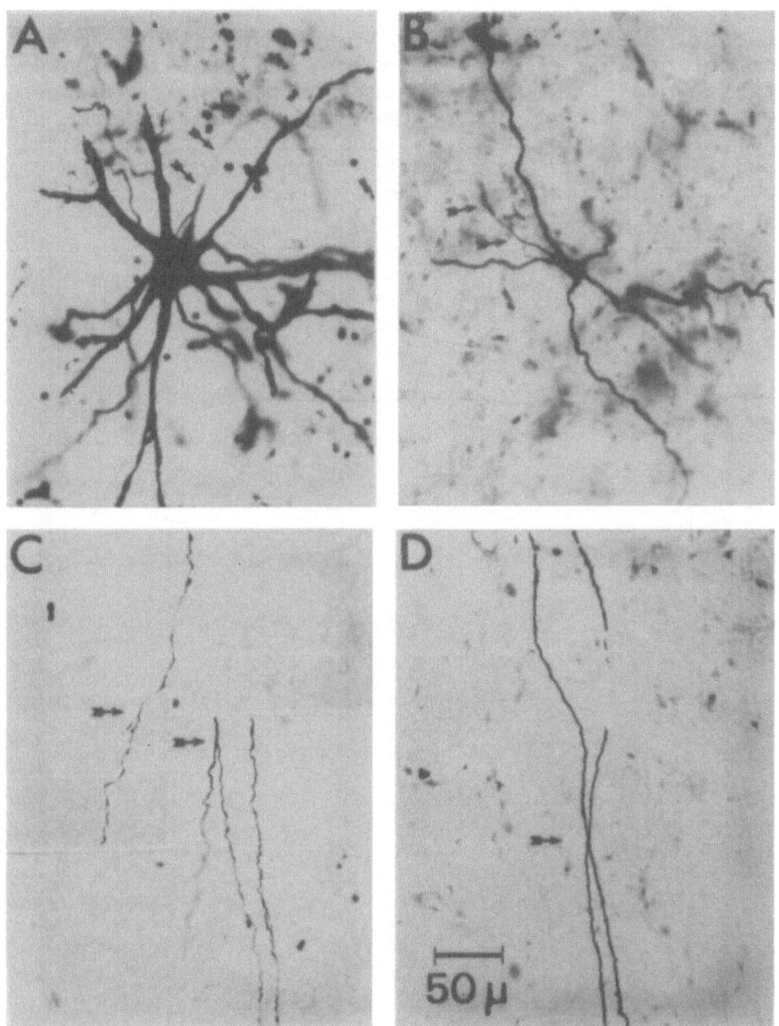

FIGURE 4. Photomicrographs of an abducens motoneuron
soma and proximal dendrites A), an internuclear neuron
soma and dendrites B), motoneuron dendrites C), and
internuclear dendrites D). Dendrites illustrated in C)
are dorsal dendrites of the motoneuron illustrated in 2A.
The upper left arrow in C) indicates a point 1200μm from
the cell soma and the lower right arrow a point 700μm
from the soma.

The point where
the dendrites cross in D) (arrow) is 700μm below the soma
of the cell. This figure is included for a direct comparison of motoneuron and internuclear neuron dendrites.

neurons had small somas, and axons which bifurcated immediately after crossing the midline. The thicker of
the two branches ascended in the contralateral MLF to the
oculomotor nucleus, giving rise to a collateral which
terminated near the midline, just rostral to the abducens
nucleus. The thinner branch descended in the contralateral MLF, and terminated within and around the caudal
MLF and in the dorsal part of the raphe caudal to the
abducens nucleus. Figure 5 shows a reconstruction of

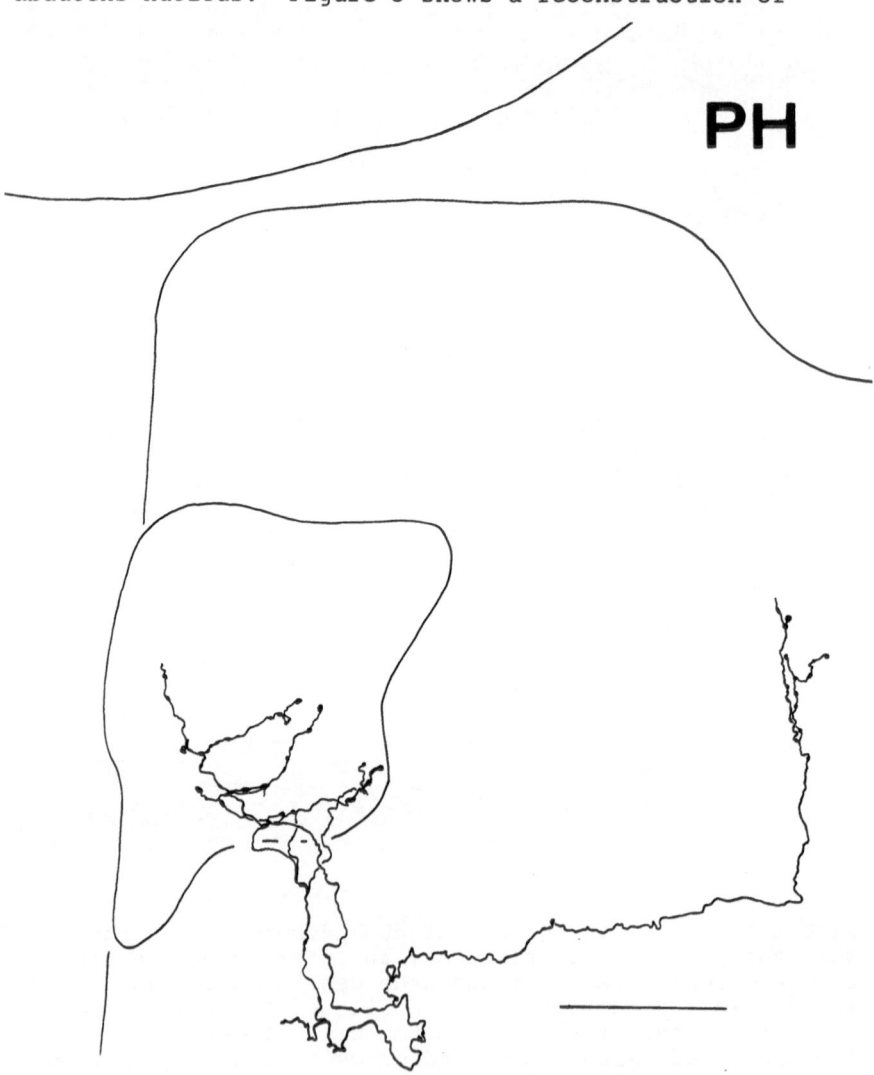

PH

Figure 5. Reconstruction of part of the terminal
arborization of the caudal collateral of an internuclear
neuron. PH: nucleus prepositus. Calibration: 100μm.

part of the caudal terminal arborization of one of this third group of cells. No terminations within the contralateral prepositus nucleus were found. Figure 6 summarizes schematically the branching pattern of each groups of internuclear neurons.

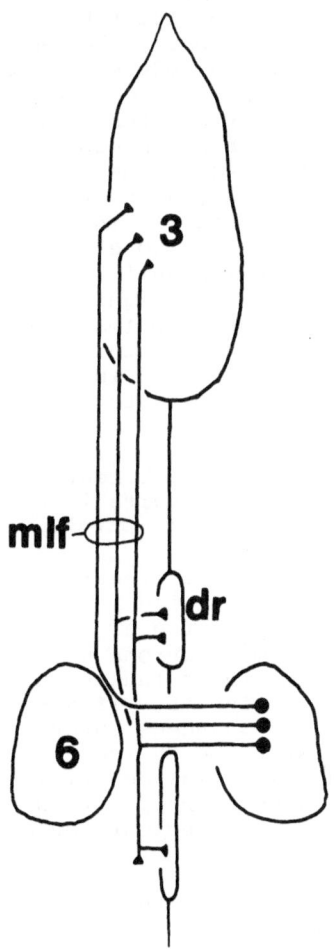

FIGURE 6. Summary diagram of axonal collateralization of squirrel monkey internuclear neurons. Three patterns of arborization were found. One group of cells projected to the oculomotor nucleus (3) without collaterals. The other two groups of cells gave rise to collaterals which terminated in the raphe rostral to abducens (6); a third group of internuclear neurons gave rise to caudally projecting collaterals which terminated near the midline caudal to 6. dr, caudal dorsal raphe n.

DISCUSSION

In similarity to the cat, the squirrel monkey abducens contains both abducens motoneurons and internuclear neurons. All of the injected internuclear neurons were confined within the boundaries at the abducens nucleus, suggesting that the origin of the internuclear pathway in primate originates exclusively from cells within the abducens nucleus. One interesting difference between the cat and primate abducens nuclei is the qualitative difference in the dendritic domain of the constituent neurons. In the cat, the abducens nucleus is an "open" nucleus; i.e., the dendrites of most of the neurons in that nucleus extend beyond the cellular boundaries. On the other hand, the primate abducens nucleus appears to be a "closed" nucleus; i.e., regardless of the position or size of the soma of an abducens neuron, its dendrites arborized completely within the cellular boundaries of the nucleus. This reflects, in part, the fact that the dendritic domain of the primate abducens neurons is considerably smaller (less than 1/2) that of the cat. One obvious consequence of this is that afferents to abducens motoneurons and internuclear neurons must terminate within the cellular boundaries of the abducens nucleus in the primate, while in the cat, axons terminating in the periabducens region but not within the boundaries of the abducens nucleus could also contact abducens neurons. While the functional significance of this observation is obscure, the practical significance is clear. The fact that afferent axons to primate abducens neurons must terminate within the boundaries of the abducens nucleus will be an important aid in determining the origin of abducens afferents if future studies.

Primate abducens motoneurons and internuclear neurons are qualitatively similar to their counterparts in the cat, both in respect to their physiological activity during spontaneous eye movements and in respect to the pattern of arborization of their dendritic trees; observations which are probably not unrelated. The smaller, less highly branched dendritic tree of internuclear neurons compared to that of motoneurons would tend to contribute to a higher total input independence and greater responsiveness to phasic inputs. If afferents are similarly distributed to abducens internuclear and motoneurons, as appears to be the case (Spencer, Sterling, '77), this differential dendritic morphology could account for the higher eye position and velocity coefficients reported for internuclear neurons in cats (Delgado-Garcia et al., '77).

The results of our experiments demonstrate that some primate abducens motoneurons give rise to terminal collaterals within the brainstem. Intracranial collaterals of abducens motoneurons have never been observed in the cat, in spite of the fact that dozens have been injected with HRP in various laboratories (see Baker et al., '81). Since only four motoneurons were injected in this study, and only one of these gave rise to a collateral, it is impossible to estimate what proportion of primate abducens motoneurons give rise to collaterals, although it is probable that most do not. The significance of the single observed collateral termination within the rootlets of the abducens nerve is obscure and requires ultrastructural analysis before the postsynaptic targets can be ascertained.

A majority of the abducens internuclear neurons in the primate appear to project not only to the oculomotor nucleus but also to other brainstem regions. An important target for internuclear neuron collateral termination appears to be cell groups lying ventromedial to the MLF in the midline raphe, both rostral and caudal to the abducens nucleus, and at the level of the abducens nuclei. Although we do not know what cells these collaterals contact, it is interesting to note that many premotor vestibular neurons also terminate in this region in the squirrel monkey (unpublished observations). In the cat, many of the cells in the rostral part of this region (the caudal part of the dorsal raphe nucleus) appears to project to the flocculus and are active during the slow phase of vestibular nystagmus (Nakao et al., '80).

In summary, the morphological and physiological characteristics of abducens motoneurons and internuclear neurons in the squirrel monkey are similar in may ways to those previously described in the cat. On the other hand, the eye position sensitivity of squirrel monkey abducens neurons appears to be higher than in the cat, and the dendritic domain of squirrel monkey abducens neurons is more restricted. Also in contrast to the cat, some squirrel monkey motoneurons appear to give rise to intracranial collaterals. Finally, we have found that many squirrel monkey internuclear neurons not only project to the oculomotor complex, but also to regions near the MLF, primarily the raphe nuclei, rostral, caudal and between the abducens nuclei.

REFERENCES
1. Baker R, Evinger C, and McCrea RA (1981) Some thoughts about the three neurons in the vestibular ocular reflex, NY Acad. Sci. 374, 171-188.
2. Baker R and Highstein SM (1975) Physiological identification of interneurons and motoneurons in the abducens nucleus, Brain Res. 83, 292-298.
3. Buttner-Ennever JS (1981) Anatomy of medial rectus subgroups in the oculomotor nucleus of the monkey. In Fuchs and Becker, eds. Progress in Oculomotor Research, pp. 247-252. New York/Amsterdam, Elsevier/North-Holland Biomedical Press.
4. Buttner-Ennever JA and Akert K (1981) Medial rectus subgroups of the oculomotor nucleus and their abducens internuclear input in the monkey, J. Comp. Neurol. 197, 17-27.
5. Delgado-Garcia J, Baker R, and Highstein SM (1977) The activity of internuclear neurons identified within the abducens nucleus of the alert cat. In Baker and Berthoz, eds. Control of Gaze by Brain Stem Neurons, pp. 219-300. New York/Amsterdam, Elsevier/North-Holland Biomedical Press.
6. Fuchs AF and Robinson DS (1966) A method for measuring horizontal and vertical eye movement chronically in the monkey, J. Appl. Physiol. 21, 1068-1070.

150

7. Glicksman MA (1980) Localization of motoneurons controlling the extra-ocular muscles of the rat, Brain
Res. 188, 53-62.
8. Graham RC and Karnovsky MJ (1966) The early stages
of absorption of injected horseradish peroxidase in
the proximal tubules of mouse kidney: ultrastructural
cytochemistry by a new technique, J. Histochem.
Cytochem. 14, 291-302.
9. Graybiel AM and Hartwieg EA (1974) Some afferent
connections of the oculomotor complex in the cat:
an experimental study with tracer techniques, Brain
Res. 81, 543-551.
10. Highstein SM, Karabelas A, Baker R, and McCrea RA
(1982) Comparison of the morphology of physiologically identified abducens motor and internuclear
neurons in the cat. A light microscopic study
employing the intracellular injection of horseradish
peroxidase, J. Comp. Neurol., in press.
11. Hikosaka O and Kawakami T (1977) Inhibitory reticular neurons related to the quick phase of vestibular
nystagmus. Their location and projection, Exp. Brain
Res. 27, 377-396.
12. Jankowska E, Rastad J, and Westman J (1976) Intracellular application of horseradish peroxidase and
its light and electron microscopical appearance in
spinocervical tract cells, Brain Res. 105, 557-562.
13. King WM, Lisberger SG, Fuchs AF (1976) Responses of
fibers in medial longitudinal fasciculus (MLF) of
alert monkeys during horizontal and vertical conjugate eye movements evoked by vestibular or visual
stimuli, J. Neurophysiol. 39, 1135-1149.
14. McCrea RA, Yoshida K, Berthoz A, and Baker R (1980)
Eye movement related activity and morphology of
second order vestibular neurons terminating in the
cat abducens nucleus, Exp. Brain Res. 40, 468-473.
15. Nakao S, Curthoys IS, and Markhan CH (1980) Eye
movement related neurons in the cat pontine reticular formation related to the quick phase of
vestibular nystagmus, Brain Res. 182-451-456.
16. Paige GD (1982) The vestibulo ocular reflex and its
interactions with visual following mechanisms in the
squirrel monkey. I. Response characteristics in normal animals, J. Neurophysiol., in press.
17. Pola J and Robinson DA (1978) Oculomotor signals in
medial longitudinal fasciculus of the monkey, J.
Neurophysiol. 41, 245-259.
18. Robinson DA (1970) Oculomotor unit behavior in the
monkey, J. Neurophysiol. 33, 393-404.
19. Robinson DA (1963) A method of measuring eye movement using a scleral search coil in a magnetic field,
IEEE Transactions on Bio-Medical Electronics, Volume
BME-10, Number 4, pp. 137-145.
20. Skavenski AA and Robinson DA (1973) Role of abducens
neurons in vestibulo-ocular reflex, J. Neurophysiol.
36, 724-738.
21. Spencer RF and Sterling P (1977) An electron microscope study of motoneurons and interneurons in the

cat abducens nucleus identified by retrograde intra-axonal transport of horseradish peroxidase, J. Comp. Neurol. 176, 65-86.

22. Steiger HJ and Buttner-Ennever JA (1975) Oculomotor nucleus afferents in the monkey demonstrated with horseradish peroxidase, Brain Res. 160, 1-15.

ANATOMY AND PHYSIOLOGY OF THE OPTOKINETIC PATHWAYS TO THE VESTIBULAR NUCLEI IN THE RAT

W. PRECHT*, L. CAZIN**, R. BLANKS, J. LANNOU**
*Institut für Hirnforschung, Universität Zürich;
**Laboratoire de Neurophysiologie, Université de
Rouen, and Dept. of Anatomy, Univ. of California,
Irvine

1. INTRODUCTION

Neurons in the vestibular nuclei (Vn) have been shown in
a variety of species to respond not only to vestibular
but also to pure optokinetic stimuli, i.e. rotation of
large visual patterns (cf. ref. Precht, 1981). Vestibular
and optokinetic inputs are synergistic and expand the
working range of Vn (Keller, Precht, 1979). In this context, the vestibular nuclei may be considered as an important premotor structure having direct and indirect
access to ocular and spinal motoneurons. At the behavioral level the importance of the transvestibular optokinetic path is stressed by the findings that optokinetic
nystagmus (OKN) and afternystagmus (OKAN) are severely
affected by bilateral (Cohen et al.,1973) and unilateral
(Maioli et al.,1982) labyrinthectomies for long periods
of time. More specifically, the transvestibular path has
been considered part of the velocity storage mechanism or
indirect path which, after the initial fast rise (direct
path), provides the additional slower rise of OKN slow
phase velocity to steady state values during prolonged
stimulation (Cohen, et al. 1977). The relative contribution of the indirect pathway varies among species, being
large in cat (Keller, Precht, 1979; Maioli et al.,1982),
moderate in man and monkey (Cohen, et al. 1977) and virtually absent in frog (Dieringer, Precht, 1982). The purpose of the present paper is to review the functional and
morphological organisation of the transvestibular optokinetic pathway and to describe the optokinetic and vestibular response properties of single units located in
various nuclei along the pathway. Since the most complete
study of this kind has been performed in the rat horizontal optokinetic path, the paper will focus on this work.
Comparative aspects have been reviewed elsewhere (Precht,
1981; Precht, 1982). Those parts of our work that have
already been published will be reviewed only briefly and
emphasis will be on unpublished material.

Supported by *grants nos. 3.505.79 and *3.616.80 from the
Swiss National Science Foundation and the *Dr. Eric Slack-
Gyr Foundation; USPHA no. EY 03018, RCDA EY 00016 from NEJ
and NATO grant (1918)/1047(79)AG

Roucoux, A. and Crommelinck, M. (eds.): Physiological and Pathological Aspects of Eye Movements.
© *1982, Dr W. Junk Publishers, The Hague, Boston, London.* ISBN-13: 978-94-009-8002-0

2. PROCEDURE

Details have been published elsewhere (physiology:Cazin et al., 1980a,b,c; anatomy: Blanks et al., 1982). Of relevance in this context is that all single unit studies employing natural stimulations have been performed in paralyzed, unanesthetized DA-HAN pigmented rats prepared under ether anesthesia for chronic recording. Electro-physiological experiments were done under Nembutal (30 mg/kg) or chloral hydrate (35%, 0.1 ml/100 g.b.w.). Pure vestibular stimulation was achieved by applying horizontal angular accelerations with a Toennies turn-table in the dark; it served to identify the units as type I or type II neurons of the horizontal canal system. Pure optokinetic stimuli (velocity steps of 0.2-60°/sec) were produced by a Toennies shadow projector generating a stripe pattern on a cylinder surrounding the animal. Recording-, lesion- and stimulating sites were identified in serial sections stained with the Nissl technique. The signal from the glas microelectrode was amplified by conventional electronics, displayed on an oscilloscope, and played over an audiomonitor. The same signal, after amplitude discrimination with a window detector, was converted to instantaneous frequency and smoothed with a first-order filter and displayed on a brush recorder together with table position or pattern velocity. In the electrophysiological study intracellulary recorded PSPs and extracellulary recorded spikes were fotographed on film and/or averaged by a Nicolet computer for latency measurements. Horizontal eye movements in response to vestibular or optokinetic stimuli were recorded with EOG electrodes placed on the outer canthi of both eyes.

3. RESULTS AND DISCUSSION

3.1. Horizontal OKN

In the pigmented rat full-field optokinetic stimulation evoked symmetrical OKN only when both eyes were open; in monocular condition a vigorous OKN was evoked on temporo-nasal stimulus direction only, whereas nasotemporal stimuli generated no detectable OKN within our experi-mental situation (Cazin et al., 1980b). By contrast, bidirectional responses were evoked in cats under mono-cular conditions (Montarolo et al., 1981). It is of interest to note that in albino rats even binocular sti-muli failed to generate OKN (Precht, Cazin, 1979).Visual-vestibular interactions in the VOR occurred readily in pigmented rats but were strongly deficient in the albino strain (Lannou et al., 1982).

3.2. Responses of Vn to optokinetic stimuli

Nearly all horizontal type I and type II Vn responded to optokinetic stimulation in a direction-selective,velocity-related manner (Cazin et al., 1980a) and these responses were synergistic with the responses to pure vestibular stimuli. With both eyes open, type I (type II) neurons increased (decreased) firing on optokinetic stimulation

BOTH EYES OPEN

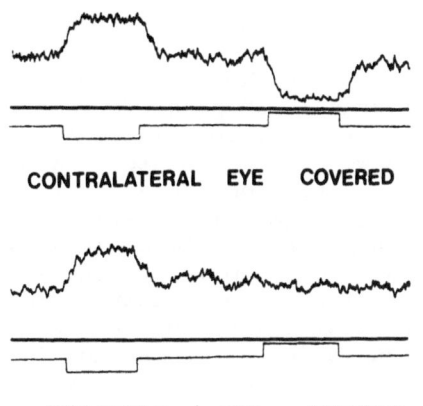

CONTRALATERAL EYE COVERED

IPSILATERAL EYE COVERED

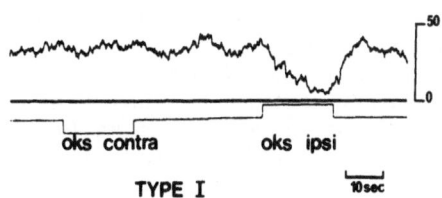

oks contra   oks ipsi

TYPE I   10sec

FIGURE 1
Optokinetic responses
of type I Vn. Upper,
middle and lower traces
in each record give
smoothed instantaneous
frequency, zero dis-
charge level and stimu-
lus velocity (1°/s).
Rat immobilized.

directed away from the recording side and decreased
(increased) firing on stimulation towards the recording
side (Fig.1, Table 1). Covering one eye, abolished the
decrease in firing of type II and excitation of type I
on the ipsilateral side and removed type II excitation
and type I inhibition on the opposite side (Fig.1,
Table 1). Note that this lack of responses of Vn to
nasotemporally directed stimuli in monocular condition
were paralleled by the absence of OKN in this direction.
Parenthetically it should be added that in albino rats
Vn did not respond to optokinetic stimulation, nor was
there any OKN (see 3.1) evoked.
The time course of Vn responses to velocity steps of
surround motion was characterized by a slow rise or fall
in firing (apparent incremental time constants of type I
and type II Vn responses were 5.4 + 2.6 s and 3.0 $\pm$ 1.7 s)
indicating significant central processing of the input
signal (see below). As shown in Fig.2 peak responses of
Vn occurred at retinal slip velocities of ca. 1°/s.

3.3. <u>Effects of central lesions on Vn responses</u>
The first experimental step in defining the optokinetic
pathways to the Vn was to place lesions in various nuclei
and fiber tracts and to compare Vn responses in these

lesioned animals with those of controls (Cazin et al., 1980b).

3.3.1. Lesions in the pretectum. Previous work in the rabbit (Collewijn, 1975a,b) suggested that the pretectum particularly the n. of the optic tract (NOT) was the first central relay in the horizontal OKN path. To test the importance of the pretectum (Pt) for optokinetic responses of Vn and OKN in rats we placed unilateral and bilateral lesions in this area and recorded Vn activity and OKN thereafter. Bilateral lesions abolished OKN and all optokinetic Vn responses, and with unilateral lesions Vn responses to binocular stimuli were similar to those of control animals to monocular stimulation (Cazin et al., 1980b). In addition, monocular viewing with the ipsilateral eye gave no responses of Vn in these rats suggesting that uncrossed retino-pretectal fibers cannot drive Vn and that all effects are produced by crossed fibers originating in the eye ipsilateral to the lesion. The optokinetic tuning curves of Vn responses in the lesioned animals were comparable to those of controls indicating that no effective crossing between the bilateral pretecta occurred in control animals via crossed connections (see 3.6.1). Midbrain reticular lesions ventral to the Pt had very similar effects on optokinetic Vn responses as Pt lesions suggesting fiber passage or further relays in this area.

3.3.2. Lesions of the n.reticularis tegmenti pontis (NRTP) Since no direct fibers are known to connect Pt and Vn, optokinetic effects recorded in Vn must be relayed by at least one other structure. We found that unilateral and bilateral lesions in the NRTP had effects on OKN and Vn responses to optokinetic stimuli very similar to those described for Pt lesions (Cazin et al., 1980b). Whether the effects were due to lesions of NRTP neurons or fibers passing through the area or both cannot be decided on the basis of lesion work. Anatomical and recording studies are needed; they will be described below.

3.3.3. Lesion of the vestibular commissure. As shown in Table 1, monocular stimulation leads to an increase in type II and a decrease in type I Vn firing in the contralateral vestibular nuclei and the reverse response pattern is noted ipsilaterally. Following midsagittal section of the vestibular commissure, Vn on the side ipsilateral to the eye stimulated no longer responded, whereas contralaterally, Vn responses remained as described above. This finding indicates that no effective transfer of optokinetic signals occurs rostral to Vn, and that in the rat, the bilateral mirror image responses of Vn are mediated by the commissure. It also explains why in the binocular condition a given Vn responds with an increase in one and decrease in the other stimulus direction.

3.3.4. <u>Other lesions</u>. Lesions of descending tracts such as the tectospinal tract, medial longitudinal fascicle and central tegmental tracts had no appreciable effects on Vn responses to optokinetic stimuli. Likewise, removal of the bilateral visual cortices or large lesions of the superior colliculi, total removal of the cerebellum and lesions of the inferior olive did not abolish these responses. This is not to imply that these lesions may not affect at all Vn responses but with the criteria used in our study we could not detect any significant changes (Cazin et al., 1980b).

To summarize the results obtained from the lesion studies it appears that Pt, midbrainreticular and NRTP lesions as well as sections of the vestibular commissure were effective in impairing Vn responses to optokinetic stimuli as well as OKN. However, the only tentative conclusions that can be drawn from this lesion work is that - as in other mammals - the Pt serves as a primary relay in the horizontal optokinetic path and that the commissure is of importance. The other results merely serve as a useful guideline for anatomical and physiological work to be described below.

3.4. <u>Unit responses in optokinetic relay nuclei</u>
In this section the response characteristics to optokinetic stimulation of various possible relay neurons will be described and compared to those of Vn obtained under identical conditions. Furthermore, in each group of neurons responses to pure vestibular stimuli, i.e. horizontal rotation in the dark were studied in order to determine where along the path visual-vestibular interaction occurs first.

3.4.1. <u>Responses of pretectal neurons</u>. Table 1 summarizes some of the various optokinetic response types obtained in the Pt (Cazin et al., 1980c). Of particular interest is the fact that the majority (48%) of the units responding to optokinetic stimuli were excited by temporonasal stimuli presented to the contralateral eye; other stimuli showed no effects. This response pattern is compatible with the unidirectional OKN obtained with monocular stimulation (see 3.1) and suggests that these neurons may represent the prime candidates for horizontal optokinetic relay cells. A closer look at the time course of a typical response of one of these unidirectional Pt neurons to optokinetic velocity steps shows a fast rise and fall in firing after the beginning or end of the stimulus, i.e. they show a step response to a step input (Fig.3). The mean velocity tuning curve of the Pt neurons is very similar to those of Vn (Fig.2). Finally, Pt neurons never responded to rotation of the table in the dark, i.e. no visual-vestibular convergence was noted. Taken together our findings strongly suggest that the unidirectional

158

group of Pt neurons are central sensory relay neurons coding primarily direction and magnitude of retinal slip velocity.

3.4.2. Responses of NRTP neurons. Guided by our lesion studies we recorded from neurons in the NRTP during optokinetic stimuli. As in the Pt, the largest group of neurons showed responses to temporonasal stimuli of the contralateral eye only (Table 1, Fig.4) and had velocity tuning curves similar to those of Pt and Vn (Fig.2) suggesting that they belonged to the same system. Compared to unidirectional Pt units two significant differences were noted in NRTP units: 1) the mean apparent time constants of the rising phases of the firing to velocity steps were larger (2.0 $\pm$ 1.4 s), and 2) they responded to horizontal rotation in the dark in the type II mode. These differences prove that we were recording from neurons and not from pretectal fibers projecting to or running through the NRTP.

How are NRTP responses generated? As will be shown below the Pt projects monosynaptically to NRTP. This connection could, however, not explain all the response properties of NRTP units which clearly deviate from those of sensory relay cells. We must, in addition to the retinal slip input mediated by Pt neurons, postulate a head velocity input or, even more likely, an efference copy of eye velocity to these neurons to account for their response behavior outlined above. A combination of these two signals somewhere in the brain stem has been postulated (Robinson, 1977) as a basis for the central reconstruction of the velocity of the surround relative to the head.

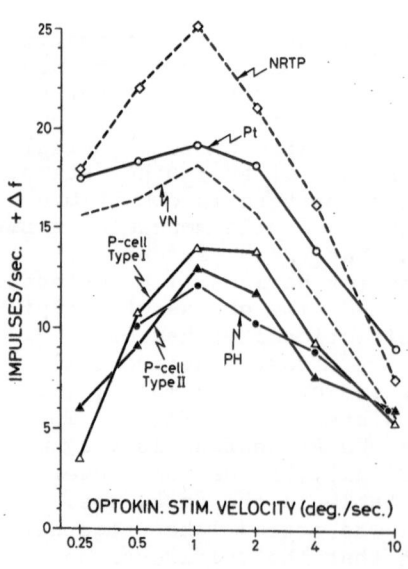

FIGURE 2
Summary of velocity tuning curves of Pt, NRTP, PH, P-cells and Vn units to optokinetic stimulation in immobilized rats. Each symbol gives mean increases of all units measured above resting level.

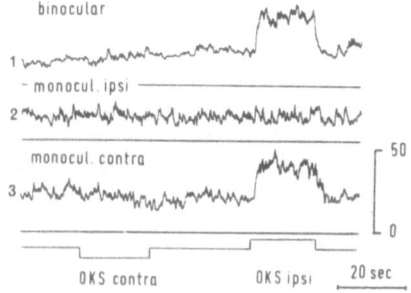

FIGURE 3
Responses of unidirectional Pt neuron to optokinetic stimulation (1°/s). Arrangement as in Fig.1. Note fast rise to peak.

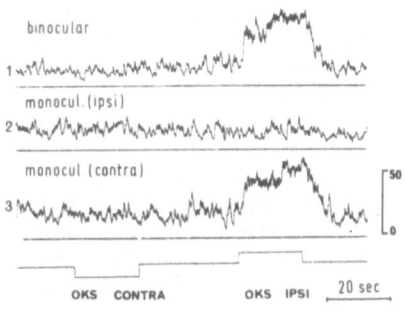

FIGURE 4
Responses of unidirectional NRTP neuron to optokinetic stimulation (1°/s). Arrangement as in Fig.1. Note slow rise to peak.

The so far unknown brain site may well be the NRTP. The NRTP signal, after passing through a yet unknown neural integrator (velocity storage network), will be fed into Vn yielding their sluggish response to optokinetic stimuli. With this model in mind we would not expect direct connections between NRTP and Vn; in fact, they do not seem to exist (3.6.4). Where then does the NRTP project? One strong projection reaches the cerebellum, particularly also the flocculus but, as shown by our lesion work, this path is not of crucial importance for optokinetic Vn responses. As will be shown below, another output reaches the n.prepositus hypoglossi (PH) which, on other grounds, has been implicated in velocity storage networks (Blanks et al., 1977).

3.4.3. Responses of PH neurons. For reasons given in the preceding paragraph optokinetic responses of PH neurons were studied under the same conditions as Pt, NRTP and Vn neurons. Only those PH neurons were considered which responded to horizontal rotation in the dark. As in the vestibular nuclei type I and type II neurons were found; they were mainly located in the rostral part of the nucleus. Again, the unidirectional response group deserves particular attention (Table 1). These units respond only

160

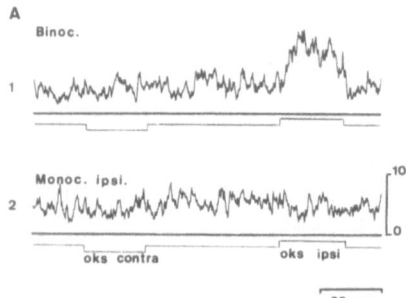

A

Binoc.

FIGURE 5
Responses of unidirecti-
onal PH neuron to optoki-
netic stimulation (1°/s).
Arrangement as in Fig.1.
Note similar rise time
as Fig.4.

to temporonasal stimulation of the contralateral eye
(Fig.5) and thus were similar to the majority of Pt and
NRTP neurons. Their velocity-tuning curves were likewise
similar to those of the other units (Fig.2). Whereas in
most neurons the apparent time constants were similar to
those of NRTP and Vn or even much larger, some units had
extremely rapid rise times. It is possible that these
units received strong direct Pt-inputs (see below).
Finally, it should be emphasized that vestibular stimuli
evoked a type II response pattern in unidirectional neurons. About 25% of PH neurons responding to optokinetic
stimuli showed a clear rhythmic modulation of firing that
may have been caused by a concomitant OKN.
The results presented above are compatible with the
notion that PH neurons are probably the final prevestibu-
lar relays in the OKN-path. Their strong projections to
the vestibular nuclei (see 3.6.5) certainly would provide
a structural basis.

3.4.4. Responses of floccular Purkinje cells. The involvement of the flocculus in OKN was first demonstrated
in lesion experiments in which impairment of smooth pursuit to the ipsilateral side and loss of fixation suppression of the VOR along with slowing of OKN at high
stimulus velocities and an absence of immediate fast rise
in OKN slow phase velocity with velocity steps was reported (cf.ref. Waespe, Henn, 1981). These experiments, together with data obtained from single unit recording from
the flocculus in several species, indicate that the flocculus is an important link in the "direct" OKN path and
not of crucial importance for the 'indirect' path or optokinetic responses of Vn. In fact, lesion of the cerebellum did not affect Vn responses (3.3.4).
Purkinje cells in the rat flocculus also respond to both
vestibular and optokinetic stimuli (Blanks, Precht,1981).
Optokinetic responses were generally bidirectional, asymmetrical (increase/decrease in rate) and synergistic to
vestibular responses in both Type I and Type II P-cells.
The latter resulted in a significant enhancement of

Optokin. response pattern		Ipsil. eye T→N	Ipsil. eye N→T	Contral. eye T→N	Contral. eye N→T	% of units	Vestib. resp.
Pretectum	Unidirectional*	—	—	↑	—	48	—
Pretectum	Bidirectional selective	↓	—	↑	—	16	—
Pretectum	Bidirectional selective	—	—	↑	↓	6	—
Pretectum	Bidirectional selective	↑	—	↓	—	3	—
NRTP	Unidirectional*	—	—	↑	—	43	Type II
NRTP	Unidirectional*	↑	—	—	—	8	Type I
NRTP	Bidirectional selective	↓	—	↑	—	16	Type II
NRTP	Bidirectional selective	↑	—	↓	—	33	Type I
PH	Unidirectional*	—	—	↑	—	25	Type II
PH	Bidirectional selective	↓	—	↑	—	32	Type II
PH	Bidirectional selective	↑	—	↓	—	37	Type I
VN	Bidirectional selective	↓	—	↑	—	40	Type II
VN	Bidirectional selective	↑	—	↓	—	60	Type I

TABLE 1. Summary of unitary responses to optokinetic stimuli in various relay nuclei. Only directionally selective responses shown. Upward and downward arrows indicate frequency increase or decrease, line indicates no response. Abbrev.s.text.

vestibular gain and phase when the animal was rotated, against a lighted, fixed-world environment. In paralyzed animals, there was a broad range in the time course of P-cell responses to optokinetic velocity steps as shown in Fig.6. At the one extreme were units whose response to optokinetic stimuli rose slowly and outlasted the stimulus 10-12 s (Fig.6A) the responses resembled those of Vn (Cazin et al., 1980a). At the other end were P-cells whose responses showed a brisk rise and fall at the onset and termination of the stimulus, respectively (Fig.6C). Interestingly, the latter units responded only to opto-kinetic stimuli and showed no vestibular responses. However, the vast majority of units had optokinetic re-sponses which consisted of a fast rise of simple spike firing followed by a smaller tonic response of the same polarity (Fig.6B).
One of the characteristic differences in the velocity step responses of P-cells compared to other elements in the OKN pathway in rat was the time constants. As shown in Fig.6E, P-cell time constants were significantly shorter than those of type I and type II Vn but similar

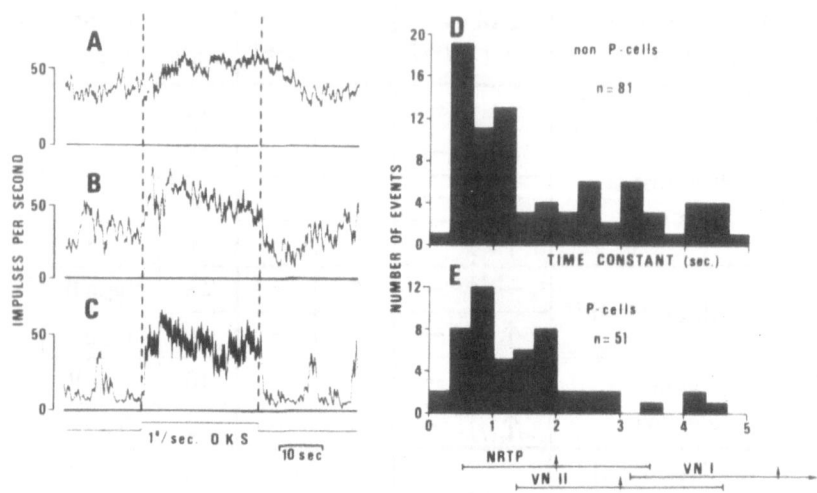

FIGURE 6 A-E. Response time constants to optokinetic
velocity steps (1°/s). A and B, Type I and Type II
P-cells, respectively. C, P-cell not responsive to horizontal rotation but showing a brisk optokinetic response.
The incremental time constants to optokinetic steps
(measured as 1/3 the time to maximum peak) is shown for
31 non P-cells (D) and for 51 P-cells (E). Note that
time constants for P-cells and non P-cells are shorter
than those for Type I (VNI) and Type II (VNII) Vn and
NRTP neurons. The mean and s.d. for VNI, VNII and NRTP
are given in E (see also text).

in value to those of NRTP neurons (Cazin et al., 1980a).
Values for afferent fibers, termed non-P-cells in Fig.6D,
reflect the diversity of OKN information transferred to
the flocculus. Another important difference demonstrated
by these experiments was that the peaks of P-cell type I
and type II tuning curves were higher (av. 1-2°s) and
the responses to low stimulus velocities poorer than
those of the PT, NRTP and VN (Fig.2). These data suggest
that the flocculus conveys a signal which is in some way
proportional to retinal slip velocity and operates in a
higher stimulus velocity range than the Vn. In this respect, the situation in the rat is quite similar to the
one in the monkey in which P-cells show a fast rise in
firing with optokinetic stimuli, no activity related to
OKAN (Waespe and Henn, 1981) and response range exceeding
that of the Vn (Waespe and Henn, 1978).
Lastly, monocular testing revealed that approximately
half of the P-cells and non P-cells were driven from the
contralateral eye with polarities similar to Vn (Cazin
et al., 1980a) whereas the other half were excited by
temporo-nasal stimuli to the ipsilateral eye. A systematic

analysis of these data suggests that the ipsilateral projection can be explained on the basis of crossing NRTP-FLOC, PH-FLOC and/or VN-FLOC connections for which there is ample anatomical evidence in most species and in the rat (Blanks et al., 1982).

3.5. Electroanatomy of the pathway

Our lesion work and the single unit studies during opto-kinetic stimulation suggested that signals from the contralateral eye first reach the Pt. From there the signal must travel indirectly to Vn since no Pt-Vn connections exist. In this section we shall describe the electrophysiological details of the shortest possible connections between eye and Vn. As illustrated schematically in Fig. 7 stimulation of the contralateral optic nerve (ONc) evoked in the Pt presynaptic spikes and EPSPs; their mean and shortest latencies differ by 0.3 - 0.6 ms, respectively, i.e. by one synaptic delay. This monosynaptic connection between retinal ganglion cell axons and Pt neurons is well supported by anatomical

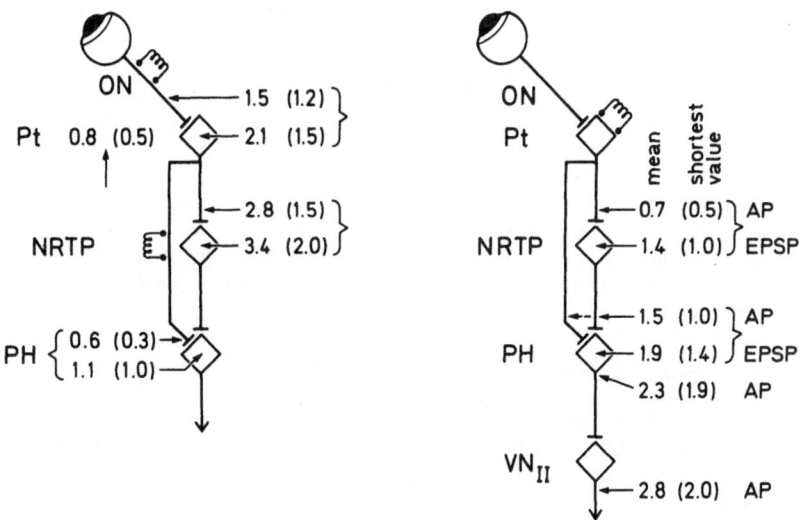

Horizontal OKN path

FIGURE 7. Schematic representation of short latency connections between optic nerve (ON) and vestibular nuclei (VN). Stimulation and recording sites are indicated; the numbers give mean latencies (1st number) and shortest latencies (2nd number) in ms. AP = action potentials; further abbrev.s.text.

findings (Scalia, Arango, 1979). Many of the neurons so
activated were also driven antidromically from the NRTP
(Fig.7,left) which had emerged as a possible mediator
of optokinetic signals. In the NRTP ONc stimulation
evoked presynaptic spikes and EPSPs with latency differences that also indicated monosynaptic delay in this
nucleus. However, it is difficult to conclude from this
that Pt neurons project directly to NRTP. To search for
such connections the Pt was stimulated and presynaptic
spikes and EPSPs were sampled in NRTP (Fig.7,right).
The short latency values for presynaptic spikes and
EPSPs and the calculated synaptic delay of 0.5 - 0.7 ms,
indeed, suggest monosynaptic impingement of Pt axons on
NRTP neurons. Anatomical work (3.6.4) showed that the
NRTP does not project directly to Vn. Based on sections
3.4.3 and 3.6.4 the PH appeared as a relay candidate.
We therefore stimulated both the NRTP and Pt areas and
recorded from PH. Both Pt (Fig.7,right) and NRTP (Fig.7,
left) seem to project monosynaptically to PH neurons.
Mean EPSP latencies in PH after Pt and NRTP stimulation
measured 1.9 and 1.1 ms, respectively, the difference
of 0.8 ms being due to the mean conduction time from Pt
to NRTP (Fig.7,left). Anatomical support for both connections exists (3.6.4).
Since the PH is known to have connections to the vestibular nuclei (3.6.5) PH neurons could mediate optokinetic
responses of Vn. Our preliminary results support this
notion, i.e. the difference in latencies of the Pt-evoked
spikes in type II PH neurons and those of type II Vn
evoked by the same stimuli was short enough (0.5 ms) to
allow for such a connection (Fig.7,right). The type I
inhibition observed with Pt and natural stimuli may be
mediated by inhibitory type II Vn located on the same
side (Precht, 1981). In addition to the shortest possible
connections between eye and Vn illustrated here, it
should be emphasized that the optokinetic responses obtained with natural stimuli may also require polysynaptic
pathways.

3.6. Anatomy of the optokinetic pathway

Although there are a number of similarities in the organization of the horizontal OKN among the mammalian species studied, there are several interspecies differences
which set the rat apart from the other species studied.
As shown above, the most dramatic difference is an almost
complete absence of an optokinetic response in the rat
Vn to nasotemporal stimulation and an absence of OKN in
this direction. In this respect, a study of the anatomical pathways of the optokinetic system is easier than
in other species (e.g. cat, monkey, man) in which both
nasotemporal and temporonasal monocular OKN can be elicited (cf.ref. Precht, 1981, 1982). In the sections that
follow, the previously mentioned electrophysiological

and lesion experiments will be discussed in relation to
the anatomy of the horizontal OKN pathways which includes critical subcortical pathways which synapse within or pass through: 1) the Pt, 2) the ventrolateral midbrain reticular formation, 3) the region of the NRTP and
4) the PH and VN. Additionally, there is experimental
evidence that other structures such as the accessory
optic system, inferior olive and cerebellum play a modulatory role in the performance of OKN (Precht, 1982).

3.6.1. The pretectum and accessory optic system (AOS)

Because of their importance as the first relay station
in the optokinetic pathways, a brief account will be
given of the anatomy of the Pt and the AOS.

The Pt in the rat consists of four nuclear groups termed
the anterior, posterior and olivary pretectal nuclei and
the nucleus of the optic tract (NOT) (Scalia, 1972).
With the exception of the anterior nucleus each of these
groups receive retinofugal projections which are primarily, though not exclusively, crossed (Scalia, Arango,
1979). Although each of these structures may be involved
with some aspect of visual-motor control, it is primarily
the NOT which has emerged as the important structure for
controlling horizontal OKN. In this regard it should be
noted that the crossed retinofugal projections to the
NOT are distributed to the superficial portions of the
nucleus, overlapping in part, the visual cortical (cf.
Linden and Rocha - Miranda, 1981) and AOS projections.
Additionally, the descending pretectal connections to
subsequent stations in the OKN pathways e.g. the NRTP and
inferior olive (IO), arise primarily from the NOT, but
more specifically its superficial part (Torigoe et al.,
1982a).

The AOS in the rat consists of three terminal nuclei,
the medial (MTN), lateral (LTN) and dorsal terminal
nucleus (DTN) which receive a crossed retinal input via
several accessory optic tracts (Hayhow et al., 1960).
In addition to the retinal projections to these nuclei
there is evidence for a large number of cortical and
subcortical afferents that cannot be mentioned here.
Considering the functional importance of the Pt and the
AOS in OKN the large number of interconnections between
these structures requires attention. Thus, the NOT has
been shown to project to the DTN, MTN and LTN in the rat
(Cazin et al., unpubl.obs.) and, in return, the MTN projects heavily upon the NOT and DTN (cf. Simpson et al.,
1978). In fact, it has been recently shown autoradio-
graphically that the heaviest projection of the MTN in
the rat is to the ipsilateral NOT (Blanks et al., 1982b).
While it could be argued that these interconnections
serve to sharpen the receptive field properties of NOT
and AOS neurons (Simpson et al., 1978), their precise
role requires further investigation. It is, however,

instructive to note that with the exception of crossing
NOT-NOT and NOT-DTN connections in rat (Terasawa et al.,
1979) most of the reciprocal connections described so
far involve nuclei on the same side.

3.6.2. Descending connections of NOT. In the rat the NOT
gives rise to several descending bundles which are distributed to the midbrain reticular formation (MRF), the
pontine nucleus, NRTP and IO (Terasawa et al., 1979).
Using the Nauta-Gygax Technique in rats, (Terasawa et al.,
1979) describe one bundle of thick axons which arises
from the NOT and is distributed to the NRTP and IO. This
group of fibers courses ventromedially to the region of
the medial lemniscus, within which (and dorsal to which)
it descends to the pontine level. The bundle then divides,
one group being distributed to the middle one-third of
the ventromedial portion of the NRTP, and the second continuing caudally to terminate within the dorsal cap of
the IO. A second group of fibers leaves the NOT and is
distributed to the pontine nuclei. These fine fibers descend through the dorsomedial part of the mesencephalic
reticular formation, medially to the parabigeminal nucleus then ventrally along the lateral border of the pons
to enter the medial one-third of the lateral pontine
nuclei.
Recent autoradiographic work showed terminal fields not
only in NRTP, IO, pons, MRF but also in the PH (Cazin
et al., unpubl.observ.). This finding is in excellent
agreement with the electrophysiological results (3.5).
The course taken by the NOT-NRTP/IO bundle is important
for interpreting electrical stimulation and lesion studies. Thus, whereas electrical stimulation of the NOT
in rabbit produced OKN, there was also a low threshold
region which extended ventromedially through the MRF
(Collewijn, 1975a). Given that the NOT-NRTP/IO and reciprocal NOT-AOS fibers in rabbit and rat (Giolli et al.,
1982) course through this region it could be assumed
that the OKN generated by electrical stimulation resulted
from stimulation of the fibers of these bundles. Similarly, lesions placed bilaterally in the ventrolateral quadrant of the midbrain which interrupted these fibers
showed effects similar to pretectal lesions (Cazin et al.,
1980b). Of additional concern in interpreting lesion
studies is that a lesion of the NRTP which interrupts
the NOT-NRTP bundle and effectively blocks OKN and the
optokinetic modulation of Vn potentially interrupts the
NOT-IO fibers. While this is a concern, the IO pathway
does not appear to be an essential part of the OKS pathway to the Vn (3.3.4).
It is also instructive to note that the NOT-pontine
fibers would be left intact with the NRTP lesions (Cazin
et al., 1980b) and although the lateral pontine nuclei
project to the vermis, paraflocculus and flocculus this

projection does not appear essential for generating OKN.
Rather, these may be important for mediating the modulatory cerebellar effects on optokinetic nystagmus.

3.6.3. <u>Afferents to the NRTP</u>. The NRTP in the cat and
monkey receives well described connections from the ipsilateral NOT, the bilateral parietal and frontal cortex
(P. Brodal, 1980), the contralateral superior vestibular
nucleus (Ladpli,Brodal, 1968) the contralateral cerebellar nuclei by way of the descending limb of the brachium
conjunctivum and the contralateral superior colliculus
(Altman, Carpenter, 1961; Ladpli, Brodal, 1968). Our recent HRP studies on the afferents to the NRTP in rat
are summarized in Fig.8 (Torigoe et al., 1982a). These
cases have confirmed each of the projections listed
above and have, in addition, demonstrated that there

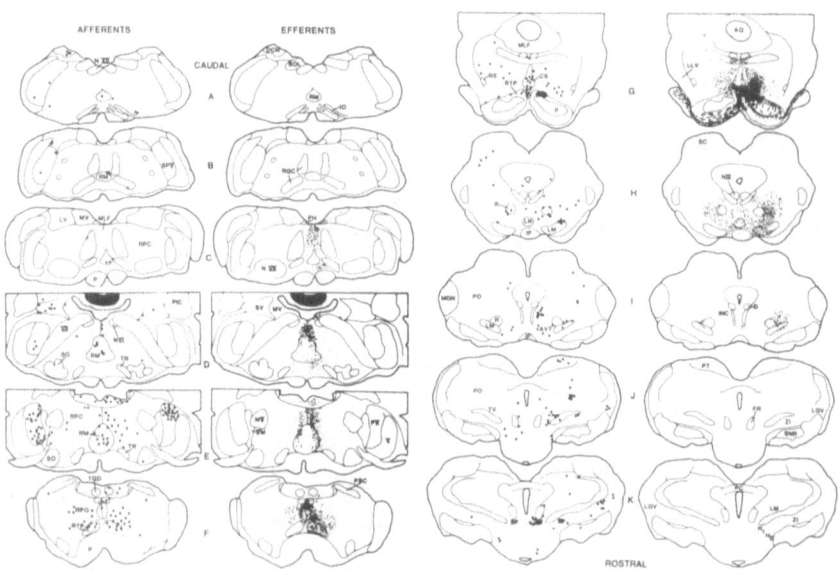

FIGURE 8. Afferent and efferent connections of the NRTP
as studied with HRP, and ^{3}H-leucine autoradiography,
respectively (A-K,left,right). Extent of HRP and leucine
injections are shown in G. All HRP-labeled cells in 3
consecutive 40 μM sections are plotted as dots on representative sections (48 h survival after injection,
substrate tetramethyl benzidine. Labeling in trigeminal
complex results from uptake into decussating axons. Axons
arising from leucine injection site are small dashed
lines, terminal fields are plotted as dots (72 h of survival). Abbrev.s.text.

are other nuclei which may serve to relay visual and
oculomotor afferents to the NRTP. One such area is
the interstitial nucleus of Cajal (INC) which in the
rat receives afferents from the NOT (Terasawa et al.,
1980) and MTN (Giolli, Blanks, 1982) and on the basis
of our anatomical data projects to the NRTP. INC neurons
are related, however, mainly to vertical eye movements
and are not of prime interest in this context. Other
areas which heavily project to the NRTP and which receive input from the NOT are the ventrolateral geniculate nucleus, the zona incerta and the H_1 and H_2 fields
of Forel. However, each of these areas will have to be
examined in more detail before a possible connection
with OKN can be established.

3.6.4. Efferent projections of NRTP. The NRTP is one of
the classical precerebellar nuclei, yet the above reviewed electrophysiological studies would suggest that
the NRTP has subcerebellar projections which indirectly
terminate within the VN. We have examined the efferent
projections of the NRTP using ^{3}H-leucine light autoradiography in rats. In a first series of experiments
(Cazin et al., unpubl.observ.) injections of isotope
into the pontine tegmentum in rats, including the area
of the NRTP, produced large numbers of labeled axons
within the middle cerebellar peduncle and terminal fields
within the entire cerebellum (especially the cerebellar
hemisphere, paraflocculus and flocculus). A second group
of axons entered the MLF to terminate ipsilaterally in
the PH and in the dorsal cap of the IO. More importantly,
there was no evidence of terminal labeling within the
VN. The injection sites in these experiments encompassed
the central and pericentral portions of the NRTP and the
overlying pontine reticular formation (PRF) and in many
respects produced results similar to PRF injections in
the cat (Graybiel, 1977) and monkey (Buttner-Ennever,
Henn, 1976). Thus it was impossible to resolve the precise cell bodies of origin for the PH and IO projection.

In another series of experiments (Torigoe et al., 1982b),
isotope injections confined to the NRTP and minimally
involving the adjacent PRF further demonstrated that the
NRTP shows extensive non-cerebellar projections but these
are largely distributed bilaterally to the tegmental reticular nuclei (N.reticularis pontis oralis; RPO, and
N.reticularis pontis caudalis, RPC, but there was evidence for a bundle to the PH. The complexity of these
projections are illustrated in Fig.8. The injection site
in this case was confined largely to the NRTP and involved minimal spillage across the midline or to the
pontine tegmental reticular nuclei. The strongest projections from this region of the NRTP are, bilaterally,
to the cerebellum via the middle cerebellar peduncles.

Additionally, however, and more important to the present discussion, are the persistent NRTP-reticular projections. These were bilateral but most heavily distributed to the ipsilateral side. The delicate axons providing the NRTP-reticular projection radiate through the ipsilateral tegmentum and provided a diffuse projection to the RPO over its full extent from the interpeduncular nucleus rostrally to its junction with the RPC caudally. Terminal labeling was also detected within the rostral portions of the RPC. The contralateral projection was provided by equally delicate axons which decussate at the rostral pole of the NRTP and were distributed to approximately symmetrical locations of the reticular formation. This series of animals also provide evidence for interconnections between the bilateral NRTP and between the NRTP and pontine nuclei. Such connections have not been described before, but they may play an important part in conveying polysynaptic information to cerebellar, reticular or PH projecting neurons.

Lastly, there were bundles of axons which ascended rostrally along the midline to provide terminal fields in the midbrain reticular formation, parvicellular portion of the red nucleus (Fig.3H,right) and posteriorly coursing fibers giving rise to dense terminal fields within the superior central nucleus of the raphe complex just ventral to the MLF. This bundle continues, giving rise to sparse terminations within the ipsilateral nucleus supragenualis and PH. It should be noted that these projections were heaviest when injections involved the midline areas between the bilateral NRTP and as such may represent a part of the ascending and descending raphe projections from neurons of the raphe pontis which are clustered along the midline and forming a cap over the dorsal medial portion of the NRTP.

In the context of the present ARG data, it is important to note that the lesions most effective in blocking the optokinetic responses of Vn were confined to the NRTP in the rat (Cazin et al., 1980b). Such a lesion would have destroyed not only the NRTP neurons but also would have interrupted the ipsilateral NRTP-PRF-PH axons as well, thereby disrupting two portions of the presumed OKN pathway.

3.6.5. Summary of Pt-NRTP-VN paths. The physiological and lesion studies and the Pt-NRTP projections mentioned earlier provided evidence that the NRTP provides a link between the Pt and the VN. How then are impulses conducted from the NRTP to the Vn? The areas to which the NRTP is shown to project are the PH bilaterally but predominantly ipsilaterally and no definite projections were found to the VN. This projection, combined with the strong reciprocal connections between the PH and VN (McCrea et al., 1979) may provide the pathway by which

the NRTP is capable of modulating the Vn. It should
also be recalled that direct Pt-PH connections were
found which could mediate optokinetic effects to Vn.
Of lesser importance are the projections via the cerebellum or IO.

Finally, it is important to emphasize that the PRF represents an important premotor area for the control of
horizontal conjugate gaze (Buttner-Ennever, Henn,1979).
Anatomical and electrophysiological data show the evidence of a direct monosynaptic pathway from the PRF to
the ipsilateral abducens nucleus (cf. Buttner-Ennever,
Henn, 1976; Highstein et al., 1976). The NRTP-PRF connections described here may imply that optokinetic information is relayed directly to abducens motoneurons
via the PRF and also offers means for polysynaptic paths
to the Vn.

Acknowledgments: I wish to thank Mrs. M. Cavegn, Mrs.
V. Schedler, Mrs. E. Schneider, Mr. B. Frey and Mr. J.
Kuenzli for extremely valuable technical assistance.

REFERENCES
Altman J and Carpenter MB (1961) Fiber projections of
the superior colliculus in the cat, J. Comp. Neurol.
116, 157-178.
Blanks RHI, Volkind R, Precht W and Baker R (1977)
Responses of cat prepositus hypoglossi neurons to horizontal angular acceleration, Neuroscience 2, 391-404.
Blanks RHI and Precht W (1981) Mossy fiber responses of
purkinje cells in the cerebellar flocculus of the alert,
pigmented rat during optokinetic and vestibular stimulation, Soc. Neurosci. Abstr. 7, 775.
Blanks RHI, Giolli RA and Sang Van Pham (1982b) Projections of the medial terminal nucleus of the accessory
optic system upon pretectal nuclei in the pigmented rat.
(Submitted to Exp. Brain Res.)
Brodal P (1980) The cortical projection to the nucleus
reticularis tegmenti pontis in the rhesus monkey, Exp.
Brain Res. 38, 19-27.
Buttner-Ennever JA and Henn V (1976) An autoradiographic
study of the pathways from the pontine reticular formation involved in horizontal eye movements, Brain Res.
108, 155-164.
Cazin L, Precht W and Lannou J (1980a) Optokinetic
responses of vestibular nucleus neurons in the rat,
Pflüg. Arch. 384, 31-38.
Cazin L, Precht W and Lannou J (1980b) Pathways mediating optokinetic responses of vestibular nucleus neurons
in the rat, Pflüg. Arch. 384, 19-29.
Cazin L, Precht W and Lannou J (1980c) Firing characteristics of neurons mediating optokinetic responses to
rat's vestibular neurons, Pflüg. Arch. 386, 221-230.

Cohen B, Uemura T and Takemori S (1973) Effects of labyrinthectomy on optokinetic nystagmus (OKN) and optokinetic after-nystagmus (OKAN), Equilibrium Res. 3, 88-93.
Cohen B, Matsuo V and Raphan T (1977) Quantitative analysis of the velocity characteristics of optokinetic
nystagmus and optokinetic after-nystagmus, J. Physiol.
270, 321-344.
Collewijn H (1975a) Oculomotor areas in the rabbit's
midbrain and pretectum, J. Neurobiol. 6, 3-22.
Collewijn H (1975b) Direction-selective units in the
rabbit's nucleus of the optic tract. Brain Res. 100,
489-508.
Dieringer N, Precht W and Cochran SL (1982) Is there a
velocity storage in the frog brain stem? (In press)

Giolli RA and Blanks RHI (1982) Projections of the medial
terminal nucleus of the accessory optic system in rat
and rabbit. (In preparation)
Graybiel AM (1977) Direct and indirect preoculomotor
pathways of the brainstem: an autoradiographic study of
the pontine reticular formation in the cat, J. Comp.
Neurol. 175, 37-78.
Highstein SM, Maekawa K, Steinacker A and Cohen B (1976)
Synaptic input from the pontine reticular nuclei to abducens motoneurons and internuclear neurons in the cat,
Brain Res. 112, 162-167.
Keller EL and Precht W (1979) Visual-vestibular responses
in vestibular nuclear neurons in intact and cerebellectomized, alert cat, Neurosci. 4, 1599-1613.
Ladpli R and Brodal A (1968) Experimental studies of commissural and reticular formation projections from the
vestibular nuclei in the cat, Brain Res. 8, 65-96.
Lannou J, Cazin L, Precht W and Toupet M (1982) Optokinetic, Vestibular, and Optokinetic-vestibular responses in
albino and pigmented rats, Pflüg. Arch. (In press)

Linden R and Rocha-Miranda CE (1981) The pretectal complex in the opossum: projections from the striate cortex
and correlation with retinal terminal fields, Brain Res.
39, 245-251.
Maioli C, Precht W and Ried S (1982) The vestibulo-ocular
Reflex after acute and chronic unilateral neurotomy. In:
Physiol. and Pathol. Aspects of Eye Movements.

McCrea RA, Baker R and Delgado-Garcia J (1979) Afferent
and efferent organization of the prepositus hypoglossi
nucleus, Prog. Brain Res. 50, 653-665.
Montarolo PG, Precht W and Strata P (1981) Functional
organization of the mechanisms subserving the optokinetic
nystagmus in the cat, Neurosci. 6, 231-246.
Precht W and Cazin L (1979) Functional deficits in the
optokinetic system of albino rats, Exp. Brain Res. 37,
183-186.

Precht W (1981) Visual-Vestibular Interaction in Vesti-
bular Neurons: Functional Pathway Organization. In:
Vestibular and Oculomotor Physiology: International
Meeting of the Bárány Society. Ed. B. Cohen. Ann. New
York Acad. Sci. 374, 230-248.
Precht W (1982) Anatomical and functional organization
of optokinetic pathways. In: Functional Basis of Ocular
Motiliy Disorders. Eds. Lennerstrand et al.
(In press)
Robinson DA (1977) Linear additon of optokinetic and
vestibular signals in the vestibular nucleus, Exp. Brain
Res. 30, 447-450.
Scalia F (1972) The termination of retinal axons in the
pretectal region of mammals, J. Comp. Neurol. 145,
223-258.
Scalia F and Arango V (1979) Topographic organization
of the projections of the retina to the pretectal region
in the rat, J. Comp. Neurol. 186, 271-292.
Simpson JI, Soodak RE and Hess R (1978) The accessory
optic system and its relation to the vestibulocerebellum.
In: Reflex control of posture and movement. Eds. R.Granit
and O. Pompeiano, Pisa. Prog. Brain Res. 50.
Terasawa K, Otani K and Yamada J (1979) Descending pathways of the nucleus of the optic tract in the rat, Brain
Res. 173, 405-417.
Torigoe Y, Precht W and Blanks RHI (1982a) Anatomical
studies on the connections of the nucleus reticularis
tegmenti pontis in the pigmented rat. I. afferent projections demonstrated by the retrograde transport of
horseradish peroxidase. (In preparation)

Torigoe Y, Precht W and Blanks RHI (1982b) Anatomical
studies on the connections of the nucleus reticularis
tegmenti pontis on the pigmented rat. II. efferent projections demonstrated by anterograde ^{3}H-leucine autoradiography and retrograde transport of horseradish
peroxidase. (In preparation)

Waespe W and Henn V (1978) Conflicting visual-vestibular
stimulation and vestibular nucleus activity in alert
monkeys, Exp. Brain Res. 33, 203-211.
Waespe W and Henn V (1981) Visual-Vestibular Interaction
in the Flocculus of the Alert Monkey. II. Purkinje Cell
Activity, Exp. Brain Res. 43, 349-360.

THE ROLE OF THE FOVEA AND PARAFOVEAL REGIONS IN THE CONTROL OF "FAST" OPTOKINETIC RESPONSES IN THE MONKEY

U. BÜTTNER * (Dept. of Neurology, Univ. of Zürich),
O. MEIENBERG (Dept. of Neurology, Univ. of Bern) and
B. SCHIMMELPFENNIG (Dept. of Ophthalmology, Univ. of Zürich, Switzerland)

It has been well established over the last few years that optokinetic nystagmus in response to high velocity stimuli consists of two components (Cohen et al., 1977): A "fast" component, which has been attributed to the pursuit system and depends on direct visual pathways, and a "velocity storage" component utilizing neural integration through indirect pathways (Robinson, 1980). In response to high velocity stimulation these components manifest themselves in the following manner (fig. 1): the sudden presentation of a high velocity stimulus leads to a rapid increase in nystagmus velocity due to the "fast" component. Next the "velocity storage" mechanism leads to a further, more gradual increase. Thus during high velocity optokinetic nystagmus (OKN) both components are activated. When the lights are turned off, eye velocity shows an immediate initial drop due to inactivation of the "fast" response. The "velocity storage" mechanism decreases more slowly during optokinetic after-nystagmus (OKAN).

Since the "fast" component has been attributed to the pursuit system (Robinson, 1980), it implies that the visual input of the "fast" component mainly derives from the fovea. To test this hypothesis OKN was investigated after retinal lesions were made in and around the fovea. It was found that "fast" responses are still present with large lesions of the central retina.

METHODS

Experiments were performed on monkeys (Macaca mulatta). Initially a receptacle for a head holder was attached to the skull under general anaesthesia. Eye position was recorded with implanted DC silver-silver chloride electrodes. During the experiments the monkey sat upright with its head fixed in a primate chair. It received small doses of amphetamine to maintain a high level of alertness. The optokinetic stimulus consisted of a cylinder covered with vertical black and white stripes (width 7,5 deg). Drum velocity was varied between 10 and 200 deg/s.

* present address: Dept. of Neurology, Univ. of Düsseldorf, Moorenstr. 5

Roucoux, A. and Crommelinck, M. (eds.): Physiological and Pathological Aspects of Eye Movements.
© *1982, Dr W. Junk Publishers, The Hague, Boston, London.* ISBN-13: 978-94-009-8002-0

Optokinetic nystagmus was recorded with both eyes open
and one eye covered. Confluent laser lesions were
placed under general anaesthesia in and around the fovea
of one eye. Animals received 2-3 successive lesions in
one eye over a period of several weeks. Responses of
the lesioned and the non-lesioned eye were then compared. The retina was photographed after each lesion to
facilitate the determination of the extent of the
lesion.
At the end of all experiments monkeys were perfused
with formalin under an overdose of pentobarbital. The
retina was embedded and serial sections were taken.

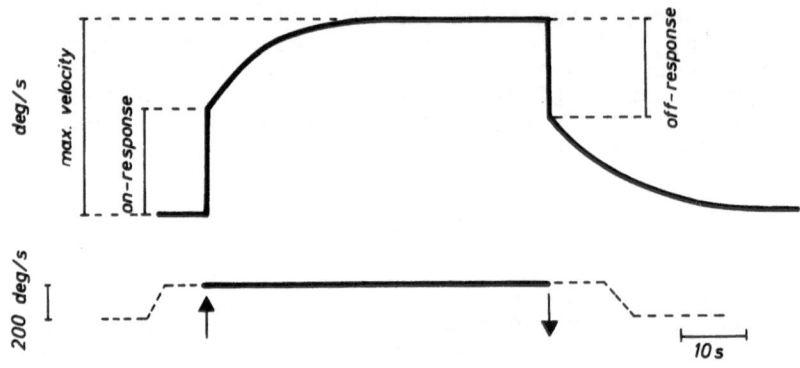

Fig. 1 Schematic drawing of OKN velocity in response
to high velocity full-field optokinetic stimulation.
Upper half shows nystagmus velocity and lower half time
course of stimulus velocity. Light-on (upward arrow)
during constant velocity rotation leads to an initial
rapid rise in eye velocity (on-response) followed by a
more gradual increase. At light-off (downward arrow),
eye velocity drops immediately (off-response), and
subsequently OKAN decreases exponentially.

RESULTS
Fig. 2 shows the responses to optokinetic stimuli at
different constant velocities, when both eyes were stimulated either simultaneously or seperately. Up to
stimulus velocities of 120 deg/s OKN velocity increased
linearly and was virtually identical for monocular or
binocular stimulation. At higher stimulus velocities
the increases were smaller, particularly during monocular stimulation. During monocular stimulation no
differences were observed between naso-temporal and
temporo-nasal stimulus directions.
    The maximal OKN-velocity during constant velocity
stimulation was only slightly affected when small
lesions were placed in and around the fovea (fig. 3).
The first lesion for the results shown in fig. 3 was
restricted to 6-7 deg and centered on the fovea.

In the monkey the fovea and the parafovea have a diameter of 6 deg (Stone, 1965). With the second lesion the retina around the first lesion was destroyed resulting in a total lesion of 2o deg diameter. As fig. 3 demonstrates there is only a small decrease of maximal velocity as a result of the 2nd lesion. The effect is slightly more pronounced for stimulation in the temporo-nasal direction (right nystagmus).

Finally the third lesion destroyed, in addition, all fibers from the temporal retina, as well as below and above the optic disc, leaving only the medial part of the retina and 5 deg below and above the optic disc intact. With this lesion no proper nystagmus was obtained from the lesioned eye in the temporo-nasal direction. However in the naso-temporal direction it was still possible to elicit a nystagmus velocity of more than 130 deg/s. These velocities, however, took a long time to build up and were more easily achieved when the stimulus velocity was increased gradually. If the maximal velocity decreased during constant velocity stimulation usually OKN stopped altogether and the monkey was not able to regain the original velocity unless the stimulation procedure was repeated. These differences in effectiveness of stimulus directions were surprising, since in lower species it is known that the temporo-nasal stimulus direction is generally more effective (see Precht and Hofmann, this volume).

ON-Responses

On-responses (see fig. 1) can reach values of 100 deg/s, particularly when both eyes are stimulated. With monocular stimulation the responses are slightly smaller. Fig. 4 shows the effect of central retinal lesions on the on-response. The first lesion, centered on the fovea, covered an area of 10-12 deg. This led to a small, but definite reduction of the on-response, both for right and left nystagmus. After the second lesion the non-functioning area covered more than 25 deg sparing the optic disc. With lesions of this size definite on-response up to 40-50 deg/s were still obtained.

OFF-Responses

The size of the off-response (fig. 1) closely correlates with the maximal OKN-velocity and the on-response. Off-responses can reach 80-100 deg/s decrease in velocity. Lesions which lead to a reduction of the on-response, also affected the maximal OKN-velocity and consequently the off-response. The exponential decay of OKAN after the off-response started at velocities of 80-120 deg/s. Thus, if the preceding OKN velocity exceeded these values an off-response could be clearly distinguished.

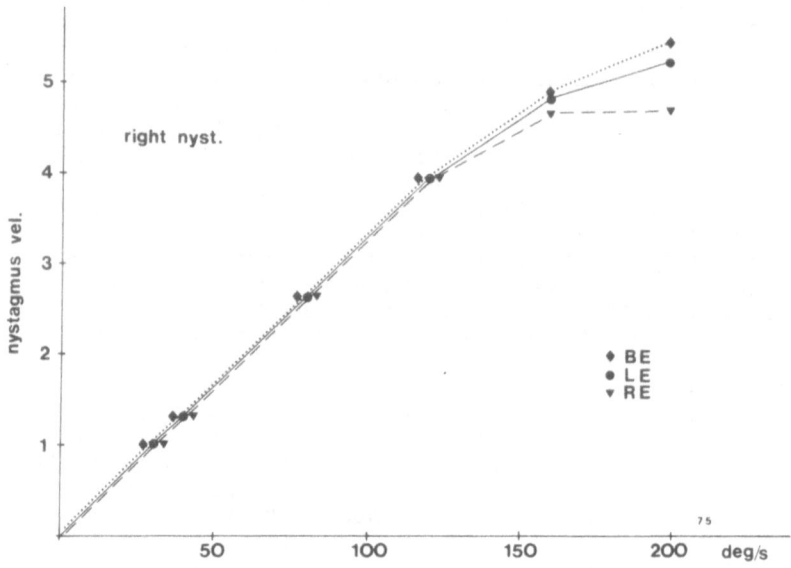

Fig. 2 Maximal OKN velocity (right nystagmus) during
constant velocity stimulation with a striped cylinder.
Abscissa: stimulus and ordinate: nystagmus velocity.
Nystagmus velocity at 30 deg/s stimulus velocity is
normalized to 1. BE: both eyes open, RE: right eye and
LE: left eye open. Nystagmus velocity increases linearly up to 120 deg/s stimulus velocity. At higher velocities the increase is smaller for monocular stimulation.

DISCUSSION
The results demonstrate that in the monkey "fast" optokinetic responses still can be elicited with large central retinal lesions exceeding 25 deg. The best manifestation of the "fast" response is the on-response
(fig. 1) which with such a lesion can be still about
50 % of the response obtained from the non-lesioned
eye (fig. 4). The other parameters (maximal OKN-velocity, off-response) are in accordance with this finding.
Since the "velocity storage" component is only affected
by extremely large lesions, the maximal velocity reflects as a first approximation the sum of the "fast"
and the "velocity storage" component. The size of the
off-response is then directly determined by the on-
response.
    As described earlier the "fast" optokinetic res-
ponse has been attributed to the smooth pursuit system.
The results show that "fast" responses can be elicited
from retinal areas, which are generally assumed not to
be involved in smooth pursuit eye movements. This finding is not necessaryly in conflict with the assumption
of Robinson (1980). It rather suggests that large retinal areas outside the fovea provide a visual input to
the smooth pursuit system. This extrafoveal visual input

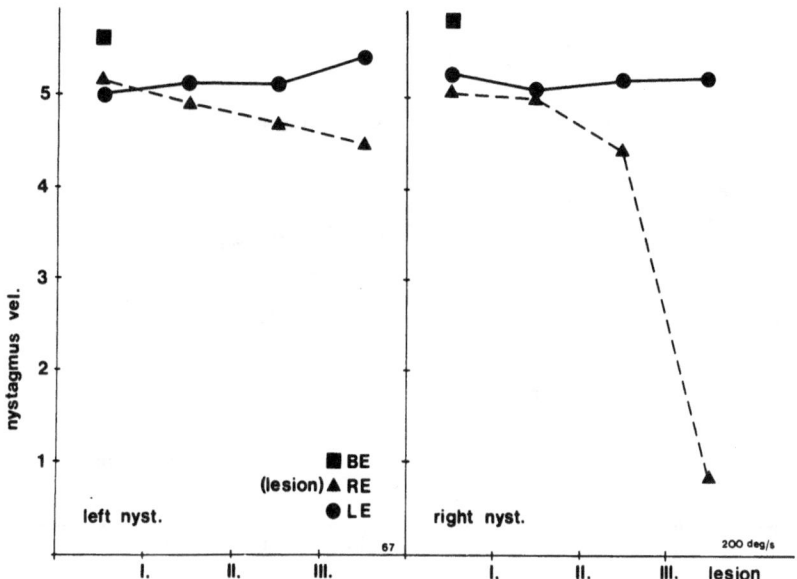

Fig. 3 The effect of central retinal lesions on maximal OKN-velocity at 200 deg/s stimulus velocity. Nystagmus velocity (ordinate) was set at 1 for 30 deg/s stimulus velocity. Before the first (I, foveal) lesion binocular (BE) stimulation leads to higher maximal velocities than stimulation of the right (RE) or left (LE) eye alone. Increasing central retinal lesions of the right eye lead to a decrease in maximal velocity, which becomes prominent only after the largest (III) lesion for stimulation in the temporo-nasal direction (right nystagmus). For further explanation see text.

probably only becomes effective, when large retinal areas are stimulated simultaneously, as during OKN.

In contrast small visual objects, as during smooth pursuit, stimulate the visual input more effectively in and around the fovea and are therefore kept there during tracking. Thus the smooth pursuit system and the "fast" optokinetic response under normal conditions share the foveal visual input and the same premotor structures in the cerebellum and the brainstem. In addition the "fast" optokinetic response relys on extrafoveal retinal areas.

That the visual inputs from foveal and extrafoveal regions with respect to smooth pursuit are not basically distinct is underlined by several reports which show that extrafoveal visual inputs can activate smooth pursuit eye movements easily when foveal stimulation is prevented (Michalski et al, 1977; Winterson and Steinman, 1978).

It should be stressed, that for the experiments all efforts were made to obtain optimal optokinetic responses. Monkeys received amphetamine to maintain a high

178

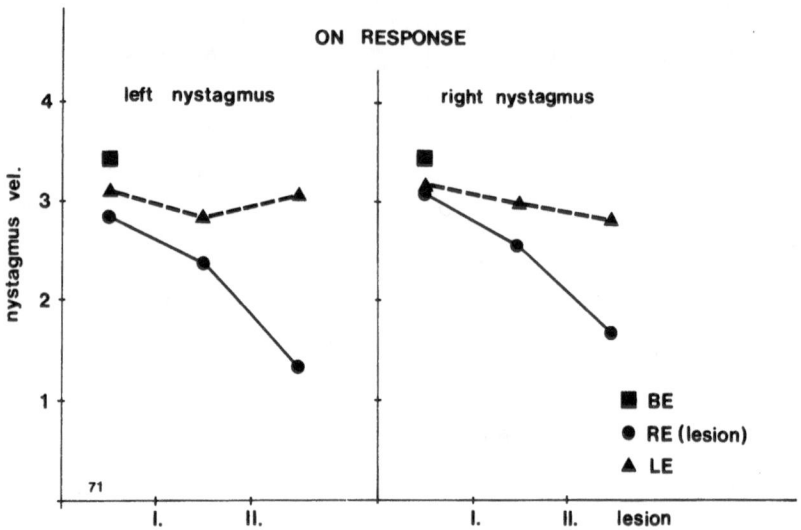

Fig. 4   Influence of central retinal lesions on the
optokinetic on-response in the monkey. Nystagmus velocity was normalized to 1 at 30 deg/s constant velocity
stimulation. The binocular (BE) on-response is
slightly larger than the monocular response of the
right (RE) or left (LE) eye. The on-response is smaller
with central retinal lesions (RE, right eye), but definite on-responses are still present after the second
(II) lesion covering more than 25 deg of central retina.

level of alertness. The stimulus consisted of a physi-
cally moving cylinder, which stimulated the whole retina. Furthermore the monkey optokinetic system is
known to be more powerful than the human system (Cohen
et al., 1977). This has to be kept in mind to allow a
comparison with reports in the literature on related
topics. Particularly the work of Cheng and Outerbridge
(1975) clearly demonstrates the effect of attention on
OKN-velocity (see their fig. 6): With high levels of
attention, OKN-velocity can be virtually unaffected,
even if 30 deg of central vision are deleted.
In recent years single unit studies in alert monkeys
demonstrated that the "velocity storage" mechanism
probably involves the vestibular nuclei (Waespe and
Henn, 1977), whereas the "fast" optokinetic response is
associated with activity changes of Purkinje cells in
the flocculus (Waespe and Henn, 1981).
   These data strongly suggest that the same Purkinje
cells can be active during smooth pursuit eye movements
and "fast" optokinetic responses (Büttner et al., 1981).
The unaffected nystagmus responses after retinal
lesions suggest that the visual input to these
Purkinje cells also originates from extrafoveal regions.

Acknowledgements: This work was supported by Swiss National Foundation 3.343 - 2.78 and Deutsche Forschungsgemeinschaft SFB 200, A2. The authors wish to thank Mrs. Kosemetzky for typing the manuscript.

REFERENCES

Büttner U, Waespe W, Henn V (1981) The role of the cerebellum and the vestibular system in the generation of slow conjugate eye movements.
in: Neurogenetics and Neuro-ophthalmology.
Eds. A. Huber and D. Klein, pp. 89-102, Elsevier North-Holland Biomedical Press, Amsterdam

Cheng M, Outerbridge JS (1975) Optokinetic nystagmus during selective retinal stimulation.
Exp. Brain Res. 23, 129-139

Cohen B, Matsuo K, Raphan T (1977) Quantitative analysis of the velocity characteristics of optokinetic nystagmus and optokinetic after-nystagmus.
J. Physiol. 270, 321-344

Michalski A, Kossut M, Zernecki B (1977) The ocular following reflex elicited from the retinal periphery in the cat.
Vision Research 17, 731-736

Robinson DA (1980) in: Visual-vestibular interaction in motion perception and the generation of nystagmus.
Eds. V. Henn, B. Cohen, L.R. Young.
Neurosciences Research Program Bull. 18, Nr. 4

Stone J (1965) A quantitative analysis of the distribution of ganglion cells in the cat's retina.
J. Comp. Neurol. 124, 337-352

Winterson BJ, Steinman RM (1978) The effect of luminance on human smooth pursuit of perifoveal and foveal targets. Vision Res. 18, 1165-1172

Waespe W, Henn V (1977) Neuronal activity in the vestibular nuclei of the alert monkey during vestibular and optokinetic stimulation. Exp. Brain Res. 27, 523-538

Waespe W, Henn V (1981) Visual-vestibular interaction in the flocculus of the alert monkey. II Purkinje cell activity. Exp. Brain Res. 43, 349-360

THE ROLE OF CENTRAL AND PERIPHERAL RETINA IN ELICITING OPTOKINETIC NYSTAGMUS IN CATS

K.P. Hoffmann, H.P. Huber, C. Markner and M. Mayr
(Ulm, German Federal Republic)

INTRODUCTION

Considerable evidence has accumulated to support the idea that the nucleus tractus optici (NTO) in the pretectum of mammals plays a major role in controlling the optokinetic nystagmus (OKN) (for review see Collewijn, 1981; Hoffmann, 1981; Precht, 1981). In recent papers we have presented a map of the density or relative strength of the retinal projection to NTO neurons in the cat (Ballas, Hoffmann, Wagner, 1981; Hoffmann, Schoppmann, 1981). This map suggests that also in the cat the central retina (area centralis) has the strongest power to elicit the OKN. For man and rabbit the superiority of the central retina in producing a high gain of OKN has been shown already by Dubois and Collewijn, 1979. We propose here that the number of receptive fields of NTO neurons overlapping at a given eccentricity of the visual field correlates with the gain of OKN which is obtained from restricted stimulation at this location.

We tested the hypothesis in two ways: First we placed retinal lesions of different size in the central and peripheral retina by photocoagulation. Second we placed optical "lesions" at various eccentricities and with various diameters onto the retina by a stabilized image method. The results from both methods show that a strong OKN can be elicited from the area centralis as well as from the periphery of the retina. A decrease of closed loop gain due to the lesions is only seen with high stimulus velocities.

METHODS

Stimulation: Eye movements were elicited by the movement of a random dot pattern (dot size approximately 1° diameter) across a 90° by 90° screen 40 cm in front of the animal. This stimulus is different from the more commonly used optokinetic drum, providing full field stimulation. We chose our condition for several reasons. Firstly and most importantly, we wanted to test OKN with stimuli more or less identical to those used to test the neuronal responses in the NTO. Secondly, it was easy to test OKN in directions other than horizontal. Thirdly, being a possibly less powerful stimulus more subtle changes in the central pathways mediating OKN could be revealed because the contrast and size of the pattern could be easiliy varied. Of course, comparison of normal and experimental conditions were always carried out

Roucoux, A. and Crommelinck, M. (eds.): Physiological and Pathological Aspects of Eye Movements.
© *1982, Dr W. Junk Publishers, The Hague, Boston, London.* ISBN-13: 978-94-009-8002-0

using the same stimulus parameters. A film loop of random dot film was projected by a slide projector into the image plane of a second objective. In this plane an aluminium ring was moved by a double galvanometer system in horizontal and vertical directions. To this ring variable masks could be attached. A motor moved the random dot film through the image plane of the first objective. This stimulus movement was then projected through the second objective onto the screen. This stimulus evoked an eye movement which was recorded by the coil attached to the eye. The signal was fed to the galvanometers which moved the aluminium ring exactly proportional to the eye movements. Any mask attached to the ring was then seen as a stabilized image by the cat. In this way we could select any desired central or peripheral area on the retina for optokinetic stimulation.

Recording: Optokinetic nystagmus was measured by implanting a magnetic search coil to one or both eyes according to the technique as described by Judge, Richmond and Chu, 1980. In addition, head restraining bolts were attached to the skull by means of dental acrylic. Some days after surgery the animals were put into a horizontal and vertical alternating magnetic field for eye movement recording. We investigated the eye velocity in relation to stimulus velocity for stimulation of the two eyes separately and binocularly. Eye velocity was calculated from the eye position signal by on-line computer analysis. Data were stored on magnetic discs and could be displayed as eye velocity frequency histograms for individual velocities tested or as velocity tuning curves for all velocities tested (figure 1 and 2).

RESULTS

Retinal lesions were placed in the eyes of four cats by photocoagulation. In two animals a circular lesion about 6° - 10° diameter was centered on the area centralis. No deficit in OKN could be detected when the lesioned and non-lesioned eyes were compared. In two animals ellipsoid lesions, 20° - 40° horizontal, 10° - 20° vertical extent, centered on the area centralis were placed in the left eyes. At velocities above 10° per second this type of lesion led to a decrease in gain when compared to the non-lesioned eye. At lower velocities, OKN was normal. Additional large peripheral lesions, leaving intact only an about 20° diameter retinal patch, including the area centralis, were placed in the normal right eyes of the cats with central lesions in the left eye. The gain of OKN elicited through the eye with the peripheral lesion (right eye) was decreased at all velocities when compared to the prelesioned state and to the eye with the central lesion.
In summary, lesions of the central retina cause a small but significant decrease in gain of OKN at high stimulus velocities, whereas lesions of the peripheral retina cause a small but significant decrease at all velocities. The main result is, however, that possibly after a short recovery period a close to normal OKN can be elicited despite substantial retinal damage.

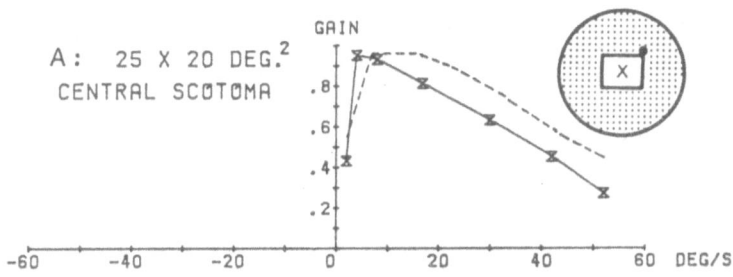

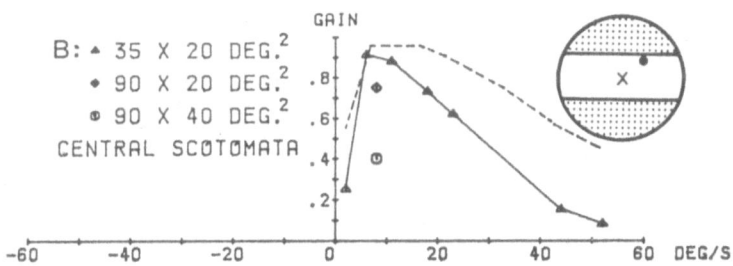

Figure 1: The effect of peripheral optokinetic stimulation (excluding the area centralis) on the gain of OKN at different velocities. The velocity of a random dot pattern moving in temporo-nasal direction across a 90° x 90° frontal screen is plotted on the X-axis. Gain of OKN (eye velocity : stimulus velocity) is plotted on the Y-axis.
A: An area of 25° horizontal and 20° vertical extent centered on the area centralis is excluded from optokinetic stimulation. The gain at velocities above 20°/sec (full line) is only about 75 % of the gain with full field stimulation (broken line).
B: An area of 35° x 20° stabilized and centered on the area centralis is excluded from optokinetic stimulation. The gain at velocities above 20°/sec is only 50 % of the gain with full field stimulation. If central areas with 90° horizontal and 20° or 40° vertical extent are not stimulated the gain decreases already at velocities below 20°/sec.

The only way to exclude fast recovery and to have continuous control by comparison to the normal performance is the placement of reversible "lesions" by masking or exposing various parts of the retina to an optokinetic stimulus.

In figure 1 we compare the effects of various central scotomata on the gain of OKN. A scotoma of less than 20° x 20° produced no difference in closed loop gain when compared to the OKN gain with full field (90° x 90°) stimulation. A central scotoma of 25° or 35° horizontal and 20° vertical extent produced clear deficits at higher (> 10°/sec) stimulus velocities (A, B). Leaving a horizontal streak 20° high across the entire retina unstimulated led to a clear drop in gain even at the optimal velocities. Extenting the unstimulated area to 40° vertical extent reduced the gain at the best velocity to 0.4 compared to close to 1 with full field stimulation (B).

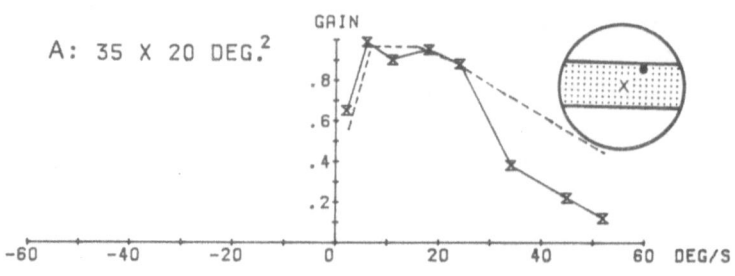

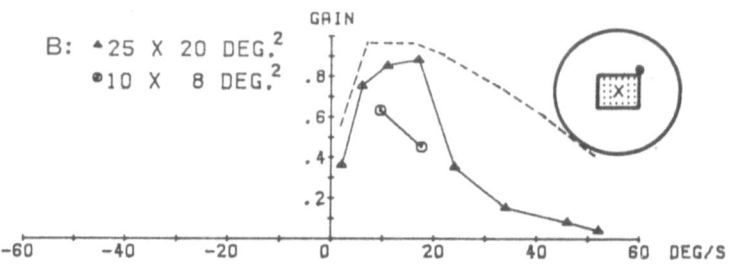

Figure 2: The effect of central optokinetic stimulation (exclu-ding the peripheral retina) on the gain of OKN at different velocities: X-axis represents stimulus velocity. Y-axis repre-sents closed loop gain (eye velocity : stimulus velocity).
A: The optokinetic stimulus is presented only in an area of 35° horizontal and 20° vertical extent stabilized and centered on the area centralis. At velocities above 30°/sec there is a decrease in gain compared to full field stimulation (broken line).
B: Areas of 25° x 20° and 10° x 8° extent centered on the area centralis OKN elicit only a low OKN gain. Again the clearest deficit is at high velocities.

Figure 2 demonstrates the effectiveness of pure central stimu-lation tested in the same eye in which the measurements of figure 1 were done. A 10° x 8° stimulated area centered on the area centralis evoked a weaker than normal OKN even at the optimal velocities. A 25° horizontal 20° vertical stimula-ted area evokes a good though still subnormal OKN at low velo-cities and shows a clear drop in gain at higher velocities (B). A 35° x 20° stimulated area evokes a normal OKN of velo-cities below 25°/sec but is deficient at higher velocities when compared to full field stimulation (A).

In a second type of experiment we tested for monocular viewing the contribution to OKN when a stimulus field of constant area is projected onto various retinal eccentricities. Figure 3 presents the results of such an experiment. The area centra-lis is the most effective OKN generator. The gain of OKN elici-ted from a 20° x 20° area shows a steep fall off when the area centralis is not included in the stimulated area. When the area centralis is included, however, in the stimulated area, OKN can be elicited in both horizontal directions almost

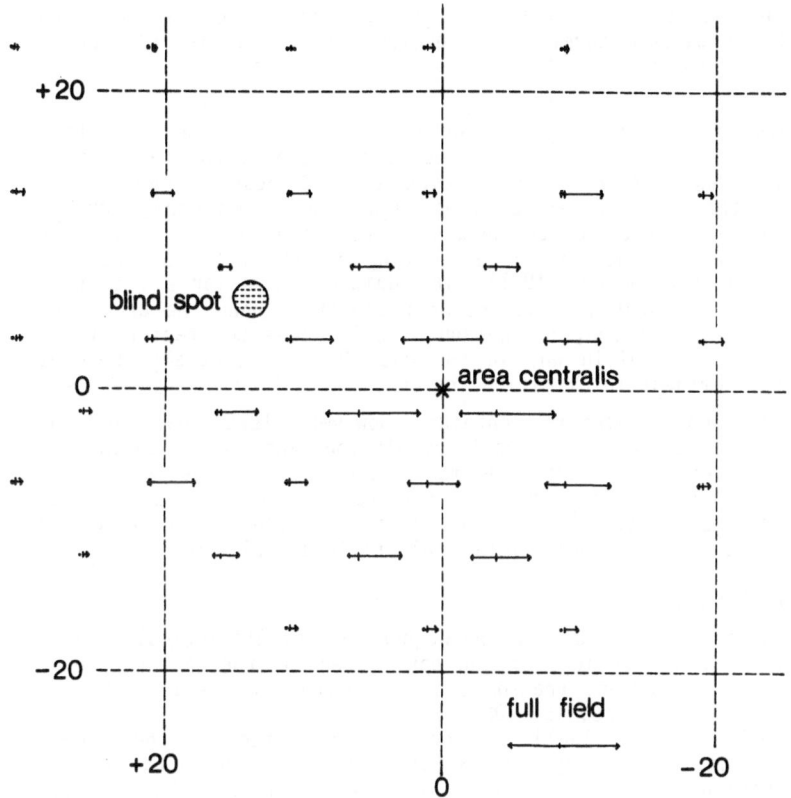

Figure 3: Map of the most effective locations on the retina for eliciting an optokinetic nystagmus. The stimulated area stabilized on the retina was 20° x 20°. The stimulus consisted of a random dot pattern moving at 20°/sec horizontally through this stimulus area. The arrows representing the gain of OKN (eye velocity : stimulus velocity in the closed loop condition) start at the center of the stimulated area and point to the right for the gain in response to temporo-nasal stimulus direction and to the left for naso-temporal stimulus direction. The gain for full field stimulation is presented at the lower right. It can be clearly seen that the most effective site to elicit OKN is around the area centralis.

equally well. On the other hand a clear assymetry, i.e. a higher gain for stimulus movement from temporal to nasal appears for peripheral stimuli, irrespective whether the stimulated area is in the nasal or temporal retina.

DISCUSSION

These results fully confirm the observation with retinal lesions placed by photocoagulation and indicate that restricted central stimulation as well as only peripheral stimulation elicits a close to normal OKN at low velocities. At higher velocities area centralis and peripheral retina have to be stimulated together to develop a high gain for slow phase eye movements in OKN.

The gain of OKN with temporo-nasally directed stimulus movement as indicated in figure 3 by the rightward pointing arrows at various eccentricities corresponds to the relative frequency of receptive fields of NTO neurons overlapping in the area stimulated (see figure 4a in Hoffmann, Schoppmann, 1981) or to the number of ganglion cells from various retinal eccentricities projecting to the NTO (see Ballas, Hoffmann, Wagner, 1981). In addition, the large receptive fields of NTO neurons are most sensitive near the area centralis (Hoffmann, Schoppmann, 1981). These two factors together may explain why in the cat the area centralis becomes so prominent in eliciting the OKN.

The area centralis contains, however, less than 10 % of the total ganglion cell population and large peripheral stimulus areas activate many more ganglion cells than a 10° central stimulus. Therefor it is not astonishing that lesions of the area centralis have little or no effect on OKN under the condition of whole field stimulation.

REFERENCES

Ballas, I, Hoffmann KP and Wagner, H-J (1981) Retinal projection to the nucleus of the optic tract in the cat as revealed by retrograde transport of horseradish peroxidase, Neurosci. Letters, 26, 197-202.
Collewijn, H (1981) The oculomotor system of the rabbit and its plasticity, in: Studies of Brain Function, Vol. 5, (Barlow, Bullock, Florey, Grüsser, van der Loos, eds.) Springer, Berlin, Heidelberg, New York.
Dubois, MFW and Collewijn, H (1979) Optokinetic reactions in man elicited by localized retinal motion stimuli, Vision Res., 10. 1105-1115.
Hoffmann, KP (1981) Neuronal responses related to optokinetic nystagmus in the cat's nucleus of the optic tract, in: Progress in Oculomotor Research (Fuchs, Becker, eds.), Elsevier North Holland, 443-454.
Hoffmann, KP and Schoppmann, A (1981) A quantitative analysis of the direction-specific response of neurons in the cat's nucleus of the optic tract, Exp. Brain Res., 42, 146-157.
Judge, SJ, Richmond, BF and Chu, FC (1980) Implantation of magnetic search coils for measurement of eye position: an improved method, Vision Res., 20, 535-538.
Precht, W (1981) Functional organization of optokinetic pathways in mammals, in: Progress in Oculomotor Research (Fuchs and Becker, eds.), Elsevier North Holland, 425-433.

POSSIBLE CONTRIBUTION OF THE CORTICAL AREAS 17, 18 and 19
TO THE OPTOKINETIC RESPONSE IN THE CAT

G.A. ORBAN, J. DUYSENS, H. KENNEDY (Katholieke Universiteit
te Leuven, Lab. Neuro- en Psychofysiologie, Campus Gasthuisberg,
B-3000 Leuven, Belgium)

According to Wood et al. (1973) ablation of areas 17, 18 and 19
of the cat, produces a marked reduction in the gain of the
monocular OKN in the naso-temporal direction. Such a deficit can
also be produced by rearing conditions such as dark rearing
(Harris et al. 1980) and strobe rearing (Amblard et al. 1981),
which are known to disturb visual cortical cell functions
(Leventhal, Hirsh 1980; Orban et al. 1978). From these results,
it has been suggested (Harris et al. 1980; Hoffmann 1981) that
the visual afferences of OKN, reach the motor stages both through
a cortical loop (movement in the naso-temporal direction) and a
subcortical loop (movement in the temporo-nasal direction. Since
the OKN requires information on the direction of motion of the
visual field over the retina, we have investigated the direction
selectivity of areas 17, 18 and 19 of the cat (Orban et al.
1981b; Duysens et al. 1982).
Single cells were recorded in areas 17, 18 and 19 of
paralyzed and lightly anesthetized cats using standard electrophysiological techniques. The RFs of the cells were localized in
the lower contralateral quadrant. The direction selectivity was
investigated with computer-controlled stimuli rear projected on
a screen and moving back and forth on the optimal axis, determined
by hand plotting. Stimuli were narrow, high contrast (c = .85)
light slits of optimal length and orientation. Direction
selectivity was evaluated over a wide range of velocities
(.3 to 700 deg/sec) with a multihistogram technique producing
a set of interleaved post stimulus time histograms (PSTHs)
(Maes, Orban 1980). The response was defined as the maximum
firing rate evaluated from the PSTH bin (bin width 8 msec) with
the highest spike count. For each stimulus velocity, direction
selectivity was estimated by the direction index (DI) which
compares the response in the two opposite directions along the
optimal axis : $DI = \dfrac{R_p - R_{Np}}{R_p} \times 100$, where R_p and R_{Np} are net
responses in the preferred and nonpreferred direction respectively
and which have to be significant (i.e. exceed mean maximum firing
rate + 2 sd).
Since the DI changes as a function of velocity in many
cortical cells (see Fig. 1A), we used a weighted mean to
characterize the direction selectivity of a cell :

Roucoux, A. and Crommelinck, M. (eds.): Physiological and Pathological Aspects of Eye Movements.
© *1982, Dr W. Junk Publishers, The Hague, Boston, London.* ISBN-13: 978-94-009-8002-0

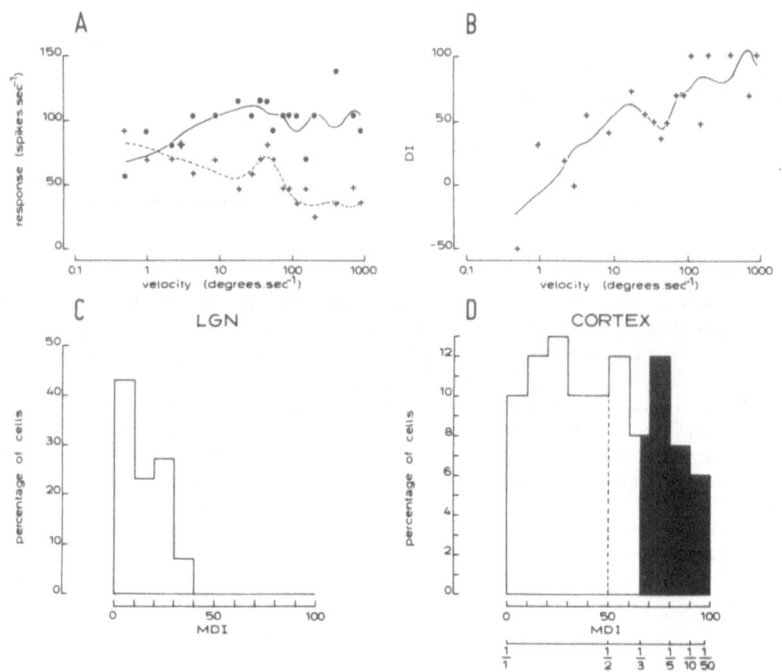

FIGURE 1. (A) Example of velocity-response (VR) curve in preferred direction (PD) (solid line) and nonpreferred direction (NPD) (dashed line) of a cell at the border of areas 17 and 18. Horizontal line : significance level (mean maximum firing rate + 2 sd). (B) DI-velocity relationship of the corresponding cell. (C) Distribution of absolute mean DI (MDI) among LGN cells (N = 44) and among cortical cells. (D) (Areas 17, 18 and 19, total = 283). Ratios between preferred direction (PD) and nonpreferred direction (NPD) are indicated below the corresponding MDIs. Open area : nondirection selective (NDS) cells, hatching : direction asymmetric (DA) cells, dark area : direction selective cells.

$$\sum_{i=1}^{n} \frac{R_{pi} \; DI_i}{\sum_{i=1}^{n} R_{pi}},$$ where R_{pi} is the net response in the preferred

direction at a given velocity and DI_i the direction index of that velocity (n = 20). Cells having a MDI below 50 were considered as nondirection selective (NDS), those with a MDI over 66 as direction selective (DS) and those with intermediate MDIs as direction asymmetric (DA). A companion study of 44 LGN cells (Orban et al. 1981), showed that none of the LGN cells had a MDI over 40, indicating that direction asymmetry and selectivity as we define it, are cortical properties (compare Fig. 1C to 1D).

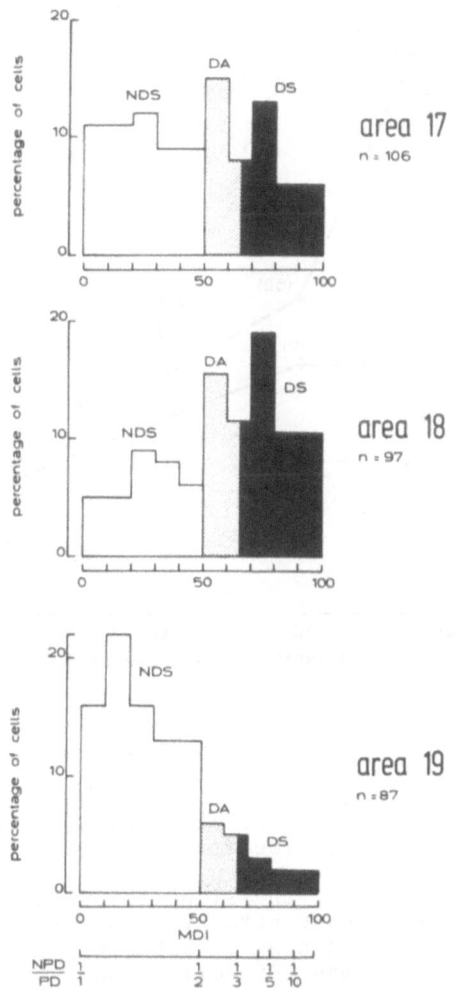

FIGURE 2. Distribution of MDIs in areas 17, 18 and 19. Same
conventions as in figure 1.

　　　Figure 2 compares the amount of direction selectivity
in about equal samples of the three cortical areas (Orban et al.
1981b; Duysens et al. 1982). Clearly the largest proportion of
DS cells occurs in area 18, while area 19 has few DS cells. These
differences hold even when one considers the different RF types,
in particular the C family cells which project subcortically
(Orban 1982). The differences between the areas are more striking
if one considers different eccentricity classes within each area
(Fig. 3). In this figure, results from recent experiments on
102 area 17 cells and 38 area 18 cells have been added to the
samples of Fig. 2. In all three areas the proportion of DS cells

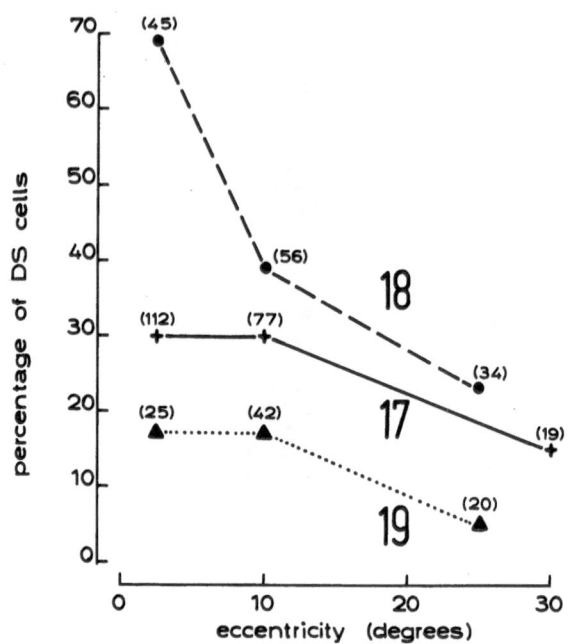

FIGURE 3. Proportion of DS cells plotted as a function of
eccentricity of the RF for 3 cortical areas (17, 18 and 19).
The three eccentricity classes are 0-5°, 5-15° and larger
than 15°. The number between brackets indicate the number of
cells used to calculate the proportions.

decreases with eccentricity, the slope being steepest in
area 18. Area 18 subserving central vision (0-5°) has more than
twice as many DS cells than area 17 subserving the same region
and more than 4 times as many DS cells than the equivalent part
of area 19. This suggests that the signals carrying information
on the direction of movement arise mainly from area 18 (and to
some extend from area 17), subserving central vision and not
from area 19.
     There are important differences between the direction
selective cells of both areas. Area 17 cells are responsive to
slower velocities than area 18 cells (Orban et al. 1981a). In
addition the preferred directions of DS cells are different in
the 2 areas. Area 17 DS cells prefer direction on the vertical
and horizontal axes whereas area 18 DS cells prefer direction
away from the fixation point into the contralateral visual
field (Fig. 4). Since the cortical loop is binocular (Hoffmann
1973) it may well be that the bias of the preferred direction
is in terms of the visual field.

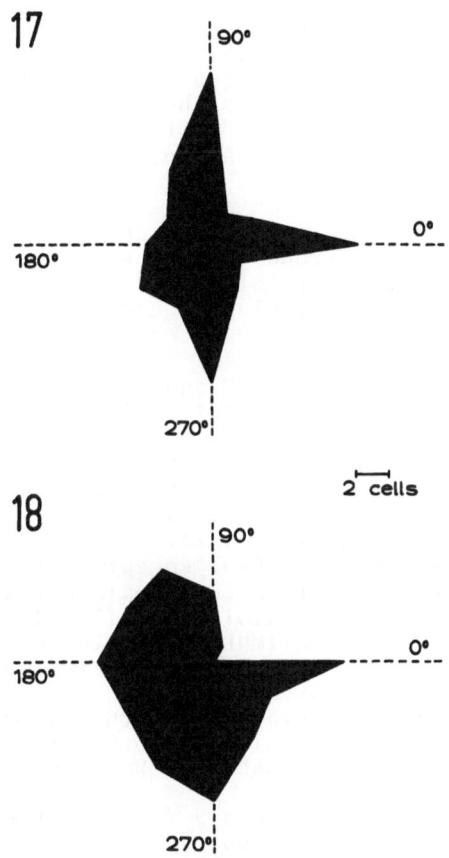

FIGURE 4. Preferred directions in the visual field of area 17 (A) and area 18 (B) DS cells of the left hemisphere. 0° indicates movements to the left and 90° upward movements. All the RFs were located in the lower contralateral (i.e. right) visual quadrant or in the contralateral horizontal meridian. The preference of area 17 DS cells for principal axes is significant ($\chi^2 = 10.7$, $p < 0.005$). The absence of area 18 cells preferring 15 to 75° directions (i.e. the direction of the fixation point, given the localization of the RFs) is significant ($\chi^2 = 10$, $p < 0.005$).

In conclusion our results show that area 18 and to a lesser extend area 17 could make a substantial contribution to the cortical afferent loop of OKN. Both areas project to the pretectum (Schoppmann 1981). The relative importance of both areas may depend on the stimulus conditions as e.g. the stimulus velocity. In addition area 18 would appear to have an overall bias in its preferred direction (naso-temporal) and it is precisely this direction which is absent in the monocular OKN of the decorticate cat. Our results further stress the importance of central vision for the cortical loop.

REFERENCES
Amblard B, Courjon JH, Cremieux J, Flandrin JM and Kennedy H (1981) The influence of stroboscopic rearing on the optokinetic nystagmus in the cat, J. Physiol. (Lond.) 316, 74P-75P.
Duysens J, Orban GA, van der Glas HW and de Zegher FE (1982) Functional properties of area 19 as compared to area 17 of the cat, Brain Res. 231, 279-291.
Harris LR, Leporé F, Guillemot JP and Cynader M (1980) Abolition of optokinetic nystagmus in the cat, Science 210, 91-92.
Hoffmann KP (1973) Conduction velocity in pathways from retina to superior colliculus in the cat : a correlation with receptive-field properties, J. Neurophysiol. 36, 409-424.
Hoffmann KP (1981) Naso-temporal versus temporo-nasal OKN in the cat, Soc. Neurosci. Abstr. 7, 23.
Leventhal AG and Hirsch HVB (1980) Receptive-field properties of different classes of neurons in visual cortex of normal and dark-reared cats. J. Neurophysiol. 43, 1111-1132.
Maes H and Orban GA (1980) STIMUL : stimulus control and multihistogram analysis of single neurone recordings, Med. & Biol. Eng. & Comput. 18, 569-572.
Orban GA (1982) Neuronal operations in the visual cortex. In Braitenberg V, Barlow HB, Bizzi E, Grüsser OJ and van der Loos H ed. Studies of Brain Function, Springer Verlag, Berlin, in press.
Orban GA, Hoffmann KP and Duysens J (1981) Influence of stimulus velocity on LGN neurons. Soc. Neurosci. Abstr. 7, 24.
Orban GA, Kennedy H, Maes H and Amblard B (1978) Cats reared in stroboscopic illumination : velocity characteristics of area 18 neurons, Arch. ital. Biol. 116, 413-419.
Orban GA, Kennedy H and Maes H (1981a) Response to movement of neurons in areas 17 and 18 of the cat : velocity sensitivity. J. Neurophysiol. 45, 1043-1058.
Orban GA, Kennedy H and Maes H (1981b) Response to movement of neurons in areas 17 and 18 of the cat : direction selectivity. J. Neurophysiol. 45, 1059-1073.
Schoppmann A (1981) Projection from areas 17 and 18 of the visual cortex to the nucleus of the optic tract, Brain Res. 223, 1-18.
Wood CC, Spear PD and Braun JJ (1973) Direction-specific deficits in horizontal optokinetic nystagmus following removal of visual cortex in the cat, Brain Res. 60, 231-237.

INFLUENCE OF BILATERAL PLUGS OF PAIRS OF SEMICIRCULAR
CANALS ON OPTOKINETIC AND VESTIBULOOCULAR REFLEXES

N. H. BARMACK (The Biological Sciences Group, The
University of Connecticut, Storrs, CT, USA)

1. INTRODUCTION
The participation of the vestibular nuclei in the
control of reflexive eye movements is emphasized by the
physiologically demonstrated convergence of vestibular,
neck proprioceptive and visual information onto
secondary neurons (Henn et al, 1974; Keller, Daniels,
1975; Rubin et al, 1977). This sensory convergence is
also reflected in the deficits in reflexive eye
movements caused by damage to the vestibular apparatus.
Bilateral labyrinthectomies and neurectomies not only
abolish vestibuloocular reflexes, but also reduce the
gain of optokinetic reflexes and shorten the duration
of optokinetic after-nystagmus in cats (Capps, Roth,
1978), monkeys (Cohen et al, 1973), humans (Zee et al,
1976) and rabbits (Baarsma, Collewijn, 1974; Barmack
et al, 1980; Collewijn, 1976). One possible
explanation for the reduction in gain of the HOKR
caused by bilateral labyrinthectomies is that the
spontaneous activity of secondary vestibular neurons is
reduced by the loss of spontaneous primary afferent
input. The consequent reduction in secondary
vestibular neuronal activity would restrict of
discharge frequencies over which this activity could be
modulated by other sensory inputs; specifically
vision. It is possible to eliminate modulated primary
afferent activity without depressing spontaneous
primary afferent activity by plugging the membranous
portion of selected semicircular canals, thereby
preventing movement of the endolymph relative to the
ampulla of the plugged canal. The present experiment
was undertaken with the purpose of testing whether the
HOKR would be influenced by this canal plugging
procedure. The second aim of this experiment was to
determine if the effects of bilateral plugs of the
horizontal semicircular canals on the gain and phase of
the HVOR were reversible.

2. PROCEDURE
2.1. Methods
Fifteen rabbits were subjected to either bilateral
plugs of the horizontal or anterior semicircular
canals. The horizontal optokinetic reflex (HOKR),
horizontal vestibuloocular reflex (HVOR), and vertical
vestibuloocular reflex (VVOR) were tested before and
after the plugging operation, and at various times
following the removal of the plugs. Plugs were
constructed from silver wire formed into a spindle
under heat. After a small opening was made in the bony
portion of the semicircular canals at least one mm from

Roucoux, A. and Crommelinck, M. (eds.): Physiological and Pathological Aspects of Eye Movements.
© 1982, Dr W. Junk Publishers, The Hague, Boston, London. ISBN-13: 978-94-009-8002-0

the ampullae in anesthetized rabbits, plugs were inserted into the semicircular canals where they compressed the membranous labyrinth. The plugs were left in place for 24-48 hr, after which the rabbits re-anesthetized and the plugs were removed (Figure 1).

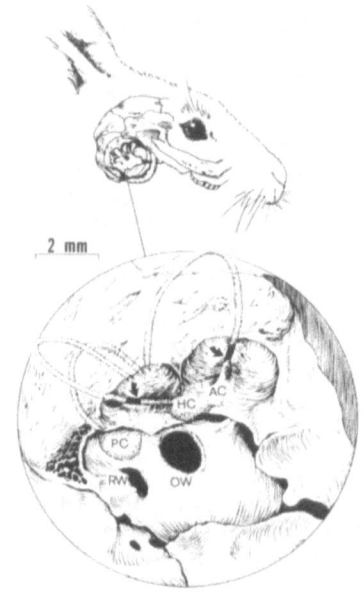

Figure 1. Illustration of the labyrinth of the rabbit. The arrows indicate where plugs are inserted into the horizontal and anterior semicircular canals. Abbreviations: AC, HC, PC - ampullae of the anterior, horizontal, and posterior semicircular canals; RW, round window; OW, oval window.

The HOKR was evoked by monocular closed-loop optokinetic stimulation with a contour-rich pattern rear-projected onto a tangent screen which subtended   72 x 72 degrees of visual angle. The HVOR was evoked by sinusoidal oscillation of the rabbit in a rate table about the earth vertical axis (Barmack, 1981).

3. RESULTS
Bilateral plugs of the horizontal semicircular canals reduced the gain of the HVOR to less than .03 over the entire range of frequencies examined, .01-.80 Hz (Figure 2). This reduction in HVOR gain was equivalent to that produced by bilateral labyrinthectomy with the exception of the residual gain of .03 present in bilaterally plugged animals at stimulus frequencies above .1 Hz. Bilateral plugs of the horizontal semicircular canals caused only a nominal decrease in the monocularly-evoked HOKR (Figure 3). This small reduction can be compared with a much larger reduction in the gain of the HOKR following bilateral labyrinthectomies (Figure 3). Bilateral plugs of the horizontal semicircular canals caused no decrement in the gain of the VVOR (Figure 4). Conversely, bilateral

plugs of the anterior semicircular canals did cause a
reduction in the gain and an increase in the phase lead
of the HVOR (Figure 5). This reduction in gain was
completely reversible following removal of the plugs of
the anterior semicircular canals. The gain of the VVOR
also returned to normal when tested 150 days after the
bilateral plugs of the anterior semicircular canals
were removed (Figure 5).

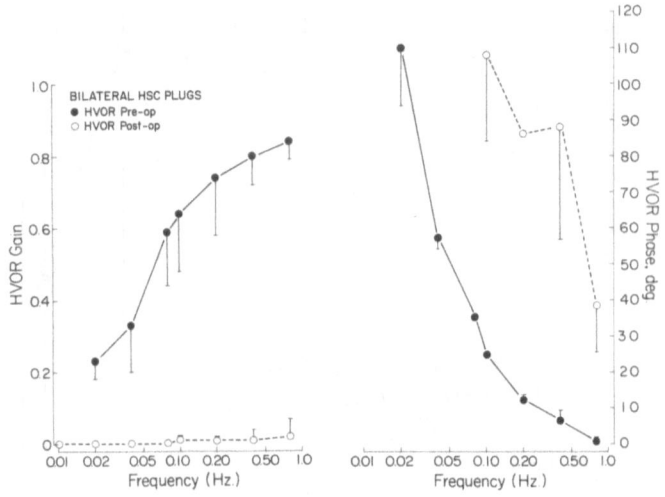

Figure 2. The influence of bilateral plugs of
the horizontal semicircular canals on the
horizontal vestibuloocular reflex (HVOR). The
HVOR of five rabbits was tested before (filled
circles) and 24-48 hr after (open circles)
bilateral plugs of the horizontal semicircular
canals were made. One standard deviation is
illustrated for each data point for this and
subsequent figures.

The time course of the recovery of the gain of the HVOR
was studied in five rabbits at two different
frequencies, .1 and .8 Hz. The recovery of the gain of
the HVOR, tested at .8 Hz, was complete within ten days
following the removal of the plugs of the horizontal
semicircular canals. However, the gain of the HVOR,
tested at .1 Hz, did not fully recover. Twenty days
after the plugs were removed, the gain of the HVOR
tested at .1 Hz recovered to about 70% of its
pre-operative value (Figure 6).

196

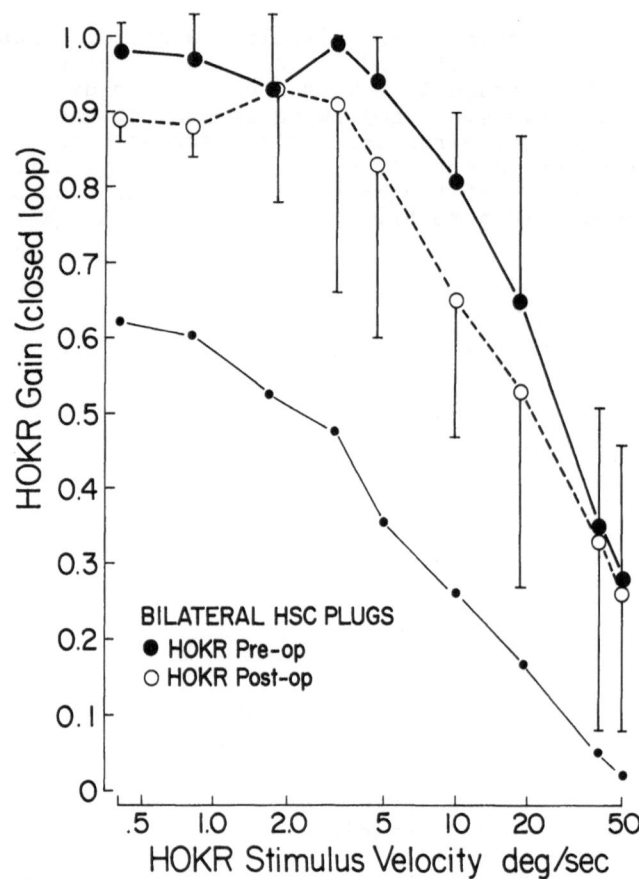

Figure 3. The influence of bilateral plugs of the horizontal semicircular canals on the HOKR. The HOKR was tested in four rabbits before (filled circles) and 24-48 hours after (open circles) bilateral plugs of the horizontal semicircular canals were made. The HOKR was also tested in four rabbits after bilateral labyrinthectomies (smaller filled circles).

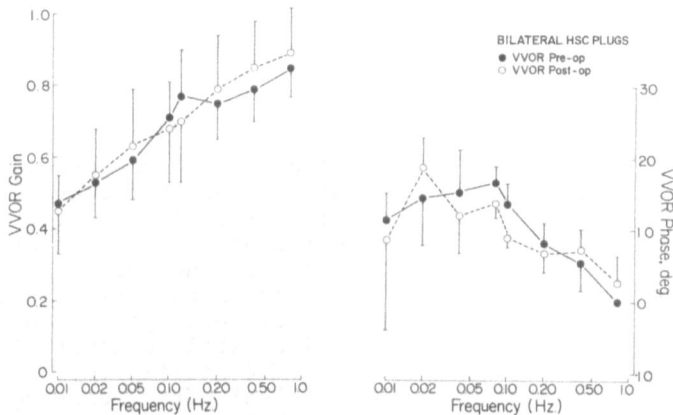

Figure 4. The influence of bilateral plugs of
the horizontal semicircular canals on the VVOR.
The VVOR of five rabbits was tested before
(filled circles) and 24-48 hr after (open
circles) bilateral plugs were made in the
horizontal semicircular canals. Note that these
plugs did not affect the gain or phase of the
VVOR.

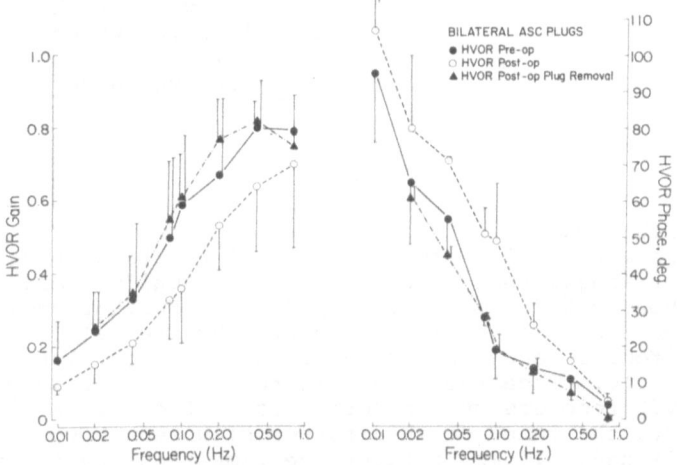

Figure 5. The influence of bilateral plugs of
the anterior semicircular canals on the HVOR.
The HVOR was measured in five rabbits before
plugs were inserted bilaterally in the anterior
semicircular canals (filled circles), 24-48 hr
after the plugs were inserted (open circles),
and 150 days after the bilateral plugs were
removed (filled triangles). Note that the
bilateral plugs of the anterior semicircular
canals caused a consistent reduction in gain of
HVOR, which recovered upon removal of the plugs.

198

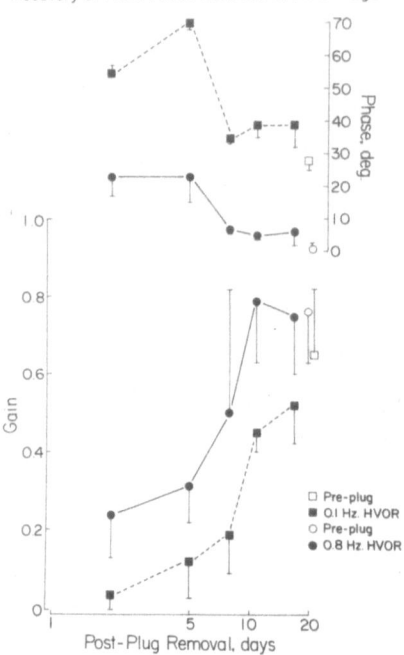

Figure 6. Recovery of the HVOR after the removal of bilateral plugs of the horizontal semicircular canals. The HVOR was tested in five rabbits at two different frequencies, 0.1 Hz (filled squares) and 0.8 Hz (filled circles) after removing the bilateral plugs of the horizontal semicircular canals. The pre-operative values for the gain and phase at these two different frequencies are illustrated by the open symbols. Note that the gain of the HVOR at 0.8 Hz recovered completely, but that the gain of the HVOR at 0.1 Hz recovered to only 70% of its preoperative value.

4. DISCUSSION

The present results demonstrate that bilateral plugs of the horizontal semicircular canals virtually abolish the HVOR, but do not impair the HOKR. Furthermore, the influence of bilateral plugs of the horizontal semicircular canals on the HVOR is almost completely reversible. Once the plugs are removed, the gain of the HVOR recovers over a period of 5-20 days. At present, the cause of this rather slow recovery remains unexplained. It may reflect the time required for the membranous labyrinth to regain its "pre-compressed" diameter, or it may reflect a form of neural adaptation of secondary vestibular neurons to the loss and subsequent recovery of a modulated primary afferent signal.

Of particular interest in the present experiment is the observation that bilateral plugs of the horizontal semicircular canals do not impair the VVOR, but that bilateral plugs of the anterior semicircular canals do cause a reduction in gain and an increase in phase of the HVOR. If the semicircular canals of the rabbit were truly orthogonal, this result would not be expected. However, the plane of the anterior semicircular canal near its ampulla forms an angle of approximately 95 degrees with respect to the plane of the horizontal semicircular canal, near its ampulla. These two semicircular canals also share a common ampullo-utricular duct which is roughly co-planar with the toroid of the anterior semicircular canal, but which is almost orthogonal to the plane of the horizontal semicircular canal. This shared ampullo-utricular duct is approximately 2.2 mm long in the rabbit. At present, it is not known whether the horizontal and anterior semicircular canals share a common membranous passage through this funnel-shaped ampullo-utricular bony duct.

The possibility that the plugging technique causes some damage to the labyrinth cannot be ruled out entirely. However, the functional evidence from these experiments, and the electrophysiological evidence from the experiments of others (Abends, 1978) suggest that the neural apparatus of the ampullae of the semicircular canals remains functionally intact if the membranous labyrinth is not ruptured by the plugging operation.

5. REFERENCES

Abend WK (1978) Response to constant angular acceleration of neurons in the monkey superior vestibular nucleus, Exp. Brain Res. 31, 459-473.

Baarsma EA, Collewijn H (1974) Vestibulo-ocular and optokinetic reactions to rotation and their interaction in the rabbit, J. Physiol. (Lond.) 238, 603-625.

Barmack NH (1981) A comparison of the horizontal and vertical vestibuloocular reflexes of the rabbit, J. Physiol. (Lond.) 314, 547-564.

Barmack NH, Pettorossi VE, Erickson RG (1980) The influence of bilateral labyrinthectomy on horizontal and vertical optokinetic reflexes in the rabbit, Brain Research 196, 520-524.

Barmack NH, Pettorossi VE, Nastos MA (1981) The horizontal and vertical cervicoocular reflexes of the rabbit, Brain Research 224, 261-278.

Capps MJ, Roth JA (1978) Visually evoked eye movements: effects of labyrinthectomy, Exp. Neurol. 58, 251-260.

Cohen B, Uemura T, Takemori S (1973) Effects of labyrinthectomy on optokinetic nystagmus (OKN) and optokinetic after-nystagmus (OKAN), Equilibrium Res. 3, 88-93.

Collewijn H (1976) Impairment of optokinetic (after-)nystagmus by labyrinthectomy in the rabbit, Exp. Neurol. 52, 146-156.

Erickson RG, Barmack NH (1980) A comparison of the horizontal and vertical optokinetic reflexes of the rabbit, Exp. Brain Res. 40, 448-456.

Henn V, Young LR, Finley C (1974) Vestibular nucleus
units in alert monkeys are also influenced by moving
fields, Brain Research 71, 144-149.
Keller EL, Daniels PD (1975) Oculomotor related
interaction of vestibular and visual stimulation in
vestibular nucleus cells in alert monkey,
Exp. Neurol. 46, 187-198.
Rubin AM, Liedgren SCR, Milne AC, Young JA, Fredrickson
JM (1977) Vestibular and somatosensory interaction in
the cat vestibular nuclei, Pflugers
Arch. ges. Physiol. 371, 155-160.
Zee DS, Yee RD, Robinson DA (1976) Optokinetic
responses in labyrinthine-defective human beings, Brain
Research 113, 423-428.

VESTIBULOOCULAR AND OPTOKINETIC REFLEX COMPENSATION
FOLLOWING HEMILABYRINTHECTOMY IN THE CAT

C. MAIOLI, W. PRECHT, S. RIED
Institut für Hirnforschung, Universität Zürich, Zürich

1. INTRODUCTION

Numerous studies have been performed on behavioral compensation following hemilabyrinthectomy (HL), but most
of them dealt mainly with compensation of the static
imbalance induced by the lesion, i.e. postural asymmetries and spontaneous nystagmus, and relatively few studies have been devoted to the modifications of the dynamic vestibular reflexes. It is well known that compensation of the postural deficits is remarkably good, especially in higher mammals (Schaefer, Meyer, 1974). By contrast, the few studies on the recovery of dynamic reflexes, e.g. the vestibuloocular reflex (VOR), indicate
that some deficits persist even many months after the
lesion when tested in the dark (Moran, 1974; Baarsma,
Collewijn, 1975; Wolfe, Kos, 1977). However, a complete
description of the long and short term modifications of
the VOR after hemilabyrinthectomy is missing. The aim
of this paper was to investigate the time course of dynamic reflex compensation, here of the VOR after hemilabyrinthectomy in the cat and to compare it with the
recovery of the postural symptoms. In addition, OKN has
also been studied, given that bilateral labyrinthectomy
strongly impaires OKN (Cohen et al., 1973).

2. RESULTS AND DISCUSSION

2.1. Compensation of dynamic reflexes

Fig.1 shows the postoperative time course of VOR gain
measured in the dark in 10 cats operated at adult ages.
Gain was computed as the ratio between maximum nystagmic slow phase eye velocity and maximum stimulus velocity. Stimuli consisted of velocity steps and sinusoidal
oscillations (0.05 to 1.0 Hz) about the vertical axis.
Data obtained from the two types of stimulations were
pooled together as they gave identical gain values. From
8 of these animals control data were also measured prior
to the lesion (not shown in Fig.1). If care was taken
not to saturate the system with too strong stimuli, the
mean VOR gain in intact animals was 0.97 (SD=0.08).
Acutely after the lesion (days 1-4) we observed: 1) a
drop in gain of more than 50% on rotations to both direc-

Supported by grants Nos. 3.505.79 and 3.616.80 from
the Swiss National Science Foundation and the Dr. Eric
Slack-Gyr Foundation and SFB45 of the German Research
Council

Roucoux, A. and Crommelinck, M. (eds.): Physiological and Pathological Aspects of Eye Movements.
© *1982, Dr W. Junk Publishers, The Hague, Boston, London.* ISBN-13: 978-94-009-8002-0

202

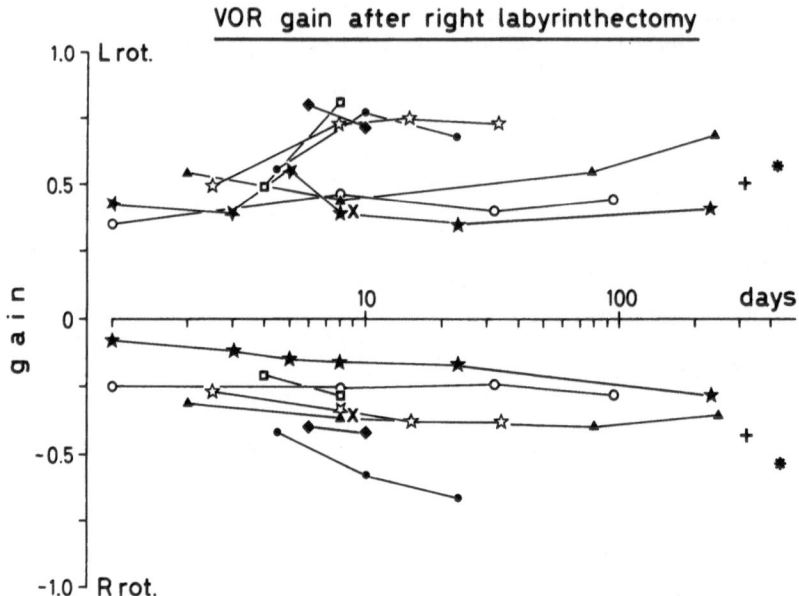

VOR gain after right labyrinthectomy

FIGURE 1. Time course of VOR gain in 10 adult cats that
underwent a labyrinthectomy on the right side. Chronically implanted EOG electrodes were used to record eye
movements. When spontaneous nystagmus was present, its
slow phase velocity was subtracted from the responses.

tions; 2) a marked VOR asymmetry, as the gain during rotation towards the lesioned side was much lower than that
to the opposite direction (mean=0.61X; SD=0.20). Between
5 and 10 days postoperatively the gain values of the
animals fell in two groups. One group increased abruptly
the gain when rotated towards the intact side, while in
the other group the gain remained low. However, this
change was not accompanied by any improvement in symmetry. From this time on, modifications occurred very
slowly. There was a small further increase in the absolute gain, but control values were never reached again.
A good degree of VOR symmetry is reached only after about
1 year.
Looking at the phase of the VOR responses to sinusoidal
oscillations we also found long-term deficits. Responses
recorded 7 to 10 days after the lesion (Fig. 2B) had a
larger phase lead of about 10° over the whole frequency
range tested as compared to control values obtained from
the same animals (Fig.2A). This larger phase lead was
still present 10 to 22 months postoperatively (Fig.2C).
The parallel phase shift typical of hemilabyrinthectomized animals showed up even more clearly when the mean
values for each frequency were plotted for each group of
animals (Fig.2D).

Considering now the responses of the hemilabyrinthectomized animals to pure optokinetic stimulation, a marked
asymmetry was noted immediately after the lesion. In
fact, when the visual scene moved towards the intact
side, almost no OKN was elicited, whereas responses to
opposite pattern rotations were basically normal. In
about half of the animals tested many months post-operatively (up to 1 year or more) this asymmetry persisted
almost unchanged (Fig.3); in the other animals OKN was
again symmetrical. It is also interesting to note that

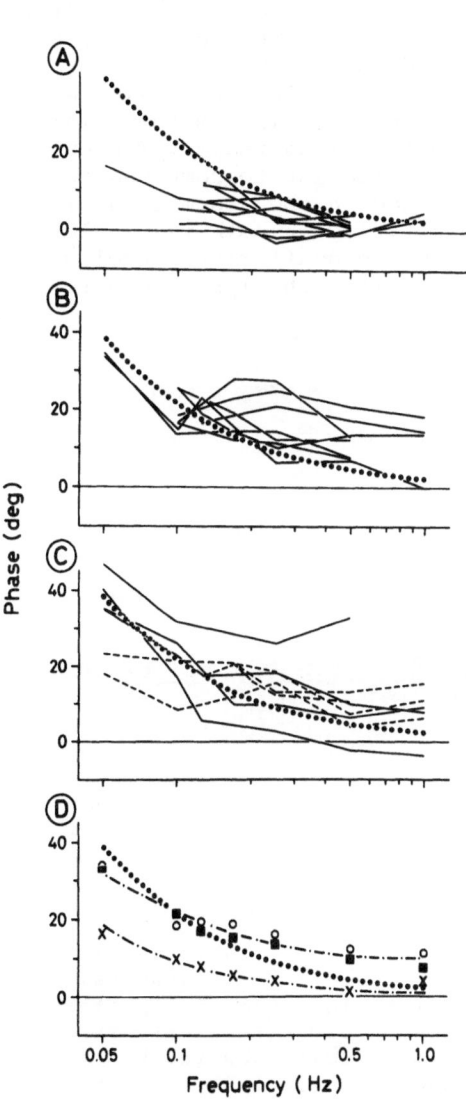

FIGURE 2. VOR phase in
relation to frequency
of sinusoidal oscilla-
tions measured at dif-
ferent times before and
after HL. The dotted
lines indicate in all
the panels the theore-
tical values that we
would observe if the
VOR were dominated by
the time constant of
the canals (4 sec).
A) Control values.
B) Values measured 7 to
10 days after the le-
sions in the same ani-
mals shown in A.
C) Values measured 10
to 22 months post-ope-
ratively. The animals
are different from A
and B except for two.
Dashed lines represent
cats lesioned at the
age of 6 weeks.
In B and C the phases
for stimuli to both di-
rections were symmetri-
cal. D) Mean values for
each frequency for each
group of animals. Cros-
ses, control; squares,
7-10 days post-operati-
vely; circles, 10-22
months post-operatively.
The curves fitting the
experimental data are
also plotted. Values
from acute and chronic
cats were pooled to-
gether.

VOR and OKN do not recover in a parallel way, i.e. a well compensated OKN may still be accompanied by a low gain and asymmetrical VOR. In our sample we never observed the opposite.

2.2. <u>Comparison of compensation of static imbalance and dynamic VOR</u>

From the above analysis it became clear that recovery of the dynamic VOR was far from being complete. However, in our cats a remarkable improvement of the postural symptoms was present already within the first week after the lesion. In particular, the lesion-evoked spontaneous nystagmus had almost completely subsided after the first 3-4 days. In remarkable contrast to this recovery no appreciable improvement in VOR gain or symmetry was observed. In general, we found no correlation at all between compensation of static and dynamic symptoms. This was quite surprising for the following reason. The current view about the mechanisms leading to compensation of postural asymmetries is based on the assumption of a rebalancing of the resting activity in both vestibular nuclei, since the activity in the deafferented nucleus is strongly depressed acutely after the lesion and re-

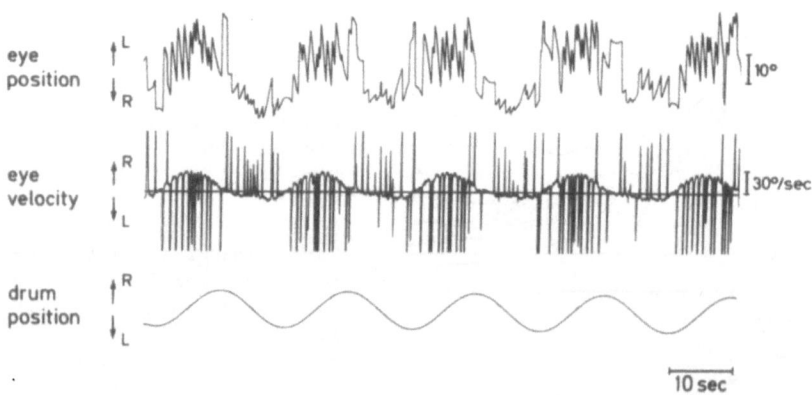

FIGURE 3. OKN recorded 10 months after right labyrinthectomy. The optokinetic drum was oscillated sinusoidally at 0.05 Hz (±25°/sec). A full field random dot pattern was used as a visual stimulus. A clear asymmetry is present even if the maximum drum velocity was reached very slowly, which normally enhances considerably the OKN performance.

turns, though not quite completely to control levels, with time elapsing after lesion (see Precht, 1974). This latter condition would then be very close to the unila- teral plugging of the semicircular canals, which renders central vestibular neurons functionally deafferented without abolishing the normal symmetrical tonic input from the canal periphery. When the VOR was studied in unilaterally canal-plugged animals (e.g. Zuckermann, 1967; Barmack, Pettorossi, 1981) it was found that the VOR gain droped approximately by half but that the responses remained - unlike with hemilabyrinthectomy - symmet- rical. Assuming similarity of the two conditions and that balance of bilateral vestibular activity is respon- sible for postural balance one would expect symmetrical VORs in both cases. That the two conditions are, in fact, very different will be shown in the last section. The explanation for the gain decrease comes from the work of Abend (1978), who studied in the monkey, the effects of unilateral canal plugging on central vestibular neurons. The results can be summarized as follows: 1) no changes occurred on either side in the absolute number of units responding to rotation; 2) a decrease of the sensitivity of neurons by half was noted; 3) the sensitivity on the plugged side is only slightly lower than that on the intact side. This shows that almost all central canal vestibular neurons receive an input from the contralate- ral labyrinth and that the 2 labyrinths have about the same weight in driving them.

Another finding incompatible with the idea of the major role of vestibular neurons for rebalancing is that bila- teral canal plugging does not affect OKN (Henn, personal communication; see also Barmack, this book). This indi- cates that vestibular neurons, even when functionally deafferented from the labyrinths, are still able to con- vey optokinetic signals to oculomotor nuclei. However, in our chronic hemilabyrinthectomized cats not only re- mained the VOR asymmetrical but also, in many cases, OKN was strongly impaired, in spite of the presence of a good balance control.

2.3. Vestibular neuron activity in hemilabyrinthecto- mized cats

In an attempt to clarify the discrepancies between re- covery of gain and balance control, we recorded single unit activity in both the deafferented and intact vesti- bular nuclei in cats hemilabyrinthectomized 30-40 days before the acute recording session. Intact animals served as controls. The experiments were done under light Ketamine anaesthesia and the midline of the cerebellum was removed in order to have a direct view of the vesti- bular nuclei and to exclude effects mediated by the cerebellar commissure. Units were identified as type I or type II neurons by rotating the animal about the

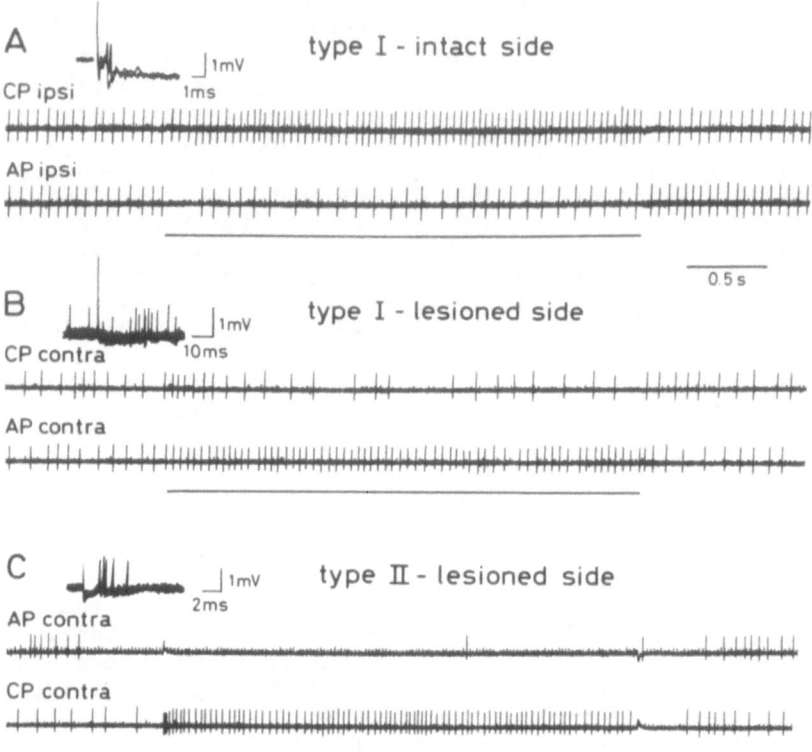

FIGURE 4. Examples of anodal (AP) and cathodal polariza-
tions (CP) in horizontal canal neurons identified by
natural and electrical stimulation. Units were recorded
in chronic HL cats from the intact (A) and lesioned side
(B-C). Insets show responses to single shock stimuli to
ipsi (A) or contralateral side (B-C). Stimulation time
with DC current is indicated by continuous lines (intensity = 1X thr. N_1).

vertical axis with the head pitched 30° nose down with
respect to the stereo-taxic position. On the lesioned
side, it was possible to record type I and II units,
while in the intact side almost exclusively type I activity was found. The latter finding can be easily understood since type II neurons receive their inputs from
the contralateral side. In comparing the number and ease
with which units could be found in the intact and deafferented sides in each animal the dearth of responding
units in the deafferented nuclei was striking. The type
I activity on the intact side was basically indistinguishable from that present in intact animals (as for
numbers of canal units and level of resting discharge).

On the other hand, the units isolated in the deafferented nuclei had, on the average, a lower resting rate (13.2 spikes/sec +10.4; N=45) than the controls (23.3 spikes/sec +14.7; N=77). The difference was less striking when comparing resting rates between intact and deafferented nuclei.

We also tested the capacity of the intact labyrinth to modulate the activity in the deafferented nuclei, to assess if changes in the efficacy of the vestibular commissure occurred after the loss of one labyrinthine input. To this end we applied polarizing DC currents to the round window (Fig.4). The intensity of stimulation was calibrated relative to the threshold for eliciting the N_1 field potential by single shock. Briefly, the main results of this study were: 1) vestibular neurons responding to horizontal rotation could be easily and consistently driven by polarization of the ipsi- and contralateral labyrinth in an opposite way; 2) in control cats both labyrinths had the same efficacy in driving horizontal central canal neurons. This finding is consistent with the already mentioned data by Abend; 3) there was no difference between the responses of control animals and those of chronically hemilabyrinthectomized cats to polarization of the contralateral labyrinth, i.e. in the efficacy of the vestibular commissure.

3. CONCLUSION

The data reported here indicate that compensation of the static symptoms following unilateral section of the VIIIth nerve (at least for the vestibuloocular system) is only partially achieved through a rebalancing of the outputs of the vestibular nuclei. It is not clear why the static and dynamic activity recorded on the deafferented side was clearly below control levels. As for the lower resting rate one possibility is that the tonic commissural inhibition, no longer counterbalanced by the exitatory input from the labyrinth, is powerful enough to keep vestibular neurons below threshold. Cell loss is an unlikely explanation for lack of type I responses, since preliminary anatomical studies showed that no significant transneuronal cell death occurred on the lesioned side. Possibly, maladaptive sprouting accounts for some of the deficiencies. Given these deficiencies of vestibular neuronal circuitry in chronic cats it is not surprising that dynamic vestibular reflexes remain likewise impaired. It should be emphasized, however, that the VOR dynamics described here only refer to the VOR proper, i.e. compensatory eye movements tested with the vestibular input only. When optokinetic and neck proprioceptive inputs are also activated during head movements in the light stabilization of gaze presumably is much improved as judged from the nearly perfect locomotory behavior of the chronically hemilabyrinthectomized cats

208

and from measurements of the VOR in the light in these
animals (Precht et al., 1981).

REFERENCES
Abend WK (1978) Response to constant angular accelerations of neurons in the monkey superior vestibular nucleus. Exp. Brain Res. 31, 459-473.
Baarsma EA and Collewijn H (1975) Changes in compensatory eye movements after unilateral labyrinthectomy in
the rabbit. Arch. Oto-Rhino-Laryng. 211, 219-230.
Barmack NH and Pettorossi VE (1981) The influence of
unilateral horizontal semicircular canal plugs on the
horizontal vestibuloocular reflex of the rabbit. In:
Lesion-induced neuronal plasticity in sensorimotor
systems. Eds. H. Flohr and W. Precht, Springer-Verlag
B.H.N.Y. pp. 231-239.
Cohen B, Uemura T and Takemori S (1973) Effects of labyrinthectomy on optokinetic nystagmus (OKN) and optokine-
tic after-nystagmus (OKAN). Equilibrium Res. 3, 88-93.
Moran WB (1974) The changes in phase lag during sinusoidal angular rotation following labyrinthectomy in the
cat. Laryngoscope 84, 1707-1728.
Precht W (1974) Characteristics of vestibular neurons
after acute and chronic labyrinthine destruction. In:
Handbook of sensory physiology, Vol.6/2, pp. 451-462.
Edit. H.H. Kornhuber. Springer Verlag Berlin Heidelberg
New York.
Precht W, Maioli C, Dieringer N and Cochran S (1981)
Mechanisms of Compensation of the Vestibulo-Ocular Re-
flex after Vestibular Neurotomy. In: Lesion-Induced Neu-
ronal Plasticity in Sensorimotor Systems, pp. 221-230.
Edit. H. Flohr and W. Precht. Springer-Verlag Berlin
Heidelberg.
Schaefer KP and Meyer DL (1974) Compensation of vesti-
bular lesions. In: Handbook of Sensory Physiology, Vol.
6, pp. 463-490. Edit. H.H. Kornhuber. Springer-Verlag
Berlin Heidelberg New York.
Wolfe JW and Kos CM (1977) Nystagmic responses of the
rhesus monkey to rotational stimulation following uni-
lateral labyrinthectomy: final report. Trans.Am.Acad.
Ophthalmol.Otolaryngol. 84, 38-45.
Zuckermann H (1967) The physiological adaptation to
unilateral semicircular canal inactivation. McGill
Med.J. 36, 8-13.

GAZE PALSIES AFTER SELECTIVE PONTINE LESIONS IN MONKEYS

W. LANG, V. HENN, K. HEPP

(Depts of Pathology and Neurology, University Hospital,
and Dept of Physics, ETH, Zürich, Switzerland)

Electrical stimulation and lesion studies in the monkey have localized
an area in the pons responsible for generating rapid eye movements to
the ipsilateral side (Bender, Shanzer, 1964). Subsequently, this area has
been defined more precisely physiologically and anatomically and has been
named paramedian pontine reticular formation, or for short, PPRF (Goebel
et al., 1971; Cohen et al., 1968). For generating vertical rapid eye movements, a corresponding area was postulated in the rostral mesencephalon.
This area was delineated in lesion studies by Kömpf et al. (1979) and
the exact anatomy has been worked out by Büttner-Ennever et al. (1982).
The region has been named the rostral interstitial nucleus of the medial
longitudinal fasciculus (rostral iMLF). This separation of immediate
premotor areas for horizontal and vertical gaze requires minimally that
either one structure dominates the other, or that another common source
exists for exact coordination and timing of rapid eye movements. Bender
and Shanzer (1964) have previously observed that a bilateral pontine
lesion can cause a complete loss of rapid eye movements in all directions.
Single neuron studies in alert monkeys support conclusions from lesions
and stimulation experiments. Specifically, neurons in the PPRF and in
the rostral iMLF were found whose activities changed in close temporal
relation to rapid eye movements. Physiological characteristics of these
neurons have been summarized in several recent publications (Keller, 1981;
Hepp, Henn, 1982). Specific differences between the mesencephalic and
pontine premotor areas are that the vertical area contains predominantly
medium-lead burst neurons with vertical on-directions. Especially conspicuous is the absence of pause cells which are thought to provide exact
timing for saccades. On the other hand, in the PPRF, pause cells are
abundant in a cluster located medially and caudally. Another class of
neurons is also typical for the PPRF, i.e. the long-lead burst neurons
which carry an early signal for rapid eye movements about to occur especially in the horizontal plane to the ipsilateral side. These neurons
are predominantly found in rostral parts of the PPRF.
Anatomical studies with anterograde or retrograde tracer substances reveal
a reciprocal connection between the PPRF and the rostral mesencephalon,
especially the area which is defined as the rostral interstitial nucleus
of the MLF (Büttner-Ennever, 1977). They also reveal a projection from
the PPRF to the ipsilateral abducens nucleus where internuclear neurons
are found which, in turn, project to the medial rectus motor neurons of
the contralateral side. These PPRF connections to abducens internuclear
and motor neurons are an important input for directing horizontal fast
eye movements.

Roucoux, A. and Crommelinck, M. (eds.): Physiological and Pathological Aspects of Eye Movements.
© *1982, Dr W. Junk Publishers, The Hague, Boston, London.* ISBN-13: 978-94-009-8002-0

The purpose of this study is to show that cells in the PPRF are responsible for generating rapid eye movements, because in previous lesion studies using electrolytic lesions fiber systems were also damaged. Another aim is to place small selective lesions in either the more rostral or caudal parts of the PPRF to observe how the differential destruction of the various neuronal populations, based on their unequal distribution in the PPRF, produces different eye movement deficits. Finally, bilateral lesions were placed to decide whether such lesions simply double the deficits of unilateral lesions or to what extent other functions are additionally involved, e.g. vertical gaze.

METHODS

Experiments were performed on Rhesus monkeys (Macaca mulatta). First, an operation was performed to implant electrodes to monitor eye position, a receptacle for a microdrive above a trephine hole in the skull, and head bolts to immobilize the head during experiments. Surgery was done under anesthesia with halothane and a gas mixture of N_2O-O_2, initiated by pentobarbital. About a week after the operation, single neuron recordings were started. In all cases these single unit studies were extended over several months. These data have been reported elsewhere. One animal was trained to fixate a stationary or moving light spot (Wurtz, 1969). In the other untrained animals, eye movements were calibrated by rotation in the light at a velocity of 30^0/sec. In this range, the optokinetic nystagmus was assumed to have a gain of unity. All relevant data were stored on magnetic tape: single unit activity, horizontal and vertical eye position, stimulus parameters, and a time code. Data were then written out on a rectilinear oscillograph or displayed on an oscilloscope. Further measurements were taken from these records.

Chemical lesions were placed stereotaxically using kainic acid (McGeer et al., 1978; Coyle et al., 1978). Prior to an injection, a region of interest was identified with microelectrode recordings. The electrode penetrated into the brain inside a guide tube which had an outer diameter of 0.9 mm. The electrode could be advanced about 12 mm beyond the tip of the guide tube. When a region whose activity was considered typical for the neuronal population under investigation had been identified, the electrode was withdrawn with the guide tube left in place. The animal then received 4 mg of dexamethasone intramuscularly. Next the microsyringe was advanced through the guide tube with a tip protruding the same amount as the previous electrode. The actual injection procedure was performed in several steps, the total amount being 0.8 to 1.6 μl. The kainic acid was concentrated 4-8 μg/μl; was dissolved in 0.2 M phosphate buffer; and had a pH of 7.4. With a successful lesion, within 20 minutes some gaze paresis was evident. To prevent further chemical activity of kainic acid, 5 mg diazepam was then injected i.m. Animals were then carefully watched over the next 12 hours. During that time possible problems involved hypo- or total akinesia with subsequent hypothermia. Monitoring rectal temperature and providing heat with an infrared lamp was sufficient to control temperature. Another possible complication was autonomous dysregulation with the most caudally placed lesion, resulting in irregular breathing and tachycardia. With a treatment of dexamethasone, followed by diazepam, this complication did not reoccur. In all cases, during the first 24 hours, oculomotor deficits were greatest. Often, even with a unilateral lesion, there was complete ophthalmoplegia. Within 24 hours, these effects subsided and reduced to symptomes which then were permanent. Clinical

testing for oculomotor and vestibular functions was done daily. More
extensive testings with eye movement recordings during vestibular
stimulation, optokinetic stimulation or combinations were done on a
weekly basis. In addition, film records were made.

After a period between one and six weeks, animals were sacrificed. They
were perfused, under deep pentobarbital anesthesia, with 4% paraform-
aldehyde, phosphate buffered to pH 7.4, after initial treatment with 2 ml
Heparin (10000 units) and 200 ml 6% plasma expander (Dextran). The brain
was left in fixative for about 16 hours and then transferred to a 0.1 M
phosphate buffered 30% sucrose solution for 48-72 hours. Frozen sections
of 30 μm thickness were cut in the coronal plane from the nucleus prepositus hypoglossus to the posterior commissure and every third section
was stained with cresyl violet and luxol for cell bodies and myelin. One
case was processed for electron microscopy with special perfusion and
fixation techniques.

RESULTS

(1) Morphopathology of kainic acid lesions revealed time-dependent changes.
With a survival time of about 2 weeks, severe neuronal cell loss and
infiltration of microglia could be observed in Nissl-stained sections,
especially in perivascular areas. With survival time of about 4 weeks,
the lesion contained predominantly macrophages and was relatively well
demarcated from surrounding tissue. With survival time exceeding 6 weeks,
proliferation of astrocytes was dominant.

In all cases there was a virtually complete loss of neuronal cells (Coyle
et al., 1978). Electron microscopy showed some myelin breakdown within
the lesion; however many myelin sheaths remained unaffected.

(2) Unilateral caudal PPRF lesions.
In two animals unilateral caudal PPRF lesions were successfully produced.
In two other animals bilateral lesion were effected in two stages, per-
mitting the study of one-sided lesions for about one week. Results are
essentially the same as those obtained with electrolytic lesions reported
by Bender and Shanzer (1964), Cohen et al. (1968) and Goebel et al. (1971).
Our data concerning chemical lesions has been reported previously (Jaeger
et al., 1981). Essentially, the clinical symptoms are: All rapid eye
movements towards the ipsilateral side are lost. These include saccades
and quick phases of optokinetic or vestibular nystagmus (even in the
contralateral hemifield). On attempted gaze straight ahead, the eyes are
in a slightly paramedian position to the opposite side. The animal seems
unable to move its eyes into the ipsilateral hemifield. In total darkness
spontaneous nystagmus towards the contralateral side is present which
increases in velocity with eccentric gaze position. During horizontal
vestibular stimulation there is normal nystagmus in one direction and it
is absent into the contralateral direction. In the right sided lesion,
during rotation to the right, the eyes fully deviate to the left and stay
in this eccentric position, as the animal cannot generate quick phases
towards the right. After the end of acceleration in complete darkness,
the eyes very slowly drift back towards midposition. The time course of
that recentering takes about 20-30 sec which is within the range of the
time constant of central vestibular neurons (Jaeger et al., 1981). During
rotation to the left, animals have normal nystagmus. It is noteworthy that
during slow phases towards the right, the eyes move into the ipsilateral
hemifield without any abnormality in slow phase velocity. Vertical

nystagmus is normal in such animals in both directions.

Single neuron activity in the caudal PPRF comprises mostly horizontal long-lead bursters, horizontal and vertical medium-lead bursters, burst-tonic neurons, and pause cells. In various models these types of units have been put together and found sufficient to generate rapid eye movements in the horizontal plane towards the ipsilateral side. The pause cells act to synchronize all burst cell activity for horizontal as well as vertical movements. The unilateral loss of all these different units seems to be consistent with the clinical deficits. Single unit recordings in the contralateral, unaffected PPRF revealed normal activity during movements to the unaffected side or in a vertical direction (Jäger et al., 1981).

Discussion: Our data fully confirm earlier reports, in which unilateral PPRF lesions were made by means of coagulation. It proves that the ability to generate rapid eye movements depends on the integrity of cells in the PPRF and not on fiber systems in that region.

(3) Unilateral rostral PPRF lesion:

In one animal a bilateral rostral lesion was made in two stages. Therefore we could observe the deficits of a unilateral rostral PPRF lesion for about one week. It had features essentially like the caudal PPRF lesion save the one observation that spontaneous nystagmus to the contralateral side was minimal and at times absent.

On a single neuron level, rostral and caudal PPRF differ in the respect that in the rostral part burst neurons are prevalent, mostly of the long-lead type without tonic activity. It is conceivable that strong spontaneous nystagmus is present only when the balance of the tonic activity in the caudal PPRF is disturbed and shifted.

(4) Bilateral caudal PPRF lesions:

Two animals received a bilateral caudal PPRF lesion. Bilateral lesions in one animal were each less than 2 mm in diameter and located immediately ventral and rostral to the abducens nuclei. The other animal had a much larger confluent lesion which is shown in Fig. 1. We have chosen to show the larger lesion to stress the extreme extent of destruction in which slow compensatory eye movements in response to vestibular stimulation are still possible. Oculomotor deficits in both cases were the same. The most striking phenomenon was the loss of all rapid eye movements in all directions. Slow eye movements in response to vestibular stimulation could be elicited. If the stimulus amplitude did not exceed the normal movement range of the eyes, the eyes followed in a compensatory fashion. This was true for sinusoidal stimulation, for amplitudes up to about 50°, or to step displacements. With high accelerations of small amplitude, compensatory movements could be induced which reached velocity ranges characteristic of saccades. When the stimulus amplitude exceeded the oculomotor movement range, the eyes were caught in an extreme eye position and remained there until the stimulus ceased or reversed its direction during sinusoidal stimulation. Essentially the same was found for stimulation in the vertical plane. Optokinetic stimulation had a similar effect, although gain was generally lower. Both animals had preserved some ability to follow moving objects (pieces of fruit, etc.). As animals were untrained, this ability could not be systematically checked or quantified.

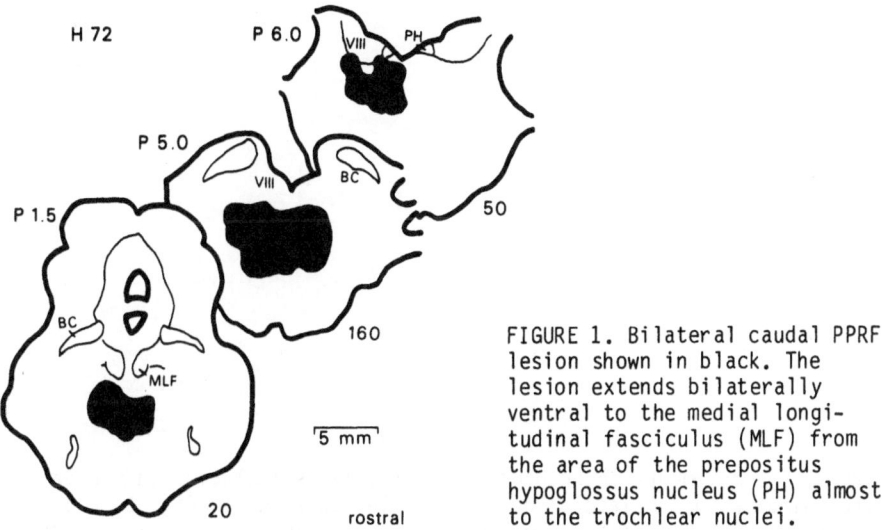

FIGURE 1. Bilateral caudal PPRF lesion shown in black. The lesion extends bilaterally ventral to the medial longitudinal fasciculus (MLF) from the area of the prepositus hypoglossus nucleus (PH) almost to the trochlear nuclei.

<u>Single neuron activity</u> in the caudal PPRF is characterized by medium-lead burst, burst-tonic, and pause cell activity. It seems that pause cells and some of the medium-lead bursters play an important role in coordinating horizontal and vertical movement components. Furthermore, the continuous high discharge rate of pause neurons during periods of fixation or slow movements seem to inhibit burst cell activity. With the elimination of inhibition and other cells in the caudal PPRF which may convey excitatory signals, burst cell activity in the rostral iMLF, the immediate premotor area for vertical rapid eye movements, becomes uncoordinated (Fig. 2). Animals can still move their eyes in a vertical direction, but the eyes cannot be held steady to fixate so that an irregular oscillatory pattern results. We observe that during these movements, presumed medium-lead bursters in the rostral iMLF discharge with high frequency bursts. <u>Discussion:</u> Results confirm the clinical observation of the dominant role of the PPRF in triggering and coordinating rapid eye movements in all directions. For movements in the horizontal plane the immediate premotor apparatus is destroyed and consequently there are no spontaneous movements. For the vertical system, the immediate premotor system in the rostral iMLF lacks coordinated input. Therefore, some spontaneous vertical movements without clear separation of the movement and fixation periods are possible. There are few clinical reports (Hoyt, Daroff, 1971; Christoff, 1974; Larmande, 1982) which have recently been reviewed (Henn, Büttner, 1982). Vestibular stimulation leads to compensatory movements with normal phase and gain relations as long as stimulus amplitudes do not exceed the oculomotor range (Fig. 2). Also, during step displacements of the head, the eyes move in a compensatory fashion and are then held in the new position. This proves that the velocity-to-position integrator is still intact. It provides the motoneurons with the appropriate tonic input to hold the eyes in eccentric positions. Even in the animal with the large lesion shown in Fig. 1, this integrator displayed no gross deficits. This poses the question whether it can be located in a single site, possibly

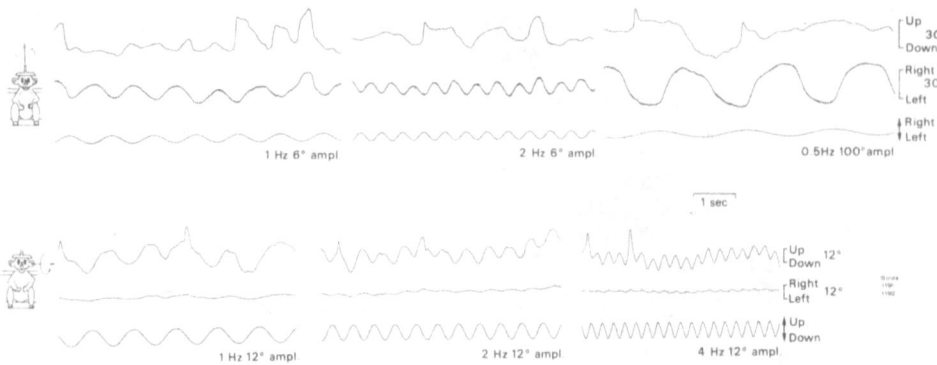

FIGURE 2. Eye movements in response to vestibular stimulation in the dark
in the animal with a bilateral caudal PPRF lesion shown in Fig. 1. From
above: vertical eye position, horizontal eye position, head position. With
6° stimulus amplitude (peak-to-peak), movements are largely compensatory
in a horizontal direction. At the same time the eyes make coordinated but
rather arbitrary excursion in the vertical plane. With a larger stimulus
amplitude the eyes move to the right or left and stay there, resulting in
a distorted sinusoidal movement pattern. With vertical stimulation (head
pitching), eye movements are also largely compensatory with some irregular
drift and movement superimposed, especially with low frequency stimulation.

in the prepositus hypoglossus nucleus, or whether it is the coordinated
action from several areas which provide this integration.

<u>(5) Bilateral rostral PPRF lesions:</u>
Lesions were placed in two animals, one of which was trained to fixate
a light spot. A scheme showing the extent of the lesion (Fig. 3), and a
sample of the nystagmus response (Fig. 4), are taken from the untrained
animal. The most prominent feature in these two animals was the complete
loss of all rapid eye movements in the horizontal plane with preservation
of rapid vertical eye movements. While inspecting these monkeys it was
apparent that the eyes moved in a vertical direction up and down with
normal fixation periods in between. However, the animals were not able
to make any rapid eye movements in a horizontal direction. Clinically,
convergence was intact, although that was not tested with oculography.
Both animals were able to follow small moving objects into either hemifield. During vestibular stimulation in the horizontal plane, movements
were compensatory, if the stimulus amplitude remained within the oculomotor range (Fig. 4). In this respect, these animals were not different
from those with a bilateral caudal lesion. In the vertical plane the
animals had normal vertical nystagmus. This was tested by placing the
animals on the side and rotating them about the vertical axis. Animals
were also tested by rotating them about a horizontal axis while sitting
upright which results in somersaulting. Optokinetic stimulation in the
horizontal plane led to tonic eye deviation in the appropriate direction

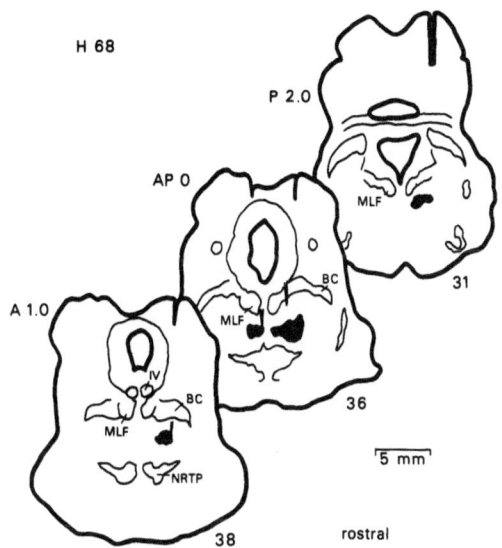

H 68

P 2.0

AP 0

MLF

A 1.0

MLF

BC

31

IV

BC

MLF

36

NRTP

38

rostral

5 mm

FIGURE 3. Bilateral rostral PPRF lesion shown in black. On the right side, the lesion extends from the level of the trochlear nucleus about 3 mm caudally. On the left side, the lesion is smaller and less than 2 mm in diameter.

without any fast phases of nystagmus. In the vertical plane, again, nystagmus was normal.

One animal which was trained to fixate a light spot could be tested further. Its lesion was smaller than that shown in Fig. 3. Over two weeks it regained the ability to make some horizontal saccades with amplitudes not exceeding a few degrees. It was placed in front of a tangent screen onto which a small light spot was projected from a laser beam via a servo-controlled mirror system. During sudden vertical displacements the animal made the appropriate saccadic jumps with normal latency and velocity. For horizontal displacements, the animal initiated a series of very small saccades until after a few seconds it finally reached the target. The eyes were held at the new target position without drifting back towards midline. For oblique eye movements the vertical movement component was executed at normal saccadic velocity whereas the horizontal movement component again took much longer and was interrupted in a staircase fashion. After vestibular stimulation with the eyes in an extreme lateral position, the animal often executed a series of large amplitude up and down movements during which it managed to bring the eyes towards midposition. The mechanism for this horizontal movement is unknown, although it appears that a saccade with a large vertical movement component also enables the eyes to move to a limited extent in a horizontal direction.

Single neuron recordings in the rostral PPRF reveal mostly long-lead bursters with on-directions towards the ipsilateral side. Other units comprise medium-lead bursters with horizontal on-directions. The absence of these neurons after lesions seems to deprive the caudal PPRF of input specifically for generating rapid eye movements in a horizontal plane. This results in a complete loss of any rapid movement component in the horizontal plane.

Discussion: Loss of all horizontal movements with vertical gaze intact has rarely been observed in patients. In most cases, this is a congenital familial disorder (review: Vetterli, Henn, 1981). Pathological data are

216

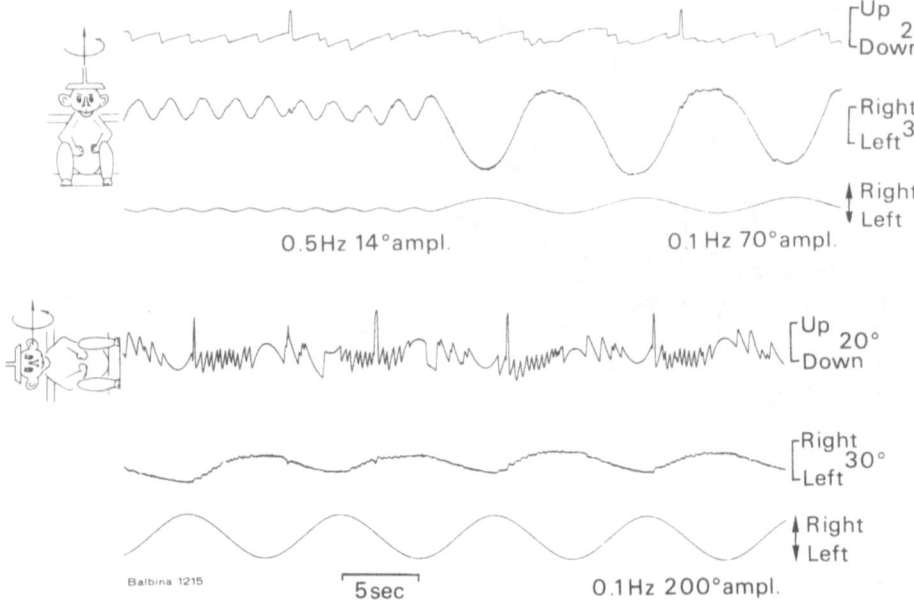

FIGURE 4. Eye movements incuded by vestibular stimulation in a monkey with a bilateral rostral PPRF lesion documented in Fig. 3. From above, vertical eye position, horizontal eye position, and turntable position. The animal had spontaneous downward nystagmus which is clearly visible during stimulation in the horizontal plane, and leads to an asymmetric response when vertical nystagmus is elicited. Eye movements in response to different amplitude stimulation (peak-to-peak values indicated) lead to compensatory movements horizontally and vertically, but quick phases are only present in the vertical direction.

not available. Our experimental data provide a possible basis for this syndrome. It suggests that the rostral PPRF generates rapid eye movement in the horizontal plane, although few long-lead burst neurons with vertical on-directions can be recorded there. It is unclear where the main input for the rostral iMLF originates to program vertical saccades. The input from the caudal PPRF seems to coordinate and trigger movements, but could not program velocity and amplitude of vertical saccades.

CONCLUSION
Chemical lesions with kainic acid prove to be a valuable tool in studying pathophysiology of gaze in regard to neuropathology, neurological deficits, and on a single neuron level. The lesions are well demarcated with complete neuronal cell loss inside the damaged region and restricted damage of extrinsic fiber systems. The extent of lesions in two animals had been documented here. Even with a large bilateral caudal PPRF lesion, the velocity-to-position integrator was not much affected. On the other hand,

a small bilateral rostral PPRF lesion led to clearly defined deficits in the generation of rapid eye movements in the horizontal plane. Neurological deficits remain stable and animals are in excellent general condition for repeated neurological testing. With this new technique we were able to reaffirm earlier lesion studies using coagulation techniques, and fully document the differential effects of bilateral caudal and rostral PPRF lesions.

REFERENCES

Bender MB, Shanzer S (1964) Oculomotor pathways defined by electrical stimulation and lesions in the brainstem of the monkey. In Bender MB, ed. The oculomotor system, pp. 81-140. New York, Harper and Row.

Büttner-Ennever JA (1977) Pathways from the pontine reticular formation to structures controlling horizontal and vertical eye movements in the monkey. In Baker R, Berthoz A, eds. Control of gaze by brain stem neurons, pp. 89-98. Amsterdam, Elsevier/North Holland Publishing Company.

Büttner-Ennever JA, Büttner U, Cohen B, Baumgartner G (1982) Vertical gaze paralysis and the rostral interstitial nucleus of the medial longitudinal fasciculus (rostral iMLF). Brain 105, 125-149.

Christoff N (1974) A clinicopathologic study of vertical eye movements. Arch. Neurol. 31, 1-8.

Cohen B, Komatsuzaki A, Bender MB (1968) Electrooculographic syndrome in monkeys after pontine reticular formation lesions. Arch. Neurol. 18, 78-92.

Coyle JT, Molliver ME, Kuhar MJ (1978) In situ injection of kainic acid: a new method for selectively lesioning neuronal cell bodies while sparing axons of passage. J. Comp. Neurol. 180, 301-324.

Goebel H, Komatsuzaki A, Bender MB, Cohen B (1971) Lesions of the pontine tegmentum and conjugate gaze paralysis. Arch. Neurol. 24, 431-440.

Henn V, Büttner U (1982) Disorders of horizontal gaze. In Lennerstrand G, Zee DS, Keller EL, eds. Functional basis of ocular motility disorders, in press. Oxford, Pergamon Press.

Hepp K, Henn V (1982) Physiology of horizontal gaze. In Lennerstrand G, Zee DS, Keller EL, eds. Functional basis of ocular motility disorders, in press. Oxford, Pergamon Press.

Hoyt WF, Daroff RB (1971) Supranuclear disorders of ocular control systems in man: clinical, anatomical, and physiological correlations. In Bach-y-Rita P, Collins CC, eds. The control of eye movements, pp. 175-235. New York, London, Academic Press.

Jaeger J, Henn V, Lang W, Miles TS, Waespe W (1981) Vestibular unit activity in monkeys with horizontal gaze palsy. In Fuchs AL, Becker W, eds. Progress in oculomotor research, pp. 89-95. Amsterdam, Elsevier/ North Holland Publishing Company.

Keller EL (1981) Brain stem mechanisms in saccadic control. In Fuchs AL, Becker W, eds. Progress in oculomotor research, pp. 57-62. Amsterdam, Elsevier/North Holland Publishing Company.

Kömpf D, Pasik T, Pasik P, Bender MB (1979) Downward gaze in monkeys. Stimulation and lesion studies. Brain 102, 527-558.

218

Larmande P, Hénin D, Jan M, Elie A, Gouazé A (1981) Abnormal vertical eye movements in the locked-in syndrome. Ann. Neurol. 11, 100-102.

McGeer EG, Olney JW, McGeer PL, eds. (1978) Kainic acid as a tool in neurobiology. New York, Raven Press.

Vetterli A, Henn V (1981) Congenital gaze palsy in two brothers. In Huber A, Klein D, eds. Neurogenetics and neuro-ophthalmology, pp. 81-88. Amsterdam, Elsevier/North Holland Publishing Company.

Wurtz RH (1969) Visual receptive fields of striate cortex neurons in awake monkeys. J. Neurophysiol. 32, 727-742.

THE ROLE OF THE PRIMATE FLOCCULUS DURING VESTIBULAR AND OPTOKINETIC
NYSTAGMUS: SINGLE CELL RECORDINGS AND LESION STUDIES

W. WAESPE*, B. COHEN, TH. RAPHAN

(Dept of Neurology, Mount Sinai School of Medicine, New York)
*Permanent address: Dept of Neurology, University Zürich,Switzerland

1. INTRODUCTION

Optokinetic nystagmus is composed of two processes: a rapid initial
increase in slow phase velocity followed by a slower rise to a
steady state level (Cohen et al., 1977). The rapid rise is believed
due to activation of direct pathways from the visual to the oculomotor system which are capable of exciting the oculomotor system at
short latencies. Indirect pathways are presumed to be responsible
for the slower changes in eye velocity during OKN and for optokinetic after-nystagmus (OKAN). A key element in the indirect pathways
is a velocity storage mechanism that is shared in common with the
vestibular system; it contributes significantly to the low frequency
characteristics of the vestibulo-ocular reflex (VOR; Raphan et al.,
1979). Recently single cell recordings in the primate vestibular
nuclei showed that all vestibular neurons which receive their vestibular information from the horizontal canals are also modulated during optokinetic nystagmus (OKN) and after-nystagmus (OKAN) (Waespe,
Henn, 1977a,b). Activity changes are compatible with those in
indirect pathways that mediate slow changes in slow phase velocity
(Raphan, Cohen, 1981).
In the following we will demonstrate that floccular Purkinje cells
(P-cells) may be part of the direct visual-oculomotor pathways that
mediate rapid changes in slow phase velocity (Waespe, Henn, 1981;
Waespe et al., 1982).

2. METHODS

Experiments were performed on Rhesus (M. mulatta) and Cynomolgus
(M. fascicularis) monkeys. Under anaesthesia, silver silver-chlo-
ride electrodes were placed in the bone around the eyes. Screws
were implanted on the skull for immobilizing the head, and a well
that accepted a microelectrode carrier was fixed to the skull. The
flocculus and parts of the paraflocculus were removed by suction
ablation under an operating microscope (Waespe et al., 1982). Single
cell recordings in the flocculus and the vestibular nuclei were made
with varnish insulated tungsten electrodes and using conventional
equipment (for details see Waespe, Henn, 1977a; Waespe et al.,
1981). Eye movements were recorded with DC-electrooculography (EOG).
The EOG's were differentiated and rectified to obtain slow phase
velocity. During testing monkeys sat in a primate chair under an
optokinetic drum. They were given steps of angular velocity or
angular accelerations about a vertical axis, or they were given
steps or ramps of surround velocity. In order to test the response
to conflict stimulation, the OKN drum was mechanically coupled to
the primate chair so that steps of velocity or acceleration could
be given in a subject-stationary, lighted visual surround. Voltages
representing eye position, eye velocity, unit recordings and the
various stimuli were recorded on FM magnetic tape. For analysis,

Roucoux, A. and Crommelinck, M. (eds.): Physiological and Pathological Aspects of Eye Movements.
© 1982, Dr W. Junk Publishers, The Hague, Boston, London. ISBN-13: 978-94-009-8002-0

unit activity was averaged over variable time periods by a computer program.

3. RESULTS
Activity of vestibular nuclei neurons
Vestibular stimulation: Firing rates of single cells were modulated bidirectionally during pure vestibular stimulation (rotation of the monkey in darkness, Fig. 1A). During acceleration to the contralateral side, the type II neuron in Fig. 1A increased its firing rate. During constant velocity rotation, frequency decayed with a time constant (T_c) between 10-30 sec. A similar time course was observed for the slow phase velocity of vestibular nystagmus (VN). During deceleration or with rotation into the ipsilateral direction, neuronal activity was silenced. During conflict stimulation peak frequency changes were diminished at low accelerations (compared to these during pure vestibular stimulation), but they were not diminished at high accelerations (above 20 deg/s^2). T_c of neuronal activity and of nystagmus velocity was always short in conflict situations with values below 6-8 sec.
Optokinetic stimulation: All neurons were modulated bidirectionally during optokinetic stimulation (Fig. 1B). At the onset of stimulation to the ipsilateral side, the type II neuron slowly increased its frequency. Maximal frequency changes were reached only after 5-20 sec and were maintained as long as the stimulus was present. Maximal frequency changes increased on average with stimulus velocities up to 60 deg/s. At higher velocities neuronal activity but not OKN slow phase velocities saturated (Waespe, Henn, 1979). During OKAN (downward arrow in Fig. 1B, lights off), firing rate slowly returned to the resting discharge level in parallel with OKAN velocity. There was no fast rise or fast decay of neuronal activity during OKN, although there were rapid changes in eye velocity especially at higher stimulus velocities (see Fig. 3, left). For all stimulation conditions type I neurons showed a mirror-like behavior to that of the type II neurons.
Activity of Purkinje cells (P-cells) in the flocculus
Vestibular stimulation: Simple spike (SS) activity of P-cells was not modulated or only slightly modulated during pure vestibular stimulation (Lisberger, Fuchs, 1978; Waespe, Henn, 1981). Activity changes were always stronger during conflict stimulation. Over 80% of P-cells were modulated during stimulation to the ipsilateral side. This corresponds to a type I response.
Optokinetic stimulation: 5-10% of the P-cells encountered modulated their SS activity during OKN. An example is shown in Fig. 2. At the onset of optokinetic stimulation to the ipsilateral (recording side) at 120 deg/s there was a rapid increase in SS activity which was maintained for the duration of stimulation. With lights off (downward arrows), SS activity returned rapidly to the resting discharge level and was not modulated during OKAN. Maintained discharges were present only at stimulus velocities above 30-60 deg/s. All type I P-cells showed a type II response during optokinetic stimulation. That is, they were activated during rotation to the ipsilateral side, but also during surround movement to the ipsilateral side. These stimuli produce nystagmus in opposite directions. In contrast, type I vestibular nuclei neurons are activated during optokinetic stimulation to the contralateral side. In this situation VN and OKN beat synergistically in the same direction to the ipsilateral side.

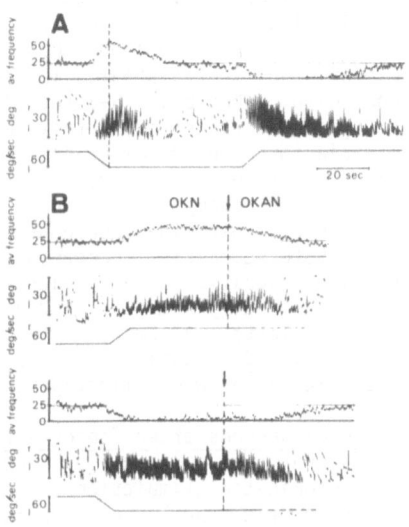

FIGURE 1. Type II vestibular nuclei neuron during pure vestibular stimulation (A), and during optokinetic stimulation (B). First trace is averaged neuronal activity, second trace horizontal EOG, third trace stimulus velocity. For description see text.

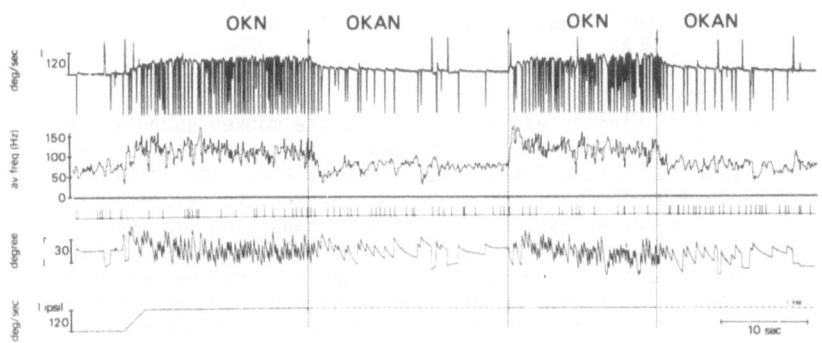

FIGURE 2. Averaged simple spike activity (second trace) and complex spike activity (third trace) of a type I Purkinje cell in the flocculus during optokinetic nystagmus with slow phases to the ipsilateral side. First trace is eye velocity, fourth trace horizontal EOG, fifth trace stimulus velocity.

Vestibular nystagmus, optokinetic nystagmus and after-nystagmus after bilateral flocculectomy

VN: Flocculectomy had little effect on VN: The gain and duration were unchanged or were only slightly reduced. During conflict stimulation, peak eye velocities could no longer be attenuated at high accelerations. However, the T_c of nystagmus in the conflict situation was still short with values below 6-8 sec. At low accelerations (5 deg/s^2) nystagmus was almost completely suppressed.

OKN, OKAN: The initial rapid increase in OKN velocity seen in the normal monkey at the onset of stimulation (Fig. 3, left) was reduced by 60-90% after bilateral flocculectomy (Fig. 3, right). The slow increase in OKN velocity had a longer time course after than before flocculectomy. OKN steady state velocities increased only up to the preoperative OKAN-saturation velocities of 50-70 deg/s. The transition of OKN to OKAN which is normally characterized by a sudden loss in eye velocity (Fig. 3, left), was smooth after flocculectomy at all stimulus velocities (Fig. 3, right). OKAN-velocities and durations were unchanged (Fig. 3) or were slightly reduced after flocculectomy.

Activity of vestibular nuclei neurons after flocculectomy

Modulation of vestibular neurons was qualitatively unchanged during vestibular, conflict and optokinetic stimulation after flocculectomy. An example of the firing rate of a type I neuron during optokinetic stimulation to the contralateral side is shown in Fig. 4. At the onset of stimulation firing rate increased slowly (a) up to a steady state level which was maintained as long as the stimulus was present. With lights off (downward arrow) the firing rate decreased slowly to the resting discharge level (b), in parallel to the slow phase velocity of OKAN. This modulation is similar to that of the neuron in Fig. 1B. During OKN all neurons were modulated bidirectionally, they increased their firing rate up to a velocity of 60 deg/s, where they saturated (Waespe, Cohen, 1982). In the light in presence of a stationary visual surround (c) neuronal activity and nystagmus were rapidly inhibited and suppressed. Thus, loss of floccular P-cells did not change the modulation of vestibular nuclei neurons during vestibular and conflict stimulation, or during OKN and OKAN.

4. SUMMARY AND CONCLUSIONS

The findings of single cell recordings in the monkey support the idea that floccular P-cells mediate activity in direct visual-oculomotor pathways. These pathways are responsible for the initial rapid increase in OKN velocity, for high OKN steady state velocities and for the fast decay in eye velocity in the transition from OKN to OKAN. They do not contribute to OKAN. After flocculectomy the contribution of the direct pathways to the OKN response was severely reduced, and animals were unable to counter rapid changes in eye velocity during conflict stimulation. However, animals retained their ability to discharge activity from the velocity storage mechanism which was modelled as a "dump" switch that is independent of the flocculus. The main features of VN, OKN, OKAN and their interaction could be simulated by a model which was homeomorphic to that proposed previously (Raphan et al., 1979), simply by removing the contribution of the direct visual pathways (Waespe et al., 1982). An important element in the model is a non-linear coupling from the visual system to the velocity storage integrator.

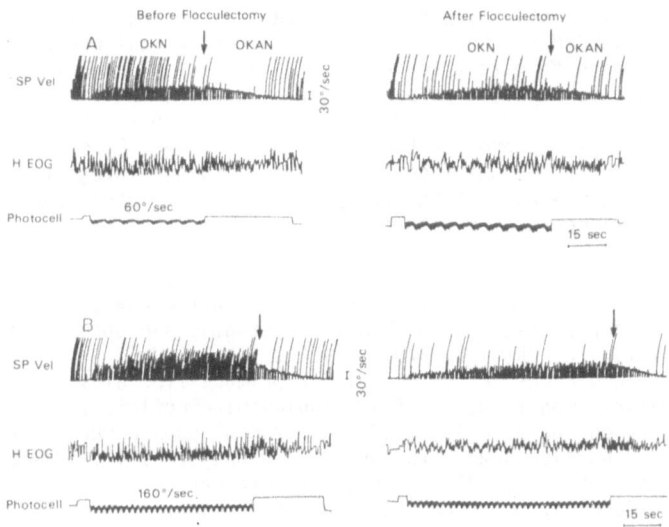

FIGURE 3. OKN and OKAN before (left) and after bilateral floccul-ectomy (right) for velocity steps of 60 deg/s (A) and 160 deg/s (B). First trace horizontal slow phase velocity, second trace horizontal EOG, third trace photocell, indicating period of stimulation. For details see text.

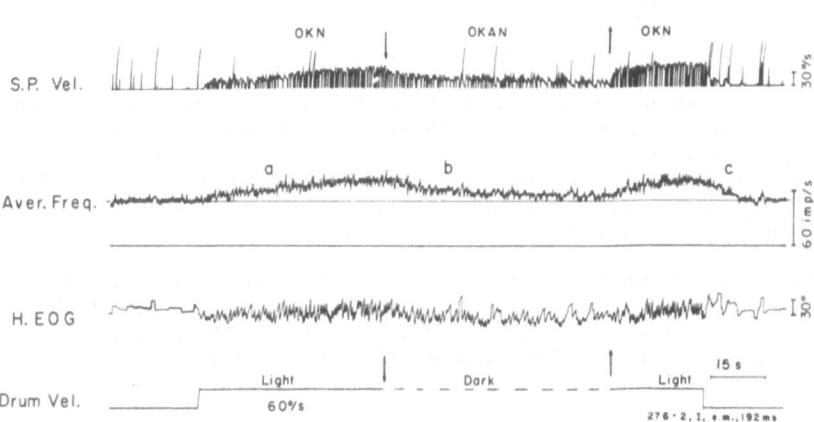

FIGURE 4. Averaged firing rate of a type I neuron (second trace) during OKN and OKAN after bilateral flocculectomy. First trace slow phase eye velocity, third trace horizontal EOG, fourth trace surround velocity. For details see text.

Vestibular nuclei activity before and after flocculectomy is similar during OKN and OKAN to that expected in indirect visual-oculomotor pathways which contain as a key element a velocity storage integrator. These pathways are responsible for the slow increase in OKN velocity, for low OKN steady state velocities up to the OKAN saturation-velocities and for the occurrence of OKAN. Flocculectomy does not change the dynamics of the velocity storage integrator, thus confirming the role of the flocculus in direct rather than indirect visual-oculomotor pathways.

REFERENCES
Cohen B, Matsuo V and Raphan Th (1977) Quantitative analysis of the velocity characteristics of optokinetic nystagmus and optokinetic after-nystagmus, J. Physiol. 270, 321-344.
Lisberger SG and Fuchs AF (1978) Role of primate flocculus during rapid behavioral modification of vestibuloocular reflex. I. Purkinje cell activity during visually guided horizontal smooth-pursuit eye movements and passive head rotation, J. Neurophysiol. 41, 733-763.
Raphan Th and Cohen B (1981) The role of integration in oculomotor control. In Zuber B, ed. Models of oculomotor behavior and control, pp. 91-109. West Palm Beach, Fla., CRC Press Inc.
Raphan Th, Matsuo V and Cohen B (1979) Velocity storage in the vestibulo-ocular reflex arc (VOR). Exp. Brain Res. 35, 229-248.
Waespe W and Henn V (1977a) Neuronal activity in the vestibular nuclei of the alert monkey during vestibular and optokinetic stimulation. Exp. Brain Res. 27, 523-538.
Waespe W and Henn V (1977b) Vestibular nuclei activity during optokinetic after-nystagmus (OKAN) in the alert monkey. Exp. Brain Res. 30, 323-330.
Waespe W and Henn V (1979) Motion information in the vestibular nuclei of alert monkeys: Visual and vestibular input vs optomotor output. Prog. Brain Res. 50, 683-693.
Waespe W and Henn V (1981) Visual-vestibular interaction in the flocculus of the alert monkey. II Purkinje cell activity. Exp. Brain Res. 43, 349-360.
Waespe W, Büttner U and Henn V (1981) Visual-vestibular interaction in the flocculus of the alert monkey. I. Input activity. Exp. Brain Res. 43, 337-348.
Waespe W, Cohen B and Raphan Th (1982) Role of the flocculus during OKN and visual-vestibular interaction: Effect of flocculectomy. Exp. Brain Res. (submitted).

This research was supported by grants of the Swiss National Foundation 3.044.76, 3.343-2.78, by a Fogarty Fellowhip to W.W. (F05 TW02768), by NIH Research Grant NS00294 and by a National Eye Institute Academic Investigator Award to T.R. (EY00157).

EFFECTS OF BILATERAL OCCIPITAL LOBECTOMIES ON EYE MOVEMENTS IN MONKEYS: PRELIMINARY OBSERVATIONS

D.S. ZEE, P.H. BUTLER, L.M. OPTICAN, R.J. TUSA, G. GÜCER
(Johns Hopkins School of Medicine and National Institutes of Health, Baltimore and Bethesda, Maryland, USA)

1. INTRODUCTION

In afoveate animals, most visually-guided ocular motor behavior is little affected by removal of visual cortex. In primates, however, the situation is less clear. To further explore the ocular motor capabilities of "cortically blind" monkeys we studied optokinetic responses, vestibulo-ocular reflex (VOR) gain adaptation, and smooth pursuit tracking in three juvenile macaques before and after bilateral occipital lobectomies.

2. METHODS AND GENERAL OBSERVATIONS

Eye movements were recorded using the magnetic field search coil technique. Animals were trained to fixate and follow targets and then, in a one-stage procedure, both occipital lobes were removed. After surgery, two of the monkeys could still orient to objects moving in the far periphery of the superior visual field although they showed no signs of central vision. In these monkeys, gross inspection of the extent of lesions after sacrifice indicated that small portions of striate cortex were probably spared. In contrast, the third monkey appeared completely blind immediately after surgery and remained so for five weeks. Subsequently it recovered the ability to orient toward and track moving objects but as yet (12 weeks post-operatively) does not appear to recognize stationary objects.

3. OPTOKINETIC RESPONSES

3.1. Optokinetic responses in afoveate animals

Before reporting our results, it will be useful to review the salient characteristics of optokinetic nystagmus (OKN) in afoveate animals such as the rabbit (Collewijn, 1981). In response to a constant velocity stimulus, eye velocity slowly climbs to a steady-state value. Eye acceleration increases when the velocity of retinal slip falls to lower values. When the lights are turned off, eye velocity slowly decays as optokinetic afternystagmus (OKAN). Higher eye velocities may be achieved with a slowly accelerating, rather than a constant velocity, stimulus. These results imply a decrease in the ability of the afoveate optokinetic system to handle increasing velocities of retinal slip. This input nonlinearity is reflected in the activity of neurons in the nucleus of the optic tract (NOT) during optokinetic stimulation (Winterson, Collewijn, 1981; Hoffman, Schoppman, 1981). During monocular viewing, afoveate animals show a better response to stimuli moving in the posterior-anterior (temporal-nasal) direction. The optokinetic responses of the rabbit appear to be mediated by subcortical pathways (Hobbelen, Collewijn, 1971).

Roucoux, A. and Crommelinck, M. (eds.): Physiological and Pathological Aspects of Eye Movements.
© 1982, Dr W. Junk Publishers, The Hague, Boston, London. ISBN-13: 978-94-009-8002-0

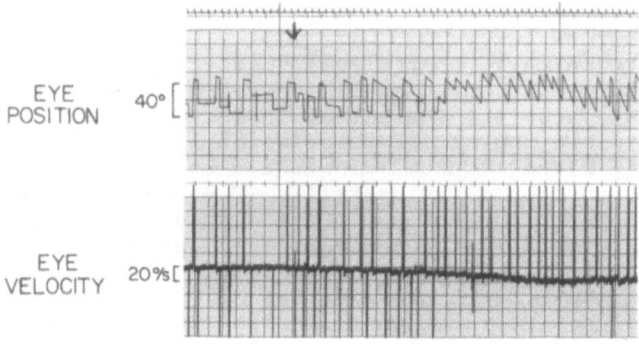

Figure 1. Response to 20 deg/sec constant velocity
full-field stimulus. Time marks at one sec intervals.
Note slow rise in eye velocity and increase in eye
acceleration as retinal slip velocity decreases.
Drum onset at arrow.

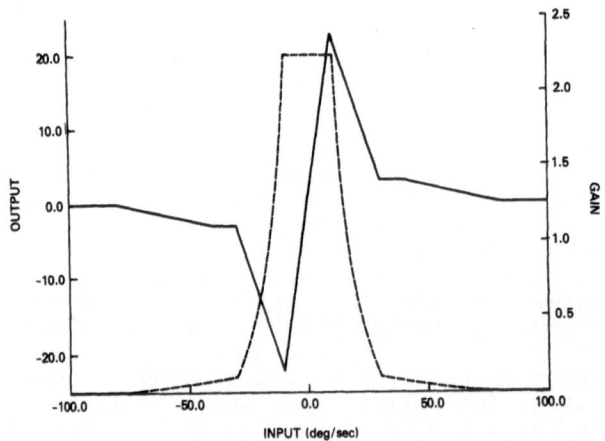

Figure 2. Nonlinearity for detection of retinal slip
velocity. Solid lines indicates shape of nonlinearity.
Dashed line indicates gain (output/input) of the
nonlinearity. Units of the ordinates are arbitrary.

3.2. Optokinetic responses in primates

In foveate animals, the response to an optokinetic
stimulus consists of two components -- a rapid,
immediate, "direct" contribution, attributed to the
pursuit system,and a slow, persistent "indirect" contribution, attributed to the "afoveate" optokinetic
system (Zee et al., 1976; Cohen et al., 1977). In
response to a constant velocity stimulus, eye velocity
immediately jumps to about 60% of stimulus velocity, and
then slowly rises to the steady-state value. When the
lights are turned off, OKAN ensues. The initial velocity
of OKAN probably best reflects the contribution of the
optokinetic (versus pursuit) system to eye velocity
during the preceding optokinetic stimulation. During
monocular viewing, there are no directional asymmetries
of OKAN or OKN. Presumably cortical inputs are
responsible for both the rapid pursuit component of OKN
and the balancing out of directional asymmetries
(Ter Braak, Van Vliet, 1963; Montarolo et al., 1981;
Hoffman, 1982; Harris et al., 1980).

3.3. Optokinetic responses in cortically-lesioned monkeys

3.3.1. General findings. After surgery, each of our
cortically-lesioned monkeys no longer responded to an
optokinetic stimulus viewed through a "tunnel" providing
only 13 degrees of binocular field. With a full-field
stimulus (velocity step), however, each animal developed
OKN with a slow rise to a steady-state value but the
initial jump in eye velocity at stimulus onset was
diminished or absent. A temporal-nasal predominance
during monocular stimulation also appeared after surgery.
3.3.2. Full-field responses. The animal that appeared
completely blind after surgery showed the most prominent
and enduring abnormalities; its behavior will be
discussed in detail. In response to a 10 deg/sec,
constant velocity stimulus, during full-field binocular
viewing, eye velocity slowly increased (rise time of
10-15 seconds) to a steady-state value nearing that of
the stimulus. Likewise, with 20 and 30 deg/sec stimuli
eye velocity nearly reached that of the stimulus but only
after a more prolonged rise time (Fig. 1). Eye
acceleration increased when retinal slip velocity
decreased to about 15 deg/sec (Fig. 1). With a 60 deg/sec
stimulus, however, eye velocity only rose to 2-8 deg/sec.
In contrast,$_2$with a slowly accelerating stimulus (about
0.25 deg/sec^2) eye velocities nearing 60 deg/sec could
be achieved.
3.3.3. Nonlinearity for retinal slip. These results imply
that the "cortically-blind" monkey, like the rabbit and
cat, has an input nonlinearity for retinal slip velocity.
Using the model described by Lisberger et al. (1981), we
have simulated a number of the optokinetic responses of
our cortically-blind monkey. We used the input nonlinearity shown in Fig. 2,and added an adaptive network
to create the reversal phases of OKAN (Leigh et al.,
1981). In intact monkeys, the nonlinearity for retinal
slip velocity appears to be affected by cortical inputs

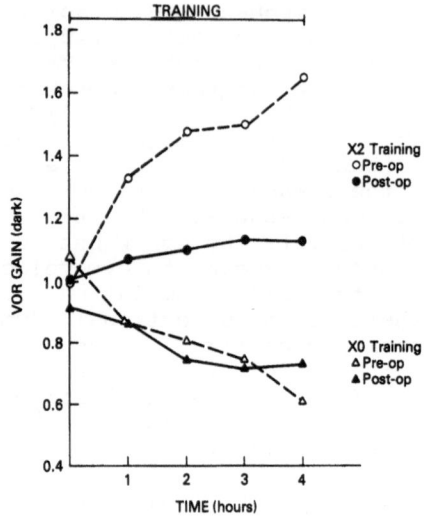

Figure 3. VOR gain adaptation. Hourly measurements in darkness. Mean of 10 cycles (S.D. about 0.1). Adaptation was decreased after the lesion, especially during X2 viewing.

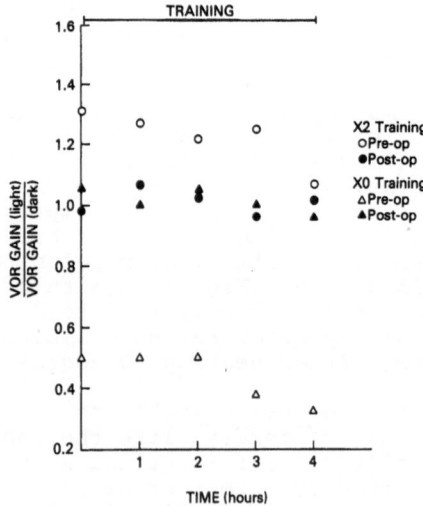

Figure 4. Immediate visual modulation of VOR gain. After the lesion, VOR gain in light and dark during training were similar.

too so that the range of retinal slip velocities, to which the optokinetic system can respond, is extended (Buettner, Büttner, 1979). The maximum value of the initial velocity of OKAN was also decreased after surgery (from 84 to 58 deg/sec); this may reflect a cortical influence on the upper limits of the range of performance of the monkey optokinetic system.

3.3.4. Responses during monocular viewing. During monocular viewing, with a slowly accelerating optokinetic stimulus, stimulation in the temporal-nasal direction elicited a maximum eye velocity of 32 deg/sec while in the nasal-temporal direction only 10 deg/sec. Therefore, cortical inputs appear to be necessary to balance inherent directional asymmetries of OKN that are revealed during monocular viewing.

3.3.5. Physiological and clinical implications. Taken together our results indicate that the monkey has an underlying and possibly subcortical optokinetic system similar to that of afoveate animals. Our results also have important clinical implications. Normally, during optokinetic stimulation, the pursuit system keeps eye velocity near stimulus velocity so the velocity of retinal slip is low and within the range of optimal performance of the optokinetic system. In patients, though, with smooth pursuit deficits due, for example, to cerebellar or cerebral lesions, constant velocity opto-kinetic stimuli may exceed the optimal range for response to retinal slip. The human optokinetic system also takes a longer time to charge and has a lower maximum velocity of OKAN than monkey (Cohen et al., 1981). Therefore, slowly accelerating stimuli may best elicit OKN and OKAN in man.

4. VOR GAIN ADAPTATION

Adaptive control of the VOR was assessed in our animals by measuring the VOR gain (peak eye velocity/peak head velocity) in darkness, before and after four hours of passive, combined, vestibular and optokinetic stimulation. The chair and drum were both oscillated at 0.25 Hz, 30 deg/sec amplitude, with the drum and chair either in phase (X0 viewing, to stimulate a decrease in VOR gain) or 180 deg out of phase (X2 viewing, to stimulate an increase in VOR gain). After surgery, the drop in VOR gain during X0 viewing was only moderately less than that before surgery while the ability to raise the VOR gain (X2 viewing) was more significantly impaired (Fig. 3). In either case, there was little ability to use vision to make immediate adjustments of VOR gain (Fig. 4). At lower frequencies and amplitudes of passive oscillation (only tested post-operatively), however, the VOR gain could be raised more effectively. Our results indicate that the cortex influences VOR gain adaptation but whether it does so solely by providing information about retinal slip during head movements or by providing the visual inputs for immediate adjustments of the VOR gain, or both, is not clear.

230

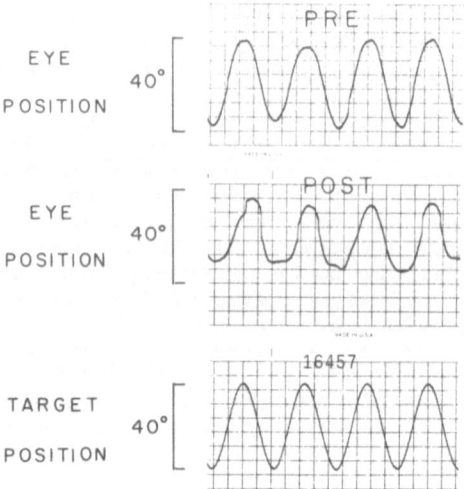

Figure 5. Smooth pursuit capability. Pre-op (top trace)
and post-op (middle trace). Target (bottom trace) moving
sinusoidally (amplitude 20 deg, peak velocity 40 deg/sec).

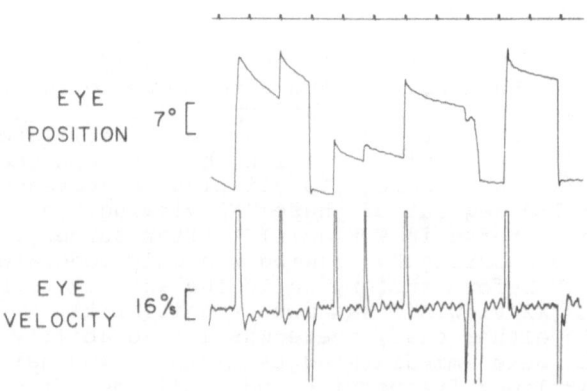

Figure 6. Spontaneous pendular oscillations in the light
that are best seen in the velocity trace. Time marks
are at one sec intervals.

5. SMOOTH PURSUIT

Four weeks after surgery none of the monkeys tracked either a jumping or smoothly moving target. After 8 weeks, though, the "cortically blind" monkey recovered the ability to follow a small (0.25 deg diameter) moving target (either with the head still or moving) using a combination of both saccades and smooth movements (Fig. 5). The latter could have gains (peak eye velocity/peak target velocity) approaching 1.0. Pursuit during monocular viewing was performed equally well in both directions. The monkey also made saccades to a jumping target though less reliably than during tracking of a moving target. Our results suggest a significant recovery of smooth pursuit capability in a "cortically blind" monkey and are compatible with other studies of restored visual function in "destriate" monkeys (Keating, 1980; Solomon et al., 1981; Denny-Brown, Chambers, 1976). In spite of the recovery of a capability for smooth tracking, pursuit responses were not sustained during optokinetic stimulation so that the slow build up of eye velocity, and the asymmetries during monocular viewing, persisted. Finally, the "cortically blind" monkey developed intermittent pendular oscillations of the eyes (about 5 Hz, maximum amplitude of about one degree) (Fig. 6). Pendular oscillations have also been reported in dark and strobe-reared cats (Harris, Cynader, 1981; Conway et al., 1981; Melville Jones et al., 1981).

6. CONCLUSIONS

Our findings, while preliminary, suggest that (1) the primate has an underlying, and possibly subcortical, optokinetic system similar to that of afoveate animals -- with a nonlinear response to retinal slip velocity and temporal-nasal predominance, (2) VOR gain adaptation is impaired but not abolished after occipital lobectomy, and (3) smooth pursuit can recover significantly in "cortically blind" monkeys.

REFERENCES
Buettner UW and Büttner U (1979) Vestibular nuclei activity in the alert monkey during suppression of vestibular and optokinetic nystagmus, Exp. Brain Res. 37, 581-593.
Cohen B, Matsuo V and Raphan T (1977) Quantitative analysis of the velocity characteristics of optokinetic nystagmus and optokinetic after-nystagmus, J. Physiol. 270,321-344.
Cohen B, Henn V, Raphan T and Dennett D (1981) Velocity storage, nystagmus and visual-vestibular interactions in human, Ann. N. Y. Acad. Sci. 374, 421-433.
Collewijn H (1981) The oculomotor system of the rabbit and its plasticity, Berlin, Springer-Verlag.
Conway JL, Timberlake GT and Skavenski AA (1981) Oculomotor changes in cats reared without experiencing continuous retinal image motion, Exp. Brain Res. 43, 229-232.

232

Denny-Brown D and Chambers RA (1976) Physiological aspects of visual perception. I. Functional aspects of visual cortex, Arch. Neurol. 33, 219-227.

Harris LR, Lepore F, Guillemot J-P and Cynader M (1980) Abolition of optokinetic nystagmus in the cat, Science 210, 91-92.

Harris LR and Cynader M (1981) The eye movements of the dark-reared cat, Exp. Brain Res. 44, 41-56.

Hobbelen JF and Collewijn H (1971) Effect of cerebro-cortical and collicular ablations upon the optokinetic reactions in the rabbit, Doc. Ophthalmol. 30, 227-236.

Hoffman K-P and Schoppman A (1981) A quantitative analysis of the direction-specific response of neurons in the cat's nucleus of the optic tract, Exp. Brain Res. 42, 146-157.

Hoffman K-P (in press) The control of the optokinetic reflex by the nucleus of the optic tract in the cat. Subcortical vs cortical nystagmus. In Lennerstrand G, Zee DS and Keller E, ed. Functional basis of ocular motility disorders, Pergamon Press.

Keating EG (1980) Residual spatial vision in the monkey after removal of striate and preoccipital cortex, Brain Res. 187, 271-290.

Leigh RJ, Robinson DA and Zee DS (1981) A hypothetical explanation for periodic alternating nystagmus: instability in the optokinetic-vestibular system, Ann. N. Y. Acad. Sci. 374, 619-635.

Lisberger SG, Miles FA, Optican LM and Eighmy BB (1981) Optokinetic response in monkeys: underlying mechanisms and their sensitivity to long-term adaptive changes in vestibuloocular reflex, J. Neurophysiol. 45, 869-890.

Melville Jones G, Mandl G, Cynader M and Outerbridge JS (1981) Eye oscillations in strobe reared cats, Brain Res. 209, 47-60.

Montarolo PG, Precht W and Strata P (1981) Functional organization of the mechanisms subserving the optokinetic nystagmus in the cat, Neuroscience 6, 231-246.

Solomon SJ, Pasik T and Pasik P (1981) Extrageniculo-striate vision in the monkey. VIII. Critical structures for spatial localization, Exp. Brain Res. 44, 259-270.

Ter Braak JWG and Van Vliet AGM (1963) Subcortical opto-kinetic nystagmus in the monkey, Psychiatr. Neurol. Neurochir. 66, 277-283.

Winterson BJ and Collewijn H (1981) Inversion of direction-selectivity to anterior fields in neurons of nucleus of the optic tract in rabbits with ocular albinism, Brain Res. 220, 31-49.

Zee DS, Yee RD and Robinson DA (1976) Optokinetic responses in labyrinthine-defective human beings, Brain Res. 113, 423-428.

ACKNOWLEDGEMENTS
Vendetta Matthews provided editorial assistance. This research was supported by National Institutes of Health Grants EY01849 and EY00158.

MODELS OF VISUAL-VESTIBULAR INTERACTION IN OCULOMOTOR CONTROL: A REVIEW

A. BUIZZA and R. SCHMID (Pavia, Italy)

1. INTRODUCTION

The crucial role of visual-vestibular interaction in determining motor reactions, motion sensation and motion sickness of onboard personnel of space vehicles has posed a series of problems to which basic and applied physiological and behavioural research has tried to give an answer through an increasing number of studies. Many of them were concerned with oculomotor responses evoked in different conditions of visual-vestibular interaction. There are at least two good reasons for fastening our attention on eye movements. First of all, the goal of oculomotor control can easily be defined in terms of fixation and visual stabilization. A great help can thus follow to interpret how sensory information is processed and in which way the different mechanisms subserving oculomotor control are used to obtain desired responses. Responses that seem not to correspond to the general goal of oculomotor control should be related to misleading interpretation in processing sensory information. The second reason for considering oculomotor responses is that eye movement can easily be measured and quantified.

In the development of knowledge on visual-vestibular interaction models have represented a constant attempt to use experimental data to make rational hypotheses. "Modeling is one of the fundamental processes in our understanding of nature. From observations of phenomena we abstract functional relations (causality) among the substantial elements of a system of interest. Whether the abstraction is intuitive or mathematical, it is the first step of modeling. The induced model is then checked against the next observation through a deductive process and, as a result, discarded, revised, or further tested. The model may be very elementary, being a verbal speculation of the cause-and-effect relations among the related elements, or it may be very formal (mathematical) expression induced from accurate observations and analytical thoughts. Although both types of modeling provide momentum for research, the more quantitative a model is, the more exact becomes the deduction and the testing. For this reason, formal modeling is preferable and modern computer tachniques make it far easier than it was decades ago."(Sagawa,1973) A progressive evolution from "verbal" to "formal" models of increasing complexity can also be observed in the description of visual-vestibular interaction. The aim of this paper is to review the main steps of this evolution and to show how experimental investigation and theoretical speculation continuously interacted to produce a progressive better understanding of the mechanisms underlying visual-vestibular interaction.

Roucoux, A. and Crommelinck, M. (eds.): Physiological and Pathological Aspects of Eye Movements.
© *1982, Dr W. Junk Publishers, The Hague, Boston, London.* ISBN-13: 978-94-009-8002-0

2. EVOLUTION OF VISUAL-VESTIBULAR INTERACTION MODELS

From the functional point of view two types of visual-vestibular
interaction in oculomotor control can be distinguished, the
interaction between the vestibulo-ocular reflex (VOR) and the
optokinetic reflex (OKR), and the interaction between VOR and the
smooth pursuit system (SP). The former is aimed to the stabilization
of the visual surround during subject motion, the latter to the
maintenance of small object fixation. This functional distinction
does not exclude a participation of SP to the generation of oculomotor responses evoked by moving visual scenes. Although the
subject is not asked to pursue any detail of the visual scene and,
therefore , SP is not voluntarily activated, nevertheless at least
some part of it can be made to participate by the fact that also
central visual receptors are stimulated by the slip of the image
of the external world on the retina.

Most of the models of visual-vestibular interaction presented in
the litterature were aimed to the interpretation of VOR-OKR
interaction, although in some of them a SP pathway was explicitly
indicated. Only models of VOR-OKR interaction in oculomotor control
will be considered in this review, and their evolution will be
discussed by making a distinction among three groups of models.

2.1. Open-loop models based on non-linear mechanisms of visual-vestibular interaction

The first group includes models that assume non-linear strategies
of visual-vestibular interaction. The progenitor of these models
is that proposed by Young in 1973 for the interpretation of both
self-motion sensations and oculomotor responses (Fig.1). Two
distinct strategies were assumed to be implemented depending on
whether the angular velocities perceived by the vestibular and by
the visual systems are in relative agreement. If the difference
between the two perceived velocities does not exceed a given
threshold, a weighted sum of them is computed to produce both
sensations and oculomotor responses. Otherwise, a hierarchical
choice program begins in which priority is given to the input
which results to be the more compelling, normally the visual input.
The hypothesee on which Young's model is based were later used to
interprete electrophysiological results obtained by measuring the
activity of vestibular nuclei (VN) neurons, evoked by pure and
combined vestibular and optokinetic stimulations (Allum et al.,
1976; Waespe, Henn, 1977). The misleading point in the interpretation of these results was probably the attempt to explain the
responses obtained in interaction conditions by a summation of the
responses obtained during separate visual and vestibular stimulation
as if VOR and OKR were working in parallel. Since they aren't, a
simple summation was immediately found to be inadequate to explain
the experimental results. Allum et al.(1976) suggested a linear
combination of the visual and the vestibular inputs consisting of
the vestibular response multiplied by a weighting factor less than

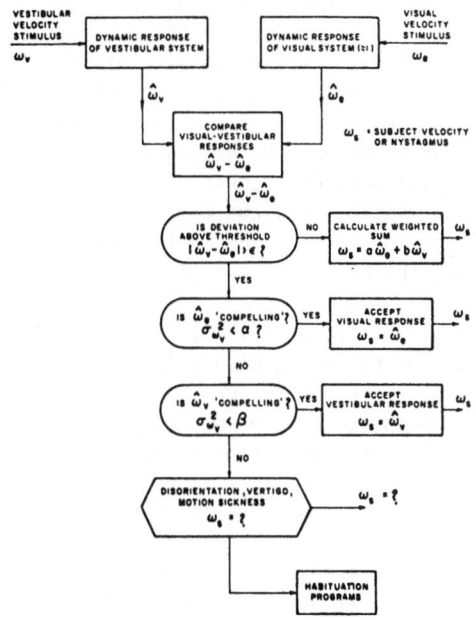

FIGURE 1. Flow-chart representation of Young's model of visual-vestibular interaction (Young, 1973)

unity, added to the optokinetic response multiplied by a weighting factor greater than unity.

After recording in the vestibular nuclei of monkeys submitted to velocity trapezoid stimuli in the light, Waespe and Henn (1977) came to the conclusion that a weighted sum of visual and vestibular responses couldn't explain the experimental results unless weighting factors were continuously changing with time. Such an adaptive control of the weighting factors was considered as to be unlikely. Since responses appeared to switch from the vestibular input to the visual input at the end of the acceleration periods, these results were considered as an electrophysiological evidence in favour of Young's switching hypothesis. With reference to a more complete set of data, two years later the same authors concluded that also the switching theory was inadequate (Waespe, Henn, 1979).

2.2. Closed-loop models based on linear mechanisms of visual-vestibular interaction

An answer to the dilemma between weighting factors and switching hypotheses came with the models of the second generation. The peculiarity of these models was the explicit statement that OKR operates as a negative feedback loop to VOR. The two reflexes do not work in parallel. An input to OKR is created only if the oculomotor response produced by VOR is insufficient or inappropriate (conflict situations) to obtain visual stabilization. OKR contribution depends on retinal slip velocity and it is automatically adjusted to the amount needed to complete vestibular compensation

or to cancel the vestibular component whenever inappropriate. As
a matter of fact, the feedback loop structure of VOR-OKR interaction
allows the system to obtain automatically that adaptive control of
the factors weighting the visual and the vestibular contributions,
which was invoked when the two systems were treated as working in
parallel. Also the switching between the vestibular and the visual
input at the end of the acceleration periods occurs automatically,
although in a gradual way. As the vestibular input to VN tends to
zero during constant velocity rotation, OKR is forced to increase
its contribution until it assumes the complete task of visual
stabilization.

The models proposed by Robinson (1977), by Lau (1978), and the
"algebraic summation" model proposed by Koenig et al.(1978) can
be considered as belonging to the second generation. In all these
models linearity was assumed for both the mechanisms of visual-
vestibular interaction and the gain characteristics of each
subsystem.

The most complete of the models of the second generation is that
proposed by Robinson (Fig.2). Head velocity $\dot{H}$ is transduced by
the semicircular canals (SCC) into $\dot{H}_c$, the canal's estimate of
head velocity. When its sign is changed it becomes an eye velocity
command to the plant. Gaze velocity $\dot{G}$ is obtained as the sum of
eye velocity in the head $\dot{E}$ and head velocity $\dot{H}$. The retina compares
$\dot{G}$ to the velocity $\dot{W}$ of the seen world to produce the input $\dot{e}_w$
(relative motion of the gaze with respect to the seen world) to
the optokinetic system. An efference copy $\dot{E}'$ of eye velocity ,
weighted by a constant k close to 1, is added to $\dot{e}_w$ to reconstruct
the motion of the world with respect to the head ($\dot{W}_h$). Since
the seen world never moves in nature, $\dot{W}_h$ is the negative of $\dot{H}_v$,
the visual system estimate of head velocity in space. The high
frequency components of $\dot{H}_v$ are filtered and the low frequency
components $\dot{H}_v'$ are added to $\dot{H}_c$ in the vestibular nuclei (vn). Their
sum, $\dot{H}'$, is the brainstem's estimate of the velocity of self-
rotation based on both visual and vestibular information. The
smooth pursuit system receives from the retina a signal $\dot{e}_T$ which
represents the relative velocity of a visual target with respect
to the gaze. This signal is added to an efference copy signal of
eye velocity to obtain the visual estimate of target velocity with
respect to the head ($\dot{T}'_h$), and then to $\dot{H}'$ to obtain the brainstem's
estimate $\dot{T}'$ of target velocity in space.

The presence of a low-pass filter in the optokinetic pathway
reaching VN and that of a faster visual pathway to the brainstem
(the SP pathway which is activated also by optokinetic stimuli)
can explain the existence of a slow and a fast build-up component
in step optokinetic responses and optokinetic afternystagmus
(OKAN)(Cohen et al., 1977).

Robinson's model can simulate the responses to many combinations
of visual and vestibular inputs. In the linear range, the entire
repertoire of monkey optokinetic eye movements reported by Cohen

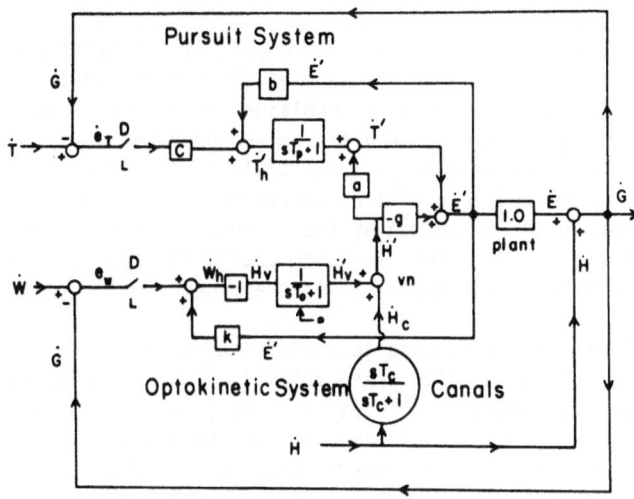

FIGURE 2. Robinson's model of visual-vestibular interaction (reproduced from Henn et al., 1980)

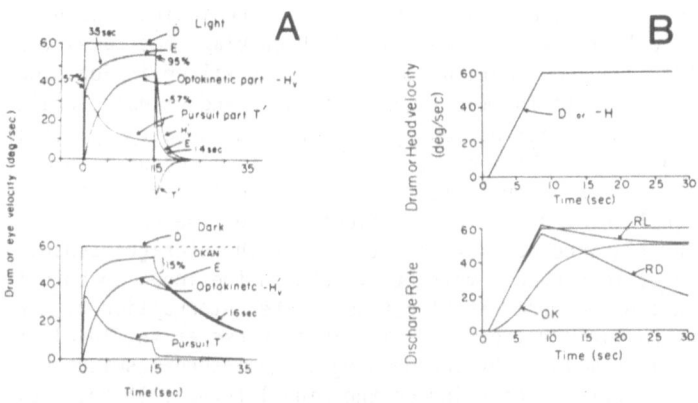

FIGURE 3. Responses predicted by Robinson's model. A: optokinetic responses (OKN and OKAN slow phase velocities). In the upper figure the drum is assumed to start rotating at 60 deg/sec and to stop in the light after 15 sec of constant velocity rotation. In the lower figure the light is assumed to be switched off while the drum is rotating at 60 deg/sec. The remaining notations are defined in Fig.2. B: discharge rate of neurons in the vestibular nuclei during rotation in the light (RL), rotation in the dark (RD), and optokinetic stimulation (OK) (reproduced from Henn et al., 1980)

et al.(1977) and the discharge patterns of many VN neurons reported by Waespe and Henn (1977) can be predicted (Fig.3). In particular the difference between the time constant of the slow build-up component of OKN and that of OKAN is explained in a simple and natural way. During OKN the optokinetic system operates as a closed loop system with a forward gain of about $1/(1-k)$. Thus the time constant T_{OKN} of OKN build-up will be approximately $T_0/(2-k)$. OKAN is produced by the discharge of the low-pass filter in open loop conditions (external visual feedback open). Its time constant T_{OKAN} will be approximately $T_0/(1-k)$ and therefore greater than T_{OKN}.

A less natural assumption is made to justify the effects of short periods of fixation on the slow phase velocity (SPV) of OKAN and of post-rotatory nystagmus (Raphan et al., 1977). A parametric control of T_0 which reduces this time constant by about 3 when the eye is going faster than the visual scene is assumed.

The model proposed by Raphan et al. in 1977 can still be considered as belonging to the second generation in spite of the presence of some asymmetric gain characteristics. As a matter of fact, asymmetries are introduced only to justify observed differences in vestibular and optokinetic responses evoked by subject or drum rotation to the right or to the left. Raphan's model is reproduced in Fig.4. Vestibular nystagmus and OKN are produced by combined activation of direct and indirect pathways. The indirect pathways include a "velocity storage mechanism" which plays the same role as the efference loop containing the low-pass filter in Robinson's model. The inputs to the model are vestibular and visual signals representing cupula deflection r_v and surround velocity r_0. It is supposed that r_0 is obtained by combining retinal error with an efference feedback of eye velocity from the oculomotor system and with a signal related to cupula deflection from the vestibular system. An efference copy of the state x of the storage mechanism is subtracted to surround velocity to obtain the input to both the direct and the indirect visual pathways. The interruption of the flow of visual information occurring in darkness at the level of the retina is simulated by the opening of an internal switch L placed in the pathway carrying on the signal (r_0-x). In this way the opening of the switch L will interrupt a negative feedback pathway to the storage mechanism with the result of increasing its time constant. The greater time constant of OKAN with respect to that of OKN is so justified. A second switch S in a further negative feedback pathway to the storage mechanism produces the same effect as the parametric control of the low-pass filter time constant T_0 in Robinson's model.

Raphan's model can predict almost the same set of experimental data as Robinson's model (Fig.5) although its structure and the hypotheses on wich it is based seem to be less justifiable than those proposed by Robinson.

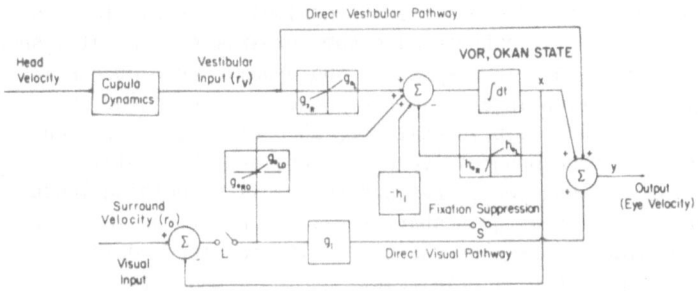

FIGURE 4. Model of visual-vestibular interaction proposed by
Raphan et al.(1977)

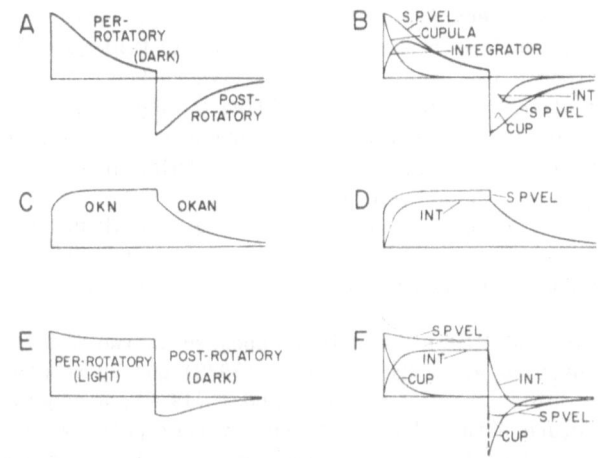

FIGURE 5. Responses predicted by Raphan et al. model. A,C,E:
model predictions of slow phase eye velocity for a step of angular
velocity in darkness (A), for a step of surround velocity (C),
and for a step of angular velocity in light (E). B,D,F: comparative
changes in slow phase velocity (S.P.VEL.), cupula deflection (CUP),
and output of the integrator (INT) for the responses shown in A,
C, and E respectively (reproduced from Raphan et al., 1979)

2.3. Closed loop models with non-linear gain characteristics

A further step in modelling visual-vestibular interaction consisted
in the attempt to interprete also some experimental results showing
a progressive change in the static and dynamic characteristics of
VOR-OKR interaction in experimental conditions bringing about
increasing retinal slip velocities (Cohen et al., 1977; Koenig et
al., 1978). Such a progressive change couldn't be explained by the
presence of switches which respond to an all-or-nothing logic.
Continuous non-linear gain characteristics had to be introduced.
The saturation of OKN slow phase velocity for large optokinetic
stimulus velocities, also in relationship to the size of the
stimulus field, was perfectly known (Dichgans et al., 1973). What
remained to be specified on both the electrophysiological and the
modelling level was: (a) are nonlinearities present in both the
direct and the indirect optokinetic pathway? (b) where do non-
linearities occur in each pathway, peripherally or centrally?
(c) how much do they differ from each other in terms of differential
gain? (d) is the presence of appropriate non-linear gain characteristics enough to justify the non-linear aspects of VOR-OKR
interaction?
A fundamental contribution on the electrophysiological plane was
given by Waespe and Henn (1979,1981) and by Waespe et al.(1981).
Two conclusions were reached by these authors in monkeys. First
of all, in response to optokinetic stimuli VN neuron activity
saturates for stimulus velocities exceeding 60 deg/sec, and
therefore much earlier than oculomotor responses. The same neurons
do not display the same saturation for vestibular inputs. Secondly,
the flocculus plays a complementary role with respect to VN, in
the sense that flocculus P-cells start firing when VN neurons
begin to saturate. Saturation in VN neurons activity during
optokinetic stimulation was observed also in cat (Keller, Precht,
1979).
Non-linear gain characteristics first appeared in two models
proposed, respectively, by Barnes et al.(1978) and by Schmid et
al.(1979), in which, as in Robinson's model (1977), a negative
feedback structure with a direct and an indirect pathway was
assumed for OKR. Nevertheless both these models were discussed
only in the linear range. Thus neither the shape of the non-linear
characteristics was quantitatively defined, nor their effects on
input-output responses was considered. In the linear range both
these models can interpret almost the same set of experimental
data as Robinson's (1977) and Raphan's (1977) models.
The first attempt to explain the non-linear aspects of visual-
vestibular interaction by the presence of non-linear gain characteristics in the forward optokinetic pathways was made by Schmid et
al.(1980) and by Buizza and Schmid (1982). The more recent and
complete formulation of their model is shown in Fig.6. VOR is
described in a simplified form as an open loop system with high-
pass characteristics. K_V and T_V denote, respectively, the gain and

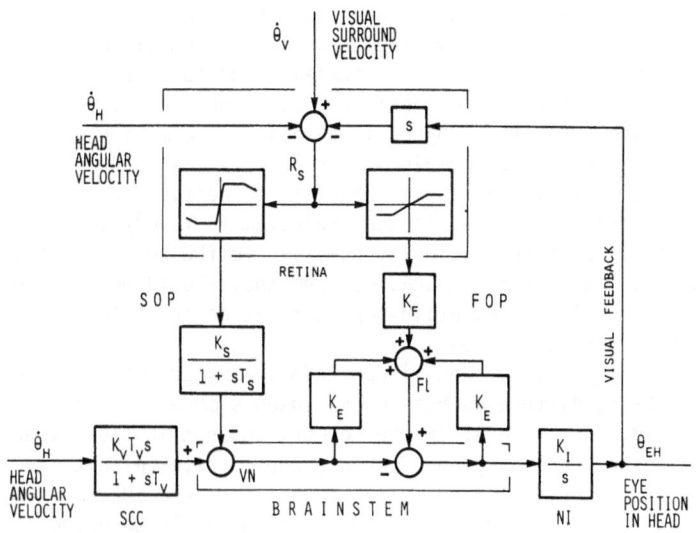

FIGURE 6. Model of visual-vestibular interaction in oculomotor control proposed by Buizza and Schmid (1982)

the time constant of the vestibular system as seen from VN. The optokinetic system is described as a closed loop system with two parallel forward pathways. A slow indirect pathway (SOP) passes through the vestibular nuclei (VN). Its dynamics is described by a low-pass filter with a time constant T_S of the same order of magnitude as the time constant T_V of the vestibular system. A fast direct pathway (FOP) passes through the flocculus (F1) and reaches the brainstem beyond the vestibular nuclei. Its dynamics has been neglected. Two additional inputs to F1 (a vestibular input and an input giving an efference copy of eye velocity) have been introduced according to the results by Lisberger and Fuchs (1978 a,b). A non-linear characteristic has been placed at the input of each visual pathway. Nonlinearities were actually observed by Collewijn et al.(1972) in the responses of rabbit retinal ganglion cells to optokinetic stimulations. The non-linear characteristics regulate the relative contributions of the two visual pathways in relation to the value of retinal slip velocity. When they were identified from data obtained in cat, monkey, and man they were found to vary significantly from species to species (Schmid et al., 1980; Buizza, Schmid, 1982). The relative contribution of the indirect pathway (SOP) decreases from cat to monkey and from monkey to man. In all these species SOP saturates for small retinal slip velocities (5 to 10 deg/sec).

As in Robinson's model, the vestibular nuclei are the centre in which sensory information about head velocity is made available in the full range of frequencies (from the visual input at low

frequencies, from the vestibular input at high frequencies, and
from the combination of the two inputs in the intermediate range
of frequencies).The output of VN in normal conditions of visual-
vestibular interaction can be considered as a central estimate
of head velocity. When the subject is fixating at a moving target,
the three inputs to Fl are combined in such a way as to provide
a central reconstruction of target absolute velocity. When Fl
output is algebraically added in the brainstem to VN output, a
central estimate of target velocity relative to the head is obtained.
This signal is actually the neural command that should be sent to
the oculomotor nuclei to maintain target fixation in spite of
subject and/or target movement.
Apart from the presence of non-linear gain characteristics, there
is only one basic difference between Robinson's model (1977) and
Buizza, Schmid model (1982). In the former, and not in the latter,
a feedback pathway bringing an efference copy of eye velocity is
used to create a positive loop common to both VOR and SOP. By
means of it Robinson could explain the experimentally observed
difference between the value of the semicircular canal time
constant as measured at the level of primary vestibular neurons,
and the value of the vestibular system time constant as measured
at the level of secondary vestibular neurons or from vestibular
nystagmus (Robinson, 1976). This difference is implicitely assumed
in the model of Fig.6, where T_V does not represent the semicircular
canal time constant but the vestibular system time constant. The
possibility of controlling VOR static and dynamic characteristics
can be created, alternatively, by a feedforward vestibulo-cerebellar-
vestibular pathway of the same type as those proposed by Ito (1972)
and by Robinson (1976) to explain plastic changes in VOR characteristics. It is enough to assume that this pathway has also dynamic
properties as some results by Llinàs et al.(1971) and by Ghelarducci
et al.(1975) seem to suggest. A gain control in such a feedforward
pathway would increase (or decrease) both VOR gain and time constant,
whereas a variation of the gain k in the positive feedback loop of
Robinson's model would decrease VOR gain and increase its time
constant or viceversa. In experimental conditions in which a
progressive variation of VOR gain was observed (Jeannerod et al.,
1976) VOR gain and time constant varied in the same way (e.g., a
progressive decrease of gain in vestibular habituation is also
accompanied by an increase of the phase lead in the frequency
response). Moreover the feedforward solution has the advantage
that all the stability problems inherent to positive feedback
loops are avoided. On the other hand, the coupling of VOR and SOP
dynamics occurring in Robinson's model can be functionally justified
in relation to the complementary roles of VOR and OKR in visual
stabilization.
In the linear range there is nothing that can be explained by one
model and not by the other for what concerns both input-output
responses and single unit activity in VN and Fl. Also smooth

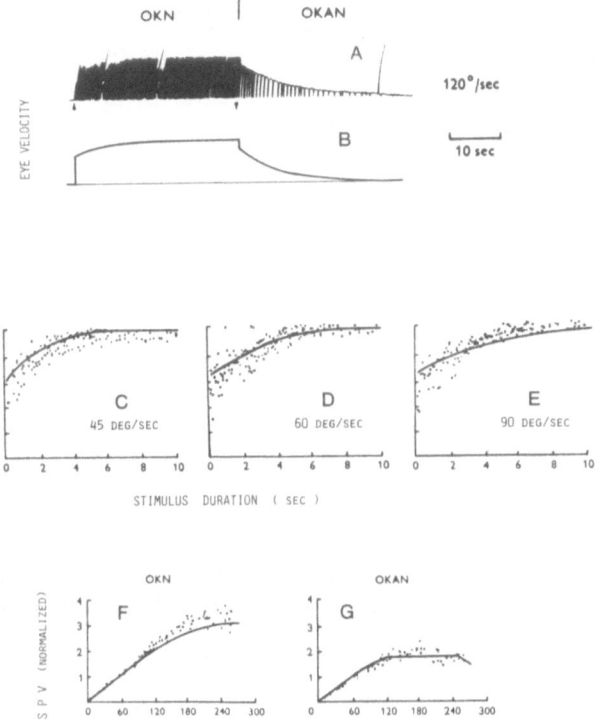

FIGURE 7. Comparison between experimental data (Cohen et al., 1977)
and model predictions (Buizza, Schmid, 1982) for monkey's optokinetic
responses (see text for explanation)

pursuit which seems to charge the low-pass filter in Robinson's
model and not in Buizza, Schmid model does not help very much in
testing the two hypotheses. Actually the charge of the filter by
a smooth pursuit input in Robinson's model will take several seconds.
Therefore the amount of the charge at the end of normal smooth
pursuit experiments will probably be too small to give appreciable
effects at the level of VN.
The model in Fig.6 was proved to be able to predict most of the
non linear aspects of visual-vestibular interaction observed
experimentally in monkey, cat, and man (Schmid et al., 1980; Buizza,
Schmid, 1982).
Figure 7 shows a comparison between experimental data in monkey
(from Cohen et al., 1977) and model predictions for the time course
of nystagmus slow phase velocity (SPV) during OKN and OKAN in a

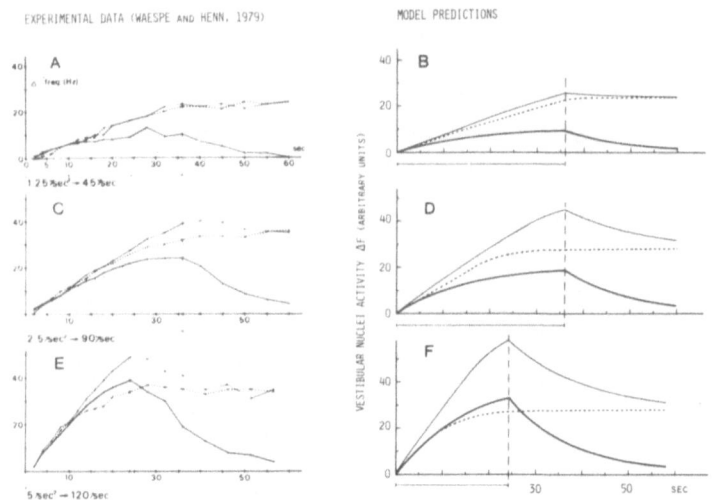

EXPERIMENTAL DATA (WAESPE AND HENN, 1979)   MODEL PREDICTIONS

FIGURE 8. Comparison between experimental data (Waespe, Henn, 1979) and model predictions (Buizza, Schmid, 1982) for the discharge rate in monkey's vestibular nuclei during rotation in darkness (heavy lines), rotation in light (thin lines), and optokinetic stimulation (dotted lines)

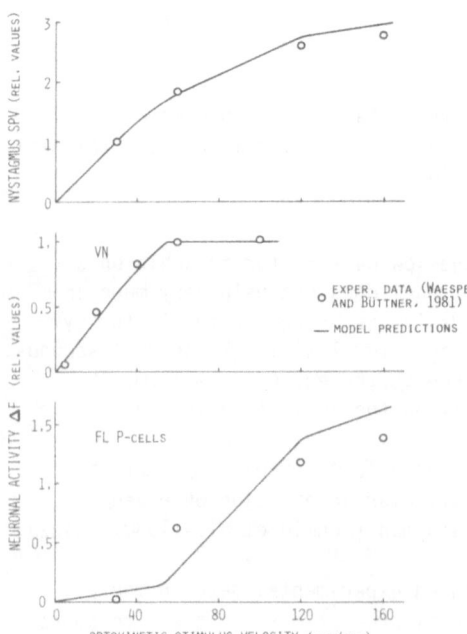

FIGURE 9. Comparison between experimental data (Waespe, Büttner, 1981) and model predictions (Buizza, Schmid, 1982) for nystagmus SPV, and for vestibular nuclei (VN) and flocculus Purkinje-cell (Fl P-cells) activity in the monkey during optokinetic stimulation

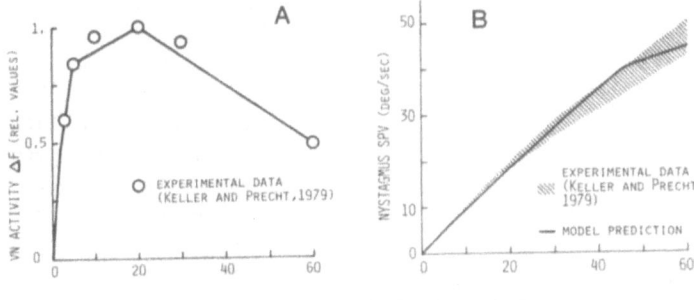

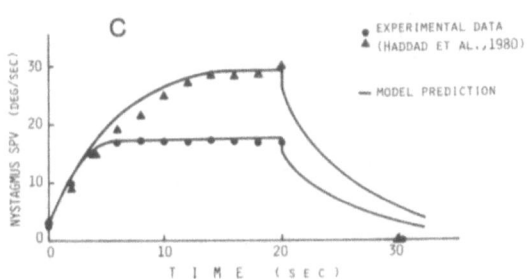

FIGURE 10. Comparison between experimental data (Keller, Precht, 1979; Haddad et al., 1980) and model predictions (Buizza, Schmid, 1982) for cat's optokinetic responses

120 deg/sec step response (Fig.7-A,B), for the pattern of SPV
build-up at different optokinetic stimulus velocities (Fig.7-C,D,E),
for the steady state gain characteristics between SPV and drum
velocity (Fig.7-F), and for the relationship between initial OKAN
velocity and drum velocity during the preceding optokinetic stimulation (Fig.7-G). The increasing duration of nystagmus build-up
for increasing stimulus velocities can be explained by the presence
of saturating gain characteristics in the slow optokinetic pathway.
As stimulus velocity increases, the working point moves within
zones of the non-linear characteristic with decreasing differential
gain (γ). Since the closed-loop time constant of OKR is given by
$T_C = T_S/(1+\gamma)$ a decrease of γ will slow down nystagmus build-up.
Figure 8 shows a comparison between experimental data (Waespe,
Henn, 1979) and model predictions for VN neurons activity during
pure vestibular stimulation (heavy lines), pure optokinetic
stimulation (dotted lines), and during rotation in a stationary
visual surround (thin lines) for different stimulus amplitudes.
The complementary roles of VN and Fl in the generation of optokinetic
responses shown by Waespe and Büttner (1981) and by Waespe and

246

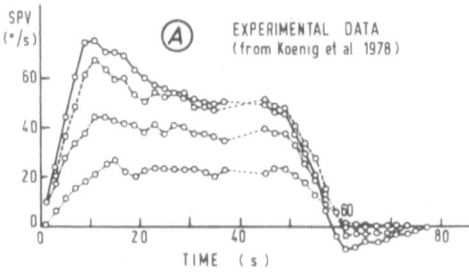

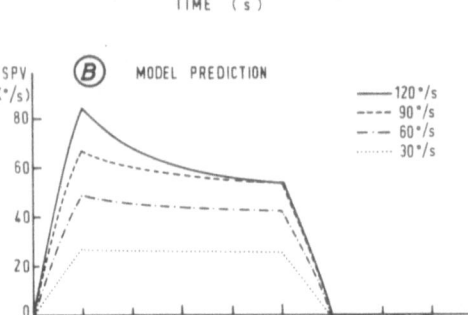

FIGURE 11.
Comparison between
experimental data
(Koenig et al., 1978)
and model predictions
(Schmid et al., 1980)
for nystagmus slow
phase velocity (SPV)
in man during rotation
in the light

Henn (1981) in monkey can be predicted by the model in Fig.6
without introducing any threshold in the fast optokinetic pathway
(Fig.9). The load distribution between the two optokinetic pathways
is actually regulated by the slope of the respective non-linear
characteristics. For small retinal slip velocities (weak optokinetic
stimuli) SOP has a much higher gain than FOP and therefore assumes
almost the entire load. Only when SOP gain decreases due to saturation, FOP contribution becomes more and more important.
The SOP non-linear characteristic in cat was constructed using the
data reported by Keller and Precht (1979) for VN activity during
optokinetic stimulations in open loop conditions (Fig.10-A). The
FOP non-linear characteristic was then adjusted in order to fit
input-output steady state data in closed loop conditions (Fig.10-B).
Afterwards also some non-linear aspects of OKR dynamics could
correctly be predicted, as shown in Fig.10-C.
Model identification for man was based on the experimental data
reported by Koenig et al.(1978). An example of model prediction is
shown in Fig.11 where the model mimics the time course of nystagmus
SPV during rotation in the light for trapezoid chair velocity
profiles of different amplitudes. At lower stimulus velocities a
complete compensation of head rotation is predicted. At higher
stimulus velocities OKR is almost saturated at the end of the
acceleration period. When an additional contribution is required
to it in order to compensate the decline of the vestibular component

during the constant velocity period, this additional contribution cannot be given. Thus nystagmus SPV is predicted to decrease exponentially with the time constant of the vestibular system to a final value which represents the maximal OKR contribution.

3. CONCLUSION

In the study of visual-vestibular interaction in oculomotor control, as in all fields of science where mathematical models are used, there is a continuous dialectic between experimental research and theoretical speculation. Models are made to give a unitary frame to the existing experimental data. They normally introduce new hypotheses and open questions pushing towards new oriented experiments. Each step in this cognitive process issues a challenge to our faculty of theoretical abstraction or to our experimental inventiveness. Sometimes the theoretical investigation runs after the experimental research, sometimes the roles of pursuer and pursued are reversed.

A brief history of models of visual-vestibular interaction in oculomotor control has been presented in this paper. At the present state of the art, the basic characteristics of the interaction between the vestibulo-ocular reflex (VOR) and the optokinetic reflex (OKR) are described in terms of mathematical models in a precise way. Oculomotor responses and single unit responses in the vestibular nuclei and in the flocculus, in both the linear and the non-linear range of visual-vestibular interaction, can be interpreted not only in a qualitative but also in a quantitative way.

Attempts were also made to use models for the interpretation of the effects of experimental lesions (Buizza, Schmid, 1982) and of pathological situations affecting visual-vestibular interaction (Lau et al., 1978; Schmid, Buizza, 1982). However the clinical applications of models were almost exclusively restricted to "a posteriori" justifications of data obtained on patients for whom a diagnosis was already available. So far, no attempt has been made to use models of visual-vestibular interaction as a diagnostic tool. In order to make it possible, further progress in our knowledge of the anatomical structures supporting visual-vestibular interaction and in our understanding of their respective roles is needed. In particular the following questions should receive more adequate answers on both the experimental and the modelling plane. What is the anatomical support of the direct and the indirect optokinetic pathways considered in the more recent models? To what extent and in which way does the cortex participate to optokinetic responses? What is the relationship between the smooth pursuit system and the direct optokinetic pathway? What are the roles of the central and the peripheral retinal receptors in the generation of optokinetic responses? Is the system invariant with respect to the conditions of visual-vestibular interaction?

New experimental data will be made available to give an answer to all these questions. Their interpretation by models will represent the only way to find essentials and to construct step by step a complete theory of visual-vestibular interaction.

AKNOWLEDGEMENT
This work has been supported by CNR, Rome, Italy

REFERENCES
Allum JHJ, Graf W, Dichgans J, Schmidt CL (1976) Visual-vestibular interaction in the vestibular nuclei of the goldfish, Exp.Brain Res. 26, 463-485.
Barnes GR, Benson AJ, Prior ARJ (1978) Visual-vestibular interaction in the control of eye movement, Aviat.Space Environ.Med. 49, 557-564.
Buizza A, Schmid R (1982) Visual-vestibular interaction in oculo-motor control: mathematical modelling and computer simulation, Biol.Cybern., in press.
Cohen B, Matsuo V, Raphan Th (1977) Quantitative analysis of the velocity characteristics of optokinetic nystagmus and optokinetic afternystagmus, J.Physiol. 270, 321-344.
Collewijn H, Oyster CW, Takahashi E (1972) Rabbit optokinetic reactions and retinal direction-selective cells. A preliminary model, Bibl.Ophthalmol. 82, 280-287.
Dichgans J, Nauck B, Wolpert E (1973) The influence of attention, vigilance and stimulus area on optokinetic and vestibular nystagmus and voluntary saccades. In Zikmund V, ed. The oculomotor system and brain function, pp.281-294, London, Butterworths.
Ghelarducci B, Ito M, Yagi N (1975) Impulse discharges from flocculus Purkinje cells of alert rabbits during visual stimulation combined with horizontal head rotation, Brain Res. 87, 66-72.
Henn V, Cohen B, Young LR 41980) Visual-vestibular interaction in motion perception and the generation of nystagmus, Neurosciences Res.Progr.Bull., Vol.18, n.4, Cambridge, Ma, MIT Press.
Ito M (1972) Neural design of the cerebellar motor control system, Brain Res. 40, 81-84.
Jeannerod M, Magnin M, Schmid R, Stefanelli M (1976) Vestibular habituation to angular velocity steps in the cat, Biol.Cybern. 22, 39-48.
Keller EL, Precht W (1979) Visual-vestibular responses in vestibular neurons in intact and cerebellectomized alert cat, Neurosci. 4, 1599-1613.
Koenig E, Allum JHJ, Dichgans J (1978) Visual-vestibular interaction upon nystagmus slow phase velocity in man, Acta Otolaryngol. 85, 397-410.
Lau CGY (1978) Modelling of visual-vestibular interaction and the fast component of nystagmus, Ph.D.Thesis, University of Califor-nia, Santa Barbara.
Lau CGY, Honrubia V, Jenkins HA, Baloh RW, Yee RD (1978) Linear

model for visual-vestibular interaction, Aviat.Space Environ. Med. 49, 880-885.

Lisberger SG, Fuchs AF (1978a) Role of primate flocculus during rapid behavioral modification of vestibuloocular reflex. I. Purkinje cell activity during visually guided horizontal smooth pursuit eye movements and passive head rotation, J.Neurophysiol. 41, 733-763.

Lisberger SG, Fuchs AF (1978b) Role of primate flocculus during rapid behavioral modification of vestibuloocular reflex. II. Mossy fiber firing petterns during horizontal head rotation and eye movement, J.Neurophysiol. 41, 764-777.

Llinås R, Precht W, Clarke M (1971) Cerebellar Purkinje cell responses to physiological stimulation of the vestibular system in the frog, Exp.Brain Res. 9, 16-29.

Raphan Th, Cohen B, Matsuo V (1977) A velocity storage mechanism responsible for optokinetic nystagmus (OKN), optokinetic after-nystagmus (OKAN), and vestibular nystagmus. In Baker R and Berthoz A, eds. Control of gaze by brainstem neurons, pp.37-47, Amsterdam, Elsevier/North Holland.

Raphan Th, Matsuo V, Cohen B (1979) Velocity storage in the vestibulo-ocular reflex arc (VOR), Exp.Brain Res. 35, 229-248.

Robinson DA (1976) Adaptive gain control of the vestibuloocular reflex by the cerebellum, J.Neurophysiol. 39, 954-969.

Robinson DA (1977) Vestibular and optokinetic symbiosis: an example of explaining by modelling. In Baker R and Berthoz A, eds. Control of gaze by brainstem neurons, pp.49-58, Amsterdam, Elsevier/North Holland.

Sagawa K (1973) Comparative models of overall circulatory mechanics. In Brown JHU and Dickson JF III, eds. Advances in biomedical engineering, Vol.3, pp.1-95, New York, Academic Press.

Schmid R, Buizza A (1982) Visual-vestibular interaction in oculomotor control: a model interpretation of pathological situations, 8th Extraordinary Meeting of the Bārāny Society, Basle, June 22-25, 1982.

Schmid R, Zambarbieri D, Sardi R (1979) A mathematical model of the optokinetic reflex, Biol.Cybern. 34, 215-225.

Schmid R, Buizza A, Zambarbieri D (1980) A non-linear model for visual-vestibular interaction during body rotation in man, Biol.Cybern. 36, 143-151.

Waespe W, Büttner U (1981) Flocculus unit activity in the alert monkey during optokinetic stimulation. In Becker W and Fuchs A, eds. Progress in oculomotor research, pp.495-502, New York, Elsevier North Holland.

Waespe W, Henn V (1977) Neuronal activity in the vestibular nuclei of the alert monkey during vestibular and optokinetic stimulation, Exp.Brain Res. 27, 523-538.

Waespe W, Henn V (1979) The velocity response of vestibular nucleus neurons during vestibular, visual and combined angular accelera-tion, Exp.Brain Res. 37, 337-347.

Waespe W, Henn V (1981) Visual-vestibular interaction in the
    flocculus of the alert monkey. II. Purkinje cell activity,
    Exp.Brain Res. 43, 349-360.
Waespe W, Büttner U, Henn V (1981) Visual-vestibular interaction
    in the flocculus of the alert monkey. I. Input activity, Exp.
    Brain Res. 43, 337-348.
Young LR (1973) On visual-vestibular interaction, in Fifth
    symposium on the role of the vestibular organs in space explo-
    ration, pp.205-210, NASA, SP-314.

NEURONAL RESPONSES IN THE PARIETO - INSULAR VESTIBULAR CORTEX OF ALERT JAVA MONKEYS (MACCACA FASCICULARIS)

O.-J. GRÜSSER, M. PAUSE and URSULA SCHREITER
(Department of Physiology, Freie Universität, 1000 Berlin 33, Arnimallee 22, Germany (West))

1. INTRODUCTION

The awake subject is aware of the space coordinates (vertical and horizontal plane) and the spatial relationship between the objects of the extrapersonal space. This percept remains approximately invariant when the subject moves or changes his position in space, a procedure requiring a continuous readjustment between personal space and extrapersonal space perception. This readjustment relies on input signals from different sensory modalities: the teleceptive modality of vision, the vestibular signals (otolith signals for static position, cupula receptor signals for dynamic position changes) and mechanoreceptor input from the body. The deep mechano-receptors from the neck region (joints, tendon organs, muscle spindles (?)) are especially important since they signal the re-lative position between head and trunk. In addition the force (pressure) gradient over the whole body is an important component in the perception of space coordinates. When this force gradient caused by the effect of gravity on the body mass is substantially altered, spatial orientation is impaired, as everybody can exper-ience when he dives for the first time. During movement or change in body position the force gradient changes and leads to a variable activation of the mechanoreceptors located in the tendons, muscles and joints as well as the mechanoreceptors of that part of the body surface touching the ground.

Several years ago we became interested in the neuronal mechanisms responsible for the perception of objects and of the structure of the extrapersonal space. We assumed that a functional analysis of cortical vestibular areas could contribute to our understanding of the perceptual constancy of space. Firstly we tried to record neuronal responses from the cortical vestibular area described by Büttner and Buettner (1978) in the Rhesus monkey. The cortical vestibular field explored by these authors is located at the later-al end of the sulcus intraparietalis and has been called area 2v (c.f. Fredrickson et al., (1966). During a year of frustrating ex-periments, however, we failed to record any vestibular responses from the cortical region of Java monkey (Maccaca fascicularis) which could correspond anatomically to 2v of the Rhesus monkey. More or less by accident, however, in one of the later experiments vestibular responses suddenly appeared as the microelectrode was penetrating into deep cortical structures. After this discovery (Pause and Schreiter, 1981 .) we performed a systematic study in 6 Java monkeys on the responses of this cortical vestibular area located deep in the parietal region bordering the sulcus lateralis. The histological analysis of the microelectrode tip position indicated that many of our recordings were obtained from an area which had been pointed out as a possible candidate for vestibular functions by Pandya and Sanides (1973) and was desig-

Roucoux, A. and Crommelinck, M. (eds.): Physiological and Pathological Aspects of Eye Movements.
© *1982, Dr W. Junk Publishers, The Hague, Boston, London.* ISBN-13: 978-94-009-8002-0

nated by these authors as <u>area retroinsularis parietalis</u> (reIpt).
Other vestibular responses were found in areas bordering reIpt.
In the following we shall tentatively designate the cortical region along the sulcus lateralis from which we obtained vestibular
responses the parieto- insular vestibular cortex (PiVeC). We will
describe the responses of neurons recorded from this cortical
region.

2. METHODS

Our report is based on the quantitative analysis of data obtained
in four of the six Java monkeys (3.0-4.5 kg body weight, two males,
four females).

<u>Preparation</u>. Under deep pentobarbital anesthesia five Ag/AgCl ball
electrodes were implanted into the bones around the orbita to record the horizontal and vertical DC-electrooculogram (EOG). The
bone of the skull was removed on one side above the parietal cortex and a cylinder 30 mm in diameter was stereotactically implanted
above the region shown in fig. 1a. The last part of the preparation
was the implantation of an aluminum corona adapted individually
to the head of the monkey.

<u>Recordings</u>. The microelectrode recordings began on the fourth day
after the operation. The awake monkey sat with the back supported
and the legs fastened in a monkey chair. The hands were either restrained or free, depending on the experimental task. The head was
fixed by the corona and two screws to a movable axis connected
with the monkey chair. A large plexiglass shield at the height of
the corona prevented the monkey from reaching the micromanipulator
or the electrodes with his hand. The plane determined by the lower
orbital rim and the outer auditory canals was inclined downwards
about 10-20 degrees from the horizontal plane. The monkey could
feed himself and was regularly rewarded for quiet cooperation
during the experiments with raisins, small pieces of chocolate,
juice etc..

The horizontal and vertical EOGs were recorded with conventional
DC-amplifiers (0-100 or 0-30 Hz bandwidth). A hydraulic micromanipulator was fixed on a XY micropositioner placed on the cylinder (Wells, Pasadena). Glass-insulated tungsten microelectrodes
with an impedance of 5-15 M were used for single unit recordings. The daily recording period lasted about 4-5 hours. Whenever
possible, the monkey's behaviour was videotaped simultaneously
with the oscilloscope display of the EOG and the single unit discharges.

<u>Anatomical localisation</u>. At the end of the experimental series
the monkey was anesthetized, received a large dose of Heparine
(1500 IU intraarterially), was then sacrificed by an overdose of
Na-pentobarbital and perfused with heparinized Ringer solution
and a fixative (10 percent Formaldehyde or Glutaraldehyde). The
brain was later examined with standard histological techniques.

During the experiments a systematic map (based on the XYZ coordinates of the micromanipulator) was constructed and during the
penetration all possible inputs affecting the activity of the
respective neuron recorded were protocolled (visual stimuli, eye
movements, head movements, body movements, somatosensory stimuli,
vestibular stimulation, attentiveness, emotional components, motor behaviour) along with the stereotaxic coordinates of the

microelectrode tip. Before perfusing the brain, guide needles were inserted into the plane at XYZ coordinate values which were later used as references for the anatomical reconstruction of the functional map from the serial histological sections.

Stimulation. The monkey chair was placed on a modified Tönnies turntable driven by a servomotor and controlled by a microprocessor unit constructed in our Institute. The turntable could be rotated sinusoidally at a constant speed to the right or the left (yaw). The position of the chair was measured by means of an optical goniometer. The monkey chair could be tilted $\pm$30 degrees in a lateral direction (roll) or anterior/posterior direction (pitch). Approximate sinusoidal movements with the same maximum amplitudes were also possible in these planes. The monkey was surrounded by a cylinder 120 cm in diameter and 80 cm high. The inner cylinder wall was covered with a precise vertical black/white stripe pattern of 1.15 degrees period. The stripe pattern was produced by means of a silk-screen printing technique. The stripe cylinder was moved by a second servomotor and could be rotated at a constant speed or sinusoidally around the monkey. Chair rotation axis and cylinder axis were aligned. It was also possible to couple the stripe cylinder directly with the chair. By disjoined control of the two servomotors, the drum and the chair were movable at variable phase angles and/or amplitudes but at the same sinewave frequency. One cylinder half was removable. For visual stimulation with single small stationary or moving visual stimuli an 80x80 cm vertical screen was placed 50 cm in front of the monkey. The single moving visual stimuli could be projected onto the screen by means of a servomotor-driven double mirror system. Larger black discs (about 5-10 degrees diameter) on long plexiglass rods could be moved in front of the monkey by hand. In addition, a large disc about 80 degrees in diameter covered by black-white stripes of 6 cm period was moved by hand at a distance of about 50 cm from the monkey in selected directions.

The head of the monkey could be rotated while the trunk was stationary. For this purpose the head was connected to the drum axis. Reversed stimulation was also possible; the monkey's head was then fixed to the stationary drum axis, while the chair was rotated sinusoidally ($\pm$30 degrees maximum).

Somatosensory stimulation was performed by hand (touching of the skin, tapping of the joints and muscles, movement of the limbs etc.). Protocols of this stimulation were the combined videotape recordings of the monkey and the unit discharges displayed on the oscilloscope.

Data analysis. The horizontal and vertical EOG, the action potential recorded from a single cell by the microelectrode, standard impulses produced from these action potentials, the chair position, the head position and the cylinder position were recorded on tape and later analyzed by means of a digital computer. In part of the recordings the corresponding velocity signals instead of chair and cylinder position were recorded. On-line computer analysis was applied during part of the experiments, but most of the data were taperecorded and analysed later. The neurobiological data and the stimuli were also recorded on a 7-channel paper oscillograph (modified Siemens Cardirex).

FIGURE 1

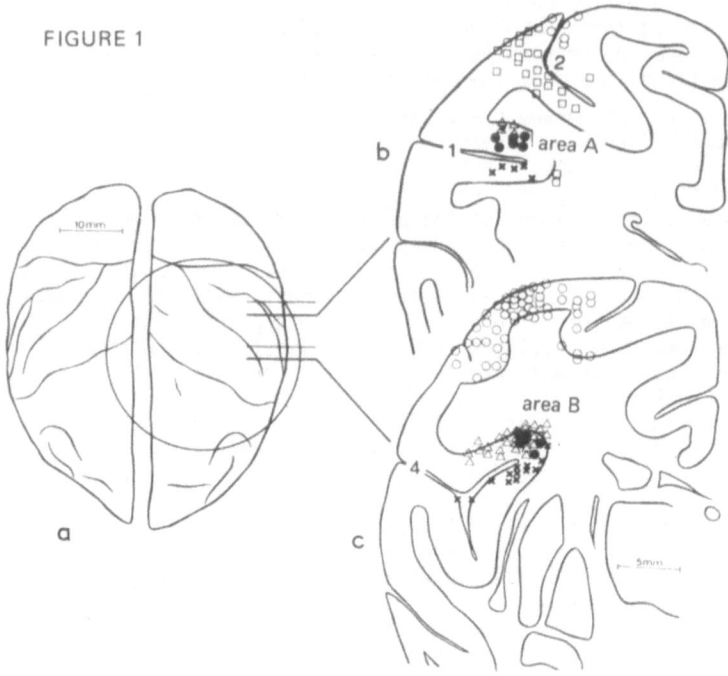

○ = somatosensory only,small receptive fields,
joint movement,muscle pressure,(presuma—
bly areae 2 and 5)
□ = complex somatosensory,attention,eye move—
ments,interesting visual objects,(presuma—
bly area 7)
△ = somatosensory only,large receptive fields,
often ipsi— and contralateral (presumably
area SII)
✗ = activation by clapping,whistling,noise (pre—
sumably auditory fields)
● = responsive to natural vestibular stimulation

FIGURE 1. Reconstruction of functional receptive field properties
of neurons recorded during 23 penetrations along two coronal planes.
Illustration of the extension of the cortical region from which
vestibular neurons were recorded in the present study.

3. RESULTS

Figs. 1b and 1c are reconstructions of 23 penetrations along two coronal planes (fig. 1a) and illustrate the cortical region from which vestibular neurons were recorded in the present study. These regions were located in deep cortical areas bordering on the posterior bank of the sulcus lateralis deep in the parietal operculum. The region where we could find units activated by vestibular stimuli extended more in an anterior-posterior than in a lateral direction. Tentatively we shall distinguish between two areas of the parieto-insular vestibular cortex. Area A is the retroinsular part, corresponding presumably to the reIpt-region of Pandya and Sanides. Area B we call the adjacent region reaching into the posterior part of the insula. From our data so far no functional differences between area A and B neurons can be determined. We cannot postulate, however, an anatomical continuity between area A and B. At present an anatomical discontinuity is more probable. In any case our recordings are from larger regions than that described as area retroinsularis parietalis by Sanides and Pandya. During our exploratory experiments vestibular responses were also observed in a few units located in area 7 and in the insular part of the temporal cortex. As mentioned, however, no vestibular responses were obtained in the cortical region described as area 2v in the Rhesus monkey.

3.1. Monomodal sensory stimulation

3.1.1. Responses to dynamic vestibular stimulation in darkness.

To date we have analyzed the responses of 160 single neurons recorded from area A or B of PIVeC which were driven by dynamic vestibular stimulation. A summary of the vestibular responses is presented in tab. 1. We tested 100 neurons by horizontal sinusoidal rotation of the turntable in darkness (head fixed to the turntable, vertical head axis and rotation axis aligned). 99 of these neurons responded to this dynamic vestibular stimulus and could be classified unequivocally according to the scheme proposed by Duensing and Schaefer (1958, 1959). Neuronal activation on movement to the contralateral side (type II) was more frequently observed than activation during movement to the ipsilateral side (type I). Only four neurons could be classified as type III, i.e. they were activated by rotation of the animal to the left and to the right side (tab. 1, figs. 2a, 3a).

The responses to sinusoidal movement (0.2 Hz, maximum amplitude 30 degrees) around an anterior/posterior axis (rotation in roll-direction) were tested in 80 neurons. From these 80 neurons 30 were activated by dynamic tilting towards the ipsilateral side (type I), 45 by movement to the contralateral side (type II) and four by movement to both sides (type III). Only 34 neurons were tested for their responses to rotation around the ear to ear transversal axis (pitch rotation). Nine neurons were activated during movement in a nose-up direction, 21 during movement in nose-down direction and 2 in both directions.

These data indicate that the neurons of the PIVeC are activated by rotation in darkness around more than one of our experimental axes of turning. Due to the differences between the planes of the semicircular canal systems and the planes of rotation in our experiments, of course, we cannot prove that these neurons receive

excitatory or inhibitory inputs from more than one of the three
semicircular canal systems. 72 neurons were tested for their responses to sinusoidal movement in two of the three different planes
(yaw, roll or pitch). All 72 neurons responded to rotation in
more than one plane. Rotation in yaw and pitch direction also
activated, of course, the otolith receptors. Since we could not
discover any activation to long lasting static tilt ($>$10 s
duration) around the anterior-posterior or the left-right head
axis, we have restricted our quantitative studies to <u>dynamic</u> vestibular stimulation and thus defined a "vestibular response" as
an activation obtained to sinewave rotation around one of the
three experimental axes. In the following we will describe data
obtained in vestibular neurons as defined by these criteria
when non-vestibular stimuli were applied.

3.1.2.<u>Visual stimulation</u>. From 59 PIVeC neurons of area A and B,
56 were found to be activated by the horizontally moving vertical
stripe pattern. We applied either continuous rotation of the stripe
cylinder to the left or the right at constant angular velocity
or a sinusoidal back and forth rotation. A few neurons were activated by visual movement in both directions. Most of the neurons,
however, increased their neuronal activity with drum movement in
one direction and decreased their activity when the drum was moving in the opposite direction. The few neurons activated by movement to the left and to the right exhibited an optimal response
vector in an oblique direction when tested with small moving visual targets or the large hand-moved stripe pattern (c.f. METHODS).
The neuronal activation increased with the speed of the stripe
pattern, but no detailed analysis of the data was performed to date.
A positive velocity step led to a transient activation when the
cylinder moved in the on-direction. A negative velocity step correspondingly was accompanied by a transient reduction of the neuronal activity as compared to the steady state activation. With
sinusoidal drum rotation at a moderate sinewave frequency (0.1-
0.5 Hz) and amplitude $\leq$30 degrees, the temporal modulation of
the neuronal impulse rate was approximately a sinewave response.
This is one requirement for response linearity of the system under investigation, but no other rigorous tests for response linearity were performed so far.

3.1.3. <u>Somatokinetic and proprioceptive stimulation</u>. 99 neurons
were tested to somatokinetic and proprioceptive stimuli. Tactile
movement across the limbs, neck and shoulder, unilateral and bilateral stretch of the arms were applied. All 99 neurons responded to at least one of these somatokinetic or proprioceptive stimuli whenever the stimulus was located around the shoulder-girdle.
A part of these neurons also responded to movement of the forearm at the elbow joint, movement of the hand or the fingers; a
few neurons also were activated by tapping the feet. The monkey's
cooperation during this procedure was variable. Depending on his
alertness and "interest" in the interaction with the experimenter,
these "passive" somatokinetic or proprioceptive stimuli were accompanied by a more or less strong motor activity (hand and arm
movements). When the monkey spontaneously grasped a raisin or
piece of apple, activation of the PIVeC neurons was also observed.
We did not have the impression that the somatokinetic or proprioceptive responses were particularly enhanced or suppressed during
active movement of the upper limbs. We did not develop any special

FIGURE 2

Java monkey , neuron of the parieto-insular vestibular cortex, area B

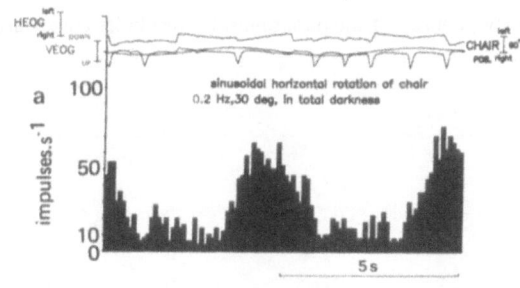

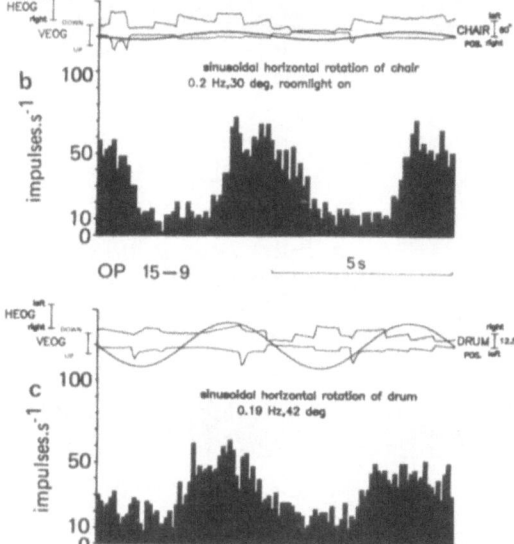

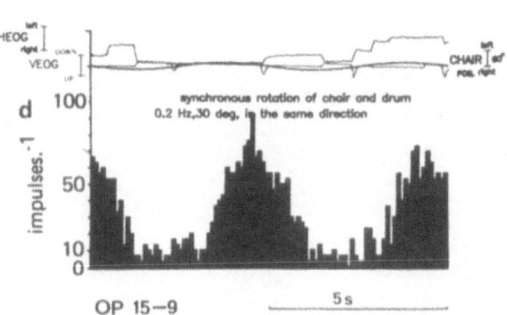

258

FIGURE 3
Java monkey , neuron of the parieto-insular vestibular cortex,area A

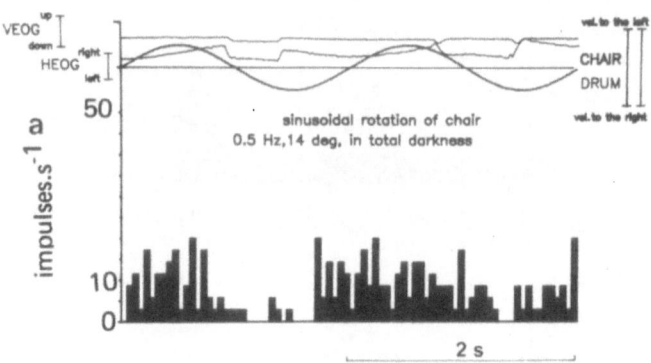

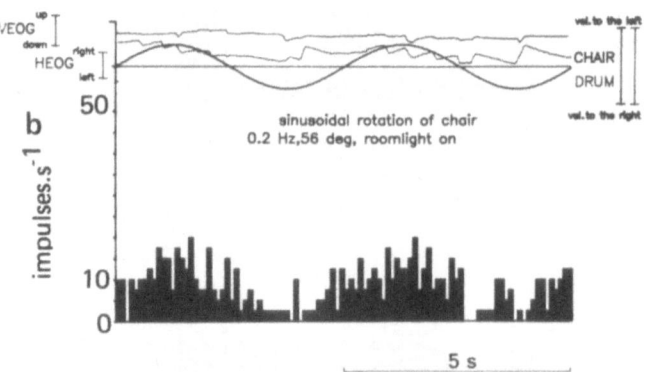

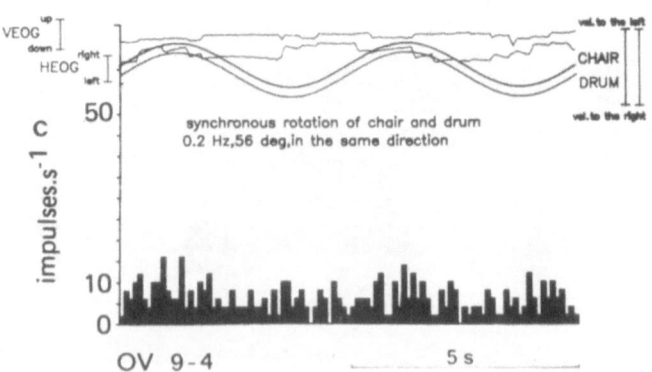

FIGURE 3
Java monkey , neuron of the parieto-insular vestibular cortex,area A

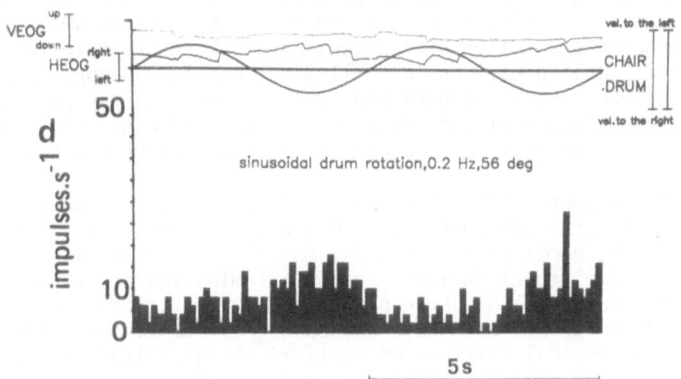

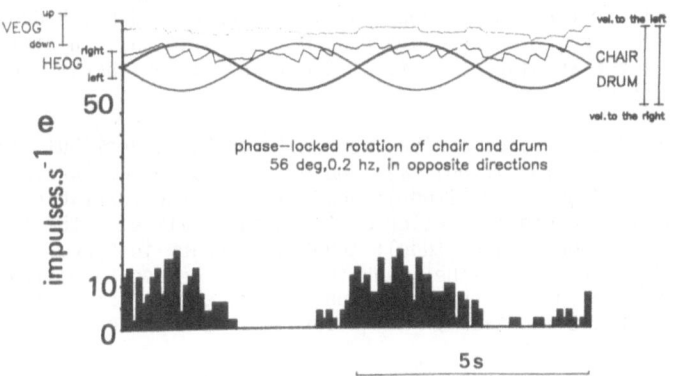

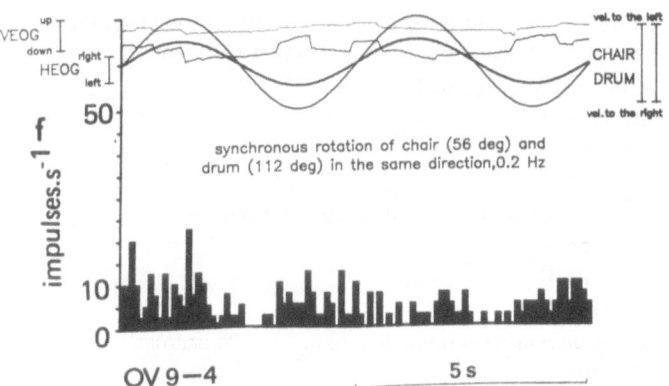

FIGURE 2. Responses of a PIVeC neuron (area B). (a) Sinusoidal horizontal rotation of the turntable (0.2 Hz, 30 degrees amplitude) in total darkness. (b) Same as in (a) but constant illumination of the stationary stripe cylinder. (c) Responses to sinusoidal rotation of stripe cylinder (0.19 Hz, 42 degrees amplitude). (d) Synchronous rotation of turntable and stripe cylinder (0.2 Hz, 30 degrees amplitude), constant illumination. In the upper parts of the figures the horizontal and vertical EOGs and the position of the turntable or stripe cylinder are recorded. Note that eye movements in the vertical EOG are recorded in reversed condition.

FIGURE 3. Responses of a PIVeC neuron (area A). (a) Sinusoidal rotation of turntable (0.5 Hz, 22 degrees amplitude) in total darkness. (b) Horizontal sinusoidal rotation of turntable (0.2 Hz, 28 degrees amplitude) during constant illumination of stationary stripe cylinder. (c) Synchronous and coupled rotation of turntable and stripe cylinder (0.2 Hz, 28 degrees amplitude). (d) Horizontal sinusoidal rotation of vertical stripe cylinder (0.2 Hz, 28 degrees amplitude). (e) Phase-locked rotation of turntable and drum (0.2 Hz, 28 degrees amplitude) in opposite directions (180 degrees out of phase). (f) Synchronous phase-locked rotation of the turntable (28 degrees amplitude) and the cylinder (56 degrees amplitude). Phase angle 0 degrees, 0.2 Hz. Note that in contrast to fig. 2 the angular velocity of the turntable or the stripe cylinder was recorded.

FIGURE 4. Responses of a PIVeC neuron (area B) to vestibular and neck receptor stimulation. (a) Sinusoidal rotation of turntable (0.2 Hz, 28 degrees amplitude); head fixed to the turntable. (b) Horizontal sinusoidal rotation of the head relative to the trunk (0.2 Hz, 28 degrees amplitude); trunk stationary in space. (c) Sinusoidal rotation of the trunk (0.2 Hz, 28 degrees amplitude); head fixed in space (trunk rotation accomplished by sinusoidal rotation of the turntable). All recordings were performed in total darkness.

Tab. 1

Neurons of the parieto - insular vestibular cortex. Responses to vestibular stimuli. 160 neurons tested. Directional selective activation was found for

(a) Horizontal rotation in 99 of 100 neurons.
   - 37 type I
   - 58 type II
   - 4 type I

(b) Left - right sinusoidal tilting (roll) in 79 of 80 neurons
   - 30 type I
   - 58 type II
   - 4 type III

(c) Nose up/down sinusoidal tilting (pitch) in 32 of 34 neurons
   - 9 nose up
   - 21 nose down
   - 2 nose up and down

experimental paradigm in the present study to separate active
and passive components of the somatosensory input.

3.1.4. Stimulation of deep neck receptors. One special somatokinetic stimulus should be mentioned here, namely rotation of the
trunk while the head was fixed in space (c.f. METHODS). From the
37 PIVeC neurons tested with this stimulus (sinusoidal, horizontal
trunk rotation with a maximum amplitude of 30 degrees) 36 were
activated by trunk rotation in one direction (fig. 4). The neuronal impulse rate was modulated more or less sinusoidally indicating
a fairly regular "neck receptor" input effect on PIVeC neurons.

3.2. Multimodal interaction

3.2.1. Vestibular-visual interaction. When the head is turned
in the light to the right, the extrapersonal world "shifts" to
the left across the field of gaze. Thus, under "natural" conditions predominant horizontal semicircular canal stimulation during
head movement to the right corresponds to "visual world movement
to the left". In the following we shall designate the response
of PIVeC neurons activated by vestibular (semicircular canal)
stimulation in one direction and by visual movement stimulation
in the opposite direction as agonistic. Correspondingly a neuron
activated by visual and vestibular stimulation in the same direction (e.g. head movement to the right, visual world movement to
the right) will be called antagonistic. We found both types of
neurons in area A and B of PIVeC. From 41 neurons tested with
horizontal optokinetic stimulation (sinusoidal to and fro movement of the vertical stripe cylinder) and horizontal sinusoidal
rotation of the animal in darkness and/or in a lighted room
(stripe cylinder stationary), 32 neurons fell into the class
"agonistic" and 9 into the class "antagonistic". Depending on the
type of visual-vestibular interaction a reduction (in some cases
cancellation) or a facilitation of the neuronal response as compared to the vestibular responses in darkness was obtained when
the room light was turned on and the cylinder was stationary.
Fig. 2 indicates the facilitation of visual and vestibular input
signals according to an agonistic response pattern of a PIVeC neuron. The responses of this unit to sinusoidal horizontal rotation
in darkness are shown in fig. 2a. The unit was activated when the
chair turned to the right. The maximum neuronal response coincided approximately with maximum velocity to the right. When the
drum was sinusoidally rotated around the animal (fig. 2c), the
neuron responded to movement to the left and the right with a
strong component towards the right. Therefore horizontal vestibular and horizontal visual stimulation did not interact optimally in this neuron during horizontal movement (yaw direction).
This fact could be easily explained by the observation that the
maximum visual movement vector as indicated by the activation
maximum was found in this neuron when a visual stimulus (a single
target 5-10 degrees in diameter) was moved from the left lower
quadrant to the right upper quadrant of the field of gaze. It is
possible that the optimum vestibular movement vector was also
not identical with the horizontal rotation plane, since this
unit also responded to tilting of the animal around the anterior-
posterior head axis (roll direction). Nevertheless, an agonistic
visual-vestibular interaction was observed as shown in fig. 2b.
The responses to sinusoidal horizontal rotation were enhanced

FIGURE 4
Java monkey , neuron of the parieto-insular vestibular cortex, area B

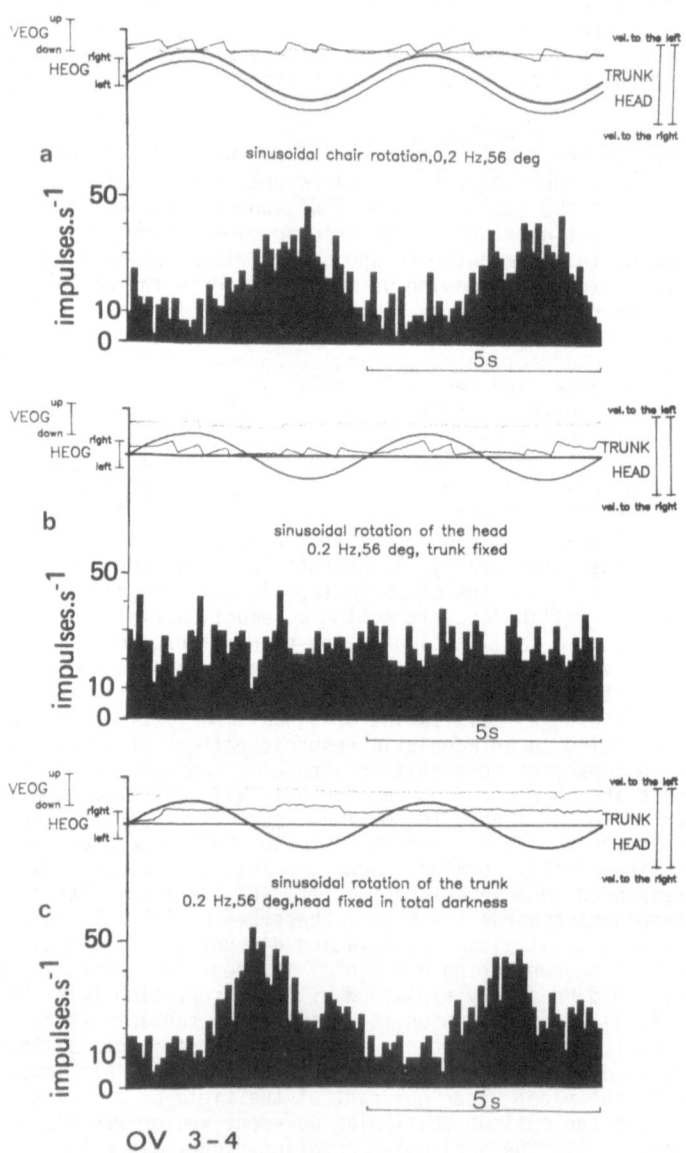

OV 3-4

(as compared to the activation during rotation in darkness) when the stationary stripe cylinder was illuminated continuously. In addition a slight shift of about 20 degrees phase angle in the vestibular response maximum towards the maximum of the visual response was visible. Otherwise the responses to horizontal rotation within a stationary visual surround were very similar to those obtained by horizontal rotation in darkness. Surprisingly the vestibular response was even stronger (and not phase shifted at all) when the continuously illuminated stripe cylinder was fixed to the sinusoidally rotating chair (fig. 2d). This observation indicates that a rotating visual input which is stationary with respect to the monkey also provides input signals facilitating the neuronal response.

Fig. 3 demonstrates a somewhat different visual-vestibular interaction of the agonistic type. The neuron from which these data were obtained was located in area A of PIVeC. In contrast to fig. 2 the velocity signals of chair and drum rotation were recorded in fig. 3 rather than the position signals. The unit was activated by horizontal sinusoidal rotation in darkness to the left. This activation became somewhat stronger when the stationary stripe cylinder was continuously illuminated (fig. 3b). The vestibular activation (fig. 3d) was again altered by non-moving visual stimuli. In contrast to the unit of fig. 2, however, the rotation of the chair and the drum coupled to the chair led to a significant reduction in the maximum neuronal discharge rate (fig. 3c). Sinusoidal rotation of the stripe cylinder around the stationary monkey elicited a neuronal activation during drum movement to the right. An increased agonistic visual-vestibular interaction was found when the drum was rotated at the same sinewave frequency as the chair but 180 degrees out of phase (fig. 3e). As one can easily see by comparing fig. 3b and 3e, this agonistic interaction (beyond normal "natural" stimulation) led to a much more pronounced alteration in the inhibitory and excitatory periods than "normal" agonistic visual-vestibular interaction (i.e. rotation inside of the stationary stripe cylinder). Fig. 3f also demonstrates the agonistic response type, but an experimental paradigm was applied from which one could expect an inhibitory agonistic interaction. The drum was rotated at a sinewave amplitude of 56 degrees, while the chair was synchronously rotated at an amplitude of 28 degrees. Thus the visual world moved faster to the right when the monkey was rotated to the right and faster to the left when the monkey was rotated to the left. As expected, the visual input led to a reduction in vestibular activation and a rather irregular and not simply phase-locked neuronal activation appeared. This PIVeC neuron also received inputs from the vertical semicircular canal system since it responded to a tilting in the saggital plane whenever the nose moved downwards (pitch rotation in the dark). This neuron also responded to movement of small visual targets across the field of gaze and the maximum movement vector pointed approximately from the left lower to the right upper quadrant.

3.2.2. Interaction of vestibular and "deep" neck receptor input. Practically all neurons of area A and B of PIVeC receiving a vestibular and visual input also responded to mechanoreceptor stimulation (presumably proprioceptive/joint type) of the neck region. The interaction of neck receptor input and vestibular

input was tested by three types of stimulation: sinusoidal rotation of the head in darkness with the trunk fixed in space, sinusoidal rotation of the trunk in darkness while the head was fixed
in space and sinusoidal rotation of the chair in darkness. In most
neurons these three tests were repeated during illumination of
the stationary surround. Fig. 4 exhibits typical responses obtained in a PiVeC neuron in area B during such an experiment.
The neuron had an agonistic response with respect to visual-vestibular interaction. It was activated when the chair was rotated
towards the right; the maximum activation coincided approximately
with the maximum angular velocity (fig. 4a). When the trunk was
sinusoidally rotated and the head fixed in space (fig. 4c), the
maximum response was obtained when the trunk in relation to the
head deviated towards the right by about 80 percent of the velocity amplitude. Thus the vestibular and neck mechanoreceptor input signals were nearly 180 degrees out of phase. It was therefore not surprising that a non-modulated neuronal impulse sequence
was observed when the head was passively rotated sinusoidally in
the horizontal plane while the trunk was fixed in space (fig. 4b).
In analyzing the data shown in fig. 4b, it became evident that the
neuronal activity under these stimulus conditions did not correspond to the sum of the neuronal activity evoked by vestibular
stimulation (fig. 4a) and by neck mechanoreceptor stimulation
(fig. 4c). The activity level aroused by combined stimulation of
the semicircular canal receptors and neck receptors corresponded
approximately to the <u>algebraic mean</u> of the vestibular and neck
receptor responses.

3.3. Responses during Sigma-optokinetic stimulation

As mentioned above, all area A and area B PIVeC neurons were activated by optokinetic stimulation when the vertical stripe cylinder rotated to the left or the right around the animal. By continuous speed rotation, as a rule, one direction led to an activation,
the other to a reduction or at least to no increase in the spontaneous neuronal activity level. Optokinetic nystagmus and movement perception are elicitable in man not only by actual rotation
of the stripe cylinder around the subject, but also by the movement perceived when a stationary stripe cylinder is stroboscopically illuminated after the subject has initiated smooth pursuit
eye movements at an angular velocity

$$V_e = P_s \cdot f_s \; [\text{degrees} \cdot s^{-1}] \tag{1}$$

whereby f_s the flash frequency and P_s the period of the stripe
cylinder (Sigma-movement, Behrens and Grüsser, 1978, 1979). Sigma-
movement and Sigma-OKN can be elicited in monkeys quite easily
and follow the same rules as found for Sigma-movement and Sigma-OKN
in man (Grüsser et al., 1979; Adler et al., 1981). In the present
experiment the <u>stationary</u> vertical stripe cylinder (stripe period
$P_s = 1.15$ degrees) was illuminated stroboscopically at a flash
frequency between 10 and 30 flashes $\cdot s^{-1}$. From the three methods
useful to lure the monkey into Sigma-OKN (Grüsser et al., 1979),
we preferentially used the technique of post-rotatory nystagmus.
The monkey was rotated for a few minutes at a constant angular
speed in darkness and then suddenly stopped. Of course, a strong
post-rotatory nystagmus appeared. Most PIVeC neurons were activated
during the post-rotatory nystagmus in one of the two directions.
After a few seconds delay from the moment the monkey was suddenly

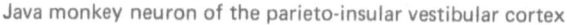

Java monkey neuron of the parieto-insular vestibular cortex

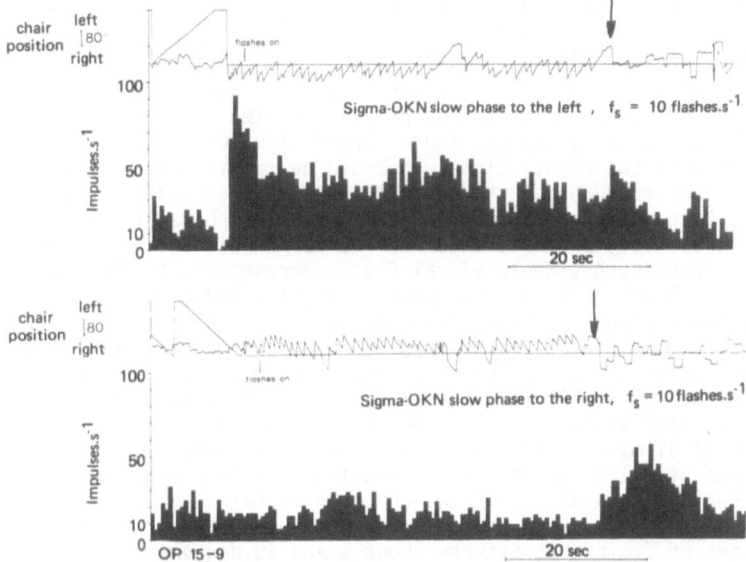

FIGURE 5. Responses of a PIVeC neuron (area B) during Sigma-optokinetic nystagmus (slow phase to the left, upper recording; slow
phase to the right, lower recording). Sigma-OKN was elicited by
stroboscopic illumination of a vertical stripe pattern of 1.15
degrees period. Sigma-OKN was aroused during post-rotatory nystagmus. Flash frequency 10 flashes . s^{-1}. The angular speed of
the Sigma-OKN slow phase was about 11 degrees . s^{-1} (corresponding
to eq.(1)). The Sigma-OKN ceased abruptly when the monkey found
something to fixate. The end of Sigma-OKN is indicated by an arrow.

stopped in darkness, the stationary stripe cylinder was stroboscopically illuminated at a flash frequency of 10 to 15 flashes
. s^{-1}. In most cases the post-rotatory nystagmus was then transformed into a longlasting Sigma-OKN for which the slow phase angular velocity V_e approximated the rule described by eq.(1). According to this rule, V_e increased when f_s was increased.

Fig. 5 demonstrates the activation of a PIVeC neuron during Sigma-
OKN when the OKN slow phase was pointing to the left, while a reduced neuronal activity was found during Sigma-OKN with the slow
OKN phase to the right. Sigma-OKN could be maintained at a constant flash frequency up to several minutes. Then suddenly the
monkey "managed" to fixate a target in his peripheral field of
gaze (presumably a part of the head holder or his own nose, because otherwise his whole visual field corresponded to the stripe
pattern). Then the Sigma-OKN ceased abruptly. Under these conditions the neuronal activity also decreased abruptly (fig. 5a) or
increased significantly above the spontaneous activity level when
the preceding Sigma-OKN led to a reduced neuronal activation.
This post-Sigma-OKN activation lasted up to 50 seconds. It might
be correlated to horizontal after-vection, which is regularly observed in Sigma-OKN experiments with human subjects tested under
the same stimulus conditions. It should be pointed out, however,
that during Sigma-OKN in man we could not obtain any horizontal
circular vection, even after minutes of Sigma-OKN and angular velocities of V_e varying between about 3 and 50 degrees . s^{-1}.
Since there is a considerable difference in monkey and man with
respect to Sigma-OKAN (very little Sigma-OKAN in man, in monkey a
longlasting Sigma-OKAN) despite identical Sigma-OKN patterns,
we have to be very cautious in comparing the responses of vestibular cortical neurons of monkeys during Sigma-OKAN with the
percepts of man. According to our hypothesis about the origin of
Sigma-OKN and Sigma-movement (Adler et al., 1981) we assume that
the neuronal activation of PIVeC neurons during Sigma-OKN indicates a directionally selective excitatory input (efference copy
signals) to PTVeC originating somewhere in the gaze motor command
structures of the parietal lobe.

4. DISCUSSION

The data presented in this report indicate the existence of an extended "vestibular" cortical area located in the retro-insular
part of the parietal cortex and stretching towards the insular
region. Our preliminary discrimination between area A and B does
not necessarily imply an anatomical separation. Further work in
more monkeys including better anatomical identification of the
recorded neurons is required before one can be sure how far the
cortical vestibular area extends beyond the area described by
Pandya and Sanides. The area is certainly distinct, however, from
the two other cortical vestibular regions described so far in the
monkey brain (area 2v, area 3a; Schwarz et al., 1971, 1973). Vestibular responses were also found in some of the neurons of area 7,
but no special vestibular region could be identified. The PTVeC
region is presumably the homologue of the vestibular cortex of
cat explored with evoked potential techniques by Mickle and
Ades (1954). The neurons of this cortical vestibular area of cats
respond to electrical polarization of the labyrinth with a short-
latency (8-20 ms) activation or inhibition depending on the direc-

tion of polarization (Grüsser et al., 1959). These neurons are
also activated or inhibited by natural vestibular stimulation
and, similar to the neuronal responses described for the PIVeC
region of the monkey, the cat vestibular cortex neurons respond
to neck receptor input and to somatokinetic stimulation (Becker
et al., 1979; Mergner, 1979; Mergner et al., 1981).

The PIVeC area is bordered by two distinctly different cortical
regions: Towards the insular part of the cortex an auditory field
is the immediate neighbour. Neurons in this field responded to
any type of auditory noise (clapping the hands, speech sounds,
whistling etc.). Towards the parietal part of the operculum the
PIVeC area is bordered by a somatosensory region dominated by
neurons having very large somatosensory receptive fields including inputs from deep mechanoreceptors and joint receptors. The
somatic receptive fields were predominantly located on the head,
neck, shoulder and forearm region. Thus it seems fairly probable
that PIVeC neurons receive an input from this neighbouring somatosensory cortical region. In contrast, auditory signals (stationary or moving) do not seem to activate PIVeC neurons.

A survey of the literature on human neuropathology reveals a considerable amount of data indicating that a cortical vestibular
field exists on both sides of the human cortex in the insular
region (e.g. Penfield and Rasmussen, 1957). Corresponding to our
finding in monkey that PIVeC is bordered by auditory cortex, clinical observations revealed that a considerable percentage of
vestibular epileptic aura phenomena observed in man was accompanied by auditory sensations. Thus one can cautiously presume that
an area homologue to PIVeC also exists in the brain of man. This
view is supported by the findings of Friberg et al. (1981) who
measured an increased cerebral blood flow in the insular cortex
during vestibular stimulation in man.

Functional properties. In the light of the neurophysiological data
described in the present report, the denotation of a "vestibular"
cortical area seems, of course, rather arbitrary, since practically
all PIVeC neurons also responded to visual and neck receptor input.
In addition, further somatosensory input from the shoulder and
arm region not directly due to secondary activation of neck receptors is at least probable. We think, however, that the desig-
nation "vestibular" cortical region is justified since a fairly
specific vestibular input is present. As far as we can see from
the data collected, it is a dynamic vestibular input related to
head movement in any direction of space which activates the neurons. The static vestibular signals (otolith input) seem rather
ineffective. The data further indicate that each neuron recorded
is activated during dynamic vestibular stimulation (rotation)
within a fairly large vectorial "response cone", while rotation in the
opposite region of the vectorial stimulation space inhibition is
aroused. From the responses of the neurons activated predominantly in the horizontal rotation direction (these neurons were selected on the basis of our experimental paradigm in searching for
vestibular cortical neurons) we can imply that at least two types
of visual-vestibular neck receptor interactions seem to be present
in the neuronal network of PIVeC neurons. In one group of the neurons the responses aroused by semicircular canal receptor activation are facilitated by the visual signals when the monkey's head

is actively or passively moved towards the right or the left. The
neck receptor input, however, leads to a suppression of the vestibular responses in these neurons. When the neck receptor signals
cancel the vestibular signals, the relative shift of the visual
surround across the field of gaze during active head movement is
signalled by these neurons.

In other neurons, however, the responses aroused by visual movement signals as well as the neck receptor input reduce the vestibular activation during head movements (antagonistic response).
A neuronal system composed of these two classes of neurons would
be able to contribute to the discrimination between visual movement caused by self-moving visual structures of the extrapersonal
space and visual movement due to active head movements. Such a
system would, however, not be able to discriminate these two different movement conditions by itself. Nevertheless, by the response
properties of these two neuronal systems, the brain could extract
information as to whether the head is moved on the trunk in darkness
or in an illuminated surround or whether the head is moved with the
trunk (no relative head-trunk movements) in darkness or within the
illuminated surround. To separate head movements and surround movements, however, one would require another class of visual-vestibular
neck receptor interaction, namely one in which the vestibular response is facilitated by neck receptor input when the head is moved
on the trunk.

The effect of eye movements. From the analysis of horizontal and
vertical EOGs we can say that saccades do not affect the activity
of the PIVeC neurons. In some of the PIVeC neurons, however, pursuit eye movements seemed to modify the responses aroused by vestibular and/or visual stimulation. In addition, the responses obtained during Sigma-OKN (fig. 5) indicate that a directionally
selective excitatory input from gaze command structures (smooth
pursuit system) exists in PIVeC neurons. A further modification
of our experimental paradigm (working with trained monkeys fixating a stationary or moving visual target) will be necessary, however, to clarify these points.

No conclusions, of course, are possible on the basis of the data
available as yet on the location of the essential multimodal interactions. In the light of data obtained in other laboratories
(e.g. Henn et al., 1974), it seems fairly probable that essential
components of visual information (and presumably also neck receptor signals) are integrated into the afferent vestibular system
at the level of the brainstem vestibular nuclei.

5. SUMMARY
(1) In Java monkeys (Maccaca fascicularis) single units were recorded from a cortical "vestibular" area which, at least in part,
coincides with the area retroinsularis parietalis (reIpt) of
Pandya and Sanides. Part of our recordings indicate the extension
of a vestibular area into the insular regions bordering reIpt.
Further work is necessary for a detailed correlation between cyto-
architectonic structure and neuronal response properties.
(2) The neurons were defined as "vestibular" since they responded
to dynamic vestibular stimulation of the animal in darkness (sinusoidal rotation or velocity steps). The majority of vestibular neurons responded to rotation in more than one of the three experi-

mental rotation planes (jaw, roll or pitch direction). With horizontal rotation (jaw) or tilting in the roll direction, class II neurons (Duensing and Schaefer classification) were more frequently found than class I neurons. Dynamic tilting nose-downwards activated more neurons than tilting nose-upwards. Prolonged static tilt did not affect the neuronal activity.

(3) All PIVeC neurons were activated by optokinetic stimulation when a vertical stripe cylinder was moved horizontally around the animal. A considerable part of the PIVeC neurons was also activated by single targets moving across the field of gaze. All neuronal responses then exhibited directional selectivity and the preferred visual movement vector was about 180 degrees in the opposite direction to null. Two types of visual-vestibular interaction were found, denoted "agonistic" and "antagonistic" responses.

(4) All neurons activated by dynamic, horizontal semicircular canal input also responded to deep mechano-receptor input from the neck region (joints or tendons). The vestibular responses of some of these neurons were antagonistic to the neck receptor input signals. Movement of the head on the trunk stationary in space led to no modulation of the neuronal impulse rate, while horizontal rotation of the whole animal and horizontal rotation of the trunk while the head was fixed in space aroused a sinusoidal modulation of the neuronal impulse rate. The neuronal responses to vestibular and neck receptor stimulation were about 180 degrees out of phase.

(5) Nearly all PIVeC neurons were activated by somatokinetic stimulation of the upper limbs and the skin region of the shoulder-girdle.

(6) Two functional possibilities for interpreting the neuronal data are discussed: the neuronal network investigated might provide information of visual movement related to the extrapersonal space; it can be argued, however, (tab. 2) that by means of two different classes of visual, vestibular and neck receptor interaction the neuronal network can discriminate between the different conditions of head and body movement in the dark or during illumination of the extrapersonal space.

(7) The responses of PIVeC neurons during horizontal Sigma-optokinetic nystagmus (activation in one direction, reduction of the neuronal activity in the other Sigma-OKN direction) indicate that the PIVeC receives efference copy signals from other brain structures related to gaze motor control.

ACKNOWLEDGEMENT. The work was supported by grants of the Deutsche Forschungsgemeinschaft (Gr 161). We thank Mrs. J. Dames for her help in the English translation of the manuscript, Mr. J. Lerch for building part of the experimental equipment and Mrs. B. Hauschild for careful typing of the manuscript.

REFERENCES

Adler B, Collewijn H, Curio G, Grüsser O-J, Pause M, Schreiter U and Weiss L (1981) Sigma-movement and Sigma-nystagmus: A new tool to investigate the gaze-pursuit system and visual movement perception in man and monkey, Ann. New York Acad. Sci. 374, 284-302.

Becker W, Deecke L and Mergner T (1979) Neuronal responses to natural vestibular and neck stimulation in the anterior suprasylvian gyrus of the cat, Brain Res. 165, 139-143.

Behrens F and Grüsser O-J (1979) Smooth pursuit eye movements and optokinetic nystagmus elicited by intermittently illuminated stationary patterns, Exp. Brain Res. 37, 317-336.

Büttner U and Buettner UW (1978) Parietal cortex (2v) neuronal activity in the alert monkey during natural vestibular and optokinetic stimulation, Brain Res. 153, 392-397.

Duensing F and Schaefer K-P (1958) Die Aktivität einzelner Neurone im Bereich der Vestibulariskerne bei Horizontalbeschleunigungen unter besonderer Berücksichtigung des vestibulären Nystagmus, Arch. Psychiatr., Z. Neurol. 198, 225-252.

Duensing F and Schaefer K-P (1959) Über die Konvergenz verschiedener labyrinthärer Afferenzen auf einzelne Neurone des Vestibulariskerngebietes, Arch. Psychiatr., Z. Neurol. 199, 345-371.

Fredrickson JM, Figge U, Scheid P and Kornhuber HH (1966) Vestibular nerve projection to the cerebral cortex of the rhesus monkey, Exp. Brain Res. 2, 318-327.

Friberg L, Skyhoj T, Paulson OB and Lassen NA (1981) Cortical activation during vestibular stimulation and rCBF measurement, J.Cerebral Blood Flow and Metabol. 1 Suppl. 1, 473-474.

Grüsser O-J, Grüsser-Cornehls U and Saur G (1959) Reaktionen einzelner Neurone im optischen Cortex der Katze nach elektrischer Polarisation des Labyrinths, Pflüg. Arch. 269, 593-612.

Henn V, Young LR and Finley C (1974) Vestibular nucleus units in alert monkeys are also influenced by moving visual fields, Brain Res. 71, 144-149.

Mergner T (1979) Vestibular influences on the cat's cerebral cortex. In Granit R, Pompeiano O, eds. Reflex control of posture and movement, Progress in Brain Research 50, 567-579.

Mergner T, Deecke L and Wagner H-J (1981) Vestibulo-thalamic projection to the anterior suprasylvian cortex of the cat, Exp. Brain Res. 44, 455-458.

Mickle WA and Ades HW (1954) Rostral projection pathway of the vestibular system, Amer. J. Physiol. 176, 243-246.

Pandya DN and Sanides F (1973) Architectonic parcellation of the temporal operculum in Rhesus monkey and its projection pattern, Z. Anat. Entwickl.-Gesch. 139, 127-161.

Pause M, Hoppmann V and Schreiter U (1981) Neurons in the insular cortex of Java monkeys activated by vestibular stimulation, Pflügers Arch. 389 Suppl. R31.

Penfield W and Rasmussen T (1957) The cerebral cortex of man. A clinical study of localization and function, New York, Macmillan.

Schreiter U, Hoppmann V and Pause M (1981) Different vestibular projection fields in the monkey's cortex: single unit recordings and analysis of functional difference, Neurosci. Lett. Suppl. 7, S488.

Schwarz DWF and Fredrickson JM (1971) Rhesus monkey vestibular cortex: a bimodal primary projection field, Science 172, 280-281.

Schwarz DWF, Deecke L and Fredrickson JM (1973) Cortical projection of group I muscle afferents to areas 2, 3a and the vestibular field in the Rhesus monkey, Exp. Brain Res. 17, 516-526.

LINEAR INTERACTION OF VESTIBULAR AND OPTOKINETIC NYSTAGMUS

E. Koenig and J. Dichgans (Neurological Clinic, Univ.
of Tübingen, W.-Germany)

SUMMARY
In humans interaction of a prior vestibular stimulus
(chair acceleration for 10 s) with an immediately following optokinetic stimulus (full field stimulation)
was quantitatively studied to determine the change of
slow phase velocity (SPV) of nystagmus elicited by the
addition of the optokinetic stimulus. This change was
compared to the SPV during pure optokinetic stimulation
on the basis of the magnitude of the optokinetic input
(retinal image motion) at the onset of the optokinetic
stimulus. When measured shortly (0.7s) after optokinetic
stimulus onset visual vestibular interaction is in fact
linear i.e. the optokinetic reflexes are as effective
in changing SPV during vestibular nystagmus as with pure
optokinetic stimulation. As the optokinetic stimulus
affects the charge in the visual vestibular integrator
interaction cannot be expected to be linear after longer
intervals of optokinetic stimulation.

INTRODUCTION
Interaction of vestibular and optokinetic nystagmus under
natural conditions was first demonstrated by Maurer
(1935) who showed that optokinetic stimulation reduces
postrotatory nystagmus. Thus additional optokinetic stimulation results in a better correspondence of stimulus
velocity and slow phase velocity (SPV) of nystagmus than
pure vestibular stimulation. Quantitative measurements
of interaction lead to contradictory assumptions on how
the outputs of the vestibular and optokinetic system are
combined to yield a common slow phase velocity output.
Allum et al. (1976) suggested a variable gain in both
the vestibular and the optokinetic system before their
summation. A switching between the vestibular and optokinetic input was first suggested by Waespe and Henn
(1977) and recently assumed by Bock (1982) who used
sinusoidal stimuli. Linear interaction was proposed by
Robinson (1977) on the basis of the data from Waespe
and Henn (1977) and, on the basis of experimental data,
by Lau et al. (1978) and Koenig et al. (1978). In the
latter paper we studied the modulation of optokinetic
nystagmus by additional vestibular stimuli and found
rather accurate linear interaction when the vestibular
and optokinetic stimuli added. But when the vestibular
stimulus was opposite to the optokinetic one OKN-SPV
was reduced more strongly than was expected on the basis
of linear interaction. These data were used as the basis
of a model of nonlinear interaction by Schmid et al.
(1980). In this paper vestibular and optokinetic reflexes
were again activated sequentially, but in reversed order:
first the vestibulo-ocular reflex (VOR) by a body acceleration (velocity ramp) and then the optokinetic

272

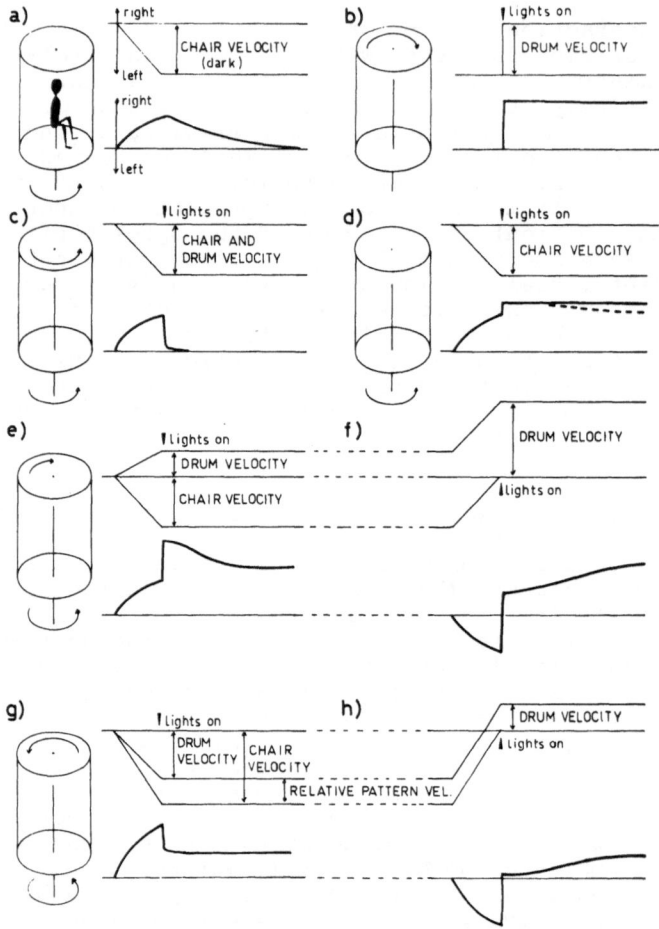

FIGURE 1. The vestibular and optokinetic stimuli used
and their combinations as well as a schematic illustration of the observed slow phase of nystagmus; a) pure
vestibular stimulation; b) pure optokinetic stimulation;
c) fixation-suppression of vestibular nystagmus (chair
and drum rotating at the same velocity); d) natural
combination (chair acceleration, surround stationary);
e) Combination of a weak acceleration and a high optokinetic pattern velocity, eliciting nystagmus into the
same direction after the acceleration and (f) into opposite directions after deceleration; g), h) combination
of a strong acceleration with a low optokinetic pattern
speed, resulting in a decrease of slow phase velocity
after the onset of the optokinetic stimulus.

reflexes by a step in surround velocity. It will be shown that the change in SPV elicited by the optokinetic stimulus during vestibular nystagmus is dependent on retinal image motion in the same way as during pure optokinetic stimulation.

METHODS

Four subjects were seated on a rotatory chair with their head restrained in a head rest. The chair was surrounded by a cylindrical drum (1.4 m in diameter) serving as the visual surround. The inner wall of the drum was covered with 48 alternating black and white vertical stripes and a band of comic strip figures at eye level as an additional foveal stimulus. Both chair and drum could be rotated about the same axis at servo controlled velocities up to 180 °/s. Eye movements were recorded by electro-oculography using d-c coupling and were calibrated by voluntary saccades repeated between each trial. Acoustic cues from the motors were masked by presenting music by earphones. Horizontal and vertical eye movements as well as drum and chair acceleration were recorded on paper charts. Measurements of slow phase velocity (SPV) of nystagmus were done manually.

EXPERIMENTAL PROCEDURE

The stimuli used and the typical responses of SPV obtained are schematically depicted in Fig. 1. For comparison pure vestibular stimulation (chair acceleration of 3, 6, 9, 12 and 18 °/s^2 for 10 s in the dark, Fig. 1a) and pure optokinetic stimulation (pattern motions of 30, 60, 90, 120 and 180 °/s, Fig. 1b) were applied, too. To test the influence of zero pattern velocity (fixation suppression, Fig. 1c) chair and drum were rigidly coupled and accelerated with 3,6, 9, 12 and 18 °/s^2 for 10 s. Within the first second after the end of the acceleration the light was switched on to present the pattern, which was stationary relative to the subject.
A "natural" visual vestibular stimulation was achieved by only accelerating the chair with 3, 6, 9, 12 and 18 °/s^2 for 10 s to final velocities of 30, 60, 90, 120 and 180 °/s and by presenting the earth-stationary drum to the subject immediately after the end of the acceleration (Fig. 1d).
To test interaction the chair was accelerated (or decelerated after an extended period of constant velocity in the dark) for 10 s (3, 6, 9, 12 and 18 °/s^2). Then within 1 s after the end of the acceleration, the light was switched on to illuminate the drum. The speed of the drum was adjusted to generate a velocity difference (faster and slower) between drum and chair of 30, 60, 90,120 and 180 °/s. The subject thereby was exposed to an optokinetic stimulus eliciting nystagmus either toward the same direction as the previous vestibular stimulus (Fig. 1e, g) or to the opposite direction (Fig. 1 f, h). For technical reasons (limited maximal speed of the drum) vestibular and optokinetic nystagmus had the same direction in the first part of each trial, whereas in the second part (deceleration) they were

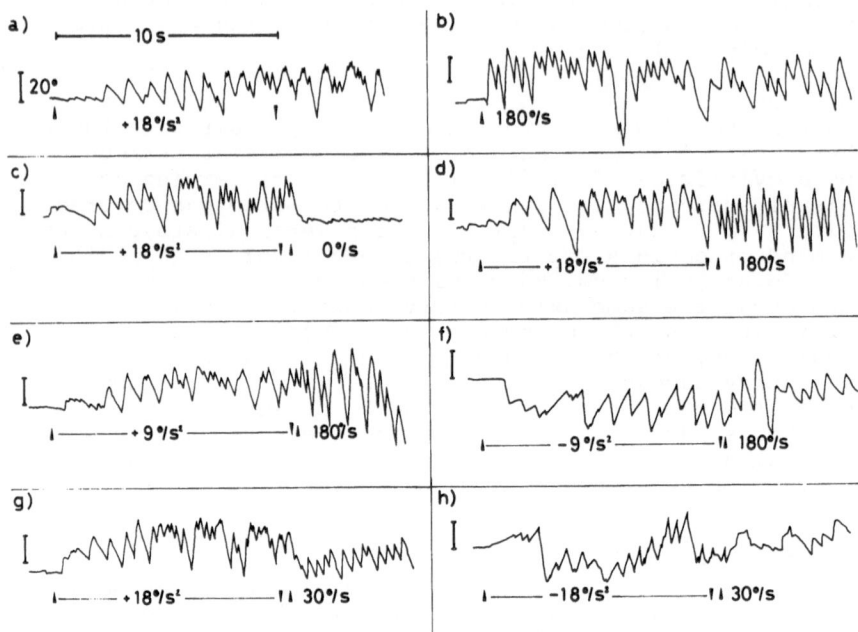

FIGURE 2. Original recordings (acceleration phase and the onset of the optokinetic stimulus) of one subject using the stimuli depicted in Fig. 1.

opposite. To balance sequential effects, the order of the trials was reversed for two subjects. All values of SPV in the paper are averages of the 4 subjects measured 0.7 s after the onset of the optokinetic stimulus (usually the second beat of nystagmus).

RESULTS
Pure vestibular stimulation for 10 s (Fig. 1a, original recording Fig. 2a) results in perrotatory and postrotatory nystagmus with a maximum at the end of the vestibular stimulus. The perrotatory nystagmus was usually somewhat stronger than the postrotatory. Averages for perrotatory (open symbols) and postrotatory (dark symbols) SPV of nystagmus measured 0.7 s after the end of the stimulus are shown in Fig. 3. The average gain of the VOR at the end of the acceleration was 0.61 with perrotatory and 0.48 for postrotatory nystagmus.
Pure optokinetic nystagmus (Fig. 1b, original recording Fig. 2b) is dependent on visual surround velocity. Average values for OKN SPV measured about 0.7 s after the start of optokinetic stimulation are shown in Fig. 3 and, to compare them with the results of the interaction

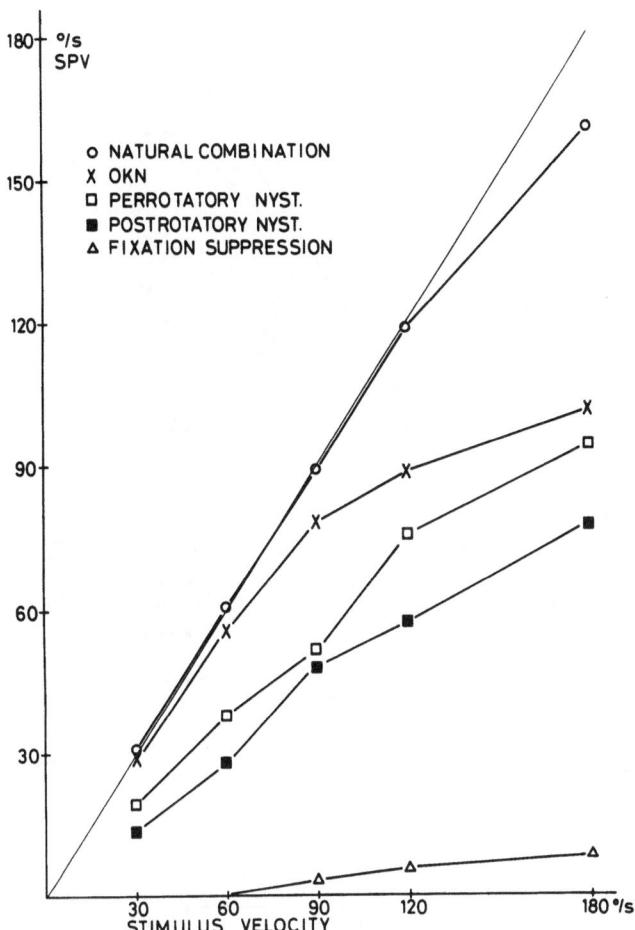

FIGURE 3. Average slow phase velocity (SPV) of 4 subjects measured 0.7 s after the onset of optokinetic stimulation; per- and postrotatory nystagmus was measured at the end of vestibular stimulation.

trials,also in Fig. 4. The gain of OKN decreases with increasing stimulus velocity (0.97, 0.92, 0.87, 0.75 and 0.59 for the five velocities tested).
Fixation suppression of vestibular nystagmus by presenting a pattern which is stationary relative to the subject (Fig. 1c, original recording Fig. 2c) results in a complete suppression of vestibular nystagmus (as measurable by EOG) within 0.7 s up to accelerations of 6 °/s². With higher accelerations SPV drops sharply after the onset of the visual stimulus, but there is

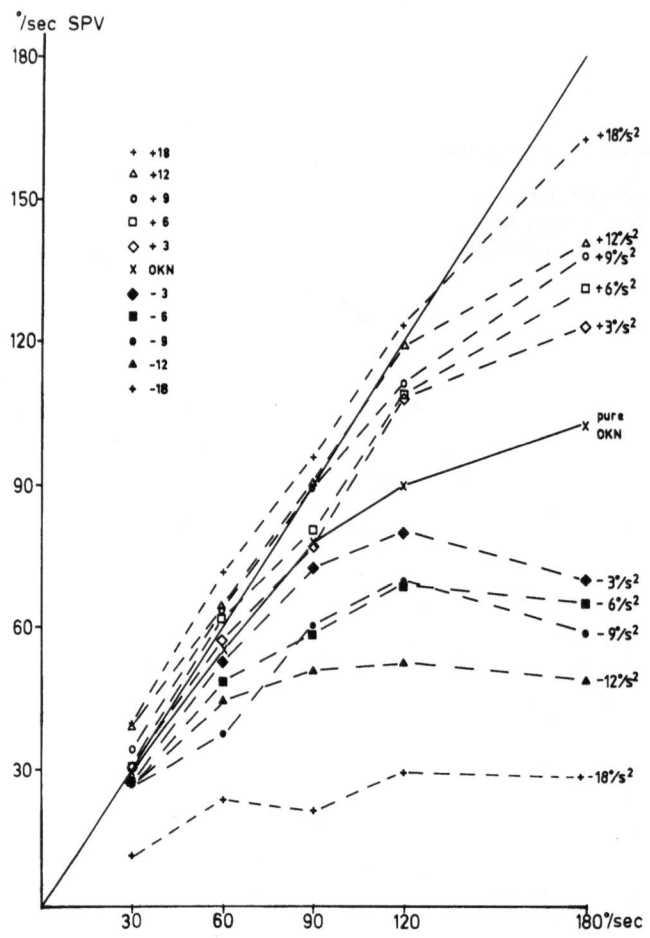

FIGURE 4. Average slow phase velocity of 4 subjects measured 0.7 s after the onset of the additional opto-kinetic stimulus in enhancing (open symbols) and de-pressing (dark symbols) interaction trials.

still a small amount of vestibular nystagmus (Fig. 3).

The "natural" combination of vestibular and optokinetic stimulation (Fig. 1d, 2d) results in a linear increase of SPV with a gain of 1 up to a stimulus velocity of 120 °/s (acceleration 12 °/s², Fig. 3).
With enhancing interaction (vestibular and optokinetic nystagmus into the same direction, Fig. 1e,g; 2e,g) SPV of nystagmus in general exceeds that with pure optokine-tic stimulation (Fig. 4). With high vestibular and slow

optokinetic stimuli SPV surpasses even optokinetic stimulus speed. This phenomenon is equivalent to the incomplete suppression of vestibular nystagmus with high
body accelerations in the fixation suppression experiment. The influence of the preceeding vestibular stimulus increases with increasing optokinetic stimulus
velocities.
Depressing interaction (vestibular and optokinetic stimuli elicit nystagmus into opposing directions, Fig.
1f,h; 2f,h) leads to a lower SPV than pure optokinetic
stimulation. Again this vestibular effect increases with
increasing optokinetic stimulus velocities. With low
optokinetic stimuli (30 °/s) the effect of the vestibular stimulus may be completely compensated by the optokinetic system (Fig. 4).
In order to determine whether the enhancing and depressing vestibular interaction is a linear addition of
both inputs (multiplied by their respective gain factors)
we tried to eliminate the effect of the vestibular stimulus by comparing the change in SPV elicited by the
additional optokinetic stimulus with the slow phase obtained by pure optokinetic stimulation. As retinal image
motion initially is the input to the optokinetic reflexes
we computed it at the onset of the optokinetic stimulus
as the difference between optokinetic stimulus velocity
and slow phase velocity of vestibular nystagmus at the
end of body acceleration. We also determined the change
in SPV by the additional optokinetic stimulation by
subtracting the SPV of vestibular nystagmus (just prior
to the onset of the optokinetic stimulus) from the combined response. Fig. 5 shows average changes in SPV related to retinal image motion at the onset of the optokinetic stimulus. When the vestibular nystagmus is opposite to the optokinetic stimulus retinal image motion
faster than 180 °/s may result. With a vestibular SPV
faster than the optokinetic stimulus retinal image motion reverses direction (negative values on the abscissa
in Fig. 3). For comparison SPV elicited by pure optokinetic stimulation is also shown. The figure demonstrates that an additional optokinetic stimulus during vestibular nystagmus changes SPV in the same way as a pure
optokinetic stimulus with the same initial retinal image
motion. This is especially convincing for enhancing
interaction (open symbols). For depressing interaction
(dark symbols) this linearity is less accurate as many
values for the change in SPV are somewhat higher than
for pure optokinetic stimulation.

DISCUSSION
We were able to demonstrate linear interaction of vestibular and optokinetic inputs when measured immediately
after the onset of the additional optokinetic stimulus.
Especially during depressing interaction the correspondence between the data and the assumed linear interaction
is much better than in our previous experiments on the
modulation of optokinetic nystagmus by a 10 s vestibular
stimulus (Koenig et al., 1978).

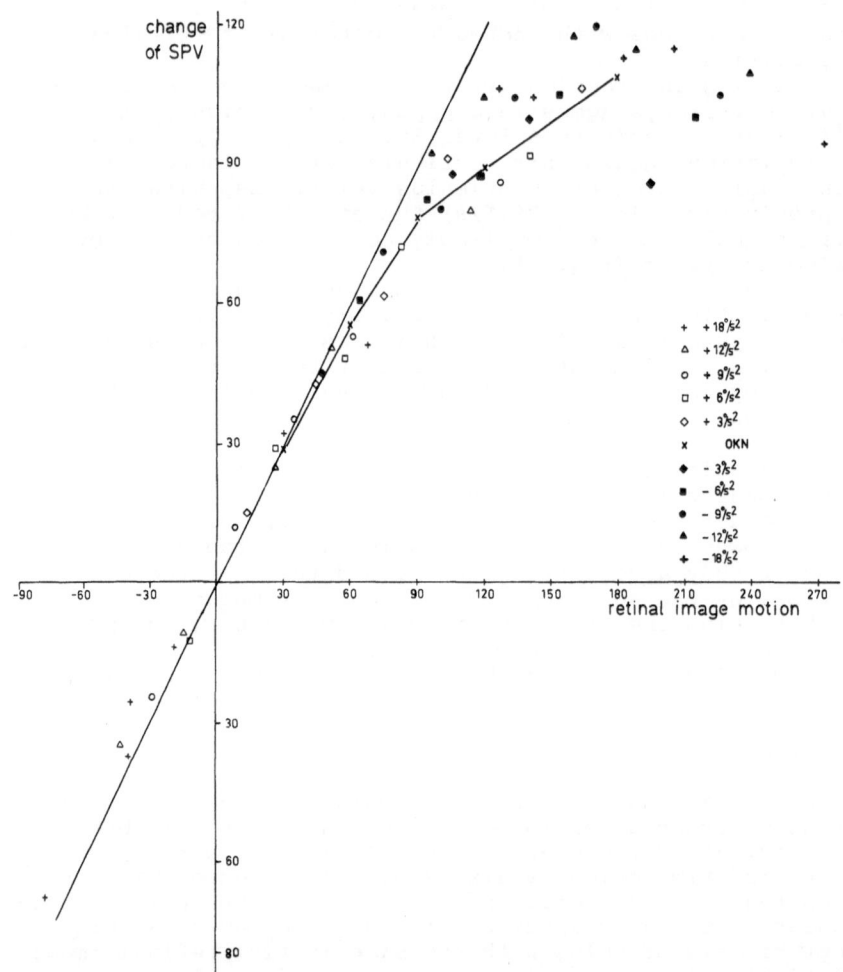

FIGURE 5. Change of slow phase velocity elicited by the additional optokinetic stimulus as dependent on retinal image motion at the onset of the optokinetic stimulation (open symbols-enhancing interaction, dark symbols depressing interaction). For comparison average OKN response is also shown (see text for details).

The basic advantage of these experiments is that we
used a velocity step instead of a ramp for the additional stimulus. This made it possible to measure the immediate effect of the additional stimulus not allowing
to storage mechanisms eliciting afternystagmus (Raphan
et al., 1979) to change their charge to a greater extent. It is, however, not possible to exclude such a
change of charge completely even in such a short interval as 0.7 s. Discharge of the visual vestibular in-
tagrator by a stationary visual surround was earlier
demonstrated in humans (Collins, 1968; Cohen et al.,
1981; Koenig et al., 1981). So it should also be discharged by an optokinetic stimulus slower than vestibular SPV, especially when vestibular SPV and optokinetic
stimulus are of opposite directions. Therefore linear
interaction cannot be expected after longer intervals
of optokinetic stimulation. The fact that during depressing interaction the change in SPV is slightly greater
than expected on the basis of linear interaction may be
due to such a slight discharge of the vestibular integrator, allowing the optokinetic input to be relatively more effective.
In general, however, there is a very good correspondence
of the SPV observed with pure optokinetic stimulation
and the change in SPV by the additional optokinetic stimulus. Thus the optokinetic reflexes, predominantly the
pursuit system, modulate SPV in the same way during
combined visual vestibular stimulation as during pure
optokinetic stimulation.
When both systems are stimulated in a quasi natural
combination the range of stimulus velocities with fully
compensatory SPV is extended up to 120 °/s, which is
almost as high as the SPV measured in Rhesus monkeys
under similar conditions (Waespe et al., 1980).
The considerably higher optokinetic gain and the more
effective fixation suppression in these experiments
compared to our earlier ones (Koenig et al., 1978) probably has to be attributed to the additional colored
stimulus on the wall of the drum, which improves pursuit. This demonstrates that the frequently applied
optokinetic stimulation by rather coarse black and white
stripes may be a good stimulus for the retinal periphery dependent OKN-system, but not for the pursuit
system.

REFERENCES
Allum JHJ, Graf W, Dichgans J and Schmidt CL (1976)
Visual-vestibular interactions in the vestibular nuclei
of the goldfish, Exp. Brain Res. 26,463-485.
Bock O (1982) Personal communication
Cohen B, Henn V, Raphan T and Dennett D (1981) Velocity
storage, nystagmus and visual-vestibular interactions
in humans, Ann. N.Y. Acad. Sci. 374,421-433.
Collins WE (1968) Special effects of brief periods of
visual fixation on nystagmus and sensations of turning,
Aerospace Med. 39,257-266.

Koenig E, Allum JHJ, Dichgans J (1978) Visual-vestibular interaction upon nystagmus slow phase velocity in man, Acta Otolaryngol. 85,397-410.
Koenig E, Dichgans J (1981) The influence of fixation on vestibular afternystagmus I and II In Fuchs and Becker, eds. Progress in oculomotor research, 509-515. New York, Elsevier North Holland.
Lau CGY, Honrubia V, Jenkins HA, Baloh RW and Yee RD (1978) Linear model for visual-vestibular interaction, Aviat. Space Environ. Med. 49,880-885.
Maurer OH (1935) Some neglected factors which influence the duration of post-rotational nystagmus, Acta Otolaryngol. 22,1-23.
Raphan T, Matsuo V, Cohen B (1979) Velocity storage in the vestibulo-ocular reflex arc, Exp. Brain Res. 35,229-248.
Robinson DA (1977) Linear addition of optokinetic and vestibular signals in the vestibular nucleus, Exp. Brain Res. 30,447-450.
Schmid R, Buizza A and Zambarbieri D (1980) A non-linear model for visual-vestibular interaction during body rotation in man, Biol. Cybernetics 36,143-151.
Waespe W and Henn V (1977) Neuronal activity in the vestibular nuclei of the alert monkey during vestibular and optokinetic stimulation, Exp. Brain Res. 27,523-538.
Waespe W, Henn V and Isoviita V (1980) Nystagmus slow-phase velocity during vestibular, optokinetic and combined stimulation in the monkey, Arch. Psychiat. Nervenkr. 228,275-286.

THE EFFECTS OF RETINAL LOCATION AND STROBE RATE OF HEAD-FIXED VISUAL
TARGETS ON THE SUPPRESSION OF VESTIBULAR NYSTAGMUS

G.R. BARNES (RAF Institute of Aviation Medicine, Farnborough, Hants.)

1. INTRODUCTION

There has been considerable interest in recent years in the
degree to which man is able to suppress reflex eye movements of
vestibular origin. The mechanisms by which this suppression is
carried out appear similar to those normally used during the visual
control of eye movement. Thus, Barnes et al (1978) were able to show
that the breakdown in suppression exhibited similar frequency characteristics to the breakdown of the pursuit reflex for a similar set
of stimulus conditions. Neurophysiological evidence also tends to
support the hypothesis that there is direct visual-vestibular interaction within the brainstem and cerebellum (Henn et al 1974, Fuchs,
Kimm 1975, Waespe,Henn 1977), although it has become clear that this
interaction is by no means a straightforward one (Buettner,Büttner
1979, Cohen et al 1977).

In man, the two principal factors which affect the degree of
suppression are the amplitude and frequency of the stimulus (Barnes
et al 1978, Guedry 1968, Benson,Guedry 1971), variables which are
also known to have similar effects upon the behaviour of the pursuit
reflex (Fender,Nye 1961, Stark 1971). One of the most important
factors in achieving complete fixation suppression appears to be the
acuity with which the display can be seen, and its position on the
retina. The relative effects of peripheral and foveal vision on eye
movement control have been investigated for both the pursuit
(Michalski et al 1977), and optokinetic reflexes (Hood 1967, Dichgans 1977, Dubois,Collewijn 1979), with the general conclusion that
reduction of the peripheral field can lead to a substantial lowering
of the peak velocity attainable. Clinical experience indicates that
lesions which affect the pursuit reflex also generally affect both
optokinetic nystagmus and suppression of the vestibulo-ocular reflex
(Dichgans 1979) but, as yet, there appears to be no quantitative evidence about the relative contribution of foveal and peripheral mechanisms on suppression.

In the following experiments, two main questions have been
addressed. First, is it possible to show graded effects on suppression of the vestibulo-ocular reflex according to the peripheral location of the visual stimulus in a manner similar to that of the optokinetic response? Second, is there any modification of suppression
when visual image slip information is degraded by tachistoscopic
presentation of visual targets?

2. APPARATUS

The same apparatus was used for each of the three experiments
reported here. The subject was seated on a large turntable to which
he was firmly harnessed and his head clamped. He viewed a display
which was also rigidly coupled to the turntable so that there was no
relative movement between the head and the display. The display
consisted of 9 red light-emitting diode (LED) target lights, placed
on a periphery at $0°$, $±2.5°$, $±5°$, $±10°$, $±20°$ from the centre line in
the horizontal plane. The target lights were placed at a distance of
0.95m from the subject; the diameter of each target light subtended
an angle of 12 min arc at the eye and each had a luminance of

Roucoux, A. and Crommelinck, M. (eds.): Physiological and Pathological Aspects of Eye Movements.
© 1982, Dr W. Junk Publishers, The Hague, Boston, London. ISBN-13: 978-94-009-8002-0

282

8 cd/m^2. The experiment was carried out in a completely darkened
room so that the target lights appeared against a featureless black
background.

Eye movements were recorded using an infra-red recording
apparatus (see Abadi et al, 1981) for details. The recording system
was incorporated into a helmet-like system which could be rigidly
coupled to the head by a dental bite-bar. The resolution with which
the eye movement could be recorded was approximately 10-20 min arc.

3. EXPERIMENT I
3.1. Method

The subject was exposed to sinusoidal motion about the yaw axis
of the body, at six discrete frequencies between 0.25 and 2.0 Hz.
The peak velocity of the stimulus was maintained constant throughout
the frequency range at ±60°/s. Six subjects were each exposed to
six experimental conditions at each of the stimulating frequencies.
In one condition the subject was presented with a single central
target light and was instructed to maintain constant fixation on the
target. In a second condition, eye movements were recorded whilst
the subject was in complete darkness. In the remaining four conditions the subject was presented with a pair of target lights at one
of four peripheral locations (±2.5°, ±5°, ±10° or ±20°). In these

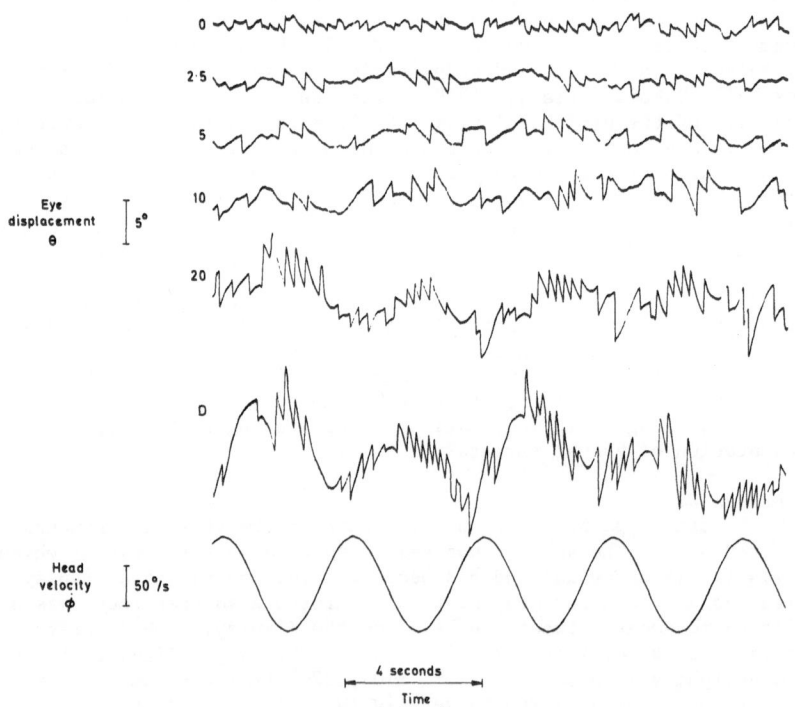

FIGURE 1. Examples of eye movements recorded whilst viewing a head-
fixed display during oscillation in yaw at 0.25 Hz. Conditions of
visual stimulation: 0 – centre target; 2.5 – 20 – targets located
at ±2.5°, 5°, 10°, 20°, from centre; D – darkness.

conditions there was no central fixation light but the subject was
instructed to look fixedly at the black featureless space midway
between the two peripheral target lights. The subjects were asked
to report any particular observations regarding image movement and
blur which occurred during the experiment.

3.2. Results
3.2.1. Qualitative features of the oculomotor response. The most
significant finding of this experiment was that the degree of
suppression of the vestibulo-ocular reflex decreased in a graded
manner when the target lights were moved from the central position
to the furthermost peripheral location. This effect was consistently
found in all the subjects and is evident in the sample records of raw
eye displacement waveforms shown in Fig. 1. Several subjects voluntarily reported that at the lower frequencies (0.25 and 0.5 Hz)
there was little or no image smear when the centre light was illuminated, but that the peripheral lights often appeared to be blurred
and to 'jump about' in an unpredictable manner. This latter observation would appear to be associated with the presence of large saccadic components in the partially suppressed vestibular response
(Fig. 1). There was no evidence of any complete cancellation of the
vestibular response under these visual conditions, even at the lowest
stimulus frequency (0.25 Hz). Rather, it appeared that the presence
of a fixation point led to a restriction of the overall amplitude of
nystagmus by a reduction in the amplitude of saccades and an increase
of saccadic frequency. At the highest frequencies (1.5, 2.0 Hz) the
light sources appeared blurred under all visual conditions, as
reported previously (Barnes et al, 1978).

Even when the eye movements were heavily suppressed at the lowest stimulus frequency, they still retained a nystagmic form similar
to that observed when recording in darkness. The fast-phases normally exhibited a sharp onset, as shown by the examples in Fig. 1.
On the other hand the slow-phases often showed considerable distortion, the actual velocity between fast-phases fluctuating in a manner
not related to the stimulus. This finding indicates that the attenuation of the vestibular response had undoubtedly taken place
upstream of the mechanism of saccadic generation. In earlier experiments (Barnes et al, 1978), the lack of sensitivity in the electro-
oculographic recording technique frequently gave the impression that
the saccades were rounded in form or indeed that suppression was more
complete because small saccades were not detected.
3.2.2. Slow-phase eye velocity. The recorded eye movements were
analysed by computer (Barnes 1982b), employing an interactive procedure to extract fast-phases and to calculate the ratio of slow-phase
eye velocity to turntable velocity (gain). Analysis of variance
indicated that there was a highly significant ($P < .001$) increase in
gain as the target sources were moved further into the periphery, and
an equally significant ($P < .001$) increase with increase of stimulus
frequency. However, the effect of the peripheral location of the
target changed with the frequency of stimulation. At the lowest frequency (0.25 Hz) even the target lights at ±20° were able to exert a
considerable degree of suppression (65% on average), whereas at the
higher frequencies only the centrally located targets (0° and ±2.5°)
had any significant effect. In other words, the frequency response
of the peripheral mechanisms exhibited a breakdown at a lower frequency than that of the central mechanisms. In darkness the gain
exhibited a gradual increase with frequency, the mean levels ranging

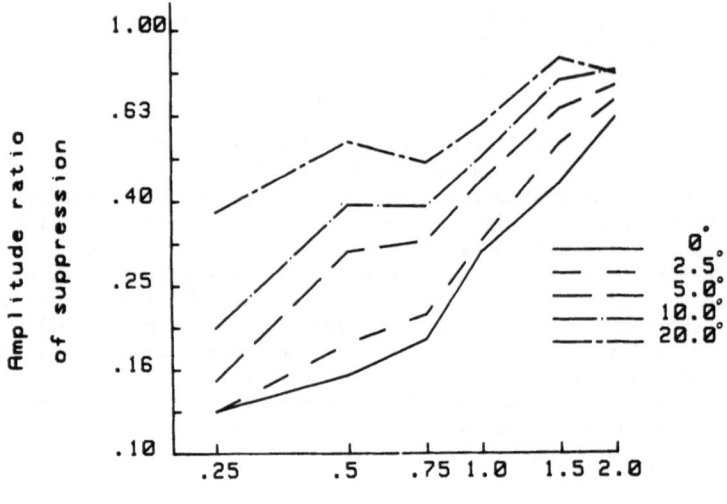

FIGURE 2. The ratio of slow-phase eye velocity during suppression
of vestibular nystagmus to slow-phase eye velocity in the dark for
the five target locations defined in Fig. 1. Mean of 6 Ss.

from 0.44 at 0.25 Hz to 0.90 at 2.0 Hz.

The effect of target location is illustrated in Fig. 2, where
the amplitude ratio of suppression is defined by the ratio of slow-
phase eye velocity during the target presentation conditions to the
slow-phase velocity in darkness. This ratio gives a measure of the
efficiency of suppression (see Barnes et al 1978 and discussion).
It can be seen that the response to the central target and the ±2.5°
targets was very similar; indeed, there was no statistically significant difference between these two conditions at any of the frequencies of stimulation. In contrast, the other visual conditions
evoked responses which were highly significantly different (P < .001)
from each other.

3.2.3. Eye displacement during suppression. As mentioned earlier,
the changes in gain of the slow-phase eye velocity were accompanied
by changes in the amplitude of overall eye displacement. One way of
assessing the magnitude of such eye displacement is to take the raw
recorded eye position signal, including both the fast and slow-phase
components, and assess the variance about the mean position by correlation with the stimulus waveform; this procedure allows the ratio of
eye displacement to head velocity to be obtained. It is evident from
the averaged values of eye displacement gain, which are plotted in
Fig. 3, that there was a highly significant trend of increasing
amplitude of eye movement as the target lights were moved further
into the periphery, with greatest overall displacement appearing in
darkness. The most marked difference occurred between the centre
light and 2.5° light conditions, where there was an average 52%
increase at the lowest frequency of stimulation (0.25 Hz), despite

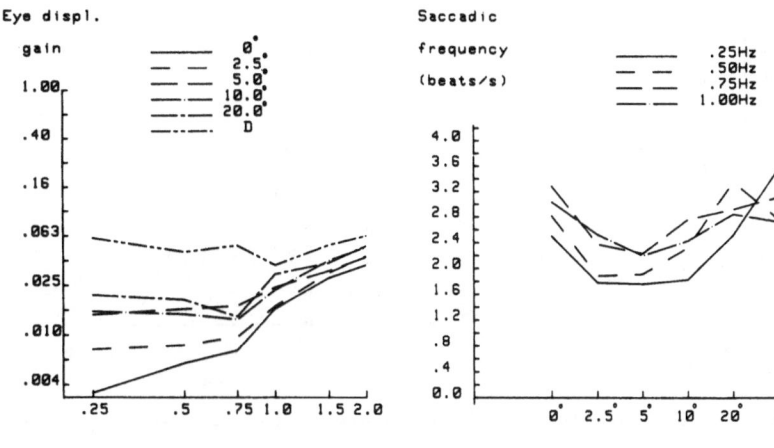

Frequency (Hz)

Visual display condition

FIGURE 3. The ratio of overall eye displacement to head angular velocity for six conditions of visual stimulation defined in Fig. 1. Mean of 6 Ss.

FIGURE 4. The frequency of saccadic activity for each frequency of stimulation (excluding 1.5 & 2.0 Hz). Visual display conditions as in Fig.1. Mean of 6 Ss.

the fact that there was no significant change in slow-phase eye velocity between these two visual target conditions. These effects are evident in the oculographic records (Fig. 1), where it can be seen that the reduction in amplitude is achieved by an increase in saccadic frequency and a reduction in saccadic amplitude.

3.2.4. <u>Frequency of saccadic activity</u>. The changes in saccadic frequency as a function of visual stimulus condition are shown in Fig. 4. This measure becomes less meaningful for the higher frequencies of stimulation (1.5 and 2.0 Hz) because of the relative paucity of saccadic activity and consequently they have been omitted from Fig. 4; but for the lower frequencies there is a trend of increasing saccadic frequency as the targets are moved from the 2.5° to the 20° position. However, for the centrally located target there is an abrupt up-turn in the curve, the average beat frequency being 1.36 times that for the 2.5° targets, with an average increase in slow-phase velocity of only 9%. For the lowest frequency alone (0.25 Hz) the beat frequency increased by a factor of 1.4 without any change in average velocity.

4. EXPERIMENT II
4.1. <u>Method</u>

In the second experiment the visual stimulus conditions were identical to those of Experiment I. However, the oculomotor response was induced by a postrotational stimulus to the horizontal semicircular canals. The subject was brought to an abrupt halt after a 120s period of constant rotation at 120°/s to the left.

4.2. <u>Results</u>

After the cessation of rotation the subjects reported that the target lights appeared blurred for a period of some 5-10s and that they were aware of movements of the visual image for considerably longer periods. However, most subjects also reported that the

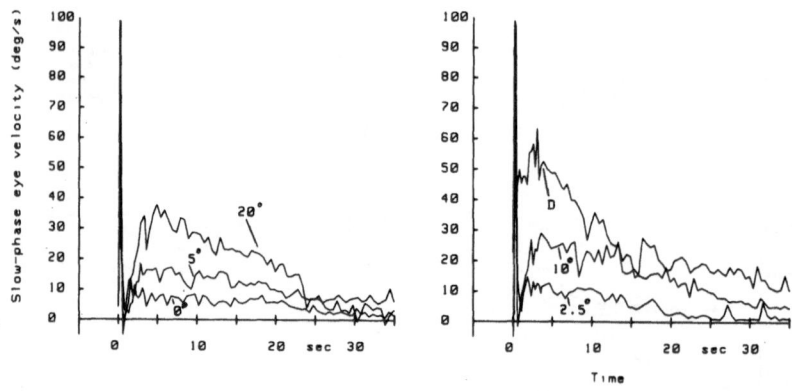

FIGURE 5. Typical oculomotor responses of one subject following a sudden stop from rotation at 120°/s. Visual stimulus conditions as defined in Fig. 1.

targets were much less blurred immediately after the stop. This effect is reflected in the slow-phase eye movement records shown in Fig. 5. When the subject was stopped, the eye initially made a rapid compensatory movement in the direction opposite to that of the head velocity signal. However, this slow-phase component was rapidly reduced to a very low level, even reversing direction in some examples. The initial transient phase was normally over within 0.5s and thereafter the slow-phase eye velocity built up to reach a peak value after 4-5s. The peak slow-phase velocity was lowest for the condition in which the subject viewed the central target light (mean 13.1°/s) and progressively increased as the targets were moved further into the periphery (means of 13.6, 16.5, 21.6, 24.3 and 67.7°/s for 2.5°, 5°, 10°, 20° and darkness respectively). However the initial dip in slow-phase eye velocity was seen in all stimulus conditions, although the eye velocity did not approach zero for the more peripherally located targets.

After reaching the peak value the slow-phase velocity decayed with a time constant which was not significantly less than that of the unmodified vestibulo-ocular response recorded in the dark (means of 9.8, 10.6, 12.6, 11.7, 13.9 and 12.4s for 0°, 2.5°, 5°, 10°, 20° and darkness, respectively). Interestingly, the response recorded in the dark also showed an initial dip in slow-phase velocity immediately after stopping the subject although this never reached a level less than 80% of the subsequent peak slow-phase velocity. However, it seems probable, as discussed later, that this feature is the source of the initial rapid drop in velocity during suppression.

An important feature of the responses which was also noted in the sinusoidal responses, was an increase in frequency and decrease in amplitude of fast-phases when the subject viewed a central target. By this means the eye movements were accurately located within the foveal area during central target fixation, whereas during suppression with the more peripherally located target sources, the eyes deviated widely from centre.

5. EXPERIMENT III
5.1. Method
     In the third experiment the target lights used in the previous
experiments were not presented continuously, but were illuminated
in a tachistoscopic manner. In an initial experiment the duration
of the light pulse was maintained at 100μs whilst the inter-pulse
interval was varied between 10 and 3000ms. The effect of peripheral target location in these conditions was assessed by comparing
the response to the centre light and a pair of lights at ±10° from
centre as in experiments I and II. In the second experiment the
centre light alone was used to assess the effect of pulse durations
between 20 and 1000μs. The inter-pulse interval was maintained at
two levels, 50 and 250ms. The stimulus for both these experiments
was a sinusoidal oscillation in yaw at a frequency of 0.5 Hz, with
a peak velocity of 60°/s.

5.2. Results
5.2.1. Qualitative features of oculomotor response. The most significant feature of the oculomotor response was that the degree of
suppression of the vestibulo-ocular reflex was decreased in a
graded manner as the inter-pulse interval was increased. During
the experiment the subjective impression was that there was no
apparent blurring of the target sources either in the centre or
±10° position, so that there was no visible source of retinal slip.
At the shortest pulse intervals (10 and 30 ms) the targets appeared
to be continuously illuminated, whereas at an interval of 100 ms
they were seen to flicker and successive images were overlaid and
slightly displaced from each other. At intervals of 300 ms and
above there was no residue of the previous pulse but the targets
appeared to jump about in a rather unpredictable manner. This
effect was probably attributable to the presence of saccadic activity in the oculomotor response, which was similar to that shown in
Fig. 1. When the centre target was strobed at the lowest frequency
the amplitude of the overall eye movement was large, with predominantly large amplitude fast-phases. In contrast when the target
was strobed at the highest rate the eye movements were confined
within the area of the fovea, but still exhibited a nystagmic form
with no evidence of any complete cancellation of the eye movement,
as noted in Experiment I.
5.2.2. Slow-phase eye velocity. Figure 6 shows the ratio of slow-
phase eye velocity to head velocity averaged over all six subjects
for each of the inter-pulse intervals. Analysis of variance was
carried out on the data and indicated a highly significant
($P < .001$) increase of gain with increase of inter-pulse interval.
There was also a highly significant ($P < .001$) increase of gain for
the targets at ±10° compared with the centre lights, a finding which
was in accord with the results of Experiment I.
     The eye velocity gains obtained at an inter-pulse interval of
3000ms for both the centre and ±10° targets were not significantly
different from each other, nor were they significantly different
from the response in darkness. The mean level for eye velocity
gain in the dark was 0.65. This value was somewhat higher than
that recorded in Experiment I, but this was probably attributable
to individual differences in the two groups of subjects; nevertheless, the mean level was well within the range recorded in other
experiments (Barnes, 1980), with individual values varying between
0.44 and 0.89.

288

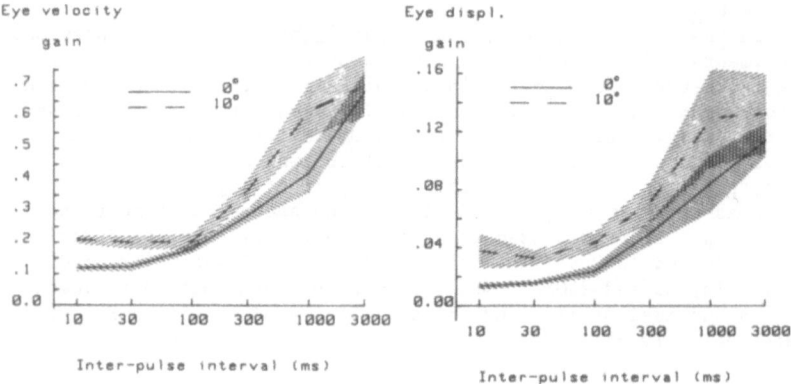

Eye velocity gain

Eye displ. gain

Inter-pulse interval (ms)

Inter-pulse interval (ms)

FIGURE 6. The effects of inter-pulse interval on the ratio of eye velocity to head velocity during tachistoscopic presentation of head-fixed targets. Peak head velocity = ±60°/s at 0.5 Hz. Mean of 6 Ss ±1 S.E.

FIGURE 7. The effects of inter-pulse interval on the ratio of eye displacement to head velocity during tachistoscopic presentation of head-fixed targets. Peak head velocity = ±60°/s at 0.5 Hz. Mean of 6 Ss ±1 S.E.

5.2.3. Eye displacement. The changes in suppression of the slow-phase eye velocity were accompanied by changes in the amplitude of overall eye displacement. The ratio of eye displacement to head velocity is shown in Fig. 7. Analysis of variance revealed a highly significant (P < .001) increase in gain as the inter-pulse interval was increased and a significant difference (P < .01) between the responses to the central target light and the ±10° lights. The levels of gain were somewhat higher than those recorded in Experiment I, but this was almost certainly due to the inter-population differences and is in accord with the higher levels of eye velocity gain shown in Fig. 6.

5.2.4. Frequency of saccadic activity. Although the overall eye displacement and the slow-phase eye velocity both increased as the inter-pulse interval was increased the frequency of saccadic beats exhibited the opposite trend as shown in Fig. 8. Analysis of variance indicated a significant (P < .01) decrease of saccadic frequency with increasing inter-pulse interval for presentation of both the centre and ±10° light sources. These effects were somewhat different to those observed in Experiment I, where the decrease in suppression associated with the more peripheral targets led to an increase in saccadic frequency. There was also a highly significant (P < .001) decrease in saccadic frequency for the response to the ±10° target sources.

5.2.5. Effect of pulse duration. One of the primary aims of varying the duration of the pulse in the second part of this experiment was to establish whether the possible smearing of such a briefly presented image on the retina was, of itself, likely to give rise to image slip information. The results indicate that it was not, since analysis of variance revealed no significant effect of pulse duration on eye velocity gain (see Fig. 9), eye displacement gain or the frequency of saccadic beats. For each of these variables there

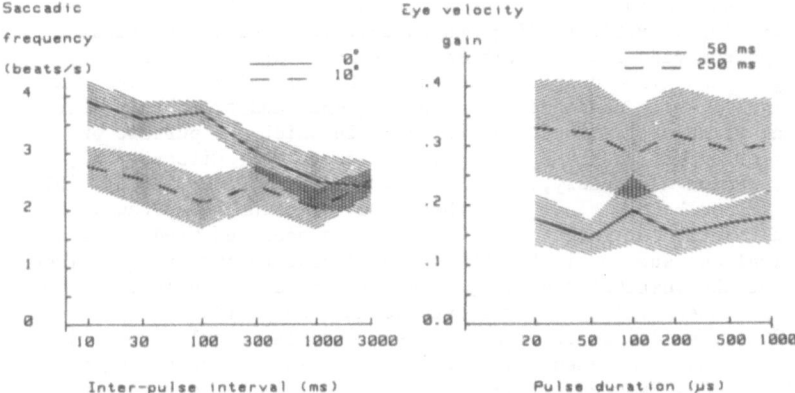

FIGURE 8. The effects of inter-pulse interval on the frequency of saccadic beats during tachistoscopic presentation of head-fixed targets. Peak head velocity = ±60°/s at 0.5 Hz. Mean of 6 Ss ±1 S.E.

FIGURE 9. The effects of pulse duration on the ratio of eye velocity to head velocity during tachistoscopic presentation of head-fixed targets. Inter-pulse interval = 50 & 250 ms. Mean of 6 Ss ±1 S.E.

was a highly significant (P < .001) difference between the two inter-pulse intervals as expected from the results of Experiment I.

6. DISCUSSION
6.1. Changes in gain of visual feedback
In the experiments described here an attempt has been made to separate the effects of foveal and peripheral retinal stimuli on suppression of the vestibulo-ocular reflex. It is apparent that visual feedback of retinal error information is essential in order to achieve optimum suppression. The results have demonstrated that graded levels of suppression are achieved if the retinal error information is degraded by moving the target sources further into the periphery or if the target lights are presented tachistoscopically. The exact manner by which this comes about is unclear at present, but it is possible that both the retinal location and strobe rate of the visual stimuli determine the gain of the feedback mechanisms responsible for suppression. Such a variation in feedback gain implies that the information about relative velocity of the image moving across the retina becomes attenuated as the image moves further away from the fovea or when the targets are presented at decreasing strobe rates. That this should be so is not surprising when evidence for the possible mechanisms involved in visual-vestibular interaction is considered. In the following discussion the findings will be assessed in relation to current neurophysiological evidence and to modelling of oculomotor control.

6.2. Neurophysiological mechanisms of visual-vestibular interaction
The mechanisms responsible for suppression of the vestibulo-ocular reflex are similar in many ways to those responsible for the response to optokinetic and pursuit stimuli. It has been appreciated

for some time that visual stimuli can induce strong sensations of
both linear motion (Berthoz et al, 1975) and rotation (Dichgans,
Brandt, 1972, 1978), findings which indicate a close relationship
between the visual and vestibular systems. Various experiments
using a head-fixed display have shown that visual performance can
be significantly degraded when the frequency and/or velocity level
of the stimulus lies outside the range in which the pursuit or
optokinetic reflexes are effective (Guedry, 1968; Gilson et al,
1970; Benson and Guedry, 1971; Barnes et al, 1978; Lau et al, 1978).
     It has become clear that there are two principal pathways of
visual-vestibular interaction. These have been referred to as the
cortical and sub-cortical pathways and appear to involve the flocculus and the vestibular nuclei, respectively, as the principal centres of interaction. Several authors have shown that units in the
vestibular nuclei which respond to semicircular canal stimulation
also respond to movement of a full-field visual scene (Dichgans,
Brandt, 1972; Henn et al, 1974; Waespe,Henn, 1977; Buettner,Büttner,
1979). Waespe and Henn (1977) reported that units within the
vestibular nuclei of the monkey responded to both vestibular and
optokinetic stimuli and that the response was attenuated during
suppression of the vestibular reflex. However, interaction was not
complete. During optokinetic stimulation the response of the vestibular units saturated when the stimulus velocity exceeded $60^o/s$,
whereas the nystagmus reached much higher velocities. The units
were active during optokinetic after-nystagmus and in response to
a transient vestibular stimulus decayed fairly slowly in comparison
with the decay in slow-phase eye velocity.
     These characteristics of the pathway through the vestibular
nuclei may be observed in foveate animals after removal of the
flocculus, which suggests that the visual input is relayed, at
least in part, by direct brainstem pathways (Keller,Precht, 1979;
Cazin et al, 1980). It is probable that the input arises from
'W-type' motion sensitive ganglion cells in the retina, relayed
through the nucleus of the optic tract to the brainstem (Collewijn,
1975; Hoffman,Schoppmann, 1975,1981; Hoffman et al, 1976; Precht,
1981). This pathway is specifically more sensitive to temporo-
nasal movement of images on the retina, the naso-temporal component
being provided by pathways through the visual cortex. In patients
with loss of the cortical pursuit pathway, such asymmetry is
evident in the optokinetic response (Honrubia, 1979; Dichgans, 1979).
A feature of the optokinetic response of these patients is a slow
build-up of nystagmus in comparison with the rapid rise to peak
velocity observed in normal subjects. This feature serves to
illustrate the manner in which the cortical and sub-cortical
mechanisms normally cooperate during an optokinetic response.
     The cortical pathways are less well known, but almost certainly
involve pathways relayed via the visual cortex to the flocculus,
probably by way of the inferior olive (Maekawa,Simpson, 1973).
Waespe et al (1981) have shown that a proportion of floccular
Purkinje cells in the monkey are activated during both optokinetic
stimulation and suppression of vestibular nystagmus. These units
respond with a signal proportional to image slip and their response
is much more rapid than units within the vestibular nuclei. These
units do not become active until the eye velocity reaches that level
at which the vestibular units start to saturate and they do not
respond during optokinetic after-nystagmus. On this basis it has
been suggested that such units normally act in a complementary manner

to the vestibular units and form the mechanism by which the rapid increase in eye velocity is achieved in response to a constant velocity optokinetic stimulus (Cohen et al, 1977) . The input to such Purkinje cells and their destination within the oculomotor pathways have yet to be determined.

Other units within the vestibular nuclei and other areas of the brainstem respond specifically during pursuit tracking and not to full-field stimulation (Keller,Daniels, 1975; Fuchs,Kimm, 1975). Although such units are appropriately responsive during fixation suppression of vestibular nystagmus, the interaction is by no means straightforward and may need to be explained in terms of the interaction with other pathways.

6.3. Modelling of visual-vestibular interaction

In an earlier experiment (Barnes et al, 1978) a comparison was made between the dynamic behaviour of the pursuit reflex and the suppression of the vestibulo-ocular reflex which led to the development of a model of visual-vestibular interaction (Barnes, 1976; Benson,Barnes, 1978). A slightly modified version of this model is shown in Fig. 10. The basic concept of the original model was that the control of eye movement, both during tracking of moving objects and during suppression of vestibular nystagmus was brought about by at least two, fundamentally different, pathways for the control of smooth eye movements. These were in addition to the saccadic

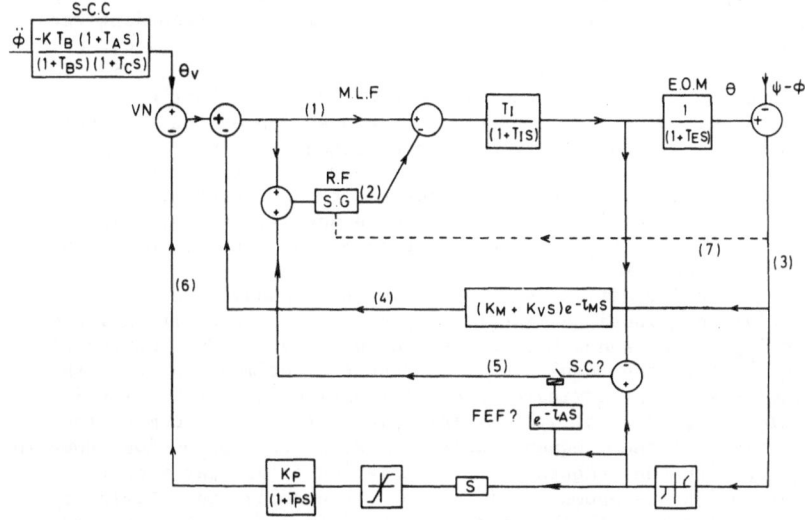

FIGURE 10. A proposed mechanism by which oculomotor control is achieved through the interaction of various visual and vestibular pathways: 1) Basic V-O.R., 2) Secondary V-O.R. pathway through saccadic generator (SG), 3) Retinal error processor, 4) Cortical smooth pursuit pathway, 5) Peripheral saccadic pathway, 6) Sub-cortical 'velocity storage' pathway, 7) Saccadic threshold control. Variables are: θ_V-vestibular afferent signal; θ-eye position; ϕ-head position, ψ-target position in space. Approximate values of parameters are $T_I \approx 10$ s; $T_E \approx 0.15$ s; $\tau_M \approx 0.05$ s; $K_M \approx 0$-5; $K_V \approx 5$; $K \approx 0.7$; $T_A \approx 0.25$ s; $T_B \approx 15$ s; $T_C \approx 0.01$ s; $K_P \approx 1$-10; $T_P \approx 10$ s; $\tau_A \approx 0.15$ s.

pathway responsible for foveation of peripherally located targets
(pathway (5) in Fig. 10). It was suggested that the usage of these
two pathways could be differentiated on the basis of the location of
the visual stimulus of interest to the subject. If it was within
the central parafoveal area (say ±2-3° from foveal centre) this
would lead to a smooth pursuit type response; if it lay on the peripheral retina and was a large field moving stimulus, it would lead
to optokinetic nystagmus. In the following discussion the function
of the separate pathways in the model will be described and justified by reference to recent experimental work.

6.3.1. The 'smooth pursuit' pathway. In the original model it was
suggested that smooth pursuit of a single moving object was carried
out by a combination of positional error and velocity error feedback. It was assumed that tracking of a small object was primarily
carried out by continual attempts to align the image of the pursued
object on the fovea. One of the advantages of this mechanism is
that it allows a possible explanation for the ability of human subjects to track stabilised retinal images (e.g. an after-image) with
a smooth eye movement (Kommerell,Taumer, 1972). In such conditions
the steady-state positional error forms the necessary source of
information required to generate a smooth eye movement in the
absence of retinal velocity error. Such stimuli are able to produce smooth eye movements up to eccentricities of 5° from foveal
centre. The rôle of this foveal mechanism in suppression of vestibular nystagmus was originally thought to be one of enabling complete suppression of the response (Barnes et al, 1978). The experiments carried out with more sensitive eye movement recording techniques now show that this conclusion was not altogether correct and
this has led to the modifications of the original model (Fig. 10).
It is evident from the recordings shown in Fig. 1 that none of the
feedback mechanisms responsible for suppression of the vestibular
response interacts downstream of the mechanism of saccadic generation, since there does not appear to be any modification of the
'sharpness' of fast-phase trajectories, as suggested by earlier
electro-oculographic recordings. Consequently, pathway 4 is now
assumed to interact with the vestibulo-ocular pathway before the
saccadic mechanism.

A second modification must be in the emphasis placed on the
relative contributions made to suppression by the positional and
velocity error feedback components of pathway 4. Two sources of
evidence from the results of the present experiments suggest that
velocity error predominates and positional error information is
little used, if at all. The first piece of evidence comes from a
comparison of the frequency characteristics of suppression shown in
Fig. 2, with the frequency characteristics of pathway 4 of the
model, which are shown in Fig. 11(b). A combination of velocity
and positional feedback leads to a steadily decreasing amplitude
ratio as the frequency of stimulation is decreased; the gain (Km) of
the positional error feedback determines the frequency at which the
steady decrease in amplitude ratio begins. On the other hand,
velocity feedback alone does not give zero velocity error and the
amplitude ratio reaches a plateau value at low frequency. It is
evident from the results depicted in Fig. 2 and from previous
results (Barnes et al, 1978) that the amplitude ratio of suppression
exhibits a plateau below 0.5 Hz, indicating that positional feedback
is not in evidence at frequencies above 0.25 Hz. In more recent
experiments (Barnes,G.R.,Edge,A., unpublished) it has been demonstrated that even at a frequency of 0.05 Hz, the amplitude ratio was

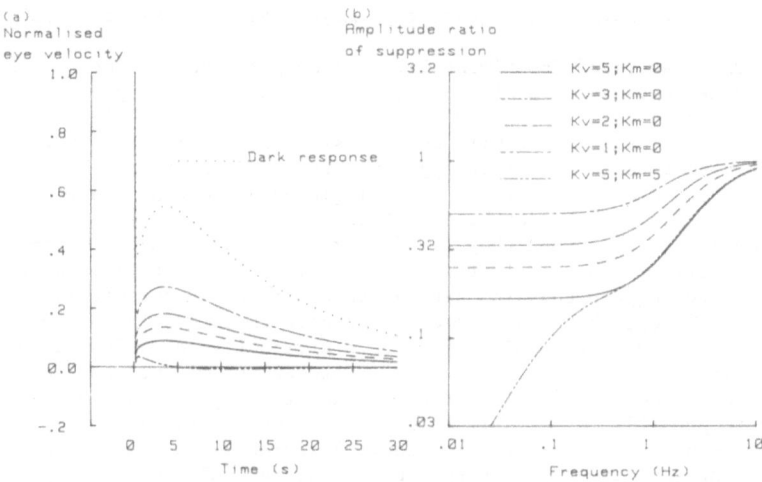

FIGURE 11. Response of the model of visual-vestibular interaction to various levels of velocity feedback gain (K_V) and positional feedback gain (K_M). (a) Ratio of post-rotational eye velocity to per-rotational head velocity. (b) Frequency response of amplitude ratio of suppression.

not appreciably lowered below that at 0.25 Hz, suggesting that positional feedback plays little part in the suppression of the slow-phase eye movement.

The second piece of evidence in favour of the predominance of velocity feedback comes from a comparison of the temporal decay of the post-rotational nystagmus shown in Fig. 5 with that of the model shown in Fig. 11(a). As stated earlier, careful examination of the vestibulo-ocular response in darkness revealed that the slow-phase eye velocity did not exhibit a simple exponential decay. During the initial period of the post-rotational response the velocity was high but dropped rapidly to 40–50% of stimulus velocity before rising again to a peak value after some 3–4s. This effect is realistically simulated by the model responses depicted in Fig. 11(a); the solid curve shows the response of the model to velocity feedback alone (Km = 0; Kv = 5), whereas the lowermost broken line indicates the effect of adding positional feedback (Km = 5; Kv = 5). It is evident that velocity feedback more accurately represents the slow-phase velocity trajectories found experimentally (Fig. 5). Positional feedback leads to a much more rapid decay of slow-phase velocity and a reversal of the direction of eye velocity, features which were not observed in the experimental records (Fig. 5).

However, before abandoning the concept of positional feedback it should be borne in mind that its primary function would be that of centering the eye. It is evident from the foregoing arguments that the positional feedback mechanism, if it exists, operates only at relatively low frequency. This precludes the possibility of its acting as a centering mechanism between fast phase beats of a prevailing nystagmus of the type which is observed during fixation suppression. Such positional information would have to be derived from overall eye position and might serve simply to steer the

nystagmic eye movements so that the image remains close to foveal
centre.

The results of Experiment III also support the concept of the
predominance of velocity feedback, since tachistoscopic presentation degrades velocity information but leaves positional information intact. This point will be discussed in more detail later.

Another feature that is apparent from the results of the
experiments described here is that single point sources can induce
a suppression of the vestibular reflex and also initiate pursuit
eye movements even when they lie far from the fovea in the peripheral retina. Thus, a further modification to the original model
must be to suggest that the pathway responsible for pursuit is not
necessarily one which only involves macular receptors, although
these may provide the only source of positionally sensitive receptors, if such exist. At this stage, without any direct proof of
positional feedback it would seem prudent to suggest that the pathways responsible for pursuit have a small positional component (Km)
which is non-zero only over the central retinal area. The velocity
component (Kv) is a decreasing function of retinal eccentricity, an
effect which is convincingly simulated by the model (Fig. 11).
Reduction of velocity gain (Kv) leads to an increase in the amplitude ratio of suppression in accord with the results of Fig. 2 and
an increase in the slow-phase eye velocity following the post-
rotational stimulus, as shown in Fig. 5. In fact, such changes in
velocity gain do not completely simulate the results of Fig. 2 for
which there appears to be a further decrease in amplitude ratio at
frequencies below 0.5 Hz for targets placed at ±5° and ±10° in the
periphery. Such an effect may be explained by the influence of
positional error feedback, but clearly, when the stimuli are in the
periphery there is little opportunity for a foveal centering
mechanism to operate. It is possible that under such circumstances
an imaginary percept of eye centre serves as a source for a rather
coarse positional error mechanism.

6.3.2. Positional influence on saccadic control. The overwhelming
feature observed in the present experiment is that there is an
alternative mechanism for foveating the image which operates by
controlling the size and frequency of the saccadic eye movements
during suppression (Fig. 4). When recordings of eye movements are
made in darkness the saccadic activity appears to be predictive of
the following slow-phase movement and the eye thus becomes biased
in the direction of head movement (Mishkin, Melvill-Jones, 1966,
Barnes, 1979). Under such circumstances the saccades are not limited by a positional threshold but, rather, appear to be governed by
a velocity threshold mechanism (Barnes, 1979,1981). On the other
hand, during suppression of vestibular nystagmus with a central
fixation point this mechanism is clearly modified to become one
which appears to be governed by a positional threshold. This
change leads to the provision of saccades that drive the eye
towards, rather than away from, orbital centre and consequently
modifies the phase relationship between eye displacement and the
stimulus waveform (Barnes, 1982a). These changes of saccadic amplitude have been accounted for in the model by an hypothesized influence of positional error on the mechanism of saccadic generation
(pathway (7), Fig. 10), although the exact mechanism has yet to be
determined.

6.3.3. The peripheral 'optokinetic' pathway. When the peripheral
retina is stimulated by a large moving visual field optokinetic

nystagmus is initiated. There is now considerable evidence to suggest that the feedback of retinal velocity error generated during an optokinetic stimulus interacts with vestibular afferent information after passing through a stage of integration. This was indicated by the experiments of Koerner,Schiller (1972), who showed that during open-loop stimulation the response to a constant velocity optokinetic stimulus was a nystagmus, having a slow-phase velocity which increased in an exponential manner to reach a peak level over a period of 20-30s. The peak velocity was greater than the stimulus velocity by a gain factor which decreased with increasing retinal velocity error. A similar study in humans (Dubois, Collewijn, 1979) showed that the gain factor had a value of approximately 10 at low velocities (<0.2°/s) but decreased below 1 at high velocities (<10°/s). These effects led to the inclusion in the original model of the dynamic characteristics shown in pathway 6 (Fig. 10). Subsequently, this pathway has been termed the 'velocity storage' pathway by Cohen et al (1977) who devised a similar dual pathway model to explain the findings relating to the persistence of optokinetic after-nystagmus. Schmid et al (1980) have also produced a similar model which, by incorporating details of the saturation effects within this apparently sub-cortical pathway, is able to explain the varying responses to optokinetic stimulation and combined vestibular and optokinetic stimulation.

In the experiments described here it is unlikely that this velocity storage pathway was activated since evidence suggests that a large structured visual field is required, rather than the point sources used here (Dubois,Collewijn, 1979). However, it is of interest to assess the likely contribution of such a pathway in the response of the suppressed vestibular reflex and to compare the results of the post-rotational stimuli shown in Fig. 5 with those obtained previously.

The frequency characteristics of the velocity storage mechanism (pathway 6) are shown in Fig. 12(b). In calculating this frequency response the non-linear saturation effects have been ignored, but their influence can be demonstrated by considering the effects of two levels of feedback gain ($Kp = 10$ and $Kp = 1$). The suppression achieved by the high feedback gain, which is appropriate only for low eye velocities (<1°/s), is negligible at frequencies above 0.1 Hz, whereas that due to the velocity feedback pathway becomes inoperative at frequencies above approximately 5 Hz. The lower value of feedback gain (Kp), which is appropriate for eye velocities up to approximately 10°/s, gives a much lower frequency range of suppression. Patients who lack a pursuit reflex response, because of the absence of the cortical velocity feedback pathway, would thus be unable to suppress vestibular nystagmus except at low frequencies and low velocities of head movement. Such patients can develop a slowly increasing response to a low-level constant velocity optokinetic stimulus but cannot suppress vestibular nystagmus at normal test frequencies of sinusoidal oscillation (Dichgans,1979). The ability of this velocity storage mechanism to suppress post-rotational vestibular nystagmus is shown in Fig.12(a) for the two levels of feedback gain. The initial decline in slow-phase velocity is much slower than that for the pursuit pathway even for the higher gain value ($Kp = 10$) and suppression is much reduced for the lower gain ($Kp = 1$). Without the pursuit pathway to bring about the rapid reduction in initial eye velocity there would be little chance of any suppression at all if the initial relative image velocity across

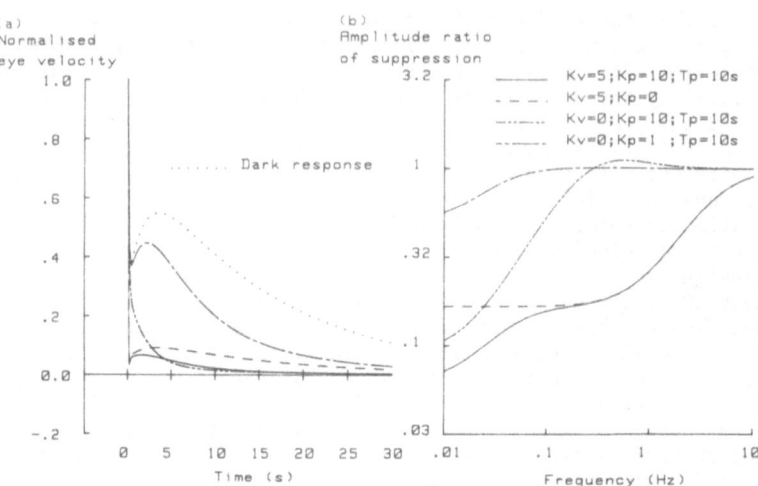

FIGURE 12. Response of the model of visual-vestibular interaction
to various combinations of velocity feedback gain (K_V) and velocity
storage feedback gain (K_p). (a) Post-rotational response.
(b) Frequency response of suppression.

the retina were greater than $10-20°$/s because the time constant of
suppression would be less than the time constant of the vestibular
response.

In the normal subject the combination of the smooth pursuit
and optokinetic pathways should have the frequency characteristics
shown by the solid line in Fig. 12(b). At low frequencies the
velocity storage pathway would contribute a further decline in the
amplitude ratio of suppression. As yet there is little evidence
from oscillation experiments to support this suggestion, but some
information can be gleaned from the expected post-rotational
responses shown in Fig. 12(a). As described earlier, the velocity
feedback pathway brings about a rapid fall in slow-phase eye velocity followed by a steady exponential decay with a time constant
similar to that of the response recorded in darkness. This model
seems to fit the responses observed in Fig. 5, but in a previous
experiment, Guedry (1968) observed a somewhat more rapid decay of
eye velocity with a time constant in the range of $3-5$s. However,
in this experiment the subject was required to read a large Snellen
chart, which is a visual stimulus much more likely to invoke the
velocity storage pathway in addition to the smooth pursuit pathway.
The solid trace in Fig. 12(a) shows the expected response of the
combined pathways. The response accords with Guedry's observations,
as it decays more quickly than that for the pursuit pathway alone.

6.4. The basis of changes in feedback gain
6.4.1. Peripheral target location.
It is a widely accepted hypo-
thesis (Grüsser, Grüsser-Cornhels, 1973) that motion detection in
the visual system is achieved by the temporal summation of the output of spatially separated retinal receptors converging upon ganglion cells. Evidence suggests that such motion sensitive ganglion
cells are less numerous and have larger receptive fields in the

peripheral retina (Hoffman, 1972, Hoffman,Schoppman, 1975, Hoffman et al, 1976, Stone,Fukuda, 1974; Fukuda,Stone, 1974); thus they will respond to a greater range of relative image velocities but with less sensitivity than those in the foveal area. It is probable that this combination of a decline in density and a decrease in sensitivity of motion-sensitive receptors in the human visual system is the basis of the decline in gain of the feedback mechanism with target eccentricity.

6.4.2 The effects of tachistoscopic presentation. In normal cir-cumstances an image passing across the retina at constant velocity would sequentially excite all retinal receptors within its path. The response of a motion sensitive ganglion cell receiving its input from spatially separated retinal receptors would be a pulse train with constant inter-pulse interval. Increasing the velocity of the image would lead to an increase in the firing rate of the ganglion cell and thus a signal proportional to image velocity would be derived. If the target were pulsed on in such a way that, in its passage across the retina, its illumination coincided with only a proportion of the total number of receptors, the firing rate of the ganglion cell would be reduced. Further increases in the inter-pulse interval would lead to further reductions of the gang-lion cell firing rate. If it is assumed that the velocity informa-tion derived from such ganglion cells forms the basis of the velo-city feedback mechanism responsible for suppression of the vesti-bular response, then strobing the target sources should lead to a decrease in the amplitude ratio of suppression. Thus, it would be expected that the suppression would become less effective as the inter-pulse interval was increased as indicated in the experimental results (Fig. 6).

6.5. Visual and non-visual mechanisms of suppression
    It is particularly noteworthy that, although there was no sub-jective impression of image blur when viewing the centre target light at the lowest frequencies (Experiment I; 0.25 Hz), the eye movement was never completely suppressed in any of the subjects. In such conditions the slow-phase eye velocity (approximately 2-3°/s) was sufficiently low that it was unlikely to cause signi-ficant blurring of the image (van Nes, 1968, King-Smith,Riggs, 1978, Barnes,Smith, 1981) and thus there was no incentive to achieve further suppression even if it were possible.
    The results of the suppression experiments described here are of interest in relation to the results of experiments by Barr et al (1976) concerning the ability of subjects to achieve high levels of suppression in darkness by imagining the presence of a head-fixed target. Firstly, when conducting the initial pilot experiment, it was found that if the subjects were not brought to a halt during the period when the visual conditions were changed there was fre-quently a carry-over effect from one condition to another. For example, if the subject was fixating a central light which was then extinguished, the gain of the response was frequently lower than would be expected. Stopping the subject, even for only a few sec-onds, was sufficient to cause this effect to disappear. Secondly, when the subject viewed the paired targets in the periphery the conceptual effort required to imagine a point midway between the peripheral light sources was minimal, and yet, as shown here, this was not sufficient for the subject to be able to achieve optimum suppression. However, the levels of velocity gain for the response

298

in darkness obtained in Experiment I were comparable to those
obtained by Barr et al (1976) for an imagined head-fixed target and
lower than their gains for the untasked response. Leaving aside any
consideration of different stimulus levels and subject populations
in these different experiments it would appear that mental set can
affect the gain of the vestibular-ocular reflex to a certain extent
but that further decreases in gain below a certain level rely on
visual feedback. The simulation studies suggest that the major part
of this suppression is provided by cortical pathways giving feedback
of the retinal velocity error: the sub-cortical 'velocity storage'
pathway probably makes but a small contribution to suppression
commensurate with its minor rôle in the genesis of the optokinetic
response.

7. REFERENCES
Abadi,R.V., Carden,D. and Simpson,J. (1981). Listening for eye movements. Ophthal. Physiol. Opt. 1: 19-27.
Barnes,G.R. (1976). Vestibulo-ocular responses to head turning movements and their functional significance during visual target acquisition. Ph.D. Thesis. Univ. of Surrey, Guildford, Surrey, U.K.
Barnes,G.R. (1979). Vestibulo-ocular function during co-ordinated
head and eye movements to acquire visual targets. J. Physiol. 287:
127-147.
Barnes,G.R. (1980). Vestibular control of oculomotor and postural
mechanisms. Clin. Phys. Physiol. Meas. 1: 3-40.
Barnes,G.R. (1981). Visual-vestibular interaction in the co-ordina-
tion of voluntary eye and head movements. In Fuchs,A.F., Becker,W.,
ed. Progress in Oculomotor Research. Developments in Neuroscience
Vol.12 p.p. 299-308. N. Holland, Elsevier.
Barnes,G.R. (1982a). The effects of retinal location on suppression
of the vestibulo-ocular reflex (In press).
Barnes,G.R. (1982b). A procedure for the analysis of nystagmus and
other eye movements. Aviat. Space Environ. Med. (In press).
Barnes,G.R., Benson,A.J. and Prior,A.R.J. (1978). Visual-vestibular
interaction in the control of eye movement. Aviat. Space Environ.
Med. 49: 557-564.
Barnes,G.R. and Smith,R. (1981). The effects on visual discrimina-
tion of image movement across the stationary retina. Aviat. Space
Environ. Med. 52: 466-472.
Barr,C.C., Schultheis,L.W. and Robinson,D.A. (1976). Voluntary, non-
visual control of the human vestibulo-ocular reflex. Acta Otolaryngol
81: 365-375.
Benson,A.J. and Barnes,G.R. (1978). Vision during angular oscilla-
tion: the dynamic interaction of visual and vestibular mechanisms.
Aviat. Space Environ. Med. 49: 340-345.
Benson,A.J. and Guedry,F.E. (1971). Comparison of tracking perform-
ance and nystagmus during sinusoidal oscillation in yaw and pitch.
Aerospace Med. 42: 593-601.
Berthoz,A., Pavard,B. and Young,L.R. (1975). Perception of linear
horizontal self-motion induced by peripheral vision (Linearvection).
Basic characteristics and visual-vestibular interactions. Exp. Brain
Res. 23: 471-489.
Buettner,U.W. and Büttner,U. (1979). Vestibular nuclei activity in
the alert monkey during suppression of vestibular and optokinetic
nystagmus. Exp. Brain Res. 37: 581-593.
Cazin,L., Precht,W. and Lannou,J. (1980). Firing characteristics of
neurons mediating optokinetic responses to rats' vestibular neurons.
Pflugers Arch. 386: 221-230.

Cohen,B., Matsuo,V. and Raphan,T. (1977). Quantitative analysis of the velocity characteristics of optokinetic nystagmus and opto- kinetic after-nystagmus. J. Physiol. 270: 321-344.

Collewijn,H. (1975). Direction-selective units in the rabbit's nucleus of the optic tract. Brain Research. 100: 489-508.

Dichgans,J. (1977). Optokinetic nystagmus as dependent on the retinal periphery via the vestibular nucleus. In Baker,R. and Berthoz,A., ed. Control of gaze by brain stem neurons. Developments in Neuroscience. Vol. 1. pp 261-267. N. Holland, Elsevier.

Dichgans,J. (1979). Visual-vestibular interaction in the control of eye movement. In Schmid,R. and Zambarbieri,D., ed. Eye movement analysis in neurological diagnosis. pp 123-155. Italian National Research Council, Univ. of Pavia, Italy.

Dichgans,J. and Brandt,T. (1972). In Dichgans,J. and Bizzi,E., ed. Cerebral control of eye movements and motion perception. pp 327-338. Basel, New York: Karger.

Dichgans,J. and Brandt,T. (1978). Visual-vestibular interaction: Effects on self-motion perception and postural control. Handbook of Sensory Physiol. Vol VIII. pp 756-804. Berlin: Springer-Verlag.

Dubois,M.F.W. and Collewijn,H. (1979). Optokinetic reactions in man elicited by localized retinal motion stimuli. Vision Res. 19: 1105-1115.

Fender,D.H. and Nye,P.W. (1961). An investigation of the mechanisms of eye movement control. Kybernetik. 1: 81-88.

Fuchs,A.F. and Kimm,J. (1975). Unit activity in vestibular nucleus of the alert monkey during horizontal angular acceleration and eye movement. J. Neurophysiol. 38: 1140-1161.

Fukuda,Y. and Stone,J. (1974). Retinal distribution and central pro- jections of Y-, X-, and W-cells of the cat's retina. J. Neuro- physiol. 37: 749-772.

Gilson,R.D., Guedry,F.E. and Benson,A.J. (1970). Influence of ves- tibular stimulation and display luminance on the performance of a compensatory tracking task. Aerospace Med. 41: 1231-1237.

Grüsser,O.J. and Grüsser-Cornhels,U. (1973). Neuronal mechanisms of visual movement perception and some psychophysical and behavioural correlations. In Jung. R. ed. Central Visual Information (A). Handbook of Sensory Physiology. Vol VII/3. pp 333-429. Berlin: Springer-Verlag.

Guedry,F.E. (1968). Relations between vestibular nystagmus and visual performance. Aerospace Med. 39: 570-579.

Henn,V., Young,L.R. and Finley,C. (1974). Vestibular nucleus units in alert monkey are also influenced by moving visual fields. Brain Res. 71: 144-149.

Hoffman,K.P. (1972). Conduction velocity in pathways from retina to superior colliculus in the cat: A correlation with receptive-field properties. J. Neurophysiol. 36: 409-424.

Hoffman,K.P., Behrend,K. and Schoppmann,A. (1976). A direct afferent visual pathway from the nucleus of the optic tract to the inferior olive in the cat. Brain Res. 115: 150-153.

Hoffman,K.P. and Schoppmann,A. (1975). Retinal input to direction selective cells in the tractus opticus of the cat. Brain Res. 99: 359-365.

Hoffman,K.P. and Schoppmann,A. (1981). A quantitative analysis of the direction-specific response of neurons in the cat's nucleus of the optic tract. Exp. Brain Res. 42: 146-157.

Honrubia,V. (1979). Optokinetic nystagmus. In Schmid,R. and Zambarbieri,D. ed. Eye movement analysis in Neurological Diagnosis. pp 71-96. Italian National Research Council, Univ. of Pavia, Italy.

Hood,J.D. (1967). Observations upon the neurological mechanism of optokinetic nystagmus with special reference to the contribution of peripheral vision. Acta Oto-laryngologica. 63: 208-215.

Keller,E.L. and Daniels,P.D. (1975). Oculomotor related interaction of vestibular and visual stimulation in vestibular nucleus cells in alert monkey. Exp. Neurol. 46: 187-198.

Keller,E.L. and Precht,W. (1979). Visual-vestibular responses in vestibular nuclear neurons in the intact and cerebellectomized alert cat. Neuroscience 4: 1699-1613.

King-Smith,P.E. and Riggs,L.A. (1978). Visual sensitivity to controlled motion of a line or edge. Vision Res. 18: 1509-1520.

Koerner,F. and Schiller,P. (1972). The optokinetic response under open and closed loop conditions in the monkey. Exp. Brain Res. 14: 318-330.

Kommerell,G. and Taumer,R. (1972). Investigations of the eye tracking system through stabilized retinal images. In Dichgans,J. and Bizzi,E. ed. Cerebral control of eye movements and motion perception. pp 288-297. Basel: Karger.

Lau,C.G.Y., Honrubia,V., Jenkins,H.A., Baloh,R.W. and Yee,R.D. (1978). Linear model for visual-vestibular interaction. Aviat. Space Environ. Med. 49: 880-885.

Maekawa,K. and Simpson,J.I. (1973). Climbing fibre responses in vestibulocerebellum of rabbit from visual system. J. Neurophysiol. 36: 649-666.

Michalski,A., Kossut,M. and Zernicki,B. (1976). The ocular following reflex elicited from the retinal periphery in the cat. Vision Res. 17: 713-736.

Mishkin,S. and Melvill Jones,G. (1966). Predominant direction of gaze during slow head rotation. Aerospace Med. 37: 897-901.

van Nes,F.L. (1968). Enhanced visibility by regular motion of retinal image. Am. J. Physiol. 81: 367-374.

Precht,W. (1981). Visual-vestibular interaction in vestibular neurons: Functional pathway organization. In Cohen,B. ed. Vestibular and Oculomotor Physiology. Ann. N.Y. Acad. Sci. Vol 374: pp 230-248.

Schmid,R., Buizza,A. and Zambarbieri,D. (1980). A non-linear model for visual-vestibular interaction during body rotation in man. Biol. Cybernetics. 36: 143-151.

Stark,L. (1971). The control system for versional eye movements. In Bach-y-Rita,P. et al. ed. The Control of Eye Movements. pp 363-428. New York: Academic Press.

Stone,J. and Fukuda,Y. (1974). Properties of cat retinal ganglion cells: A comparison of W-cells with X- and Y-cells. J. Neurophysiol. 37: 722-748.

Waespe,W. and Henn,V. (1977). Neuronal activities in the vestibular nuclei of the alert monkey during vestibular and optokinetic stimulation. Exp. Brain Res. 27: 523-538.

Waespe,W., Büttner,U. and Henn,V. (1981). Input-output activity of the primate flocculus during visual-vestibular interaction. In Cohen,B., ed. Vestibular and Oculomotor Physiology. Ann. N.Y. Acad. Sci. Vol: 374 pp 591-503.

A STOCHASTIC MODEL OF CENTRAL PROCESSING IN THE GENERATION OF FIXATION SACCADES*

R. SCHMID, G. MAGENES, D. ZAMBARBIERI (Istituto di Informatica e Sistemistica, Università di Pavia, I-27100 Pavia, Italy)

1. INTRODUCTION

Fixation saccades evoked by the presentation of external targets are the results of three distinct processes: acquisition of sensory information, central reconstruction of target position, and execution of eye movement. Most of the models of the saccadic system presented in the literature (Young, 1962; Young et al., 1968; Robinson, 1973, 1975; Jürgens et al., 1981) were mainly concerned with the execution process. They were basically aimed to the interpretation of the amplitude-duration and amplitude-peak velocity characteristics of saccades elicited by the presentation of visual targets. An appropriate reference signal was assumed to be available at the execution level. Depending on whether a retinotopic or a craniotopic (spatial) saccade organization was assumed, the reference signal was target position relative to the eyes or target position relative to the head.

The measure of target position by retinal receptors was always assumed as a deterministic variable. Under this assumption, very simple operations were needed to generate an appropriate reference signal both in the retinotopic and in the craniotopic hypothesis. The deterministic assumption on the acquisition of target position was quite acceptable for the interpretation of the basic characteristics of visual saccades. Nevertheless, the existence of multiple saccade responses with hypometric as well as hypermetric primary saccades, and the observed latency distributions of both primary and corrective visual saccades could hardly be explained by models based on that assumption. The introduction of samplers (either deterministic or stochastic), of complex nonlinear characteristics and of logic circuits represented an attempt to overcome the difficulties created by the initial assumption of a deterministic process. The need of removing this assumption became more dramatic when saccadic responses elicited by non-visual targets were considered (Zambarbieri et al., 1982). The aim of this paper is to present a model of saccade generation in

---

* Work supported by CNR, Rome, Italy.

Roucoux, A. and Crommelinck, M. (eds.): Physiological and Pathological Aspects of Eye Movements.
© *1982, Dr W. Junk Publishers, The Hague, Boston, London.* ISBN-13: 978-94-009-8002-0

which both acquisition and central reconstruction of
target position are stochastic processes. The model is
here described in functional terms and some results of
computer simulation are presented. A more formal definition of the operations that are assumed to be performed
will be reported elsewhere.

2. MODEL

Any information we receive from our sensory organs about
the external space is more or less affected by noise.
Thus, central processing in the generation of fixation
saccades can be viewed as a running estimate of target
position through a procedure (algorithm) that progressively reduces the effect of noise. For the sake of simplicity, we shall assume that acquisition is a time discrete process, i.e. the central nervous system (CNS)
receives from sensory receptors a sequence of samples.
Each sample represents the measure of target position
at a given instant. Under the assumption of a white and
gaussian noise, samples will belong to normal distributi
ons with a mean value representing the real target position. The variance of sample distributions will depend
on both the type of target considered and target position in space. The position of a visual target projecting on the macula will be detected more accurately than
that of a visual target projecting on the retinal periphe
ry. In constrast, the position of an auditory target pre
sented near the midline is acquired with a greater uncer
tainty than that of a more lateral target.
Each sensory system has a topographically organized
receptive field within CNS giving an internal representation of the external space in a specific reference fra
me (a retinotopic representation for the visual receptive field and a craniotopic representation for the audito
ry receptive field). Each sample coming from the sensory
periphery will produce on the relevant receptive field
an excitation centered around the point representing
target position as measured by that sample.
As samples come from the periphery an excitation surface
will develop on the relevant receptive field due to the
superposition of the effects produced by the individual
samples. This process is schematized in Fig. 1, where
the receptive field is represented as unidimensional.
The target is assumed to be placed at 10 deg on the
right. The first sample gives a measure of target position of 8 deg and excites a zone of the receptive field
centered around the point 8 deg right. The second sample
produces an excitation around the point 12 deg right,
and this new excitation will add to that remaining after

the first sample. After the third sample, giving a measure of target position of 7 deg, the excitation surface (in this case, the excitation curve) will present the shape shown at the bottom of Fig. 1.

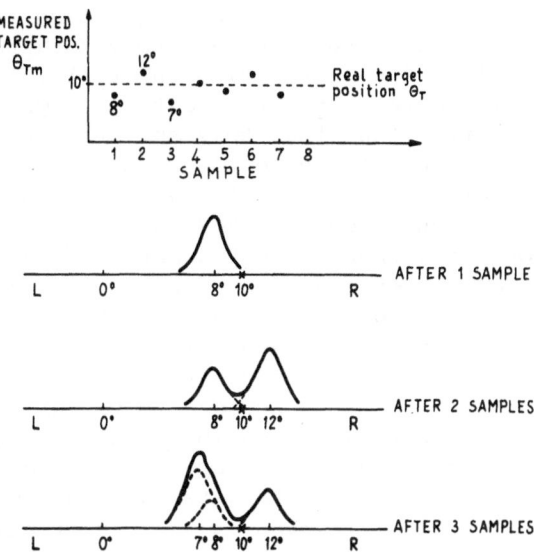

FIGURE 1. Growing of excitation on a receptive field.

At any instant of the acquisition process, the maximum of the excitation surface can be assumed to represent the central estimate of target position at that instant. This estimate will converge on the real target position. In order to avoid that an oculomotor command is generated when the estimate of target position is not yet enough accurate, it can also be assumed that the maximum of the excitation on a receptive field should reach a threshold value to produce an output to the saccade motor field. The most general hypothesis that can be made is that thresholds are different for different receptive fields, vary from point to point on the same receptive field, and can be controlled according to the degree of accuracy required to the saccadic response . The latency of saccadic responses is therefore function of the time needed to reach the threshold level, and will increase with the variance of the samples received from the periphery. The influence of the processing time on saccade latency will increase with the threshold level and, thus, with the degree of accuracy inherent to the task the sub

ject is performing(*). If some inaccuracy is tolerated,
thresholds can be maintained low, and differences in
processing time due to differences in the acquisition
noise become negligeable. In this condition the differen
ces observed in the latency of saccades evoked by different sensory stimuli will mainly reflect differences in
the detection time. This seems to be the case of monkeys
trained to fixate at visual and auditory targets with an
accuracy of only ± 5 deg (Whittington et al., 1981).
The latency of the responses to auditory targets was
found to be shorter than that to visual targets, according to the fact that the detection time of an auditory
stimulus is shorter than that of a visual stimulus
(Rupert et al., 1963; Gouras, 1967; Zambarbieri et al.,
1982). In contrast, when a great accuracy is asked to
motor responses, thresholds are maintained high. The pro
cessing time becomes dominant and the latency of motor
responses will be extremely sensitive to the level of
the acquisition noise. This seems to be the case of human subjects asked to make saccades to visual and audito
ry targets as accurately as possible. The latency of the
saccadic responses to auditory targets was found to be
greater than that to visual targets, and to decrease
with target eccentricity (Zahn et al., 1978; Zambarbieri
et al., 1982). As a matter of fact, the signal to noise
ratio is likely to be smaller in the acquisition of the
position of a sound source than in that of a light source. Moreover, according to the physiological mechanisms
of sound localization, it can also reasonably be assumed
that the signal to noise ratio in the acquisition of auditory target position increases with target eccentricity, at least up to 30-40 deg.
The variations observed by Prablanc and Jeannerod (1974)
in the latency of saccades to visual targets in relation
to light intensity can also be explained in terms of
processing time related to the signal to noise ratio in
the acquisition process.
If the receptive fields are organized in specific reference frames and the saccade motor field is organized
in head coordinates (craniotopic or spatial organization
of saccades), coordinate changes should occur somewhere

(*) This does not imply any relationship between the latency of saccades and their actual precision. Under the
assumption of a white and gaussian acquisition noise, no
correlation is expected between these two parameters.
This expectation was confirmed by the results of the
simulation experiments.

between the receptive fields and the motor field. Such changes can easely be done by using efference copy signals.

The generation of a saccadic response by the presentation of a visual target is illustrated in Figs. 2A and B. The target is presented 20 deg right with respect to subject's head. For the sake of generality, the initial eye position in the head is assumed to be different from zero. A deviation of 5 deg right is assumed (Fig. 2A). Thus, the retinal error is 15 deg, and the visual receptive field in CNS will receive samples distributed around this value. Let us assume that due to noise the threshold is exceeded in the point corresponding to the position 12 deg right. In order to obtain a reference signal in head coordinates as needed by the motor field, the output signal of the visual receptive field (12 deg) is added to an efference copy signal giving the initial eye position (5 deg). The point 17 deg will thus be excited on the motor field, and the command to the execution mechanisms will be: drive the eyes to 17 deg right in the orbit. A saccade of 12 deg to the right will be made. After the execution of this primary saccade the retinal error will be of 3 deg (Fig. 2B). A more central part of

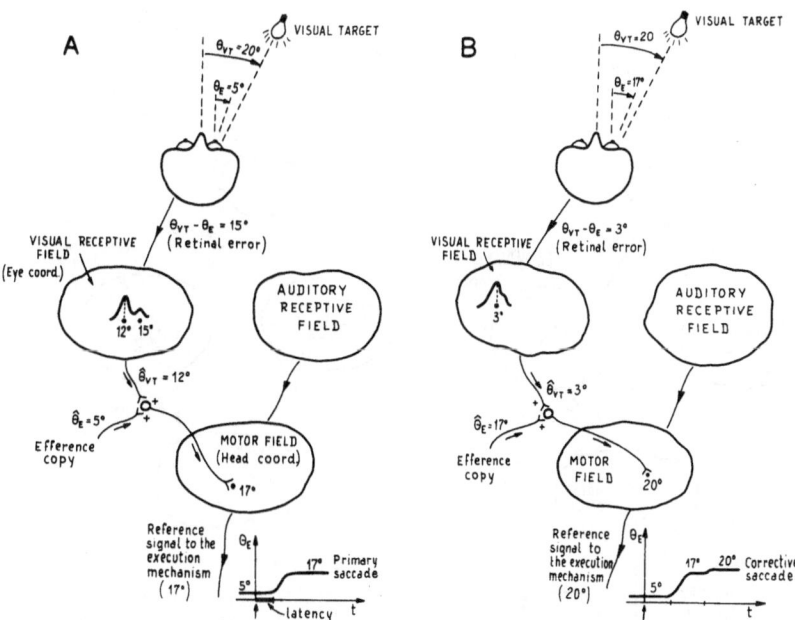

FIGURE 2. Generation of a saccadic response by the presentation of a visual target.

306

the retina is therefore involved in the acquisition
process, with an improvement of the signal to noise ratio. Thus, it is assumed that the threshold on the recep
tive field is exceeded just in the point 3 deg right.
The neural command to the motor field after addition of
the efference copy signal of eye position (17 deg) will
be 20 deg. In order to reach this position in the orbit
the eyes will make a saccade of 3 deg from 17 to 20 deg
right.
Figs. 3A and B illustrate the same process for an auditory target presented at the same position as in the
previous case (20 deg right) with the same initial position of the eyes. It is assumed that the threshold is
reached on the auditory receptive field at the point cor
responding to an estimate of target position of 15 deg
right (Fig. 3A). Since this field is organized in head
coordinates, there is no need of a coordinate change before reaching the motor field. A primary saccade driving
the eyes from 5 to 15 deg right is thus produced. Afterwards the situation is that reproduced in Fig. 3B. Since
the relevant input signal for the auditory system is
target position with respect to the head, the eye movement produced by the primary saccade does not change the

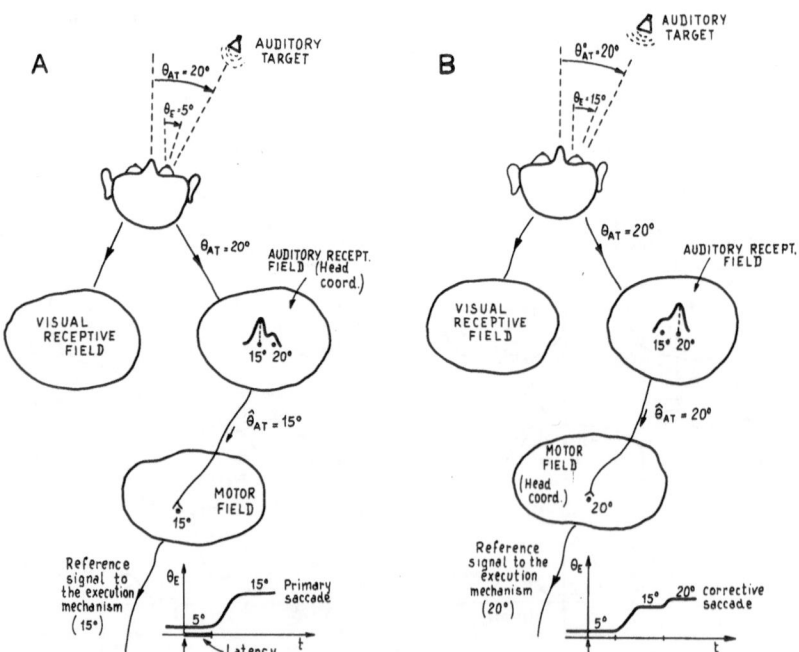

FIGURE 3. Generation of a saccadic response by the presentation of an auditory target.

zone of the auditory receptive field excited by the incoming sensory signals as it occurred for the visual
receptive field. Thus, there is no improvement of the
signal to noise ratio after the primary saccade. Nevertheless, a better estimation of target position can be
obtained since further sensory information is received
from the periphery. The probability than more than one
corrective saccade is needed to drive the eyes right on
the target is therefore greater in the auditory than in
the visual case. For the sake of simplicity, in Fig. 3B
only one corrective saccade has been assumed to occur.

3. SIMULATION RESULTS

The model described in the previous section was implemen
ted on a digital computer to simulate central processing
in the generation of saccadic responses following the
presentation of auditory targets.
The following hypotheses about the statistical characteristics of the input signal, the excitation process on
the central receptive field and the threshold values on
the same field were made.

i) Input samples belong to normal distributions with
a mean value corresponding to the real target position. The variance of these distributions decreases with target eccentricity (auditory case).

ii) Each input sample produces a bell shaped excitation on the receptive field. The volume under each
bell is the same for all points of the field, but
the broadness of the excitation increases with the
distance from the center of the field.

iii) There is a spatial and temporal superposition of
the effects produced by successive samples. The
effect produced by each sample decays linearly
with time.

iv) The threshold decreases almost exponentially with
the distance from the center of the receptive
field.

Model predictions were compared to the experimental results obtained in a previous study (Zambarbieri et al.,
1982). A general agreement was found as shown in Fig. 4,
where experimental and theoretical values for response
latency, percentage of single saccade responses and
overall response accuracy are plotted versus target
position.

308

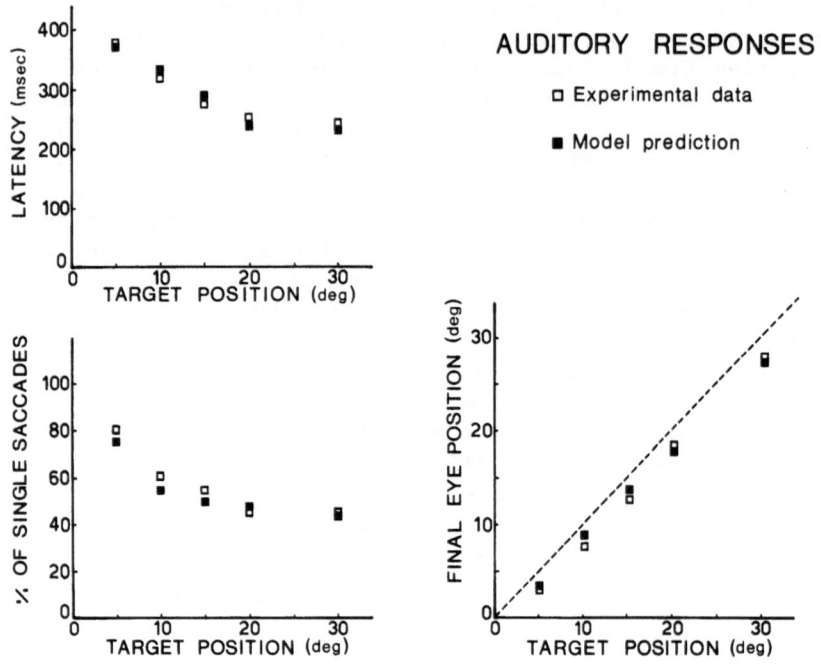

FIGURE 4. Results of simulation experiments.

4. CONCLUSIONS

A stochastic model for central processing in the generation of fixation saccades to visual and non-visual
targets has been presented. The assumption of a discrete
acquisition process was introduced only to simplify the
description of the model, but it was unessential to the
theory on which the model is based. Central processing
of sensory information is considered as a running estimate of the real target position through a procedure
which progressively reduces the effect of the noise super
posed on signals coming from the sensory periphery. Although the formal description of this procedure may appear rather complex, its implementation by neural circuits is quite simple and corresponds to classical principles of sensorimotor physiology.
The model is congruent with some experimental results
obtained by recording the neural activity in the superior
colliculus (SC) during saccadic eye movements or by recording the eye movements produced by SC stimulation
(Robinson, 1972; Schiller, Stryker, 1972; Roucoux,
Crommelink, 1976; Sparks, Mays, 1982).
Figs. 5 and 6 show the saccadic responses predicted by
the model for a short (Fig. 5) and a prolonged (Fig. 6)

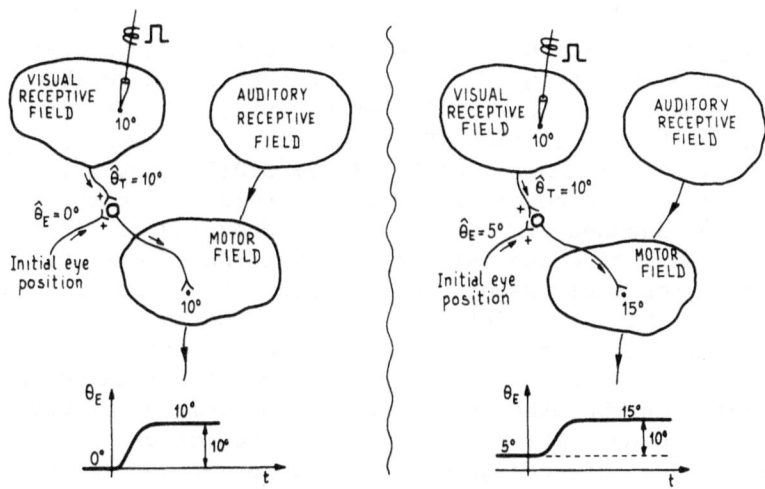

FIGURE 5. Saccadic responses evoked by a short stimulation of the visual receptive field.

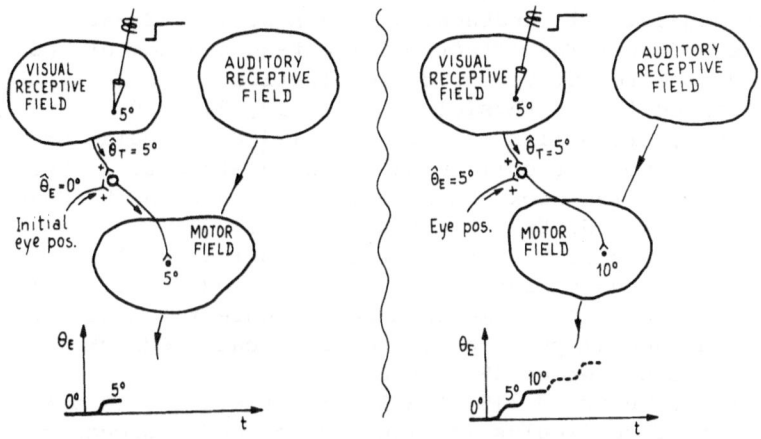

FIGURE 6. Saccadic response evoked by a prolonged stimulation of the visual receptive field.

stimulation of the visual receptive field. A short stimulation will produce a single saccade whose amplitude depends on the point of the receptive field being stimulated and not on either the intensity of stimulation beyond a given threshold and the initial eye position. A prolonged stimulation will evoke a staircase response made of saccades of the same amplitude. Similar responses were actually observed after short and prolonged SC stimulations (Robinson, 1972; Schiller, Stryker, 1972;

Guitton et al., 1980).
The superior colliculus is certainly one of the neural
structures supporting the central processing described
in this paper. Since visually evoked saccades are not
abolished by SC ablation (Pasik et al., 1966; Wurtz,
Goldberg, 1972; Mohler, Wurtz, 1977; Schiller et al.,
1980) the existence of parallel or alternative pathways
should be assumed at least for the processing of visual
information. Also the existence of internal loops that
are used for rapid saccade corrections (Prablanc, Jeanne
rod, 1975; Becker, 1976) and that of a short term memory
keeping the information on the position of targets presented for a little while (Sparks, Mays, 1982) cannot be
excluded. On the other hand, the aim of this paper was
to indicate only the main characteristics of central
processing in saccade generation and to stress the in-
trinsic stochastic nature of it.

REFERENCES
Becker W (1976) Do correction saccades depend exclusive-
    ly on retinal feedback? A note on the possible role
    of non-retinal feedback. Vision Res. 16, 425-427.
Gouras P (1967) The effects of light-adaptation of rod
    and cone receptive field organization of monkey gan-
    glion cells. J. Physiol. (Lon.) 192, 747-760.
Guitton D, Crommelink M, Roucoux A (1980) Stimulation
    of the superior colliculus in the alert cat. I. Eye
    movements and neck EMG activity evoked when the head
    is restrained. Exp. Brain Res. 39, 63-73.
Jürgens R, Becker W, Kornhuber HH (1981) Natural and
    drug-induced variations of velocity and duration of
    human saccadic eye movements: evidence for a control
    of the neural pulse generator by local feedback.
    Biol. Cybernetics 39, 87-96.
Mohler CW, Wurtz RH (1977) Role of striate cortex and
    superior colliculus in visual guidance of saccadic
    eye movements in monkeys. J. Neurophysiol. 40, 74-94.
Pasik T, Pasik P, Bender MB (1966) The superior colliculi
    and eye movements. Arch. Neurol. 15, 420-436.
Prablanc C, Jeannerod M (1974) Latence et précision des
    saccades en fonction de l'intensité, de la durée et de
    la position rétinienne d'un stimulus. Societé EEG et
    Neurophys. Clinique de Langue Française, 484-488.
Prablanc C, Jeannerod M (1975) Corrective saccades:
    dependence on retinal reafferent signals. Vision
    Res. 15, 465-469.
Robinson DA (1972) Eye movements evoked by collicular
    stimulation in the alert monkey. Vision Res. 12,
    1795-1808.

Robinson DA (1973) Models of the saccadic eye movement control system. Kybernetik 14, 71-83.

Robinson DA (1975) Oculomotor control signals. In Lennerstrand G, Bach-y-Rita P, eds. Basic Mechanisms of Ocular Motility and their Clinical Implications, pp. 337-374, Pergamon Press, Oxford.

Roucoux A, Crommelink M (1976) Eye movements evoked by superior colliculus stimulation in the alert cat. Brain Res. 106, 349-363.

Rupert A, Moushegian G, Galambos R (1963) Unit responses to sound from the auditory nerve of the cat. J. Neurophysiol. 26, 449-456.

Schiller PH, Stryker M (1972) Single-unit recording and stimulation in superior colliculus of the alert rhesus monkey. J. Neurophysiol. 35, 915-924.

Schiller PH, True SD, Conway JL (1980) Deficits in eye movements following frontal eye field and superior colliculus ablations. J. Neurophysiol. 44, 1175-1189.

Sparks DL, Mays LE (1982) The role of the monkey superior colliculus in the spatial localization of saccade targets. In Hein A, Jeannerod M, eds. Spatially Oriented Behavior, Springer, New York, in press.

Whittington DA, Hepp-Reymond MC, Flood W (1981) Eye and head movements to auditory targets. Exp. Brain Res. 41, 358-363.

Wurtz RH, Goldberg ME (1972) Activity of the superior colliculus in behaving monkey. IV. Effects of lesions on eye movement. J. Neurophysiol. 35, 587-596.

Young LR (1962) A Sampled Data Model for Eye Tracking Movement. Sc. D. Thesis. Cambridge, Mass: M.I.T.

Young LR, Forster JD, Van Houtte N (1968) A revised stochastic sampled data model for eye tracking movements. Fourth Annual NASA-University Conference on Manual Control, Un. of Michigan, Ann Arbor, Mich.

Zahn JR, Abel LA, Dell'Osso LF (1978) The audio-ocular response characteristics. Sensory Processes 2, 32-37.

Zambarbieri D, Schmid R, Magenes G, Prablanc C (1982) Saccadic responses evoked by presentation of visual and auditory targets. To be published.

RESPONSES OF THE SACCADIC SYSTEM TO SUDDEN CHANGES IN TARGET DIRECTION

J.A.M. VAN GISBERGEN, F.P. OTTES and J.J. EGGERMONT

Laboratory of Medical Physics and Biophysics
University of Nijmegen
6525 EZ Nijmegen, The Netherlands

1. INTRODUCTION

Little is known on how the brain derives a motor-command signal for initiating and directing a saccade from the visual information on the retina. Often two subsystems are distinguished. One system, called the WHERE system in this study, determines the metrics of saccades. Another system, denoted here as the WHEN system, initiates the saccade. An interesting property of the WHERE system was discovered by Becker and Jürgens (1979). They showed that saccades are directed at a delayed and filtered (or time-averaged) version of the stimulus trajectory. Several groups have observed rapid eye movements which abruptly changed course when the stimulus reversed direction. These responses have been interpreted as the sum of two separate saccades (Becker and Jürgens, 1979) or as a single saccade modified in midflight (Robinson, 1975). Recently Georgopoulos et al. (1981) found that hand-movement trajectories were curved while saccade trajectories were straight when monkeys tracked a stimulus which suddenly changed direction. Using essentially the same type of stimulus we did find curved saccade trajectories. Saccades to single step stimuli had approximately straight trajectories. These results are discussed in terms of a two-dimensional version of Robinson's model.

2. METHODS

Two rhesus monkeys were trained, for apple juice reward, to track a spot of light moving on a screen at 57 cm. Eye movements were measured with a magnetic field method. In one monkey (10) a thin ring surgically implanted beneath the conjunctiva induced a secondary magnetic field which was picked up with a coil rigidly mounted on the monkey's crown. The signal from this coil was fed into two phase-sensitive amplifiers which were tuned to the frequencies of the two primary magnetic fields (30 and 40 kHz). Their output signals were directly related to horizontal and vertical eye position in a range of $\pm$ 35 deg in all directions. This method will be described more fully elsewhere (Reulen, 1982). A static nonlinearity inherent in this method was corrected. In monkey 11 we used the system described by Fuchs and Robinson (1966). The system including low-pass filtering had a band-width of 0-200 Hz (-3 dB). The eye movement signals were sampled at at least 500 Hz in each channel. Sensitivity in both methods was 0.25 deg, or better, up to 25 deg. In the double-step experiments the spot (2.2 deg; 1.2 cd/m^2) was first presented for a variable period 20 deg to the left. It then either jumped 45 deg in the ϕ_1 = -30 deg direction followed by a vertical jump at ϕ_2 = +30 deg or vice versa. These trials (which occurred 1-3 times each in a set of 40 trials) were mixed with single steps in all directions.

3. RESULTS

Curved saccade trajectories were observed under certain conditions, e.g. for ϕ_1 - ϕ_2 = 30 deg or 60 deg at 45 deg eccentricity. The

Roucoux, A. and Crommelinck, M. (eds.): Physiological and Pathological Aspects of Eye Movements.
© *1982, Dr W. Junk Publishers, The Hague, Boston, London.* ISBN-13: 978-94-009-8002-0

phenomenon was observed more seldomly for smaller saccade sizes. As a control, we checked the trajectories of saccades to single-step stimuli in various directions. These trajectories were approximately straight in both monkeys (see Fig. 1A). In the double-step experiments the amount of saccade curvature depended on response latency as well as interstep time τ. For a given value of τ, the rapid eye movement elicited by the stimulus led the eye in one continuous movement to a position near the path of the second step depending on latency. Longer-latency responses resulted in final eye positions closer to ϕ_2. Considerable scatter in final eye position was still observed for responses with about the same latency, especially when τ was short (52 msec). The relation between the effect of the second stimulus on final vertical eye position and the time lapse between its occurrence and the onset of the eye movement was approximately linear. The correlation coefficient was 0.75 (N = 43). The effect of the second step was first visible in saccades which started 40 msec later and reached its final magnitude (i.e., final eye position was near ϕ_2) in eye movements which began 130 msec after the stimulus changed direction. When offset latency was taken as the independent variable the correlation coefficient was 0.79. The first effect of the second step could be noticed in eye movements ending 105 msec after its occurrence but was not complete until 100 msec later (offset latency 205 msec after the second step).

Typical trajectories of monkey 10 to a stimulus jumping first to $\phi_1 = -30$ deg and subsequently to $\phi_2 = 30$ deg are shown in Fig. 1 (left hand column) for various τ values. The second monkey showed the same general trend but was less extensively tested. A good impression about the onset of the curvature was obtained by computing the instantaneous direction, θ, of the trajectory ($\theta = \operatorname{arctg} \dot{E}_v/\dot{E}_h$) as a function of time. The arrows in the θ profiles (Fig. 1, righthand column) indicate when θ started deviating from the profile observed in ϕ_1 single steps. The point in time when this happened depended on τ. When τ was 92 msec, the eye movement was initially directed at ϕ_1 and about 100 msec after the target changed direction curved toward ϕ_2 until the eye stopped. When τ was smaller the direction change was again first visible about 100 msec after the target jumped to ϕ_2. As latency in the examples shown remained typically near 140 msec, the point of first direction change shifted toward saccade onset. When τ was 52 msec the saccade showed the influence of the second target step already at its start. With this stimulus, we sometimes observed responses which seemed to oscillate between ϕ_1 and ϕ_2 (Fig. 1D). This phenomenon was not observed with other stimuli.

To further characterize the dynamics of the eye movements we also computed the velocity of the eye along its path (Fig. 1, middle column). When compared to the velocity profiles of single step saccades to ϕ_1, it appeared that when the eye made a large turn it first slowed down and accelerated again immediately after it changed direction. The "slow-down" effect could be seen as early as 90-100 msec after the second target step especially when τ was 52 msec. Since the second target step was purely vertical, the possibility that the horizontal component was not modified by the second step should be considered. When τ was 92 or 72 msec, horizontal eye velocity often dropped less rapidly in the late phase of the movement than during single step responses to $\phi = -30^\circ$. When τ was 52 msec, the horizontal component sometimes had a lower peak velocity and became prolonged in time, which means that, at

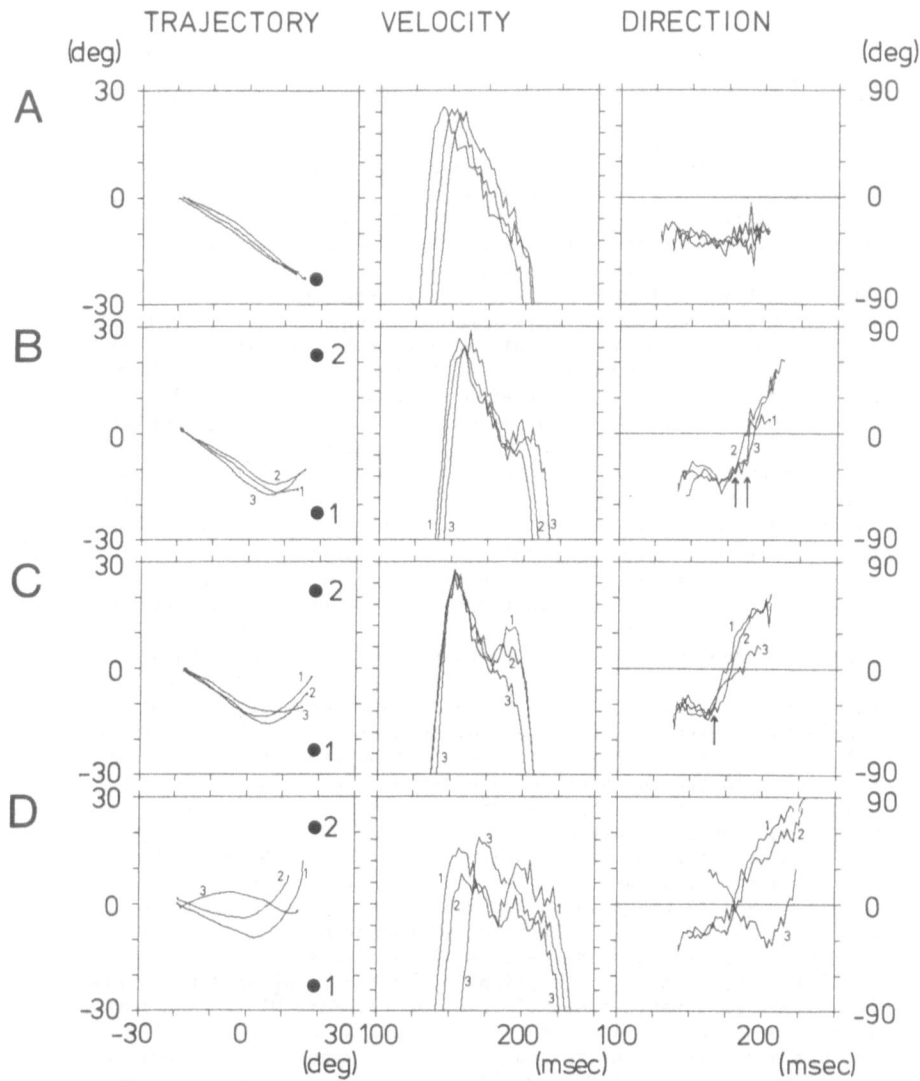

FIGURE 1. Eye movements to single steps (A) and double steps with interstep times of 92 msec (B), 72 msec (C) and 52 msec (D). Left-hand column: trajectories in H-V plane. Small numbers in B, C and D allow identification in columns on the right. Middle column: velocity of the eye along its path. Vertical scale: 0-1000 deg/sec. Horizontal scale: time since first step. Righthand column: instant-aneous direction in eye movements (drawn when velocity exceeded 150 deg/sec). Arrows indicate when the eye started deviating from its initial course (B and C). Horizontal axis as in middle column.

least in these cases, the second step did influence the horizontal component.

3. DISCUSSION

Should the responses in Fig. 1 be interpreted as single saccades whose course changed in midflight or as the sum of two separate saccades elicited by the two stimulus steps? The correction move-ment was clearly rapid. The two-saccade hypothesis does not explain why the mean latency of the eye movement was about 40 msec longer than the delay of the second-step effect. On the other hand, the distinct late acceleration in many curved eye movements seems nicely compatible with this hypothesis.

An alternative is that the curved eye movements we have observed should be regarded as a single saccade which is under continuous guidance of incoming visual information (Robinson, 1975). To test this idea, simulations must be made to see if the model can mimic the monkey data. It is not straightforward how this should be done since Robinson's model is one dimensional and it is not immediately clear how the extension to a two-dimensional model should proceed. One problem encountered in this effort is that signals in visuo-motor areas such as the superior colliculus and the frontal eye fields are spatially encoded whereas at the premotor level signals are temporally encoded and organized in horizontal and vertical subsystems. Therefore, as has been recognized before, somewhere a translation from spatially to temporally encoded information must occur.

A further problem which must be dealt with is that horizontal and vertical components of saccades are not generated independently. Although the precise nature and the amount of the cross-coupling remain to be established, data from Evinger et al. (1981) and our-selves indicate that the time courses of horizontal and vertical components in oblique saccades are synchronized. In our first simulation attempts with a two-dimensional version of Robinson's model, we have assumed simply that the nonlinear relationship be-tween motor error and eye velocity, initially proposed for hori-zontal saccades, is valid in all directions. In this tentative scheme (Fig. 2A) the signals desired eye position (T'), actual eye position (E') and their difference (motor error, M') are spatially encoded and represented as vectors (heavy lines). The transformation of $\vec{M'}$ into horizontal and vertical eye velocity signals takes place in system STT (spatio-temporal translator). Here $\vec{M'}$ is transformed into a new vector ($\dot{\vec{E}}'$) which points in the same direction (Fig. 2B) and has a magnitude related to motor error magnitude as specified by the nonlinearity in Fig. 2C. The signals $\dot{E}'_h$ and $\dot{E}'_v$ are the orthogonal components of the eye velocity vector and thought to be embodied by horizontal and vertical medium lead burst cells. Thus, the eye is driven to the target until the efference copy signal $\vec{E}'$ and T' match. Quasi-visual cells in the superior colliculus have been proposed as candidates for coding motor error (Mays and Sparks, 1980). Since eye-movement induced changes in motor error are represented in the activity of these cells even when there is no retinal-error signal available, it has been suggested that they receive a motor signal. Our scheme suggests that this motor signal and the internal feedback signal proposed to account for the beha-viour of medium lead burst cells (van Gisbergen et al., 1981) is the same (cf. Keller. 1981).

The system STT is switched on and off by a system (WHEN) which de-termines when $\vec{M'}$ gets access to STT and starts moving the eye. The

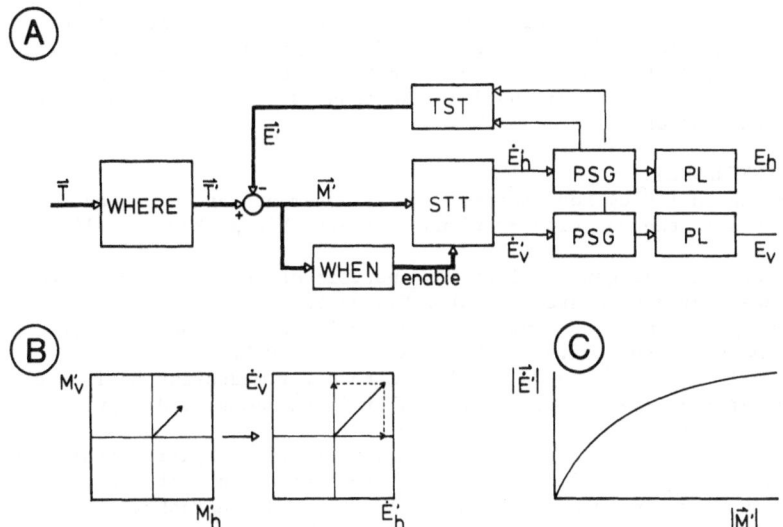

FIGURE 2. Two-dimensional version of Robinson's internal feedback model. For explanation see text. Abbreviations: $\vec{T}$ = target position; $\vec{T}'$ = neural representation of $\vec{T}$; $\vec{E}'$ = neural eye position signal; $\vec{M}'$ = motor error; $\dot{E}'_h$ = horizontal eye velocity command; E_h = horizontal eye position (vertical signals have subscript v); STT = spatio-temporal translator; TST = temporal to spatial translator (see discussion in Keller, 1981); PSG = pulse-step generator; PL = plant. All signals except input and outputs are neural.

system is switched off again when the magnitude of $\vec{M}'$ has fallen below a certain level. Note that because of the properties of STT and the presence of a single initiation system the model produces straight saccades to single step targets in all directions. The WHERE system in the scheme transforms target position into an internal signal representing desired eye position (Robinson, 1975). To account for our finding that a sudden change in required saccade direction resulted in direction adjustments, which started after about 100 msec and gradually reached their final values, we propose that this system consists of a pure time delay and a low-pass filter. This filter may represent the averaging property of the saccadic system (Becker and Jürgens, 1979).
We have convinced ourselves that when the nonlinearity in STT is the same as in an earlier study attempting to simulate monkey saccades (van Gisbergen et al., 1981) the model can at least produce curved saccade trajectories. An important question in further simulations is whether it will be possible to explain both the relation between saccade latency and final eye position and the curved trajectories with a fixed set of parameters for the WHERE system. Since a typical value for latency in our experiments was 140 msec, the value of 100 msec for the WHERE delay would mean that it takes about 40 msec after the first sign that an eye movement is needed, before the WHEN system initiates the saccade. This would explain why more time is needed for a stimulus to initiate a saccade than to modify an ongoing movement (cf. Barmack, 1970).

318

5. ACKNOWLEDGEMENT
This research was supported by the Netherlands Organization for
the Advancement of Pure Research (ZWO). We thank N. van den Berg,
J. Braks, J. Bruijns, J. Daanen and D. Stegeman for their help
and for stimulating discussions. We thank D.A. Robinson for helpful suggestions.

6. REFERENCES
Barmack NH (1970) Modification of eye movements by instantaneous
changes in the velocity of visual targets. Vision Res. 10, 1431-
1441.
Becker W and Jürgens J (1979) An analysis of the saccadic system
by means of double step stimuli. Vision Res. 19, 967-983.
Evinger C, Kaneko CRS and Fuchs AF (1981) Oblique saccadic eye
movements of the cat. Exp. Brain Res. 41, 370-379.
Fuchs AF and Robinson DA (1966) A method for measuring horizontal
and vertical eye movement chronically in the monkey. J. Appl.
Physiol. 21, 1068-1070.
Georgopoulos AP, Kalaska JF and Massey JT (1981) Spatial trajecto-
ries and reaction times of aimed movements: effects of practice,
uncertainty, and change in target location. J. Neurophysiol. 46,
725-743.
Gisbergen JAM van, Robinson DA and Gielen S (1981) A quantitative
analysis of generation of saccadic eye movements by burst neurons.
J. Neurophysiol. 45, 417-442.
Keller EL (1981) Brain stem mechanisms in saccadic control. In
Progress in oculomotor research, eds. Fuchs AF and Becker W,
pp 57-62. Elsevier North Holland, New York.
Mays LE and Sparks DL (1980) Dissociation of visual and saccade-
related responses in superior colliculus neurons. J. Neurophysiol.
43, 207-232.
Reulen JPH (1982) The measurement of eye movement using double
magnetic induction. IEEE Trans. Biomed. Eng. (accepted for publication).
Robinson DA (1975) Oculomotor control signals. In Basic Mechanisms
of ocular motility and their clinical implications, ed. Lennerstrand G and Bach-y-Rita P, pp 337-374. Pergamon Press, Oxford.

SPATIO-TEMPORAL RECODING IN THE GENERATION OF RAPID EYE MOVEMENTS

K. HEPP, V. HENN

(Physics Dept, E.T.H., and Neurology Dept, University, Zürich,
Switzerland)

One of the interesting problems of oculomotor organization is to understand
how a visual signal, coded in retinotopic coordinates, like in the superior
colliculi, is transformed into a temporal signal to drive the medium lead
burst neurons and in turn the motoneurons. Many medium lead bursters
(M-bursters) in the PPRF or rostral mesencephalon (Büttner et al., 1977)
display a one-to-one correspondence between their firing rate and vector
parameters of rapid eye movements. They therefore can be considered the
final common pathway for all rapid eye movements. Concerning the input
which drives the M-bursters, there are two opposing theories. In the
position feedback model by Robinson (1975) the difference between a
desired eye position signal and a neuronal copy of present eye position,
both in head coordinates, drives the M-bursters and hence the eyes to the
target. Such a model lends itself to computer simulation (van Gisbergen et
al., 1981) and predicts the observed fact that in visually evoked saccades
the desired eye position is reached even after violent perturbations (Mays,
Sparks, 1981). One problem of this model is that neurons coding desired
eye position with the required precision have not been found; another
difficulty is that it cannot easily be generalized for oblique saccades.
The second model (see e.g. Keller, 1981) postulates that the neuronal input
to the M-bursters is by an eye displacement signal independent of eye
position in the head. One possible input channel in the superior colliculus
could be the saccade-vector related long-lead bursters (V-bursters) in
the intermediate layer. Such V-bursters can also be found in the rostral
PPRF. The recoding from the spatial map of V-bursters to the temporally
coded M-bursters in the PPRF and rostral iMLF could involve directed
long-lead bursters (L-bursters), which have already been described in the
PPRF (Luschei, Fuchs, 1972; Keller, 1974; Henn, Cohen, 1976). Since the
quantitative coding properties of L-bursters have not been determined,
this recoding scheme has never been mathematically modeled.
First we shall briefly describe the result of a systematic study of
L-bursters in the PPRF and their coding and abundance relative to V- and
M-bursters. These results will shed some light on the structure of a model
for rapid eye movements in all directions using the V-burster input. We
shall present a model based only on neuron populations which have actually
been recorded.
V-bursters can be clearly identified by their coding properties, usually
by their movement field around an optimal saccadic vector with weaker
burst for all smaller and larger saccades. If the movement field extends
to the periphery, the neuron is only active within a narrow angular range
of less than a quadrant. Most of the V-bursters in the rostral PPRF are
conditionally saccadic: Strong bursts always correspond to saccades into
the center of the movement field. Weak bursts usually occur for movements

Roucoux, A. and Crommelinck, M. (eds.): Physiological and Pathological Aspects of Eye Movements.
© *1982, Dr W. Junk Publishers, The Hague, Boston, London.* ISBN-13: 978-94-009-8002-0

into the periphery of the movement field but can also correspond to saccades
into the center field (see Fig. 1). We have defined burst onset $t(1/3)$ as the
time the frequency in the on-direction reaches 1/3 of the maximal frequency
relative to the onset of the saccade. Rise time $r = t(2/3) - t(1/3)$. All
V-bursters are "long lead" in the sense that $t(1/3) \leq - 12$ ms and $r \geq 4$ ms.

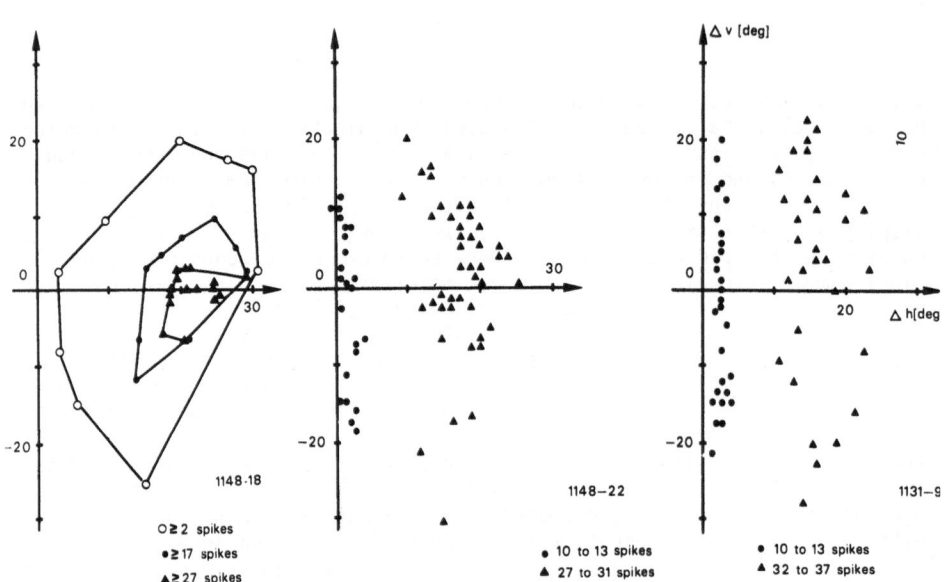

FIGURE 1. Isoburst "curves" for a V-burster (left), L-burster (middle) and
M-burster (right) in the PPRF. For the V-burster the triangles represent
all bursts, where the number of spikes is maximal, the dark dots denote
the convex hull of all above half-maximal burst events and the light dots
the just visible burst-events. Maximal bursts correspond to saccadic
vectors in a narrow movement field, but the converse is not true. The two
isoburst curves of the L- and M-burster with on-direction to the right are
well separated and qualitatively similar, although the on-latencies and
rise times of these units are very different ($t(1/3) = - 14$ ms, $r = 4$ ms
for L; $t(1/3) = - 5$ ms, $r = 1$ ms for M). For these directed burst neurons
there is an almost one-to-one relation between the number of spikes in the
burst and horizontal eye displacement Δh for all saccades with $\Delta h \geq 0$.

All other burst neurons are <u>directed</u>, i.e. the number N of spikes in the
burst increases monotonically with the size of the vector component in
a horizontal or vertical direction. Directed bursters can have short or
long on-latencies and rise times. However, there is no unique separation
by that criterium. Medium lead bursters <u>(M-bursters)</u> have latencies $t(1/3)$
shorter than -12 ms. The maximal frequency of the burst is often at its
very beginning, and they have a steep rise time, $r \leq 3$ ms. Long lead

bursters (L-bursters) have latencies t(1/3) ≤ - 12 ms; r increases
linearly with t(1/3) and there is significant early activity, which
varies with the behavioral state of the animal.
From the PPRF of 3 Rhesus monkeys we have quantitatively analyzed 157
saccade-related burst neurons with a maximal frequency ≥ 600 Hz. Our
sample comprises 16 L-bursters (all with an ipsilateral horizontal
on-direction) 45 horizontal M-bursters (and 12 with an additional weak
eye position signal), 17 vertical M-bursters (and 11 with an additional
weak eye position signal), and 56 V-bursters mainly in the rostral PPRF.
In a qualitative manner the firing patterns of L- and M-bursters are
similar. Some L-bursters encode the components of saccades with a gain
and precision comparable to the M-bursters (see Fig. 1). Some L-bursters
fire maximally with movements into one half-field and have little or no
activity with movements into the opposite direction. They could serve a
trigger function for all movements in one half-field. The fluctuations
in the encoding of saccadic parameters are greater in the L-bursters
than in the M-bursters.

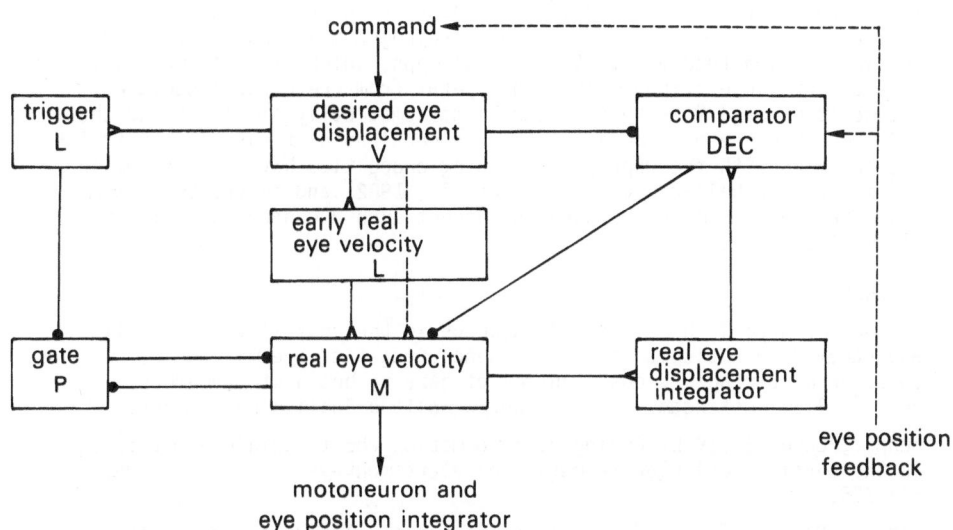

FIGURE 2. Flow diagram for the spatio-temporal recoding from V- to
M-bursters. A main pathway from V to M is qualitatively consistent with
the firing patterns of both neuron populations, since the average high
frequency burst duration is identical for spontaneous saccades into the
movement field. However, maximal V-burst events (in our experimental set
up interpreted as visually evoked saccades) last longer than in M-bursters,
in particular for small saccades, and this requires the deceleration
network using local feedback. The PPRF pausers and L-bursters with trigger
coding form the coordinating network for horizontal and vertical saccades.

Our results are compatible with the model of Fig. 2. For spontaneous eye
movements V-burster activity in the rostral PPRF (in addition similar
activity in the superior colliculus and other places) represent the
desired eye displacement input, which by graded synaptic strength is
transmitted into M-bursters populations which in turn project directly
and indirectly to the motoneurons of the six eye muscle pairs. They also
activate trigger L-bursters which inhibit the pause neurons. The latter
form an inhibitory gate for the M-bursters and filter out the early rising
and the post-saccadic activity of the V- and L-bursters. The average high
frequency discharge of the V-bursters keeps the M-bursters firing and (via
inhibitory M-bursters) the P-neurons silent.
To execute eye movements with high precision the V-bursters can activate a
local feedback circuit: The M-bursters give in good approximation a real
eye displacement signal via a leaky integrator to a family of deceleration
burst neurons (DEC). They are kept silent due to the appropriate V-input
until real eye displacement reaches desired eye displacement. Then they
shield the M-bursters from further V-input. Such a model has already been
proposed by Jürgens et al. (1981). It can explain a limited amount of
feedback which can cope with inflight deceleration of saccades (i.e. by
pause stimulation, Keller, 1974; King, 1977), the generation of stair-case
saccades by continuous V-stimulation (Robinson, 1972; Schiller, Stryker,
1972), and, more physiologically, the occurrence of a refractory period
for rapid eye movements. More dramatic reprogramming can be effected by
an eye position feedback to the central maps, which also can modify the
DEC-bursters in distinguishing centripetal from centrifugal saccades.
The merit of Fig. 2 is that it can be mathematically simulated and that
all "boxes" correspond to identified neuronal populations. In particular,
DEC-bursters with the appropriate coding properties have been found in
the medial cerebellar nuclei (Hepp et al., 1982) and in the brain stem.
Localized lesions might be used to connect such a control circuit to
clinical syndroms.

REFERENCES

Büttner U, Hepp K, Henn V (1977) Neurons in the rostral mesencephalic
and paramedian reticular formation generating fast eye movements.
In Baker R, Berthoz A, eds. Control of gaze by brain stem neurons,
pp. 309-318. Amsterdam, Elsevier/North-Holland Publishing Company.

Henn V, Cohen B (1976) Coding of information about rapid eye movements
in the pontine reticular formation of alert monkeys. Brain Res. 108,
307-325.

Hepp K, Henn V, Jaeger J (1982) Eye movement related neurons in the
cerebellar nuclei of the alert monkey. Exp. Brain Res. 45, 253-261.

Jürgens R, Becker W, Kornhuber HH (1981) Natural and drug-induced
variations of velocity and duration of human saccadic eye movements:
evidence for a control of the neural pulse generator by local feedback.
Biol. Cybern. 39, 87-96.

Keller EL (1974) Participation of medial pontine reticular formation
in eye movement generation in monkey. J. Neurophysiol. 37, 316-332.

Keller EL (1981) Brain stem mechanisms in saccadic control. In Fuchs AL,
Becker W, eds. Progress in oculomotor research, pp. 57-62. Amsterdam,
Elsevier/North Holland Publishing Company.

King WM, Fuchs AF (1977) Neuronal activity in the mesencephalon related to vertical eye movements. In Baker R, Berthoz A, eds. Control of gaze by brain stem neurons, pp. 319-326. Amsterdam, Elsevier/North Holland Publishing Company.

Luschei ES, Fuchs AF (1972) Activity of brain stem neurons during eye movements of alert monkeys. J. Neurophysiol. 35, 445-461.

Mays LE, Sparks DL (1980) Saccades are spatially, not retinocentrically coded. Science 208, 1163-1165.

Robinson DA (1972) Eye movements evoked by collicular stimulation in the alert monkey. Vision Res. 12, 1795-1808.

Robinson DA (1975) Oculomotor control signals. In Lennerstrand G, Bach-y-Rita P, eds. Basic mechanisms of ocular motility and their clinical implications, pp. 337-374. Oxford, Pergamon Press.

Schiller PH, Stryker MP (1972) Single-unit recording and stimulation in superior colliculus of the alert Rhesus monkey. J. Neurophysiol. 35, 915-924.

Van Gisbergen JAM, Robinson DA, Gielen S (1981) A quantitative analysis of saccadic eye movements by burst neurons. J. Neurophysiol. 45, 417-442.

HORIZONTAL SACCADES INDUCED BY STIMULATION OF THE MESENCEPHALIC RETICULAR FORMATION

BERNARD COHEN, VICTOR MATSUO, THEODORE RAPHAN, DAVID WAITZMAN AND JOEL FRADIN (Department of Neurology, Mount Sinai School of Medicine of the City University of New York, N.Y. 10029, U.S.A.)

INTRODUCTION

Stimulation and lesion experiments suggest that portions of the mesencephalic reticular formation (MRF) play an important role in producing horizontal eye movements (Bender & Shanzer, 1964; Komatsuzaki et al, 1972). Stimulation of the MRF produces contralateral deviation of the eyes in both cat (Szentágothai, 1943) and monkey (Bender & Shanzer, 1964). Lesions of this area induce deficits in contralateral gaze (Bender & Shanzer, 1964; Komatsuzaki et al , 1972) and in optokinetic nystagmus (OKN) (Szentágothai, 1943; Komatsuzaki et al, 1972). Preliminary studies have shown that unit activity associated with contralateral visually-induced saccades is also found in this region (Waitzman & Cohen, 1979, 1981). As yet, however, eye movements that are elicited from this area by electrical stimulation have not been characterized. The purpose of this study was to gain insight into how oculomotor information in this region is organized.

METHODS

Experiments were performed on cynomolgus (Macaca fascicularis), nemestrina (M. nemestrina) and rhesus monkeys (M. mulatta). Under anesthesia silver-silver chloride electrodes were implanted in the bone around the eyes to record horizontal and vertical eye movements. Bone overlying the MRF was removed, and a well that accepts a microelectrode carrier was implanted using dental acrylic cement. Restraining bolts were fixed to the skull. After recovery the MRF was systematically explored in vertical stereotaxic planes at a rate of 1-2 tracks/session over a period of several months. During experiments the animals sat in a primate chair with their heads restrained. The MRF was monopolarly stimulated using a tungsten microelectrode of 0.5-1.5 megohms impedance measured at 1,000 Hz. Trains were composed of constant current, 0.5 msec negative pulses. Pulse currents generally ranged between 20 and 30μA and did not exceed 40μA. Train duration and pulse frequencies were varied. Eye movements were displayed on the screen of a storage oscilloscope, registered on an oscillograph and stored on FM magnetic tape. The characteristic adduction produced by activation of the medial rectus subdivision of the oculomotor nucleus (Warwick, 1964) was used to locate the depth and laterality of the stimulating electrode. Marking lesions were made at the bottom of some electrode tracks for identification, and the tracks were later reconstructed in histological sections.

RESULTS

Horizontal eye movements were elicited from the MRF in an area that is similar to that previously described by Bender and Shanzer (1964) and Komatsuzaki et al, (1972) (Fig. 1). It roughly corresponds to nucleus cuneiformis in the human

Roucoux, A. and Crommelinck, M. (eds.): Physiological and Pathological Aspects of Eye Movements.
© 1982, Dr W. Junk Publishers, The Hague, Boston, London. ISBN-13: 978-94-009-8002-0

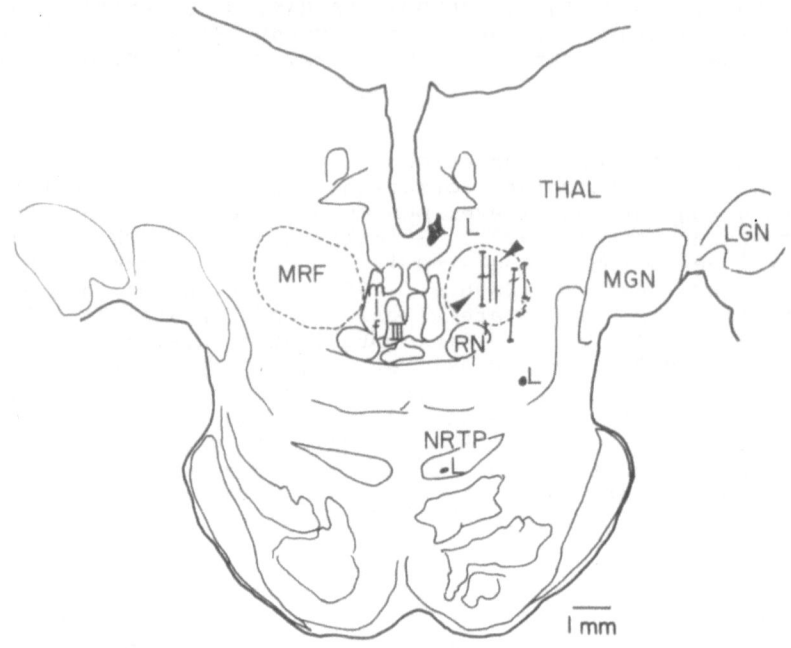

Fig. 1: Diagram of the brain stem of a rhesus monkey at about A + 3.5 (Snider and Lee, 1961). The approximate borders of the MRF are shown by the dotted lines. The vertical lines in the right MRF show 5 stimulation tracks that penetrated the MRF at this level. Three with horizontal bars at the top and bottom show the limit of the region from which contralateral horizontal eye movements were induced by stimulation. The horizontal curved lines in two of these tracks show the separation into portions from which retinotopic (dorsal) and craniotopic (ventral) saccades were elicited. Contralateral saccades were also elicited by stimulation in the other 3 tracks but as the tracks did not begin or end in this section, the transition point could not be determined precisely. The transition points are approximate because of changes due to gliosis and shrinkage, but show that retinotopic saccades were elicited from approximately the same region in different tracks. The same was true for craniotopic saccades. Abbreviations: L, lesion made to identify a stimulation track; LGN, lateral geniculate nucleus; MGN, medial geniculate nucleus; mlf, median longitudinal fasciculus; MRF, mesencephalic reticular formation; NRTP, nucleus reticularis tegmenti pontis; III, oculomotor nucleus; RN, red nucleus, Thal, thalamus .

(Olszewski and Baxter, 1954). The region is about 2.0mm wide, 1.25mm deep and 3mm from front to back. It lies lateral to the oculomotor nucleus and central gray matter, being centered at about A 3.5, L 3 and H +3 in the rhesus monkey (Snider and Lee, 1961). The laterality is the same in the cynomolgus and nemestrina monkeys, but the region is centered at about A 6.5 (Shantha et al, 1968, and unpublished data). The red nucleus is ventral and rostral to MRF. Medially the MRF is bounded by tractus retroflexus, laterally by the medial lemniscus, and dorsally by the thalamus. Caudally, the area is confluent with the superior colliculus. Rostrally, it thins and extends toward the fields of Forel. It is caudal and lateral to the rostral iMLF and adjacent regions of the MRF that have been associated with downward eye movements (Buettner et al, 1977; Koempf et al, 1979; King and Fuchs, 1979).

Only the eyes moved when stimuli were given to this region of the MRF in the restrained animal. At the borders of the area, small ear twitches or hand and leg movements were sometimes also elicited. The eye movements induced by MRF stimulation were conjugate, contralateral and horizontal. They generally had no vertical component. Only rapid eye movement, i.e. saccades or quick phases of nystagmus, were elicited by MRF stimulation. Slow movements, i.e. pursuit movements or slow phases of nystagmus, were not evoked.

Typical saccades elicited by stimulation of MRF with pulse trains are shown in Fig. 2A. The induced movements were similar in amplitude, duration and velocity to naturally-occurring saccades (Fig. 2A) and quick phases of nystagmus (Fig. 2D, E). Repetitive stimulation elicited a series of "staircase" saccades to the contralateral side with short periods of fixation in the period between saccades. This suggests that activity carried in the MRF is primarily related to generation of rapid not slow eye movements.

If the eyes were stationary when the pulse train was given, the induced movements were saccades to the contralateral side (Fig. 2A). If the eyes were pursuing a target or moving in response to movement of the visual surround, the induced movements were either opposing quick phases of nystagmus (Fig. 2D) or forward saccades superimposed on the slow eye movements (Fig. 2E). If the train repetition rate was set to about 3-4/sec during movement of the visual surround, typical OKN was produced at the frequency of stimulation. Two beats that were entrained on 5 successive sweeps are shown in Fig. 2D. Slow phases of nystagmus or pursuit velocities were unaffected by the occurrence of the induced saccades (Fig. 2D,E).

Following induced saccades there was a period of 150-200 msec when no spontaneous forward or backward saccades or quick phases of nystagmus occurred. This was true for either saccades elicited with the eyes stationary (Fig. 2A) or during nystagmus (Fig. 2D, E). A similar post-saccadic period of inhibition was found in a previous study when saccades were elicited from the paramedian zone of the pontine reticular formation (PPRF) (Cohen & Komatsuzaki, 1972). Neural networks that generate saccades in the horizontal planes are located in the PPRF (Cohen and Henn, 1972), and it is likely that activity projecting from the MRF to the PPRF was responsible for the eye movements that were elicited by MRF stimulation. The period of fixation that follows saccadic eye movements is probably also generated by pontine mechanisms (Henn and Cohen, 1973; Raphan and Cohen, 1978).

Eye movements were not induced by stimulation if the pulse train was given during a spontaneous or induced saccade in the same direction or for 50-75 msec thereafter. Following this refractory period, there was about 100 msec when a saccade could

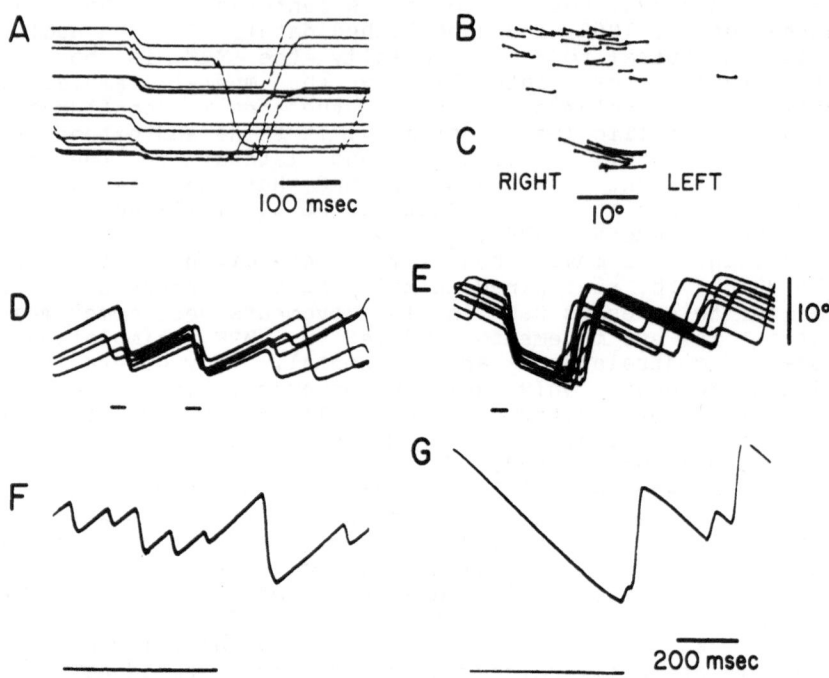

Fig. 2: A. Leftward saccades of about 2.5° induced by stimulation in the dorsal MRF on the right. The horizontal EOG was recorded bitemporally with DC coupling. Eye movements to the right caused upward trace deflections. Twelve 20 uA pulses at a frequency of 333 Hz were delivered during the period shown by the line below the EOG traces. The calibration for this and each of the EOG's shown in this figure with the exception of B and C, is given by the vertical bar next to E. The time base for D-G is shown below G. Note in A that the induced movements were followed by fixation periods of 150-200 msec when no other saccades occurred. B. Retinotopic saccades similar to those shown in A are displayed on an X-Y plot. All saccades were to the left. There was little or no vertical component to these movements. C, Variable amplitude, craniotopic saccades elicited from a stimulation site in the ventral portion of the right MRF. The eyes moved toward a restricted region of the movement field to the left of the midline. D, E, Leftward rapid eye movements elicited by right MRF stimulation during left (D) or right OKN (E). The velocity of the surround movement was 45°/sec. Two trains of pulses were delivered during D. Each train elicited a movement to the left followed by a period during which no other rapid movement occurred. F, G, Effect of a 500 msec period of MRF stimulation at 100 Hz on triggering of slow phases during left (F) and right OKN (G). This frequency was below threshold for inducing movement. Triggering was enhanced (F) or suppressed (G) when quick phases were in the same (F) or the opposite direction (G) as the movements that would be induced by higher frequencies of MRF stimulation.

be induced by another pulse train, but the amplitude of the
second movement was smaller than the first. If the stimulus was
given during a saccade in the opposite direction, the ongoing
movement was abruptly terminated and the eyes reversed direction.
This shows that there is a refractory period following saccade
generation. It suggests that the refractory period for saccade
generation in one direction is independent of that for saccade
generation in the opposite direction.

The latency of the induced deviations varied between 20 and
30 msec for trains of pulses at higher frequencies (Fig. 3A).
This is similar to latencies induced by frontal eye field and
superior colliculus stimulation (Robinson and Fuchs, 1969;
Robinson, 1972; Schiller and Stryker, 1972). Latencies were
longer at lower frequencies of stimulation (Fig. 3B, C). The
relationship between pulse frequency and latency was tested by
holding the number of pulses constant and varying the frequency.
Pulse current was held constant throughout. Trains were given
during OKN so that eye position and time after a preceding quick
phase could be controlled. Latencies of the induced movements
were close to the time it took to deliver a fixed number of
pulses to the MRF, regardless of frequency (Fig. 4). The dashed
lines of Fig. 4 show a constant product for 10 and 12 pulses.
From this it is likely that the MRF inputs to a trigger network
in the PPRF to generate saccades, and that the trigger network
integrates the spike frequency of the input signal until a
threshold is reached and a saccade is generated. The higher the
input frequency, the shorter the latency to the initiation of the
saccade.

The amplitude of eye movements induced by MRF stimulation
varied according to the region that was activated. Small
saccades were elicited from dorsal portions of the MRF and larger
saccades were evoked from regions that were more ventral in the
MRF. The saccades ranged in amplitude from about 1° in
dorsal portions to $15-20^{\circ}$ or more in deeper portions.
Examples of progressively larger saccades elicited from 4 sites
in one experiment are shown in Fig. 5. The stimulus sites were
separated by 0.25 mm. The threshold was similar at each
location.

Two classes of saccades were elicited by stimulation of the
MRF. From dorsal portions of the MRF the induced saccades were
of the same size, when a single locus was stimulated, regardless
of the position of the eye in the orbit, except for eye positions
at the limits of contralateral gaze. In contrast, in ventral
portions of the MRF saccade amplitude was dependent on the
initial position of the eyes in the orbit. The induced saccades
were larger if the eyes were on the ipsilateral side and smaller
if the eyes were on the contralateral side. Examples of these
two types of saccades from a single electrode track are shown in
Fig. 2B, C. The traces are X-Y plots of eye position on a
storage oscilloscope. The Z axis was intensified 20-100 msec
after right MRF stimulation. All induced movements were to the
left, i.e. to the contralateral side. Initial eye position
varied over a horizontal range of 40° and the vertical range
was 15°. Stimulation at a locus in the dorsal MRF induced
saccades whose amplitudes were about 2.5° (Fig. 2B). Smaller
saccades of 1° to 2° were elicited from more dorsal
positions in this track. Just below this region larger saccades
of about 5 and 10° were induced. In ventral-most portions of the

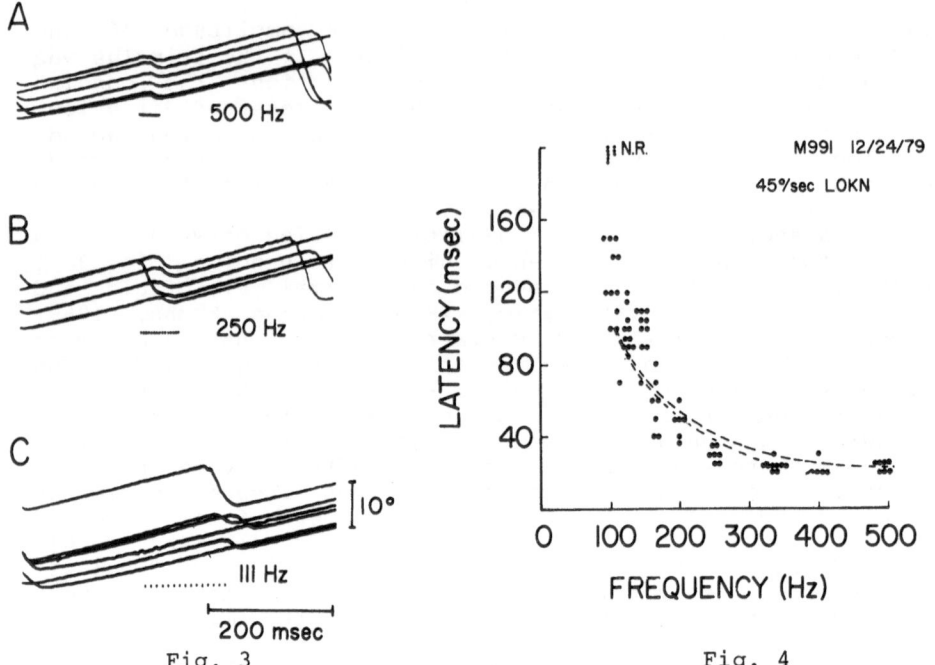

Fig. 3   Fig. 4

Fig. 3: Small saccades to the left elicited by right MRF
stimulation. In this experiment OKN to the left was induced by
surround movement at 45°/sec and the leftward quick phases
were used to trigger the sweep and stimulator. The delay to the
onset of stimulation was 200 msec. The same number of pulses in
the train was used in each instance (15), but the frequency was
varied. Note that the latency of the induced movements became
longer as the frequency of stimulation was reduced. Only the
horizontal EOG is shown.

Fig. 4: Plot of time from onset of stimulation to onset of eye
movement for stimulation at various frequencies. Data were
plotted from the experiment shown in Fig. 3. The two dashed
lines show the constant product for 10 (lower line) and 12 (upper
line) pulses. The data lay close to these constant product
lines. NR represents no reaction.

MRF, however, the induced saccades moved the eyes toward
particular regions of the contralateral field (Fig. 2C).
Consequently, the movements were larger when the original
position was farther on the ipsilateral side. The limits of the
final position varied considerably, but saccades of variable
amplitude tended to end 5-10° to the contralateral side of
the midline in a region that was itself 5-10° in diameter.
These two classes of saccades are similar to the retinotopic and
craniotopic saccades elicited from the superior colliculus by
Roucoux et al (1980) and Guitton et al (1980). Locations from
which the two types of saccades were elicited in two electrode
tracks are shown by the arrows above and below the horizontal
curved lines in Fig. 1.

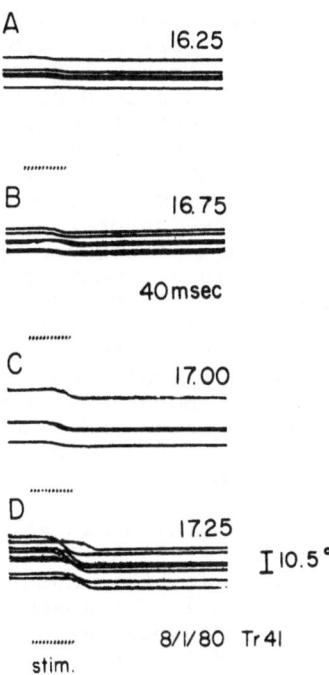

Fig. 5: Contralateral saccades induced by stimulation of the right MRF with 12 pulses at a frequency of 333 Hz. Each of the 4 stimulus sites was located in the right MRF, about 27-28 mm below the cortex. The depth of the stimulating microelectrode from the end of the guide tube is shown by the numbers to the right and above the superimposed traces; larger numbers refer to stimulation sites that were more ventral. The electrode was angled 15° from the vertical. Only the horizontal EOG is shown.

Although short bursts of pulses at high frequencies were most effective in eliciting saccades or quick phases of nystagmus, quick phase triggering was also affected by steady rates of MRF stimulation at frequencies that were themselves incapable of generating contralateral saccades or quick phases. In the monkey maximum beat frequencies of OKN are normally in the range of about 3-4 per second (Komatsuzaki et al, 1969). When the MRF was stimulated during OKN with contralateral quick phases, beat frequency rose to 5-10 beats/sec (Fig. 2F). When OKN quick phases were directed toward the contralateral side, i.e. in the same direction as the movements that would have been induced by higher rates of MRF stimulation, triggering of ipsilateral quick phases was suppressed (Fig. 2G). As a result, during MRF stimulation slow phases continued until the eyes had moved far to the contralateral side. This demonstrates that MRF activity which is below threshold for generating saccades is capable of modifying the excitability of saccade generating mechanisms.

DISCUSSION

The ability to induce saccades and quick phases of constant amplitude from the MRF by stimulation at low thresholds with relatively few pulses suggests that pathways or nuclei in MRF were activated that may contribute to production of saccades under natural circumstances. In accord with this neural activity in the MRF is associated with contralateral spontaneous saccades and is considerably enhanced when animals make visually-induced saccadic eye movements (Waitzman et al, 1979, 1981; Waitzman, 1982). The lack of effect of stimulation on the velocity of slow eye movements emphasizes the general principle of oculomotor organization that slow and fast phases are processed separately in the CNS (Westheimer, 1954; Rashbass, 1961). We would emphasize that the movements elicited from the MRF were predominantly horizontal. This implies that the MRF is "downstream" to activity arising in the superior colliculus and the frontal eye fields where stimulation often elicits oblique contralateral saccades with both a vertical and a horizontal component Robinson, 1972; Robinson and Fuchs, 1969; Schiller and Stryker, 1972). Activity responsible for vertical components of movement from these structures is apparently directed elsewhere.

The topographic dorso-ventral organization of eye movement amplitudes in the MRF bears a striking similarity to the rostro-caudal organization in the superior colliculus. In rostral colliculus small saccadic eye movements are elicited by stimulation in both cat (Rouxoux et al, 1980; Guitton et al, 1980) and monkey (Robinson, 1972; Schiller and Stryker, 1972); the amplitude of these saccades is independent of initial eye position. The movements become progressively larger as the stimulating electrode is moved caudally. In the caudal colliculus of the cat, larger saccades are elicited that move the eyes toward some portion of the contralateral movement field. These saccades are similar to the movements elicited in the ventral MRF of the monkey. The functional significance of this organization in the colliculus appears related to the size of intended gaze shifts and whether or not head movements are made with eye movements; the vestibulo-ocular reflex (VOR) is inhibited during the larger craniotopic eye movements (Guitton et al, 1980). MRF stimulation in the alert unrestrained animal also elicits head and eye movements (Wagman, 1964; Bender, Shanzer, 1964), and there are direct projections from the MRF to the cervical spinal cord (Castiglioni et al, 1978). Therefore, it seems likely that MRF is also related to producing shifts in gaze that require reorienting of the head on the neck.

Anatomic projections have been demonstrated between superior colliculus and the MRF (Harting, 1980; Grantyn and Grantyn, 1982; Cohen et al, 1981). In view of the similar topography for eye movements of different sizes in both structures, an important question is whether eye movements elicited by MRF stimulation were due to antidromic excitation of superior colliculus cells. This seems unlikely since there was no vertical component to the movements induced by dorsal MRF stimulation, whereas in the superior colliculus, vertical components are prominent. A more likely possibility is that the stimulating electrode was activating afferents projecting to MRF as well as MRF cells themselves.

It has been previously shown that the number of pulses in the burst of short and medium lead PPRF burst units is related to the component of movement in the pulling directions of the muscles that produce the deviations (Henn & Cohen, 1976). Since the amplitude of induced movement is dependent on the number of pulses in the burst, it would appear that the same set of PPRF neurons is utilized to produce movements of different sizes (Henn and Cohen, 1976). In contrast, the amplitude of the saccades induced by MRF stimulation was independent of either the frequency of stimulation or of the number of pulses in the train. Instead, the MRF stimulus appeared to act as a trigger signal. From this, it seems likely that an anatomical or "spatial-code" rather than a frequency code is utilized in the MRF to transmit oculomotor activity. If correct, then a spatial-temporal transformation of frequency must take place between the MRF and pons similar to that postulated for colliculo-reticular pathways (Robinson, 1972).

Thus results of stimulation suggest that the MRF processes activity that serves to trigger mechanisms that generate horizontal saccades. The region of the MRF that is active appears to be important for determining the size and type of the evoked saccade. The temporal aspects of the burst probably determine when the saccade will occur. In dorsal portions of the MRF activity excites trigger mechanism that elicit saccades of specific amplitudes. In ventral portions MRF activity seems directed more toward moving the eyes toward a particular sector of the field. The latter would be appropriate for being utilized during combined head and eye movements. The stimulation results indicate how activity in the MRF might be organized. Taken together with lesion and single unit data they support the idea that the MRF is an important link between the visual and oculomotor system for generation of saccades.

ACKNOWLEDGEMENTS
Supported by NIH Research Grant EY02296 and Core Center Grant EY01867. Victor Matsuo was supported by Fellowship Grant EY07014. Theodore Raphan was supported by Academic Investigator Award EY00157.

REFERENCES
Bender M B and Shanzer S (1964) Oculomotor pathways defined by electric stimulation and lesions in the brainstem of monkeys. In: Bender MB (ed) The Oculomotor System. pp 81-140, New York, Harper and Row.

Buettner U, Buettner-Ennever J A and Henn V (1977) Vertical eye movement related unit activity in the rostral mesencephalic reticular formation of the alert monkey. Brain Res 130, 239-252.

Castiglioni A J, Gallaway M C and Coulter J D (1978) Spinal projections from the midbrain in monkey. J Comp Neur 178, 329-346.

Cohen B, Buettner-Ennever J A, Waitzman D M and Bender M B (1981) Anatomical connections of a portion of the dorsolateral mesencephalic reticular formation of the monkey associated with horizontal saccadic eye movements. Soc Neurosci Abstr 7, 776.

Cohen B and Komatsuzaki A (1972) Eye movements induced by stimulation of the pontine reticular formation: Evidence for integration in oculomotor pathways. Exp Neurol 36, 101-117.

Grantyn A and Grantyn R (1982) Axonal patterns and sites of termination of cat superior collciulus neurons projecting in the tecto-bulbar-spinal tract. Exper Brain Res 46, 243-256.

Guitton D, Crommelinck M and Roucoux A (1980) Stimulation of the superior colliculus in the alert cat. I. Eye movements and neck EMG activity evoked when the head is restrained. Exp Brain Res 39, 63-73.

Harting J K (1977) Descending pathways from the superior colliculus in autoradiographic analysis in the rhesus monkey (Macaca Mulatta). J Comp Neur 173, 583-612.

Henn V and Cohen B (1973) Quantitative analysis of activity in eye muscle motoneurons during saccadic eye movements and positions of fixation. J Neurophysiol 36, 115-126.

Henn V and Cohen B (1976) Coding of information about rapid eye movements in the pontine reticular formation of alert monkeys. Brain Res 108, 307-325.

King W M and Fuchs A F (1979) Reticular control of vertical saccadic eye movements by mesencephalic burst neurons. J Neurophysiol 42, 861-876.

Koempf D, Pasik T, Pasik P and Bender MB (1979) Downward gaze in monkeys. Stimulation and lesion studies. Brain 102, 527-558.

Komatsuzaki A, Alpert J, Harris H E and Cohen B (1972) Effects of mesencephalic reticular formation lesions on optokinetic nystagmus. Exp Neurol 34, 522-534.

Komatsuzaki A, Harris H E, Alpert J and Cohen B (1972) Horizontal nystagmus of rhesus monkeys. Acta Otolaryngol 67, 535-551.

Olszewski J and Baxter D (1954) Cytoarchitecture of the Human Brain Stem. Philadelphia, J B Lippincott Co.

Raphan T and Cohen B (1978) Brainstem mechanisms for rapid and slow eye movements. Ann Rev Physiol 40, 527-552.

Rashbass C (1961) The relationship between saccadic and smooth tracking eye movements. J Physiol (London) 159, 326-338.

Robinson D A (1972) Eye movements evoked by collicular stimulation in the alert monkey. Vision Res 12, 1795-1808.

Robinson D A and Fuchs A F (1969) Eye movements evoked by stimulation of frontal eye fields. J Neurophysiol 32, 637-648.

Roucoux A, Guitton D and Crommelinck M (1980) Stimulation of the superior colliculus in the alert cat. II. Eye and head movements evoked when the head is unrestrained. Exp Brain Res 39, 75-85.

Schiller P H and Stryker M (1972) Single-unit recording and stimulation in superior colliculus of the alert rhesus monkey. J Neurophysiol 35, 915-924.

Snider D L and Lee J C (1961) A stereotaxic atlas of the monkey brain (Macaca mulatta) Chicago, Univ of Chicago Press.

Szentagothai J (1943) Die zentrale Innervation der Augenbewegungen. Arch Psychiat Nervenkrh 116, 721-760.

Wagman I H (1964) Eye movements induced by electrical stimulation of cerebrum in monkeys and their relationship to bodily movements. In: Bender M B (ed) The Oculomotor System pp 18-39. New York, Harper & Row.

Waitzman D M and Cohen B (1979) Unit activity in the mesencephalic reticular formation (MRF) associated with saccades and positions of fixation during a visual attention task. Soc Neurosci Abstr 5, 389.

Waitzman D M and Cohen B (1981) Burst neurons in the mesencephalic reticular formation (MRF) associated with visually-targeted and spontaneous saccades. Soc Neurosci Abstr 7, 132.

Westheimer G (1954) Eye movement responses to a horizontally moving visual stimulus. AMA Arch Opthalmol 52, 932-941.

TECTAL CONTROL OF VERTICAL EYE MOVEMENTS: A SEARCH FOR UNDERLYING NEURONAL CIRCUITS IN THE MESENCEPHALON

A. GRANTYN, R. GRANTYN (Leipzig, GDR), A. BERTHOZ
(Paris, France), J. RIBAS (Sevilla, Spain)

Studies of connectivity patterns underlying input from
the superior colliculus (CS) to the horizontal burst
generator in cats and monkeys led to a conclusion that
the link is established through direct or oligosynaptic
connections of collicular projection neurons with the
PPRF (Precht et al., 1974, Grantyn, Grantyn, 1976,
Raybourn, Keller, 1977). As concerns contribution of
the CS to the control of vertical saccadic eye movements, there exists only one report (King et al., 1980)
indicating the absence of any synaptic effects from the
CS on neurons in the interstitial nucleus of Cajal
(NIC), including burst and burst-tonic units discharging in relation to vertical saccades. In the present
communication we shall briefly summarize our material
bearing on the problem of synaptic connections between
the CS and preoculomotor regions of the midbrain
related to the generation of vertical components of
saccadic eye movements.

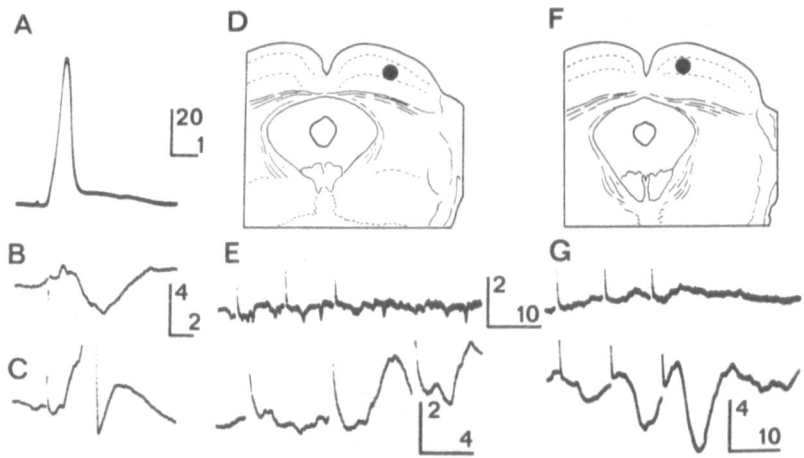

FIGURE 1. A-C) Identification of an IR motoneuron by
antidromic response to stimulation of inferior rectus
branch in the orbit (A), disynaptic IPSP from ipsilateral labyrinth (B) and disynaptic EPSP from contralateral
labyrinth (C). D) Stimulus point in the caudo-lateral
quadrant of the CS. E) EPSPs (lower trace) and extracellular field potentials (upper trace) evoked from the
point indicated in D. F-G) Reciprocal response (IPSP)
to stimulation of the rostro-medial point. Amplitude
and time calibrations in mV and ms.

Roucoux, A. and Crommelinck, M. (eds.): Physiological and Pathological Aspects of Eye Movements.
© *1982, Dr W. Junk Publishers, The Hague, Boston, London.* ISBN-13: 978-94-009-8002-0

338

Fig.1 D-G illustrates postsynaptic responses of a
physiologically identified (A-C) inferior rectus motoneuron (IR-MN) to stimulation of two different points
in the intermediate layers of the CS. About 40 IR-MNs
were studied in this paradigm using anesthetized or
encéphale isolé cats. In confirmation of the motor map
of the CS (Roucoux, Crommelinck, 1976) EPSPs were elicited from the caudo-lateral quadrant representing eye
movements with downward components and IPSPs from the
rostro-medial (upward) quadrant of the CS (Fig.2 A).
Postsynaptic responses could be induced from both ipsi-
and contralateral CS. As shown in the histograms of
Fig.2 B,C, the stimulus locked components of synaptic
responses usually appeared with latencies between 2 and
3 ms. In some motoneurons longer stimulus trains were
necessary to elicit a response which consisted of
smoothly rising de- or hyperpolarizations with latencies over 3 ms. In several preparations under Nembutal
anesthesia there was no effect of CS stimulation on
IR-MNs, even though the medial rectus motoneurons displayed normal EPSPs at disynaptic latencies.

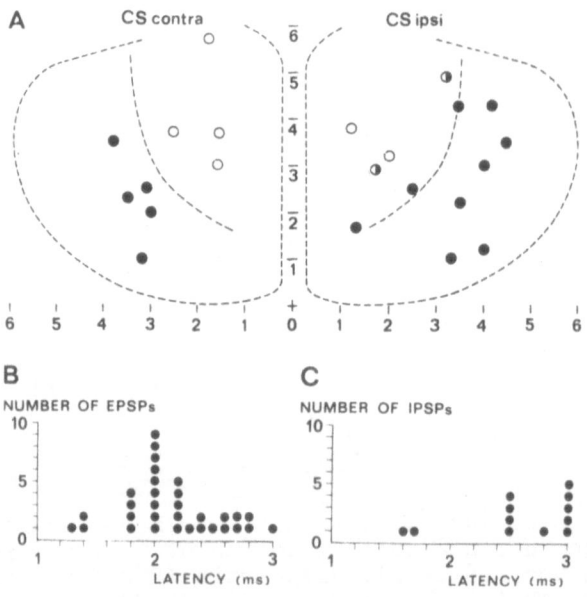

FIGURE 2. A) Dorsal view of the superior colliculi indicating the locations of stimulus points from which
EPSPs (filled circles) and IPSPs (open circles) were
elicited in IR-MNs. Interrupted line within the borders
of CS indicates approximate location of the horizontal
meridian. B,C) Histograms of EPSP and IPSP latencies
measured for stimulus locked components during ipsilateral and contralateral stimulation.

Thus, synaptic effects induced in vertical (IR) motoneurons by CS stimulation differ in important points
from those observed in horizontal motoneurons (lateral
and medial rectus)(Grantyn, Berthoz, 1977, Grantyn et
al., 1979). In contrast to the latter, transmission to
IR-MNs is predominantly tri- or polysynaptic, a contribution of disynaptic links being negligibly small. The
effectiveness and the reliability of synaptic influences on IR-MNs are, correspondingly, lower.

The paucity of oligosynaptic links makes it difficult
to trace neuronal connections underlying the observed
synaptic effects. Progress in this direction requires
detailed information on the morphological relationships
of the tectal efferent neurons with brain stem regions
containing premotor circuits responsible for vertical

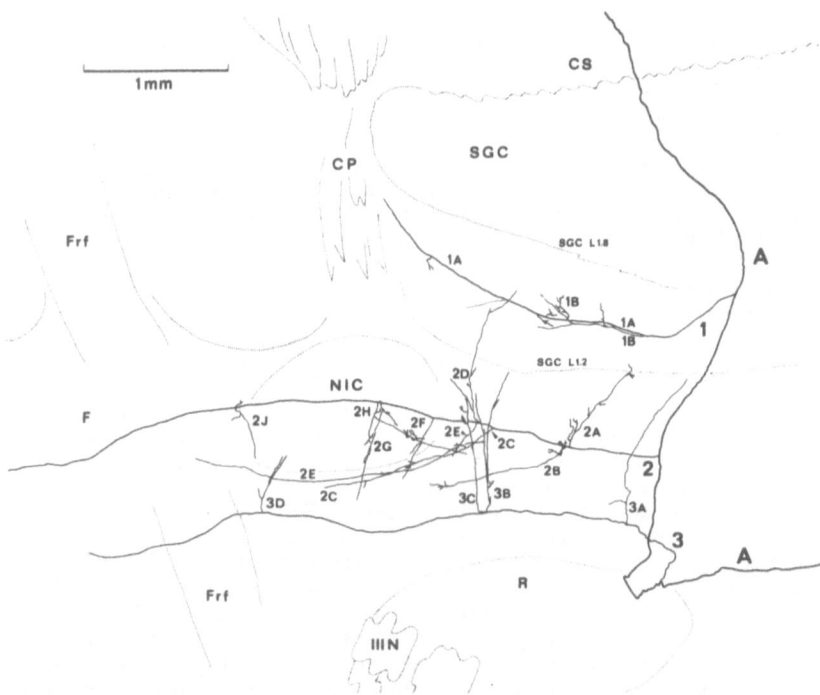

FIGURE 3. Axonal ramification of a tecto-bulbo-spinal
neuron projecting into the ventral funiculus of the
cervical spinal cord (antidromic identification). Reconstruction in parasagittal plane. Collaterals are
referred to in the text according to their numbers.
Main axon denoted by A. Abbreviations: CP - commissura
posterior, CS - colliculus superior, F - field of
Forel, Frf - fasciculus retroflexus, NIC - nucl. in-
terstitialis Cajal, R - nucl. ruber, SGC - substantia
grisea centralis.

saccades. Recently we described axonal ramification
patterns of HRP-stained tectal efferent neurons projecting in the tecto-bulbo-spinal tract (TBSN)(Grantyn,
Grantyn, 1982). Fig.3 shows the distribution of mesencephalic axonal branches which is representative for
this class of neurons. The rostrally directed longitudinal collaterals originating from the main axon before
(1,2) and after (3) the decussation issue numerous
secondary branches which ramify in the midbrain reticular formation (MRF)(e.g. 2A,B,C,3A,B), the central
grey (SGC)(1B), the rostral and caudal poles of the NIC
(2F,J,3D) and in the ventral aspect of the nuclei of
posterior commissure (NCP)(1A). Longitudinal collaterals (2,3) enter the ventral thalamus, rostrally and
ventrorostrally of the NIC. Terminal ramifications in
this region were not detected in this particular neuron
but they were present in several other TBSNs.

Relating these observations to single cell recordings
in alert animals suggests that TBSNs may establish
direct connections with vertical burst neurons in the
prestitial area (rostral interstitial nucleus of MLF)
(Büttner et al., 1977) or in the structures adjacent
to the NIC (MRF, SGC)(King, Fuchs, 1977). The situation
is ambiguous with respect to the NIC proper which, in
cats, is the site of vertical burst-tonic neurons
(King et al., 1980). In our material collaterals in the
core of the NIC were sparce in comparison with its periphery and bordering regions of the MRF (Fig.3, collaterals 2C,E,G,H,3C). Vertical burst-tonic neurons were
encountered at these locations in the monkey (King,
Fuchs, 1977) but not in the cat (King et al., 1980).

Further analysis of collicular links with vertical
motoneurons requires identification of target neurons
of the CS and clarification of their connections with
the III nucleus. Our current study has been limited to
some of the midbrain regions supplied by rostral collaterals of tecto-bulbo-spinal neurons. Cells showing
monosynaptic responses to CS stimulation (EPSPs with
latencies 0.7 - 1.2 ms) were sampled at frontal levels
corresponding to the rostro-caudal extent of the NIC.
Intracellular HRP injections were used to obtain morphological characteristics of neurons selected according
to the above criterion. As shown in Fig.4, neurons receiving monosynaptic collicular input were encountered
in the pretectum, the nuclei of posterior commissure,
the central grey and the region of the NIC. Since the
number of available pretectal and central grey neurons
is too low, we shall consider only the latter two
groups.

The ventral group includes 7 successfully stained neurons (Fig.4, A4-7, B9-11), only two of them being definitely within the borders of the NIC (A4,5). Both NIC
neurons projected via ipsilateral MLF in the interstiti-
tio-spinal tract, as revealed by antidromic response to

stimulation of the spinal cord at cervical level. Collaterals were observed in only one of them, with terminal ramifications and boutons in the NIC (recurrent
collateral), in the inferior rectus subdivision of the
III nucleus and in the SGC in front of the trochlear
nucleus. The remaining five cells were located outside
the NIC. Their axons entered the ipsilateral MLF and
descended to the cervical cord (antidromic responses).
The somadendritic profile and synaptic responses of one
of the neurons belonging to this group are shown in
Fig.5. Collaterals to the SGC and within the NIC were
observed in cells 6, 7 (Fig.4A) but were absent in more
laterally located cells 9 - 11 (Fig.4B), in spite of
strong HRP staining of their main axons. The topography
of collicular target neurons in the surroundings of the
NIC corresponds well to the branching pattern of the
rostral collaterals issued by TBSNs. A direct connection to the NIC proper seems indeed to be scanty. Main
target are the reticulo-spinal neurons located in the
adjacent MRF which, however, do not project to the III
nucleus.

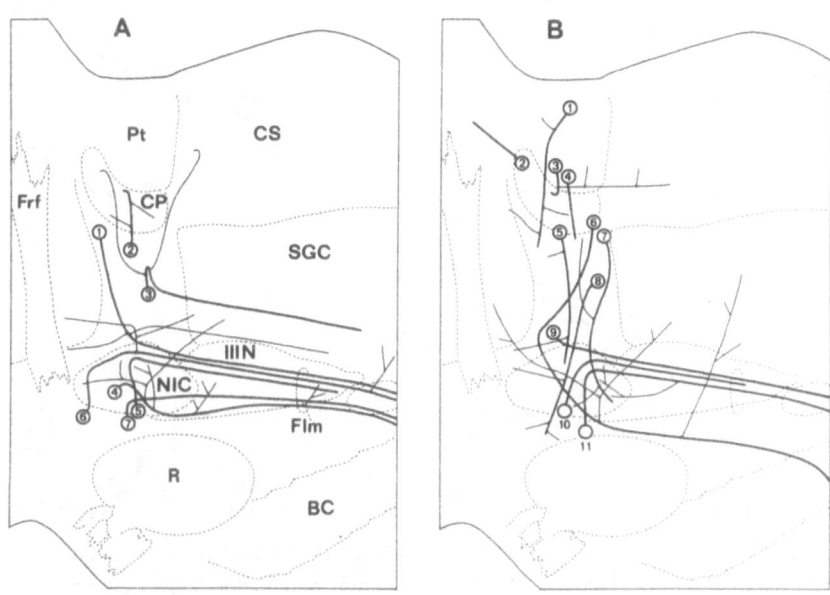

FIGURE 4. Location of neurons responding with monosynaptic EPSPs to stimulation of the ipsilateral CS and
stained with HRP. Reconstruction in parasagittal plane.
A) Cells located within 1.8 mm from the midline.
B) Cells with more lateral locations. The course of
main axon is indicated by thick lines, approximate trajectory of collaterals - by thin lines. Abbreviations
as in Fig.4. BC - brachium conjunctivum, Flm - fasciculus longitudinalis medialis, Pt - pretectum.

A high probability of recording monosynaptic responses in neurons within the nuclei of posterior commissure (NCP) was unexpected in view of anatomical data indicating quite sparse collicular projection to this region (Graham, 1977). Of particular interest are the cells whose axons do not enter the posterior commissure but course in ventral direction on the ipsilateral side. Axons of two cells were followed to the rostral pons either in the MLF (Fig.4, A1) or in the predorsal bundle (Fig.4, B6). Axons of other cells could not be traced beyond the NIC region. Collaterals with terminal ramifications were observed in the SGC (cells B6,7), in the MRF adjacent to the SGC (cells A1, B6) and dorsorostrally of the red nucleus (cell B8), in the field of Forel (cells A1, B6,8) and in the NIC (cell B7). Collaterals to the III nucleus were not detected. The NCP represent a part of the dorsorostral midbrain area which, according to clinical observations and lesion experiments, is critical for the execution of vertical eye movements. NCP neurons receiving monosy-

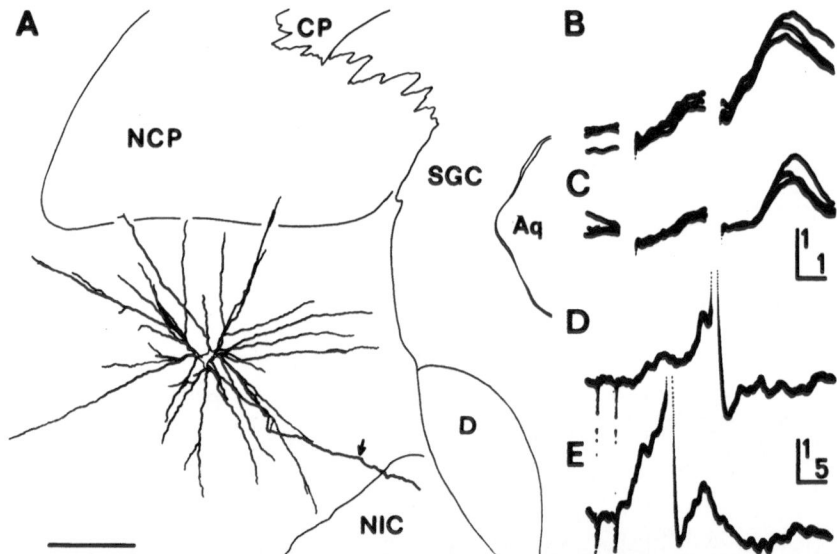

FIGURE 5. A) Mesencephalic reticular neuron stained by intrasomatic injection of HRP. Partial reconstruction in frontal plane. Axon (arrow) passes through NIC without collaterals and descends in the Flm to the spinal cord (antidromic identification). Note extremely wide dendritic field. Calibration bar - 0.5 mm. B) EPSP with monosynaptic component evoked by stimulation of rostro-medial CS. C) Disynaptic EPSP evoked from the caudo-lateral CS. D,E) Polysynaptic EPSPs evoked by stimulation of ipsi- and contralateral labyrinths, respectively. Abbreviations as in Figs. 3, 4. Aq - aqueductus, D - nucl. Darkschewitsch, NCP - nucl. commissurae posterioris.

naptic collicular input may represent a link in the
tecto-oculomotor pathway, since they show axonal ramifications in the NIC, adjacent SGC and in tegmental
regions rostral to the NIC. Preliminary observations
suggest that NCP neurons may be specifically related
to upward movement components: in the present sample
all but one neurons showed a clear preference of rostro-
medial (upward) quadrant of the CS. Monosynaptic responses could be elicited only by stimulation of this
quadrant, whereas stimulation in the caudo-lateral
quadrant either produced EPSPs of longer latencies and
higher thresholds or no response at all.

In conclusion, we have demonstrated a more complex
organization of tecto-oculomotor pathways related to
vertical eye movements, as compared to horizontal. In
the search for neuronal sets conveying tectal influences to motoneurons of the III nucleus we have presently
characterized two groups of target neurons of the CS in
the rostral mesencephalon. The ventral group includes
large reticulo-spinal neurons in the neighbourhood of
the NIC. Some of them are obviously unrelated to neural
pathways converging to the III nucleus but may represent one of additional brain stem sites at which collicular outflow gains access to the control of spinal
circuits, in parallel with the direct tecto-spinal
tract. Others are potentially capable of influencing
motoneurons of the III nucleus through their collateral
connections with the NIC and adjacent regions of the
central grey. The dorsal group is represented by neurons within the nuclei of posterior commissure. Projection of this nucleus to the contralateral NIC is well
known (Berman, 1977). In the present material, a number
of neurons projected ipsilaterally and ramified in the
NIC, adjacent central grey and in the prestitial area.
Thus, neurons of this group are appropriate candidates
for relaying collicular signals to the preoculomotor
neurons related to vertical saccades. Topographical
features of synaptic responses induced in NCP neurons
by CS stimulation suggest that this region may be specifically related to the generation of upward vector.
Similar experimental approach is now being used to
characterize other groups of mesencephalic neurons
receiving the direct tectal input.

REFERENCES
Berman N (1977) Connections of the pretectum in the
cat, J. comp. Neurol. 174, 227-254.
Büttner U, Büttner-Ennever JA and Henn V (1977) Vertical eye movement related unit activity in the rostral
mesencephalic reticular formation of the alert monkey,
Brain Res. 130, 239-252.
Graham J (1977) An autoradiographic study of the efferent connections of the superior colliculus in the
cat, J. comp. Neurol. 173, 629-654.
Grantyn A and Berthoz A (1977) Synaptic actions of the
superior colliculus on medial rectus motoneurons in

the cat, Neurosci. 2, 945-952.
Grantyn A and Grantyn R (1976) Synaptic actions of tectofugal pathways on abducens motoneurons in the cat, Brain Res. 105, 269-285.
Grantyn A and Grantyn R (1982) Axonal patterns and sites of termination of cat superior colliculus neurons projecting in the tecto-bulbo-spinal tract, Exp. Brain Res. 46, 243-256.
Grantyn A, Grantyn R, Robiné KP and Berthoz A (1979) Electroanatomy of tectal efferent connections related to eye movements in the horizontal plane, Exp. Brain Res. 37, 149-172.
King WM and Fuchs AF (1977) Neuronal activity in the mesencephalon related to vertical eye movements. In Baker R and Berthoz A, eds. Control of gaze by brain stem neurons, pp. 319-326, Elsevier, Amsterdam.
King WM, Precht W and Dieringer N (1980) Synaptic organization of frontal eye field and vestibular afferents to interstitial nucleus of Cajal in the cat, J. Neurophysiol. 43, 912-928.
Precht W, Schwindt PC and Magherini PC (1974) Tectal influences on cat ocular motoneurons, Brain Res. 82, 27-40.
Raybourn MS and Keller EL (1977) Colliculoreticular organization in primate oculomotor system, J. Neurophysiol. 40, 861-878.
Roucoux A and Crommelinck M (1976) Eye movements evoked by superior colliculus stimulation in the alert cat, Brain Res. 106, 349-363.

THE LOCALIZATION OF LARGE AND SMALL MOTONEURONS IN THE OCULOMOTOR NUCLEUS OF THE MONKEY

J.A. BÜTTNER-ENNEVER[+], P. d'ASCANIO[++], R. GYSIN (Brain Research Institute, University of Zürich, Switzerland)

INTRODUCTION

With the development of new and more sensitive neuro-anatomical tracer techniques it has become possible to reveal details which were not visible with older histological procedures. For example, the classical study of Warwick (1953) on the arrangement of moto-neurons in the oculomotor nucleus (OMN) was based on the distribution of chromatolysis after cutting individual branches of the oculomotor nerve; in this way the motoneuron pool for the medial rectus muscle was shown to lie ipsilaterally in the ventral portion of the nucleus. In contrast, subsequent experiments using retrograde tracer substances, horseradish per-oxidase (HRP) and wheatgerm agglutinin (WGA), revealed a multifocal representation for medial rectus, inclu-ding a group of small motoneurons lying outside the classical OMN (Büttner-Ennever, Akert 1981: Spencer, Porter 1981). The present article describes the location of the motoneuron pools for other muscles represented in the OMN, using HRP and WGA techniques, and demonstrates further groups of small motoneurons lying ouside the classical OMN. Since 'large and small' motoneurons can, to some extent, be related to 'phasic and tonic' muscle fibre types respectively (Büttner-Ennever, Akert 1981), the results may help the physiological interpretation of inputs into, and around, the OMN.

METHODS

Horseradish peroxidase and $[^{125}I]$ radioactive WGA were injected into the extraocular eye muscles of the monkey. After standard staining procedures for HRP reaction product (TMB) and standard autoradiographic techniques to visualise the WGA, sections were studied for labelled cells in the region of the oculomotor nucleus. Further technical details are described in Büttner-Ennever and Akert (1981). The location and diameter of labelled cells was measured only when a nucleolus could be seen, and the information stored in a PDP 11/2o computer.

Present address
+ Institute of Anatomy, University of Düsseldorf, Germany
++ Institute of Human Physiology, University of Pisa, Italy

Roucoux, A. and Crommelinck, M. (eds.): Physiological and Pathological Aspects of Eye Movements.
© *1982, Dr W. Junk Publishers, The Hague, Boston, London.* ISBN-13: 978-94-009-8002-0

346

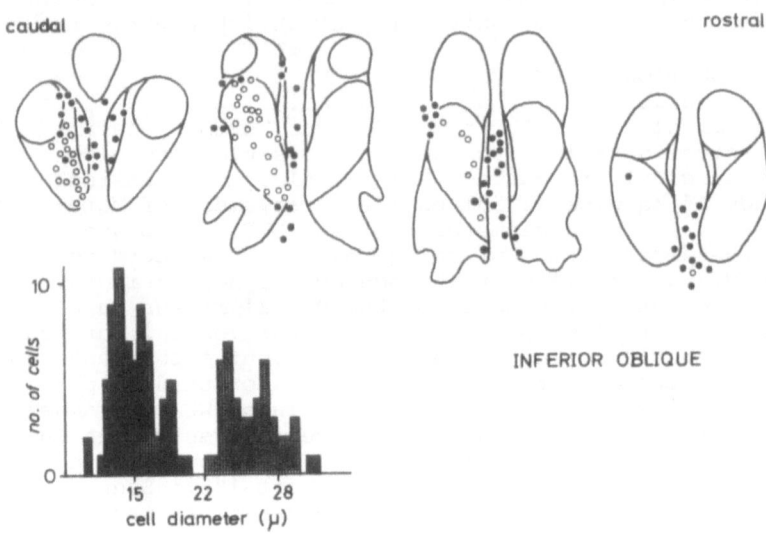

INFERIOR OBLIQUE

FIGURE 1. Drawings of the oculomotor nucleus at 4
different levels to show the location of labelled
cells after the injection of WGA into the inferior
oblique muscle. Small motoneurons ($< 22\mu$) dots:
large motoneurons ($> 22\mu$) open circles. Note that the
small motoneurons lie predominantly outside the
classical large-celled OMN.

RESULTS
After the injection of WGA or HRP into inferior rectus,
superior rectus, medial rectus and inferior oblique,
clearly labelled neurons (interpreted as motoneurons)
were found in the OMN; and the cell-body diameters were
measured. Histograms of motoneuron diameter for these
extraocular muscles were bimodal, with the minimum at
22μ (Fig. 1). Cell-bodies larger than 22μ were termed
'large motoneurons' and those less than 22μ 'small
motoneurons'. As expected the large motoneurons lay
within the confines of the classical OMN, however,
it was interesting to find that almost all the small
motoneurons lay around the perimeter, or outside, the
OMN (Fig. 1). The arrangement of large motoneurons is
shown in Fig. 2, for the muscles of one eye. The
perioculomotor region occupied by the small motoneurons
is indicated by a dashed line. This separation of large
and small motoneurons was found for all extraocular
muscles.

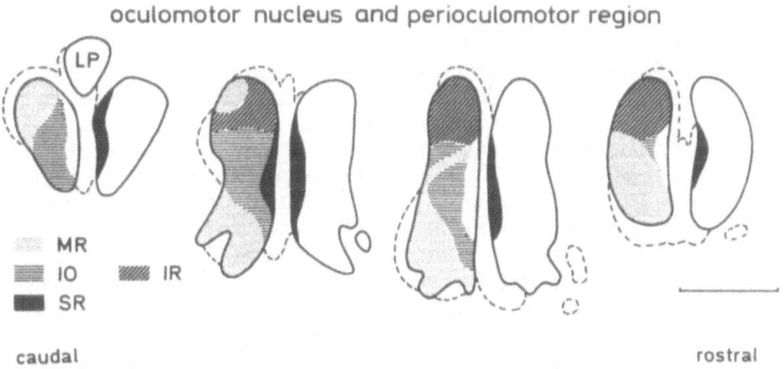

oculomotor nucleus and perioculomotor region

MR
IO   IR
SR

caudal   rostral

FIGURE 2. The arrangement of the motoneuron pools in the OMN. The shaded areas outline the groups of large motoneurons innervating different extraocular muscles of one orbit. Note the motoneurons of SR are mainly contralateral. The small motoneurons of these muscles lie predominantly within the perioculomotor region enclosed by a dashed line around the OMN. MR medial rectus, IR inferior rectus, SR superior rectus, IO inferior oblique, LP levator palpebrae. Calibration = 1mm.

Some topography could be seen in the arrangement of the small motoneurons in the perioculomotor region. Medial rectus is represented dorsally (including subgroup C), laterally and ventrolaterally, while inferior rectus lies dorsomedially; superior rectus is only found medially and inferior oblique ventro-medially and small patches lateral to OMN. The extent of the new small motoneuron border may be even more extensive than shown here because of the incomplete filling of the muscles with tracer.

DISCUSSION
Apart from the extra subgroups of medial rectus, there is not a large difference between the representation of the eye muscles inside the classical OMN proposed by Warwick (1953) and that described here. It is important to remember that some of the differences arise from the angle of section which differs in the two studies by almost 90° (Büttner-Ennever 1981, Fig. 2). The main point of this report is the description small moto-neurons of all the extraocular eye muscles which sur-round the classical OMN in a band about 300μ wide, throughout the whole rostral-caudal extent of the nucleus. This perioculomotor region must now be included in the term OMN.

A group of medial rectus motoneurons lying within the
new OMN border (subgroup C) has already been described,
and shown to innervate the orbital layer of the medial
rectus muscle (Büttner-Ennever, Akert 1981). The
orbital, as opposed to the global, layer is mainly
composed of muscle fibres which are morphologically
suited for tonic, or continous, activity. The present
results show that similar groups of small motoneurons
exist for the other extraocular muscles, and therefore
the borders of the OMN may contain predominantly tonic
motoneurons, where as the large-celled OMN is composed
of the more phasic neurons. Both types of motoneurons
have been described by Henn and Cohen (1972) in the
OMN monkey. It should be emphasised here that, unlike
the medial rectus subgroup C, the relationship of the
small motoneurons of other muscles to their respective
orbital layers has not been investigated, up to now.

Recent reports on the connectivity of the perioculomotor region have produced increasing interest in this
area. Afferents from superior colliculus and abducens
nucleus, as well as efferents to brain stem and spinal
cord are among some of the pathways already described
(Harting et al. 1978: Loewy et al. 1978: Büttner-
Ennever, Akert 1981). However the results are usually
related only to the Edinger-Westphal complex. In the
future the area between the Edinger-Westphal and the
large-celled OMN should also be carefully documented
since it is now known to be part of the OMN in monkeys.

The results described here have slightly expanded the
borders of the oculomotor nucleus and may provide a
guide to the physiological significance of different
anatomical inputs into, and around, the oculomotor
nucleus.

This work was supported by the Swiss National
Foundation for Scientific Research, Grants 3.505.79
and 3.580.79, the Dr Eric Slack Gyr Foundation and
P.d'A. was a recipient of a Fellowship in Neurobiology of the Academia Nazionale dei Lincei Roma.

REFERENCES
Büttner-Ennever JA (1981) Anatomy of medial rectus
subgroups in the oculomotor nucleus of the monkey. In
Fuchs AF and Becker W, eds. The neural control of eye
movements, pp 247-252. Elsevier/North Holland Amsterdam.
Büttner-Ennever JA and Akert K (1981) Medial rectus
subgroups of the oculomotor nucleus and their abducens
internuclear input in the monkey, J. Comp. Neurol. 197,
17-27.
Harting JK, Huerta MF, Frankfurter AJ, Strominger NL,
and Royce GJ (1980) Ascending pathways from the monkey
superior colliculus: an autoradiographic analysis. J.
Comp. Neurol. 192, 853-882.

Henn V and Cohen B (1972) Eye muscle motoneurons with
different characteristics, Brain Res. 45, 561-568
Loewy AD, Saper CB and Yamodis ND (1978) Re-evaluation
of the efferent projections of the Edinger-Westphal
nucleus in the cat, Brain Res. 141, 153-159.
Spencer RF and Porter JD (1981) Innervation and
structure of extraocular muscles in the monkey in
comparison to those of the cat, J. Comp. Neurol. 198,
649-665.
Warwick R (1953) Representation of the extra ocular
muscles in the oculomotor nuclei of the monkey, J.
Comp. Neurol. 98, 449-504.

ROLE OF VESTIBULAR AND NECK REFLEXES IN CONTROLLING EYE AND HEAD POSITION*

B.W. PETERSON, J. GOLDBERG (Department of Physiology, Northwestern University Medical School, Chicago, IL).

1. INTRODUCTION

Systems that stabilize gaze may receive afferent input from visual, vestibular or proprioceptive receptors and act upon either extraocular or neck muscles. The various combinations of these inputs and outputs thus constitute six classes of compensatory gaze reflexes. This paper will describe four such reflexes: the vestibulo-ocular, cervico-ocular, vestibulocollic and cervicocollic reflexes and describe how they interact to maintain gaze stability in normal animals and in animals with vestibular lesions.

2. VESTIBULO-OCULAR REFLEX

The neuronal substrates and physiological properties of the vestibulo-ocular reflex (VOR) have been extensively investigated and reviewed by others (cf: Wilson and Melvill Jones, 1979). In normal animals, the VOR system can generate eye movements that completely compensate for movements of the head over a wide range of velocities and frequencies (Furman et al, 1982; Keller, 1978; Pulaski and Robinson, 1981; Buettner et al, 1981). These eye movements appear to arise from a simple analog transformation of vestibular input since optimal system performance is maintained for random stimuli and stimuli at frequencies beyond the range of a predictive system such as visual pursuit (Furman et al, 1982; Keller, 1978).

The vestibulo-ocular system has also been shown to be remarkably adaptable in altering its performance in response to gaze error signals conveyed by the visual system so that accurate gaze stability is restored in visual environments modified by reversing or magnifying spectacles (Gonshor and Melvill Jones, 1973; Melvill Jones and Gonshor, 1982; Miles and Eighmy, 1980; Keller and Precht, 1979) or cross coupling of head and image rotations in different planes (Schultheis and Robinson, 1981). The modified system behavior in these situations is no longer as simple as that of the unmodified VOR, however. System performance becomes frequency-dependent, reversing toward unmodified behavior at frequencies greater than 1 Hz (Miles and Eighmy, 1980; Melvill Jones and Gonshor, 1982) and shows signs of predictive behavior, especially during active, self-generated head movements (Melvill Jones and Gonshor, 1982). The frequency of the head movement applied during the adaptation period also plays a role in determining the frequency response of the adapted VOR (Lisberger and Miles, 1981). These more complex adaptive processes presumably also play a role in the restoration of function that occurs after partial destruction of the peripheral vestibular apparatus (cf: Maioli, this volume).

With our colleagues, J. Baker and R. Schor, we have recently observed another form of modification of the VOR in cats following bilateral plugging of the horizontal semicircular canals. As described by Robinson and Schultheis, (this volume), both the

Roucoux, A. and Crommelinck, M. (eds.): Physiological and Pathological Aspects of Eye Movements.
© 1982, Dr W. Junk Publishers, The Hague, Boston, London. ISBN-13: 978-94-009-8002-0

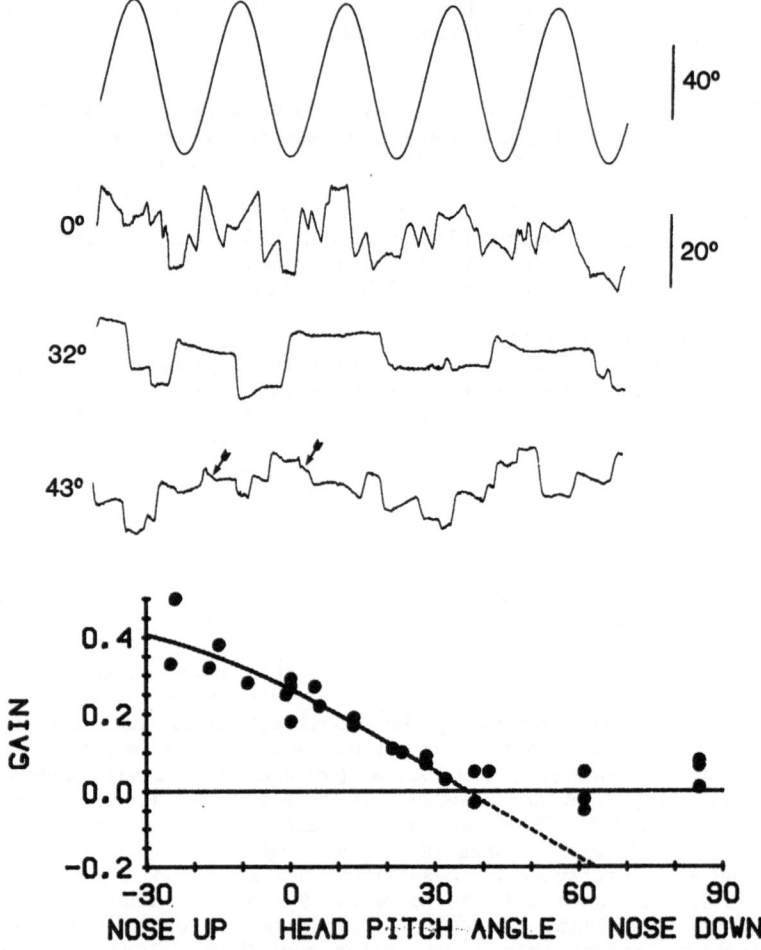

FIGURE 1. Horizontal eye movements induced by rotation in a cat with plugged horizontal semicircular canals. Cat was rotated sinusoidally (0.25 Hz, 40 deg) in a horizontal plane with its head pitched down (positive angles) or up (negative angles) from the stereotaxic plane. Records at top show the stimulus and horizontal eye position recorded at 3 pitch angles. Upward deflections indicate rightward rotation. Arrows indicate periods of compensatory eye movements in the record taken at 43 deg pitch angle. Graph plots horizontal eye movement gain (velocity of slow phase eye movement/velocity of rotation) against head pitch angle. Positive gains correspond to compensatory movements. As predicted by coupling between vertical canals and horizontal eye movers, gains obtained when the head was pitched above vertical canal null plane (here, $+36°$) vary as the sine of pitch angle (solid curve). When the head was pitched below the null plane, eye movements consisted of the anticompensatory movements expected from coupling of vertical canals to horizontal eye movers interspersed with periods of compensatory eye movement so that net gain was close to zero.

horizontal and vertical canals normally contribute to horizontal eye movements. The relative contributions of the two canal systems depends upon orientation of the head in the pitch plane. From the orientation of the semicircular canals in the cat (Blanks, et al., 1972), for instance, it can be predicted that when the animal's head is in the stereotaxic plane, the horizontal canals will contribute 83% of the gain of the vestibulo-ocular reflex while the vertical canals contribute 17%. In cats with plugged horizontal semicircular canals, a vestibulo-ocular reflex of approximately this magnitude is in fact observed when the head is in the stereotaxic plane. As shown in Figure 1, this vertical canal generated horizontal VOR increases as the head is pitched further up and decreases in a sinusoidal fashion to reach zero at an angle corresponding to the vertical canal null plane. The animal is thus using the vertical canal-induced VOR to assist in producing compensatory eye movements when its head is pitched up from the vertical canal null plane. The contribution of the vertical canals to horizontal eye movements should reverse and produce anticompensatory movements when the head is pitched below the vertical canal null plane. The data record shown in Figure 1 exhibit periods during which such anticompensatory eye movements can be observed. At other periods, indicated by arrows, eye movement direction is reversed to produce compensatory eye movements. Our preliminary observations indicate that these latter movements are of a predictive nature. As the diagram in Figure 1 shows, their net effect is to cancel the anticompensatory VOR that would otherwise be produced by the vertical canal system.

In summary, the basic, linear VOR system is able to produce optimal stabilization of gaze during head rotation in normal animals. When system performance is modified with optical devices or vestibular lesions, more complex neuronal processes involving nonlinear, predictive behavior are brought into play to modify system performance in an attempt to restore gaze stability. The performance of these systems at high frequencies is typically far inferior to that of the normal VOR.

3.   CERVICO-OCULAR REFLEX

Electrophysiological experiments have established the neuronal substrates for a cervico-ocular reflex (COR) by showing that electrical stimulation of receptors in perivertebral muscles or joints can modify transmission in vestibulo-ocular pathways (Hikosaka and Maeda, 1973) and that rotation of the neck modulates the activity of many neurons in the vestibular nuclei and in other brainstem structures related to eye movements (Anastasopoulos and Mergner, 1982; Boyle and Pompeiano, 1979; Brink et al., 1981; Kasper and Thoden, 1981). On the other hand, behavioral measurements have failed to reveal a consistent pattern of slow eye movement in normal alert animals during passive rotation of the neck at frequencies within the normal physiological range of 0.1 - 5 Hz (Barnes and Forbat, 1979; Fuller, 1980; Dichgans et al, 1973; Barmack et al., 1981). This negligible role of the COR in normal animals is not surprising since Fuller (1980) has pointed out that a COR that assisted the VOR in maintaining gaze stability during passive head rotation would act to destablize gaze under circumstances where the animal used a combination of vestibulocollic and vestibulo-ocular reflexes to compensate for body rotations. Normal animals can therefore attain better gaze stabilization by relying solely on the VOR except possibly during very slow rotations for which vestibular reflexes have low gains and where the COR may play a more important role (Barmack et al., 1981).

The situation changes when vestibular reflexes are lost bilaterally. Now a compensatory COR will improve gaze stability in all situations involving rotations of the head on the trunk. Dichgans et al (1973) and Kasai and Zee (1978) have shown that a consistent compensatory COR with a gain ranging from 0.2 to 0.7 develops in labyrinthectomized monkeys or in humans who have lost labyrinthine function due to ototoxic drugs. This adaptive development of a COR does not depend on loss of labyrinthine afferent fibers or on decrease in the vestibular afferent discharge

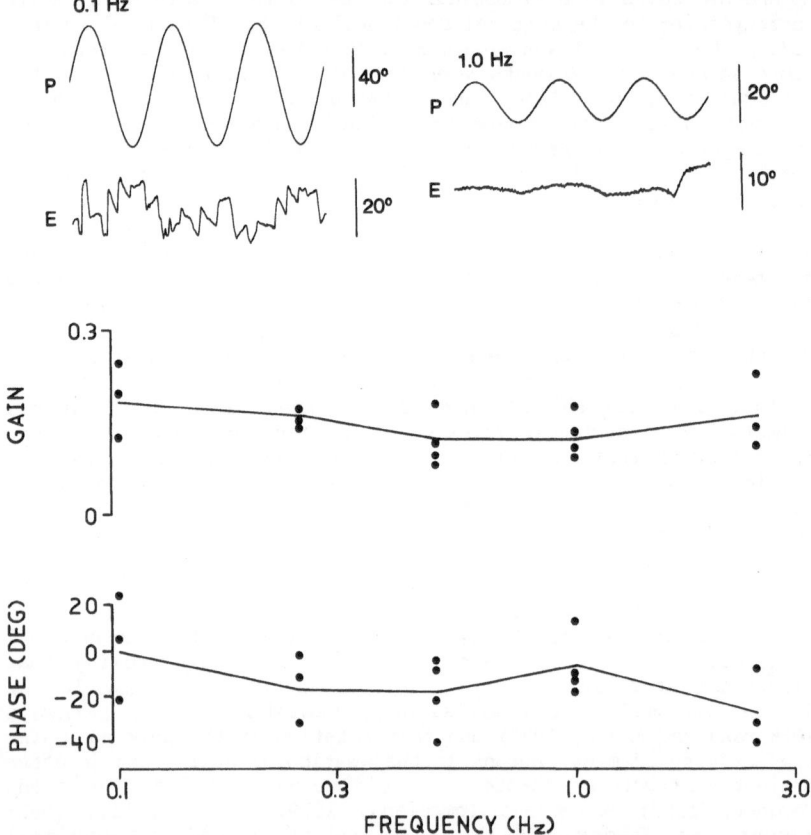

FIGURE 2. Horizontal cervico-ocular reflex in a cat 8 months after plugging horizontal semicircular canals. Records at top show modulation of horizontal eye position (E) when the body was rotated sinusoidally with the head held fixed in space (traces labeled P indicate body position) at 0.1 and 1.0 Hz. Eye movements in same direction as platform are compensatory. Graph shows that smooth eye movements produced by the cervico-ocular reflex have an approximately compensatory (0 deg) phase and constant gain from 0.1 to 2.5 Hz.

rate since it also occurs following plugging of horizontal semicircular canals. Figure 2 illustrates the COR that we (Baker et al., 1982) have observed in canal plugged cats. The reflex develops slowly reaching a gain of approximately 0.1 in the first month and 0.15 - 0.2 after 6 months. At the latter time, signal-to-noise ratio of the COR is sufficiently good to permit measurement of its frequency response. As shown in the figure, the COR maintained approximately compensatory phases and constant gains across the frequency range from 0.1 to 2.5 Hz, which indicates that central neuronal pathways are capable of transforming the neck afferent signal into the proper combination of eye position and eye velocity signals required to drive the oculomotor plant.

The COR can thus be viewed as a backup system which comes into play when the VOR is lost or severely reduced by lesion. Appearance of the COR does not require an alteration of ongoing discharge of semicircular canal afferents but instead appears to be caused by a gaze error signal, probably produced by the visual system as in the case of plastic changes of VOR. The same visual feedback may also serve to suppress the COR when the VOR is functioning normally.

4. VESTIBULAR AND NECK AFFERENT CONTROL OF HEAD POSITION

In addition to their connections with oculomotor nuclei, the vestibular nuclei also establish direct and indirect connections with neck motor nuclei thus constituting the neuronal substrates of a vestibulo-collic reflex (VCR, cf: Wilson and Melvill Jones, 1979). While it shares the labyrinthine receptor system with the VOR, the VCR is functionally different because it acts as a closed-loop system and because it must share control of head position with a second closed-loop, negative feedback system - the cervico-collic reflex (CCR). Thus, any head movement induced by the VCR will not only attenuate the vestibular signal that serves as input for this reflex but will also activate neck muscles via the CCR. To understand the control of head position, the two reflexes must therefore be treated together.

The interaction of the VCR and CCR is potentially exceedingly complex. Each system might be expected to have its own frequency-dependent response and the two outputs could interact and combine in a variety of ways to produce net neck motor activity. In fact, however, the neck motor system appears to be adapted to greatly simplify the mode of VCR-CCR interaction. The first simplification arises from the observation that both reflexes have essentially identical frequency responses above 0.2 Hz when measured in an open loop mode in either decerebrate (Peterson et al, 1981) or alert cats (Goldberg et al, 1981). As illustrated in Figure 3, the output of both reflexes, measured with respect to changes in head position, have frequency responses that can be approximated by a second order lead system. The time constants of the two zeros in the second order transfer functions that best fit the VCR and CCR data from individual cats are well correlated, which suggests that the output of the two reflex systems may be adapted to optimally match the passive mechanics of the head-neck system in each animal. Their similar time constants mean that the VCR and CCR will interact in a similar way at all frequencies of rotation, thus eliminating one potential source of complexity.

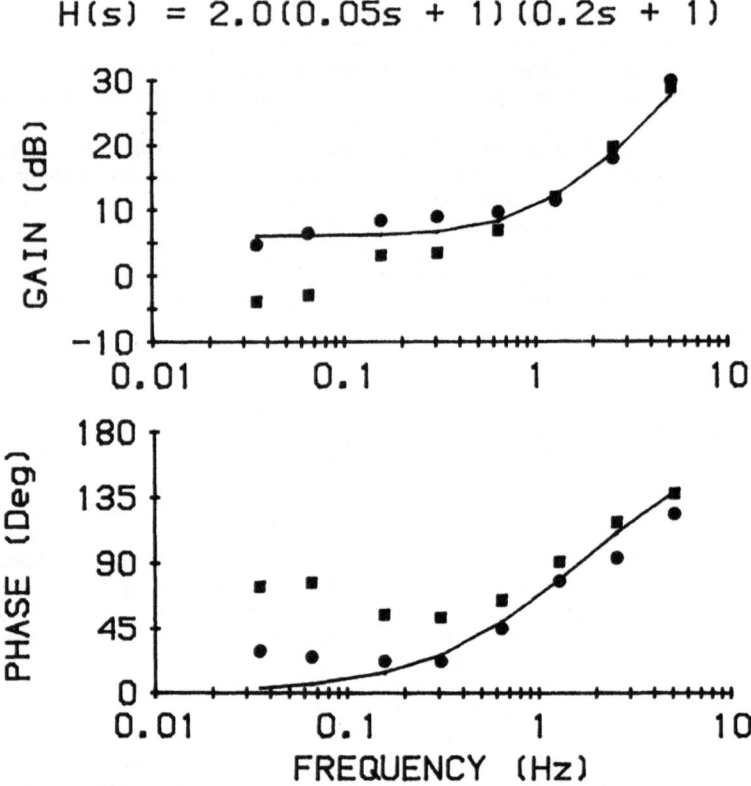

FIGURE 3. Modulation of electromyographic activity of the right complexus muscle by VCR and CCR in the same decerebrate cat. VCR (filled squares) was recorded during horizontal whole body rotation; CCR (filled circles) during horizontal rotation of the body with head held fixed in space. Stimulus in each case was the sum of 8 sinusoids with frequencies as indicated in the graph. Phase is referred to peak leftward head rotation (VCR) or rightward body rotation (CCR), so that 0 deg is compensatory. Gain is defined as percent modulation of ongoing rectified EMG activity per degree of rotation (0dB = 1% modulation/deg). Solid line shows gain and phase behavior of the second order transfer function fitted to the CCR data. Equation at top gives the transfer function in LaPlace nomenclature. Transfer function contains two zeros (frequency-dependent differentiators) with time constants of 0.05 and 0.2 sec.

A second important simplification arises from the fact that VCR—CCR interactions appear to be linear. That is, the output produced by simultaneous activation of the two reflexes is simply the sum of the output of the two systems acting alone. This is illustrated for the case of rotation of the head on a stationary trunk in Figure 4. In this situation, the VCR and CCR add linearly

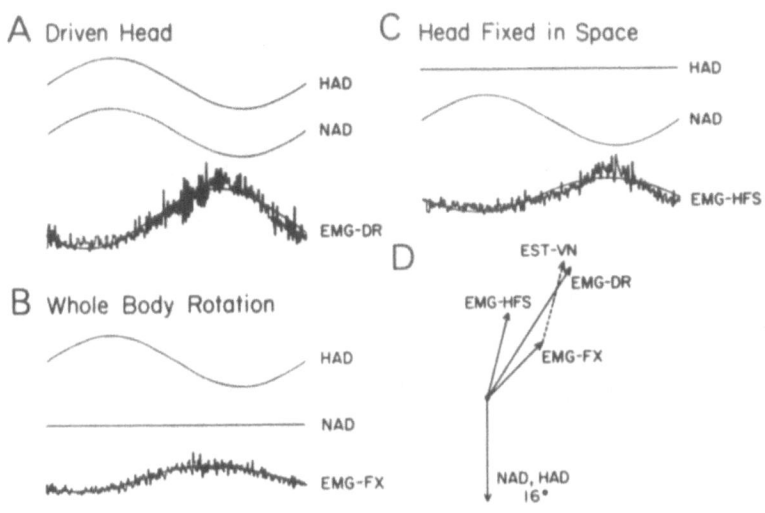

FIGURE 4. Interaction of vestibular and neck reflexes. Upper traces in A–C indicate angular deviation of the head with respect to space (HAD) and with respect to body (NAD) during three different rotational paradigms. Upward deflection indicates rightward (clockwise) rotation. Bottom traces show the averaged, rectified EMG response of the right splenius muscle together with the best fitting sinusoid at the fundamental stimulus (16 deg. 0.2 Hz sinusoid) frequency. In A, both reflexes were elicited together by rotating the head in the horizontal plane about the C_1-C_2 axis, giving rise to the EMG-DR response. In B, the same rotatory stimulus was applied to the vestibular system alone, using whole body rotation to obtain the EMG-FX response. In C, an equivalent HFS rotation was used to obtain the CCR response labeled EMG-HFS. In D, stimuli and EMG responses are represented by solid vectors with lengths proportional to amplitude and with polar angle equal to the phase of the fitted sinusoid measured from peak rightward deviation of turntable. Dotted vector EST-VN represents the vector sum of EMG-FX and EMG-HFS. Note that an increasing phase lag is plotted counterclockwise.

358

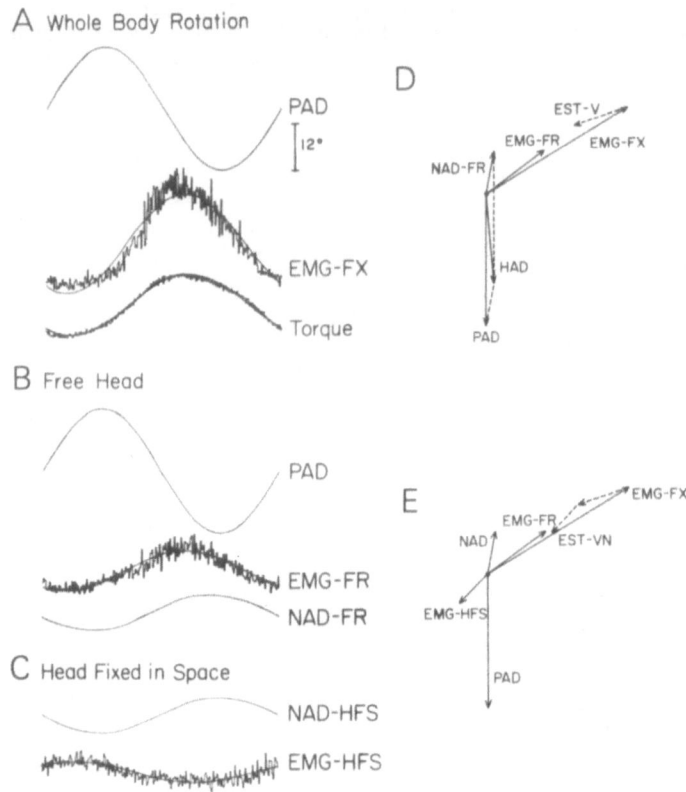

FIGURE 5. Vestibular and neck reflex contribution to the closed
loop VCR response. a) EMG activity in right splenius muscle and
horizontal head torque during 15 deg, 0.2 Hz whole body rotation
(PAD) with the head fixed to the turntable. b) Activity of the
same muscle and angular counterrotation of the head (NAD-FR) during
identical platform rotation with the head free to rotate. c) EMG
activity of the same muscle during HFS rotation with the same
amplitude and phase as NAD-FR. d) Vector diagram showing
amplitudes and phases of rotational stimuli and responses as in
Fig. 4D. Dashed lines indicate vector summation of PAD and NAD-FR
to obtain angular deviation of the head with respect to space (HAD)
during closed loop VCR. Dotted vector EST-V indicates change in
EMG response predicted as a result of the changed vestibular
stimulus in the closed loop situation. e) Similar diagram to which
the vector representing the neck reflex response (EMG-HFS) has been
added. Addition of this vector to the EST-V vector produces
EST-VN, the estimated closed loop response after compensating for
vestibular and neck reflex effects. Note the close agreement with
the measured closed loop response (EMG-FR).

to reinforce each other in damping the rotation of the head. The interaction is more complex in the case where the VCR is activated by passive body rotation. As shown in Figure 5, rotation of the body to the right induces a VCR that acts on the left neck muscles to oppose rotation of the head. When the head is restrained from the rotating, a large EMG activation occurs (A). When the head is freed, EMG activation is reduced by the closed-loop arrangement of the VCR (D) and by the opposing action of the CCR (C, E). Once again, linear summation of motor activity produced by the VCR and CCR closely predicts the neck motor output but in this case the two reflexes oppose each other, so that the overall gain of head counterrotation is reduced.

Measurements based on EMG output ignore the role played by the passive mechanical properties of the head-neck system in determining head position and leave open the possibility that these passive properties may play the dominant role in controlling head position in alert, behaving animals as suggested by Bizzi, et al (1978) for the control of voluntarily generated head movements in alert, vestibulectomized monkeys. To explore the role of reflex and passive mechanical factors in controlling head position in alert cats, Goldberg et al (1981) developed the model shown in Figure 6. The model, which is expressed as a block diagram, explores how passive rotation of the body (0) gives rise to torques (T) that act on the neck motor plant (P) to produce rotation of the head on the trunk (N). Based on measurements made in anesthetized cats, where the VCR and CCR were absent, P is modelled as a damped spring-pendulum system whose transfer function is given in LaPlace notation below the diagram. As indicated in the diagram, 0 acts on head inertia to produce a torque given by the product of head movement of inertia (I) and the second derivative of 0 (represented by s^2 in LaPlace nomenclature). The sum of 0 and N give the position of the head in space (H), changes in which generate head torques due to the VCR. Similarly, changes in N generate changes in the torque generated by the CCR. The minus signs at the summing junction indicate that inertial, VCR and CCR torques all act to oppose any change in 0, H or N respectively. Solving the block diagram gives the equation at the bottom of the figure, which relates N to 0.

We have used the model together with open loop measurements of torques produced by body rotation with the head fixed to the body or rotation of the body with the head fixed in space to analyze the role played by active (VCR and CCR) and passive elements (Is^2, Bs, K) in controlling head position during passive body rotation. The results of one such analysis are illustrated in Figure 7. The open circles indicate the head movement produced by an alert cat that was rotated in darkness using a stimulus consisting of a sum of ten sinusoids. The solid line indicates the contribution of passive elements to this response, while the crosses indicate the contribution of the active elements. At frequencies below 1 Hz, the gain of the passive term falls steeply so that head position is determined entirely by the VCR and CCR. In this case, the two reflexes have approximately equal gain, so that the transfer function reduces to N/0 = -VCR/VCR + CCR = -1/2. At higher frequencies both active and passive terms increase. Because of their differences in phase, they interact in a complex fashion to

360

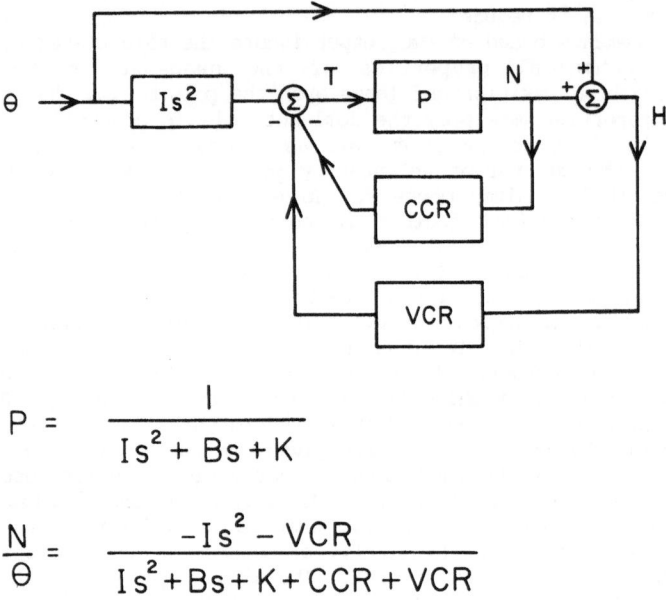

$$P = \frac{I}{Is^2 + Bs + K}$$

$$\frac{N}{\Theta} = \frac{-Is^2 - VCR}{Is^2 + Bs + K + CCR + VCR}$$

FIGURE 6. Biomechanical model of head position control system. Block diagram describes factors that determine head position during passive rotation of the body. First equation below diagram gives the transfer function of the neck motor plant. Second equation gives the overall transfer function relating rotation of the head on the body (N) to the applied rotation of the body (O). Other symbols are: B, viscosity of neck musculature; CCR, cervicocollic reflex; H, head position in space; I, head inertia; K, spring constant of neck musculature; P, neck motor plant; s, LaPlace operator; T, torque applied to head; VCR, vestibulocollic reflex.

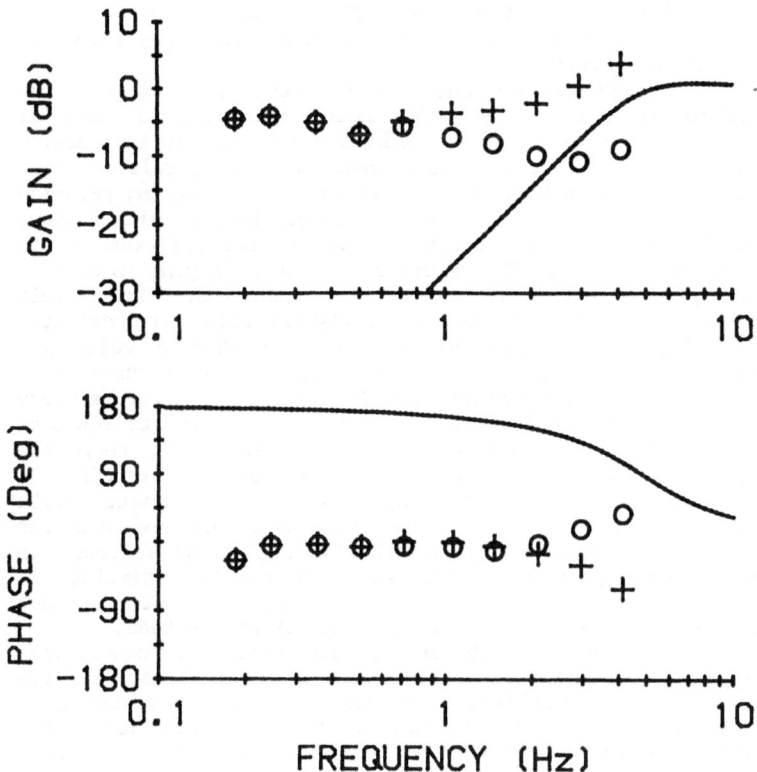

FIGURE 7. Analysis of the role played by active and passive forces in controlling head position during passive rotation of the body. An alert cat was rotated in darkness about a vertical axis passing through the C_1-C_2 vertebral joint with its head free to rotate about the same axis. Stimulus was a sum of 10 sinusoids with frequencies ranging from 0.185 to 4.1 Hz. Open circles give rotation of the head on the body recorded during 200 sec of rotation. Solid line shows contribution of passive mechanical forces; crosses indicate contribution of active forces generated by VCR and CCR to the overall response. These contributions were calculated using the model in Figure 6 and head torques measured when the same animal was subjected to an identical stimulus with its head fixed to the rotating platform or held fixed in space. Responses are plotted with respect to a perfectly compensatory neck rotation response (i.e., equal and opposite to body rotation). In this graph, such a response would have a gain and phase of 0.

determine overall head position. Eventually the passive term will approach a phase of zero and gain at one, at which point the active terms will not be necessary to stabilize the head. Our analysis indicates that this only occurs at frequencies above 10 Hz. Thus, in a normal alert animal, the VCR and CCR play the dominant role in stabilizing head position over most of the normal physiological range of head movements.

In both decerebrate and alert cats, the competitive interaction of the VCR and CCR holds the overall gain of compensatory head rotation to approximately one half during passive body rotation. Thus, it is likely that the primary role of these two reflexes is not to hold the head fixed in space during rotation of the body but rather to damp oscillation of the head with respect to a stationary body - a situation where the two reflexes act in concert as in Figure 4. The importance of such damping is seen in the canal plugged cat where the VCR is eliminated. Immediately after plugging the head becomes violently unstable and oscillates whenever displaced by passive forces or attempted voluntary movements. Head stability is regained in approximately three days. Analysis of EMG signals from neck muscles before and after recovery indicates that the animal compensates for the loss of its VCR both by co-contracting its neck muscles (thus increasing passive muscle stiffness and viscosity) and by increasing the gain of its CCR. In terms of the model shown in Figure 6, these changes would correspond to an increase in the denominator of the transfer function relating N to 0 or, in other words, to an increase in damping of head rotations. Thus, loss of the VCR stimulates a readjustment of both passive and active components of the neck motor system in order to eliminate instability of the head.

The interaction of vestibular and neck reflexes in controlling gaze may thus be summarized as follows. In a normal cat, the VCR and CCR damp out oscillation of the head and produce head counterrotations that partially compensate for the rotation of the body, while the VOR compensates for residual rotation of the head with respect to space, thus producing gaze stability. In animals with vestibular lesions such as canal plugging, the COR and CCR increase to partially compensate for the loss of vestibular reflexes and more complex predictive behaviors develop in an attempt to restore gaze stability.

*Supported by grants EY04058 & EY00231 and by funds from Bane Foundation.

REFERENCES

Anastasopoulos, D. and Mergner, T. (1982). Canal-neck interaction in vestibular nuclear neurons of the cat. Exp. Brain Res. 46: 269–280.

Baker, J., Goldberg, J., Schor, R. and Peterson, B. (1982). Oculomotor reflexes after semicircular canal plugging in cats. Soc. Neurosci. Abstr. 8, in press.

Barmack, N.H., Nastos, M.A. and Pettorossi, V.E. (1981). The horizontal and vertical cervico-ocular reflexes of the rabbit. Brain Res. 224: 261–278.

Barnes, G.R. and Forbat, L.N. (1979). Cervical and vestibular afferent control of oculomotor response in man. Acta Otolaryngol. 88: 79–87.

Bizzi, E., Dev, P., Morasso, P. and Polit, A. (1978). Effect of load disturbances during centrally initiated movements. J. Neurophysiol. 41: 542–556.

Blanks, R.H.I., Curthoys, I.S. and Markham, C.H. (1972). Planar relationships of semicircular canals in the cat. Amer. J. Physiol., 233: 55–62.

Boyle, R. and Pompeiano, O. (1979). Frequency response of characteristics of vestibulospinal neurons during sinusoidal neck rotation. Brain Res., 173: 344–349.

Brink, E.E., Hirai, N. and Wilson, V.J. (1980). Influence of neck afferents on vestibulospinal neurons. Exp. Brain Res. 38: 285–292.

Buettner, V.W., Buttner, V. and Henn, V. (1978). Transfer characteristics of neurons in vestibular nuclei of the alert monkey. J. Neurophysiol. 41: 1614–1628.

Dichgans, J., Bizzi, E., Morasso, P. and Tagliasco, V. (1973)). Mechanisms underlying recovery of eye-head coordination following bilateral labyrinthectomy in monkeys. Exp. Brain Res. 18: 548–562.

Fuller, J.H. (1980). The dynamic neck-eye reflex in mammals. Exp. Brain Res. 41: 29–35.

Furman, J.M., O'Leary, D.P. and Wolfe, J.W. (1982). Dynamic range of the frequency response of the horizontal vestibulo-ocular reflex of the alert Rhesus monkey. Acta Otolaryngol. 93: 81–91.

Goldberg, J., Bilotto, G. and Peterson, B.W. (1981). A model of the neck motor system in the alert cat. Neuroscience Soc. Abstr. 7: 482.

Hikosaka, O. and Maeda, M. (1973). Cervical effects on abducens motoneurons and their interaction with vestibulo-ocular reflex. Exp. Brain Res. 18: 512–530.

Kasai, T. and Zee, D.S. (1978). Eye-head coordination in labyrinth-defective human beings. Brain Res. 144: 123–141.

Kasper, J. and Thoden, V. (1981). Effects of natural neck afferent stimulation on vestibulo-spinal neurons in the decerebrate cat. Exp. Brain Res. 44: 401–408.

Keller, E.L. (1978). Gain of the vestibulo-ocular reflex in monkey at high rotational frequencies. Vision Res. 18: 311–315.

Lissberger, S.G. and Miles, F.A. (1981). Channels in the vestibulo-ocular reflex (VOR). Soc. Neurosci. Abstr. 7: 297.

Melvill Jones, G. and Gonshor, A. (1982). Oculomotor response to rapid head oscillation (0.5 – 5.0 Hz) after prolonged adaptation to vision reversal. Exp. Brain Res. 45: 45–58.

364

Miles, F.A. and Eighmy, B.B. (1980). Long-term adaptive changes in primate vestibulooocular reflex. I. Behavioral observations. J. Neurophysiol. 43: 1406-1425.

Peterson, B.W., Bilotto, G., Goldberg, J. and Wilson, V.J. (1981). Dynamics of vestibulo-ocular, vestibulo-collic and cervicocollic reflexes. Ann. New York Acad. Sci. 374: 395-402.

Pulaski, P.D., Zee, D.S. and Robinson, D.A. (1981). The behavior of the vestibulo-ocular reflex at high velocities of head rotation. Brain Res. 222: 159-165.

Schultheis, L.W. and Robinson, D.A. (1981). Directional plasticity of the vestibulo-ocular reflex in the cat. Ann. New York Acad. Sci. 374: 504-512.

Wilson, V.J. and Melvill Jones, G. (1979). Mammalian Vestibular Physiology, Plenum, New York.

MODIFICATION OF VOR SLOW AND QUICK COMPONENTS
BY NECK STIMULATION AND TURNING SENSATION

R. Jürgens, T. Mergner and W. Schmid-Burgk
(Sektion Neurophysiologie, Universität Ulm,
D-7900 Ulm, Federal Republic of Germany)

1. INTRODUCTION

A prominent cervico-ocular reflex (COR) can be observed in man with loss of labyrinthine function (e.g., Kasai, Zee 1978). According to Meiry (1971), a COR can also be observed in subjects (Ss) with intact labyrinths, although it is clearly weaker; the COR was found to be synergistic with the vestibulo-ocular reflex (VOR) during isolated head rotation, thus aiding stabilization of gaze in space. However, deviating results as to the direction (i.e.phase) of the COR have been reported by other authors (e.g., Barnes , Forbat 1979). Furthermore, it has been suggested in the past that the role of the neck input is mainly to reorient rather than to stabilize gaze in space, since it leads to a shift of overall eye position in the orbit ("Schlagfeldverlagerung") in the direction of head rotation (Frenzel 1928).

In a previous psychophysiological study (Nardi et al. 1981), we observed that neck stimulation also elicits prominent turning sensations. They clearly depended on the "body reference", i.e. on whether the Ss' attention was focused on their trunk in space or on their head in space. We wondered whether these different turning sensations could modify COR responses and thus explain some of the conflicting results obtained in the earlier literature. This led us to investigate quantitatively COR, VOR and the combination of both in relation to the head-in-space and trunk-in-space turning sensations.

2. METHODS

40 experiments were performed with 20 Ss. Ss were seated on a conventional Bárány chair for horizontal rotation; the head was fixed with a bite board, which was suspended from a frame pivotable with respect to the rotation chair. Four stimulus conditions were generated: Rotation of (1) whole body (labyrinthine stimulus,λ), (2) of trunk with the head remaining stationary (neck stimulus,ν), (3) of head with the trunk remaining stationary (λ,+ν), and (4) of trunk in same direction as rotation of head, but with twice the amplitude (λ,-ν). Rotation was performed sinusoidally at frequencies of 0.05 and 0.2 Hz, the peak velocity of λ and ν being 10°/sec.

Two different instructions were given to the Ss: (a) "Focus your attention on the turning of your <u>head in space</u> ("HS"-task). Estimate the magnitude of the turning sensation and signal your estimate by pressing an appropriate button on a numbered keyboard while you experience turning from right to left.", and (b) "Focus your attention on the turning of your <u>trunk in space</u> ("TS"-task). Estimate...". The estimates were to be related to a standard stimulus (λ). The estimation procedure usually guaranteed a high level of vigilance of the Ss.

Horizontal eye movements were recorded with conventional EOG and fed in a laboratory computer, together with the Ss' estimates and the

Roucoux, A. and Crommelinck, M. (eds.): Physiological and Pathological Aspects of Eye Movements.
© *1982, Dr W. Junk Publishers, The Hague, Boston, London.* ISBN-13: 978-94-009-8002-0

366

position readings of chair and head. Data analysis was performed
off-line using an interactive program, which elaborated in a
semi-automatic way the cumulative eye position separately for slow
phases (SPs) and quick phases (QPs) (for details, cf. Jürgens,
Becker 1978). Eight successive response cycles were averaged in the
0.2 Hz series and 2 cycles in the 0.05 Hz series and fitted by sine
waves. The phase and gain of these sinusoidal fits were referred to
the head-in-space (HS) position signal (stimulus conditions λ; λ,+ν;
λ,-ν) or to the head vs. trunk (HT) signal (ν-condition). Responses
elicited by the ν-stimulus were considered compensatory if they were
180° out of phase with respect to the HT signal and in phase with
the trunk-in-space (TS) signal, respectively. Also calculated was
the net displacement of the eyes in the orbit by summing the SP and
the QPs, and of gaze by further adding the HS signal.

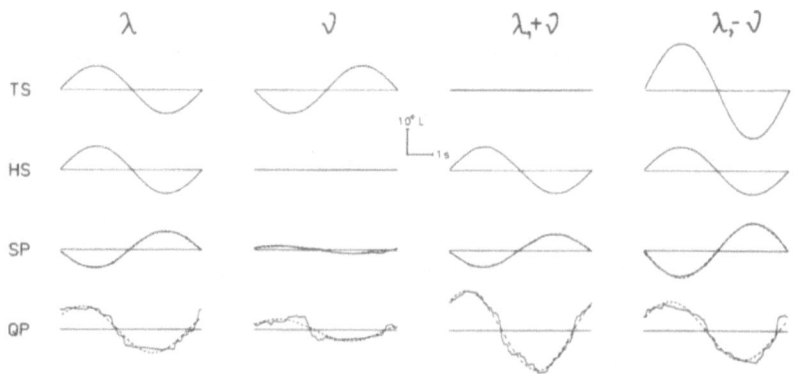

FIGURE 1. Illustration of the four stimulus conditions used and the
eye movement responses (SP and QPs) of one subject. Averages of 8
cycles; displacement left (L), upward; stimulus frequency, 0.2 Hz;
"HS"-task. Note that both SP and QPs are anticompensatory in the
ν-condition.

3. RESULTS
3.1. Turning Sensations
The turning sensations were similar to those found in previous
experiments (Nardi et al. 1981). The estimates for the TS turning
sensation, Ψ_{TS}, reflected rather well the actual trunk rotation,
i.e. $\Psi_{TS} \sim \lambda - \nu$. The estimates of the HS turning sensation, Ψ_{HS}, could
be approximated by $\Psi_{HS} \sim \lambda + a\nu$, thus they did not correspond to the
actual HS rotation (which is proportional to λ alone). The term $a\nu$
in the latter equation stands for an illusion of HS turning as it
occurred, for instance, during isolated trunk rotation (ν), where
the head, in fact, was stationary in space. In agreement with the
above equation for Ψ_{HS}, there was an increment of the magnitude
estimates with isolated head rotation (λ,+ν), and a decrement with
the reversed stimulus combination (λ,-ν).

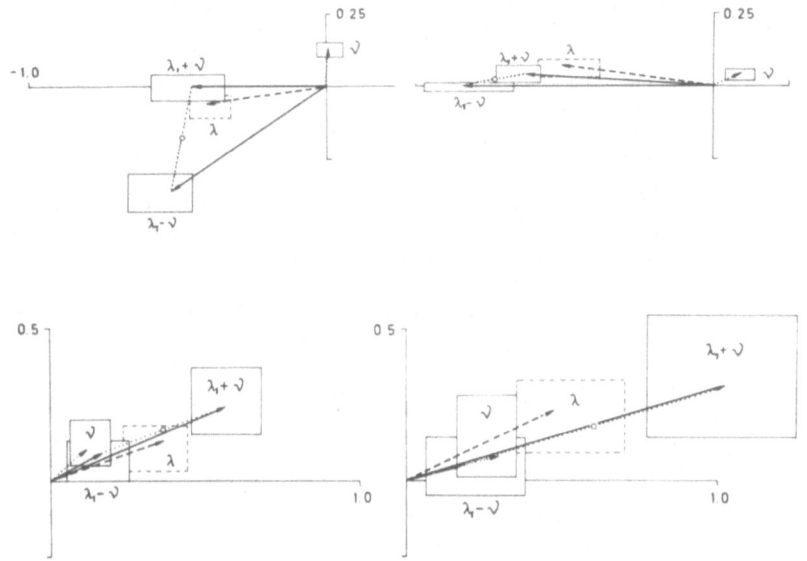

FIGURE 2. Vector plots of SPs (upper diagrams) and QPs (lower diagrams) obtained with the "HS"-task. Medians and 95% confidence ranges of 40 experiments. Stimulus frequency, 0.05 Hz (left side) and 0.2 Hz (right side). Phase lead plotted counter clockwise.

3.2. Eye Movements
3.2.1. <u>Slow Phases</u>. The SPs were basically independent from the estimation task. Thus, only responses obtained with the "HS"-task will be considered here. The corresponding median values and their 95% confidence ranges taken from 40 experiments are shown in Fig. 2 (upper diagrams).

λ-stimulation induced SPs with median gains of about 0.5 and, at 0.05 Hz stimulus frequency, with a slight phase advance relative to exact compensation of HS rotation. ν-induced SPs at 0.2 Hz stimulation frequency had a median gain of 0.1 and lagged compensation by 156° (i.e. they were roughly anticompensatory). It should be mentioned, however, that amplitude and direction of the ν-induced SPs showed considerable interindividual scatter. At 0.05 Hz, gain rose to 0.13 and phase lagged compensation by 94°.

The SP induced by the λ,+ν combination hardly differed from the λ-response. With the λ,-ν combination, by contrast, the SPs had almost 40% larger gains at both stimulus frequencies, and there was a phase lead of 35° at 0.05 Hz as compared to the pure λ-response. This asymmetric effect upon the SPs implies that the responses to combined λ- and ν-stimulations are not simply the sum of the λ- and ν-induced SPs. Consequently, the mean values calculated from the

λ,+γ and λ,-γ responses (open circles) were not identical with the actual λ-response, rather they were about 25% larger and led the λ-response in phase by about 10°. On the other hand, the difference vector between the λ,+γ and the λ,-γ responses (dotted lines) closely corresponded to twice the pure γ-response. This was consistently seen with either of the two stimulus frequencies and tasks. In contrast to the above conclusion, this would suggest that the γ-induced SPs are indeed added. A formal explanation for this contradiction is that the combination of λ- and γ-stimulations has a dual effect; one increasing the responses in gain and changing slightly their phases independently from the sign of the stimulus combination ("unspecific" effect), and the other being a linear addition of both inputs (direction specific effect).

3.2.2. <u>Quick Phases</u>. Pure λ-stimulation induced the typical "anticompensatory" QPs; they were similar with both estimation tasks as were the turning sensation. With pure γ-stimulation, by contrast, both QPs and turning sensations depended on the estimation task. With the "HS"-task, the illusion of head in space turning (ψ_{HS}~aγ) was accompanied by prominent QPs in the direction of perceived head rotation (i.e., the QPs were anticompensatory). With the "TS"-task where the turning sensation is to the opposite direction (ψ_{TS}~-γ) QPs had a reduced gain and were, in most instants, compensatory . With combined λ- and γ-stimulations, the changes of the QPs were compatible with a summation of the pure λ- and γ-responses. In particular, there were only minor changes of the QPs with the "TS"-task, while there were pronounced changes with the "HS"-task. As evident from Fig. 2 (lower diagrams), QPs obtained with the latter task were enlarged with the λ,+γ stimulus combination and diminished with the λ,-γ combination as compared to pure λ-stimulation. The amount of change corresponded approximately to the gain of the γ-induced QPs.

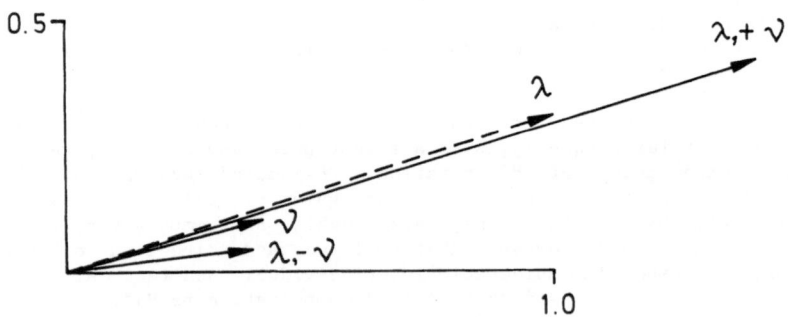

FIGURE 3. Vector plots of gaze in space obtained with the "HS"-task. Medians of 40 experiments. Stimulus frequency, 0.2 Hz.

3.2.3. <u>Gaze</u>. With pure λ-stimulation, SP and QPs had about the same amplitude. Thus, apart from some phase advance due to the QPs, the gaze was about equal to the passive displacement of head in space. This applied to either of the two tasks. The changes observed with the combined λ- and ν-stimulations were small for the "TS"-task, but pronounced for the "HS"-task. As shown in Fig. 3 for the "HS"-task and the 0.2 Hz stimulus frequency, the gaze shift in the direction of head rotation is considerable enlarged with the λ,+ν combination and reduced with the λ,-ν combination. The amount of the respective changes corresponds closely to that expected from pure ν-stimulation. A similar, but somewhat smaller effect was found at 0.05 Hz.

4. DISCUSSION

Behaviourally, neck and vestibular input may be combined in two different ways (cf. Fuller 1980): (1) Rotation of head in space with the trunk remaining stationary (λ and ν have the same direction), and (2) rotation of trunk in space with the head being partially stabilized in space by help of the vestibulo-cervical reflex (VCR) (λ is opposite to ν). A "hard wired" COR-SP adding synergistically to the VOR-SP in one condition would be antagonistic in the other. A possible solution of this dilemma could be that, depending on the particular situation, the COR-SP polarity is switched.

In our study, we tried to mimic these two behavioural situations applying both in-phase and counter phase combinations of the two inputs. We usually found a COR-SP of considerable gain mainly at the lower stimulus frequency (0.05 Hz). It hardly depended on the estimation task, and it combined with the VOR-SP such that compensation of head rotation slightly improved in the λ,+ν condition as compared to pure λ-stimulation, whereas it drastically deteriorated in the λ,-ν condition. These results indicate that the polarity of the ν-contribution is not switched according to the behavioural situation, so that its role for gaze stabilization is ambivalent. Taking also in account that the COR-SP amplitude is quite small and variable, we doubt whether the COR-SP significantly contributes to gaze stabilization, at least in healthy humans.

The COR-QPs, by contrast, did depend on the estimation task. They had a considerable gain mainly with the "HS"-task at the higher stimulus frequency (0.2 Hz) and combined linearly with the VOR-QPs. Consequently, if the head is rotated on a stationary trunk, gaze is shifted beyond the head excursion. This is in accordance with the earlier finding of Frenzel (1928), who assumed that the neck input plays a role for gaze reorientation during active as well as passive head rotation. On the other hand, when the head is turned as if to compensate for a given trunk rotation (λ,-ν), QPs are suppressed, thereby keeping gaze shifts small. In this situation, reorientation of gaze is, in fact, generally not desired.

Such modulation of the QPs clearly depended on the estimation task, which means that the cerebral cortex is involved. This raises the question how the influence upon the QPs is elaborated. Conceivably, the cortex may control the transmission from the neck to the QP generator in dependence of the body reference. Another possibility is that the QPs are elicited by the neck induced HS turning sensation and thus by the cerebral cortex itself.

REFERENCES

Barnes GR and Forbat LN (1979) Cervical and vestibular afferent control of oculomotor response in man, Acta Otolaryngol. 88, 79-87.

Frenzel H (1928) Rucknystagmus als Halsreflex und Schlagfeldverlagerung des labyrithären Drehnystagmus durch Halsreflexe, Z. Hals-Nasen-Ohrenheilk. 21, 177-187.

Fuller JH (1980) The dynamic neck-eye reflex in mammals, Exp. Brain Res. 41, 29-35.

Jürgens R and Becker W (1978) A computer program library for detecting and analyzing eye movements. BIOSIGMA 78, Vol 2. pp 187-191. Paris: Comité du Colloque International sur les Signeaux et les Images en Médecine et en Biologie.

Kasai T and Zee DS (1978) Eye-head coordination in labyrinthine-defective human beings, Brain Res. 144, 123-141.

Meiry JL (1971) Vestibular and proprioceptive stabilization of eye movements. In Bach-y-Rita P, Collins CC and Hyde JE eds. The control of eye movements, pp. 483-496. New York London, Academic Press.

Nardi GL, Mergner T, Deecke L and Becker W (1981) Vestibular-neck interaction underlying the perception of trunk and of head turning in space, Pflügers Archiv 391 (Suppl) R 30.

Supported by DFG Me 715/1-1 and Ju 163/1-1

THE RELATION OF NECK MUSCLES ACTIVITY TO HORIZONTAL EYE POSITION IN THE ALERT CAT. I: HEAD FIXED

A. ROUCOUX[1,2], P.P. VIDAL[2], C. VERAART[1,3], M. CROMMELINCK[1], A. BERTHOZ[2]

[1] Laboratoire de Neurophysiologie, University of Louvain, Brussels, Belgium.

[2] Laboratoire de Physiologie Neurosensorielle du CNRS, Paris, France.

I. INTRODUCTION

In foveate as well as in afoveate species, most displacements of the line of sight are accomplished by combined eye and head rotations. This has been demonstrated in a number of studies, among others by Bartz (1966) in man, Bizzi et al (1971) in the monkey, Gresty (1975) in the guinea-pig and Collewijn (1977) in the rabbit. Moreover, it has been shown that neck muscles are activitated in synchrony with eye saccades (Bizzi et al, 1972; Guitton et al, 1980). The torque exerted by the neck also increases together with eye saccades directed towards the ipsilateral side (Fuller, 1981). During vestibular stimulation in cats elicited by passive head rotation, Ezure and Sasaki (1978) have shown that a similar vestibular signal reached neck and eye muscles. Fuller (1981), in the rabbit, evidenced a close linkage between head torque and vestibular quick phases. Gresty (1975) had previously shown a similar phenomenon in the guinea-pig. Outerbridge and Melville-Jones (1971) in man also mentioned the same synchronization.
The aim of this study was to explore, in the alert cat, the activity of a number of neck muscles, especially small ones, in relation with eye movements induced in three conditions: spontaneous visual exploration, passive head rotation and Superior Colliculus (S.C.) microstimulation. First results obtained in head fixed animals are reported here. Some of these data have already been published (Vidal et al, 1982).

2. METHODS

Experiments were performed in alert, intact cats whose head and body were firmly restrained without signs of discomfort. Eye movements were measured with the electromagnetic technique. Calibration was performed on the anesthetized animal by rotating the field coils around the immobile eye. Moreover, the zero position of the recorded eye in its orbit was determined by bringing its visual axis into coïncidence with the field coils antero-posterior axis. The visual axis of the eye was estimated by aiming at the blind spot through an inverted image ophthalmoscope attached to the mobile field coils. Animal and field coils were placed on a turntable. Bipolar electrodes made of teflon-coated stainless steel wire were implanted chronically in a series of pairs of neck muscles. Eye movements, together with electromyograms (E.M.G.), were stored on tape for subsequent analysis.

---

[3] Research Associate N.F.S.R. Belgium

Roucoux, A. and Crommelinck, M. (eds.): Physiological and Pathological Aspects of Eye Movements.
© 1982, Dr W. Junk Publishers, The Hague, Boston, London. ISBN-13: 978-94-009-8002-0

E.M.G. could be rectified and integrated with a time constant of 10 ms. Horizontal and vertical eye position and integrated E.M.G. were sampled at a frequency of 200 Hz by
means of a LPA-11K on a PDP 11-44 computer. Eye fixations
were identified and mean value of EMG activity was computed
during these fixations. Vertical and horizontal components
of eye fixations could be plotted against EMG of left or
right muscle of a pair or the sum or difference of these
EMG's.
Eye movements were recorded in three experimental situations:
(a) during spontaneous or visually triggered exploratory
behavior; (b) during horizontal vestibular stimulation elicited by hand turning the table in a near sinusoïdal manner;
(c) during electrical microstimulation of the Superior Colliculus (S.C.). Stimulation technique and parameters were
identical to those used in previous study (Guitton et al,
1980).

3. RESULTS
Experiments were made on three cats. In one of them, 26 neck
muscles were implanted. Eight important pairs of them are
illustrated in fig.1. We shall here report results obtained
in one large muscle, the splenius, and one small muscle,
of about the size of an extraocular muscle, the obliquus
capitis cranialis. The relationship between neck E.M.G. and
horizontal component of eye movements will only be considered in this report. Analysis of data related to the vertical
component are presently in progress.
Fig.2 illustrates the activity of these two pairs of muscles
during spontaneous exploratory eye movements. Both right
splenius and obliquus muscles increase their activity in relation with eye deviation to the right. Left muscles exhibit
a reciprocal behavior. These relationships with horizontal
eye position are non linear: below a given eye eccentricity, muscles remain silent; above this threshold, muscle activity increases more or less proportionally with eye eccentricity. It is to be emphasized that the activity threshold
of a given muscle corresponds to a contralateral eye position. As a consequence, both muscles of a pair discharge
together as long as eye position remains between their respective thresholds. The threshold of the right obliquus corresponds to an eye deviation of about 4 degrees to the left
whereas the threshold of the left obliquus,to about 3 degrees to the right. This is illustrated in fig.2 by, respectively, the lower straight limit of the light hatched
areas and the upper limit of the dark hatched surfaces. The
thresholds of the splenii however, on the example shown,
are situated a few degrees in the ipsilateral half of the
oculomotor range. It is to be stressed that the activity
threshold of the splenius may vary in time within intervals
of a few minutes, whereas the threshold of the obliquus
appears to be more stable.
In order to further evaluate the proportionality of muscle
activity and eye eccentricity, beyond the threshold, we
plotted the amplitude of the rectified and integrated EMG
of the different muscles against eye position during fixation periods. The scatter of such a plot is rather high. In
order to minimize the possible effect of a variation of muscle tone , suppress the non-linearity due to thresholds and
better reflect the net balance of antagonists in a pair,
the difference between rectified and integrated EMG of both

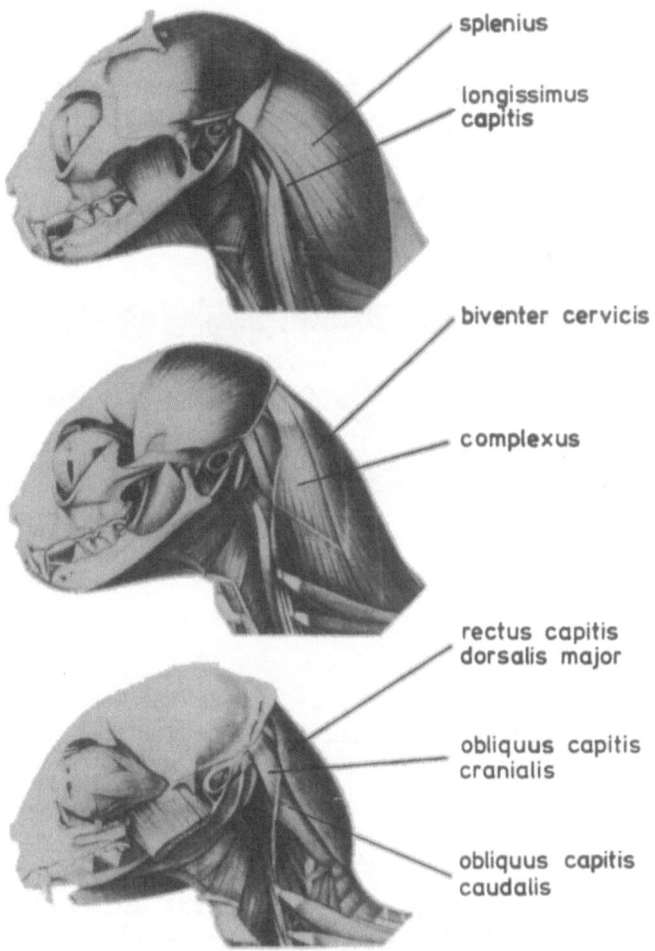

splenius

longissimus
capitis

biventer cervicis

complexus

rectus capitis
dorsalis major

obliquus capitis
cranialis

obliquus capitis
caudalis

Fig. 1. *Anatomical localization of 8 important pairs of neck muscles in the cat. Superimposed muscular layers are illustrated by three different levels of dissection. Modified from Strauss-Durckheim (1845).*

muscles of a pair was plotted against eye position. This is illustrated in fig.3 for both obliquus muscles. The relationship is almost proportional for eye positions ranging from 15 degrees to the left to 15 degrees to the right. The linear regression line is drawn. The correlation coefficient between the two variables is .82 for a sample of 802 fixations. Interestingly, this line crosses the axes close to their origin. The same relationship computed for the two splenii (not illustrated) shows a larger variability. The correlation coefficient is .59 (546 data). During vestibular stimulation, the same relationship persists, as illustrated in fig. 4. EMG of the right obliquus has been superimposed onto the horizontal eye position trace. The baseline of the EMG approximately corresponds to the muscle activity threshold. EMG of both muscles is closely related to eye position and, surprisingly, not to the vestibular signal

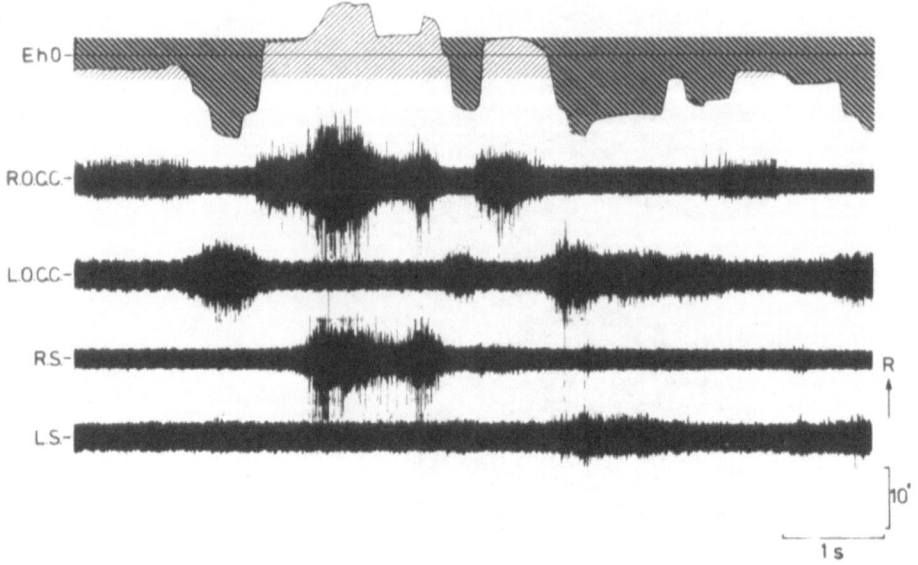

Fig.2. *Relation between EMG of the pairs of splenius (R.S. and L.S.: respectively right and left muscle) and obliquus capitis cranialis (R.O.C.C. and L.O.C.C.) and horizontal component of eye position (Eh) during spontaneous exploratory behavior.*
The dark hatched areas are delineated by the eye position trace and the activity threshold of the left obliquus, as explained in the text; the light hatched areas similarly concern the right obliquus. EhO: horizontal mid-position of the eye in the orbit; R: right deviation of the eye.

itself. No compensatory vestibulo-collic reflex (V. C. R.) appears. The two black stars indicate identical moments of two successive cycles where head velocity is close to zero and the table maximally deviated to the left: at these moments, eye position is different and muscles discharge accordingly. The same is true for the moments indicated by the white stars. In this example, muscle discharge appears to be almost exclusively modulated by eye position and not by the vestibular signal. In this recording also, thresholds of both obliquus and splenius muscles are very close to each other.
Some of us have previously shown that electrical microstimulation of the Superior Colliculus yields, together with an eye saccade, a discharge in the contralateral biventer cervicis muscle. If the stimulus is applied in the anterior collicular part, the onset of muscle discharge depends on initial eye position. We have investigated the effects of S. C. stimulation in other muscles and results obtained in obliquus and splenius are illustrated in fig. 5. A 50 ms train of stimulation was applied to the right anterior S. C. and evoked a quasi horizontal eye saccade of about 4 degrees.

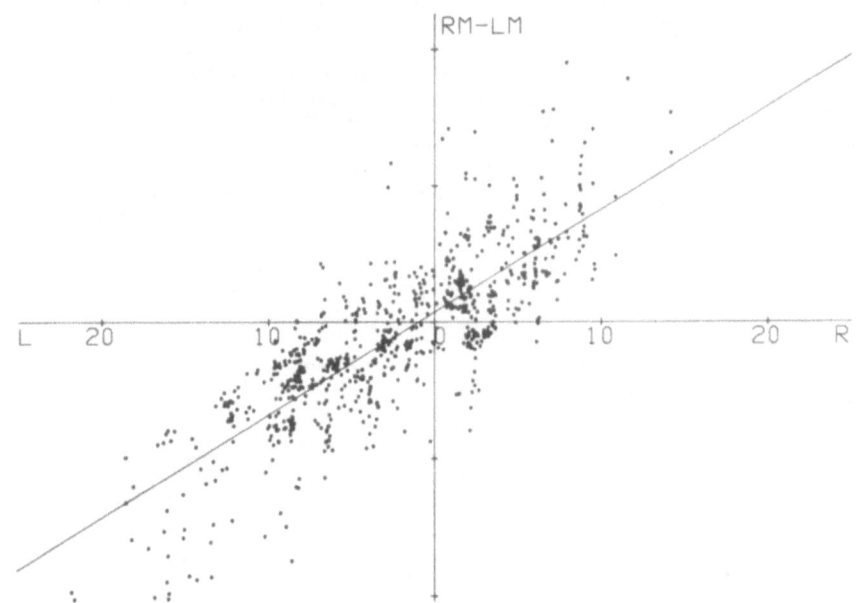

Fig. 3. *Relationship between horizontal eye position (in abscissa, L: left, R: right) and difference of right and left rectified and integrated EMG of the obliquus muscles (RM-LM, in ordinate). Eye position is calibrated in degrees. Each point represents the mean amplitude of the EMG differen- ce during fixations. The linear regression line is drawn (correl. coeff.: .82, 802 fixations).*

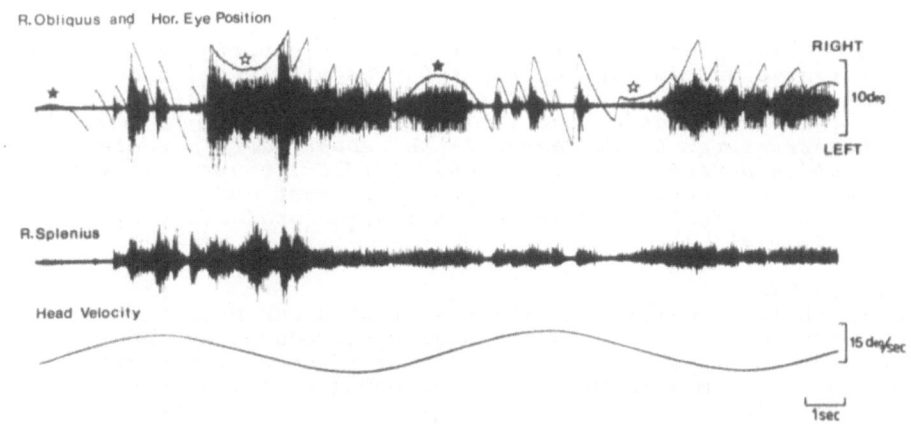

Fig. 4. *Right obliquus and splenius EMG's related to nystag- mus induced by horizontal sinusoïdal rotation of the table in the head fixed cat, in total darkness. Upward deviation of the head velocity trace corresponds to a rightward move- ment (clockwise).*

A repeated stimulation evoked a succession of retinotopic saccades as well as bursts of activity in the left muscle. As shown in the figure, the intensity of these bursts increases as the eye moves towards more eccentric positions to the left. This phenomenon clearly appears when the three successive series of stimulation are compared. Together with these phasic discharges, a tonic increase of activity, proportional to eye position, is also present. In the right muscles, the activity is antagonistic. Thresholds of right obliquus and splenius are slightly different in this example.

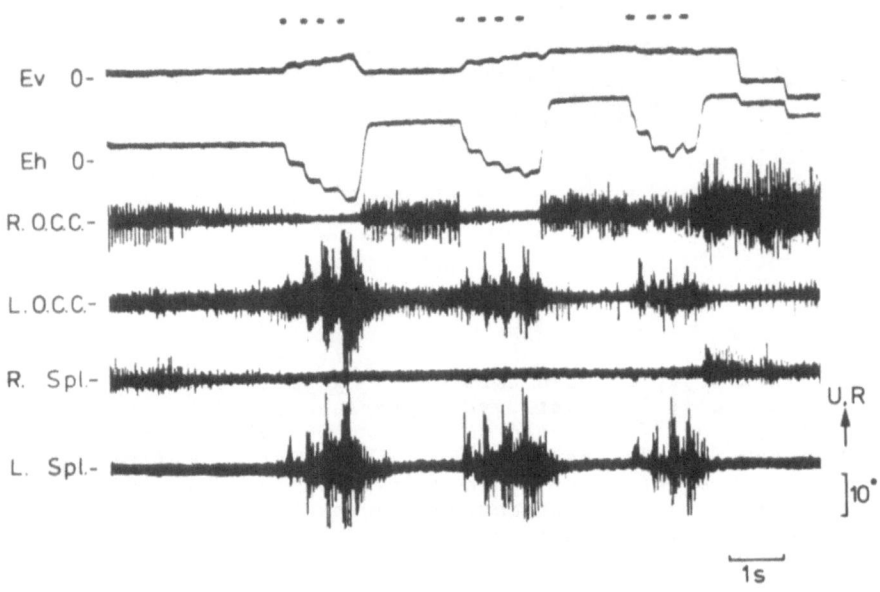

Fig. 5. *Activity of left and right obliquus capitis cranialis and splenius muscles during right Superior Colliculus deep layers microstimulation(train length: 50 ms, intensity: 60 µA). The penetration was done close to the rostral pole of the structure. Short dashes in the upper part indicate stimulation periods. R.O.C.C. and L.O.C.C.: right and left obliquus EMG traces; R.Spl. and L.Spl.: right and left splenius; Ev: vertical eye movement; Eh: horizontal eye movement; U: up; R: right.*

4. DISCUSSION

In all three conditions in which we tested our head fixed cats, neck muscle activity faithfully reproduced eye position. The activity of the two pairs of muscles illustrated here is very similar. The obliquus, however, tends to show a better relationship with eye position and a more stable threshold. The splenius behaves more like a muscle involved in neck tone and postural adjustments. Muscle pairs behave in a push-full fashion around head mid-position and the difference of EMG activity in a pair is almost linearly related to eye position up to 15 degrees of eccentricity.
In view of the previous reports of a tight linkage between eye and head movements (see introduction), these results are not surprising. Neck EMG, in our cats, behaves similarly to

head torque recorded by Fuller (1981) in alert rabbits. However, the apparent absence of a compensatory vestibulo-
collic signal in the neck muscles — the V. C. R. described by
Peterson et al (1980) and Peterson and Goldberg (this volume)
in the precollicular sectioned cat — during passive head rotations is remarkable. An explanation has been proposed
(Vidal et al, 1982) calling upon two different types of behavior. (a) When the cat is alert and visually active, the
coupling of eye and head results in a total gaze deviation
in the same direction in which the body is rotated. (b) When
the animal is not visually active or maybe not as alert,
head is stabilized with respect to external space by the
V. C. R. (eyes are stabilized by the V. O. R.) and gaze is thus
stabilized by a deviation of the line of sight in the opposite direction in which the body is turned. This hypothesis
implies the existence of a switch, enabling either the former or the latter behavior or of some sort of balance, putting emphasis on one mode rather than the other. This problem will be further discussed in the following paper
(Crommelinck et al, this volume).
The fact that S. C. stimulation evoked, in neck muscles,
bursts of activity coupled with eye saccades, modulated by a
tonic signal proportional to eye position, suggests that the
collicular command sent to the neck is adjusted according to
initial eye position. This mechanism might bring a piece of
solution to a problem already underlined by Bizzi et al (1972)
Lots of data indeed, indicate that retinal error may be
used directly to elaborate the eye saccadic command (Robinson, 1972; Schiller and Stryker, 1972; Roucoux and Crommelinck, 1976). The head motor control system, however, can
make an adequate use of the retinal error signal only if
initial eye position in orbit is taken into account. In other words, the head must receive orders in its own coordinate system (the craniotopic system) instead of a retinotopic
system. The change of coordinates might be realized by an
eye position signal permanently sent to the neck motor centers, modulating their excitability. The origin of this eye
position signal is discussed in Berthoz et al. (this volume).

5. REFERENCES
Bartz AE (1966) Eye and head movements in peripheral vision:
  nature of compensatory eye movements, Science, 152, 1644-
  1645.
Bizzi E, Kalil RE and Tagliasco V (1971) Eye-head coordination in monkeys: evidence for centrally patterned organization, Science, 173, 452-454.
Bizzi E, Kalil RE, Morasso P and Tagliasco V (1972) Central
  programming and peripheral feedback during eye-head coordination in monkeys, Bibl. Ophthal., 82, 220-232.
Collewijn H (1977) Eye and head movements in freely moving
  rabbits. J. Physiol. (London), 266, 471-498.
Ezure K and Sasaki S (1978) Frequency-response analysis of
  vestibular-induced neck reflex in cat. I. Characteristics
  of neural transmission from horizontal semicircular canal
  to neck motoneurons, J. Neurophysiol., 41, 445-458.
Fuller JH (1981) Eye and head movements during vestibular
  stimulation in the alert rabbit, Brain Research, 205,
  363-381.

Gresty MA (1975) Eye, head and body movements of the guinea pig in response to optokinetic stimulation and sinusoïdal oscillation in yaw, Pflügers Arch , 353, 201-214.

Guitton D, Crommelinck M and Roucoux A (1980) Stimulation of the superior colliculus in the alert cat. I. Eye movements and neck EMG activity evoked when the head is restrained , Exp. Brain Res., 39, 63-73.

Outerbridge JS and Melvill Jones G (1971) Reflex vestibular control of head movements in man, Aerospace Med , 42, 935-940.

Peterson BW, Bilotto G, Fuller JH, Goldberg J and Leeman B (1981) Interaction of vestibular and neck reflexes in the control of gaze. In Fuchs A and Becker W,eds. Progress in Oculomotor Research, Developments in Neuroscience, vol.12, pp. 335-342, New York, Elsevier North-Holland Biomedical Press.

Robinson DA (1972) Eye movements evoked by collicular stimulation in the alert monkey, Vision Research, 12, 1795-1808.

Roucoux A and Crommelinck M (1976) Eye movements evoked by superior colliculus stimulation in the alert cat, Brain Research, 106, 349-363.

Schiller PH and Stryker M (1972) Single-unit recording and stimulation in superior colliculus of the alert rhesus monkey, J. Neurophysiol., 35, 915-924.

Strauss-Durckheim H (1845) Anatomie descriptive et comparative du chat, T.II, Paris.

Vidal PP, Roucoux A and Berthoz A (1982) Horizontal eye position-related activity in neck muscles of the alert cat, Exp. Brain Res., 46, 448-453.

THE RELATION OF NECK MUSCLES ACTIVITY TO HORIZONTAL EYE
POSITION IN THE ALERT CAT. II: HEAD FREE

M. CROMMELINCK, A. ROUCOUX and C. VERAART [1]
Laboratoire de Neurophysiologie, University of Louvain,
Brussels, Belgium.

I. INTRODUCTION

While the preceding paper examines the activity of some neck
muscles in head fixed alert cats, this one describes first
results obtained in the head free condition. A few recordings of neck EMG have been done in free head animals.
Bizzi et al (1972) described splenius activity during orienting movements made by alert trained monkeys, showing phasi-
tonic discharges, reciprocal innervation and synchronization
of eye and neck muscles discharges. Peterson et al (1981)
studied the same muscle during passive body rotations of
precollicular-sectioned free head cats, analyzing the vestibulo-collic reflex (V.C.R.).
The question that will be addressed to here is: does the
strong correlation between eye position and neck muscles
activity, observed with head fixed, persists in the head
free condition? Is this activity translated into actual
head movement? How does the V.C.R. appear in alert cats?

2. METHODS

Methods were similar to those described in the preceding
paper. Cat's head could be freed at will while his body
was restrained in a box. Head movements were recorded with
the help of a search coil attached to the head implant,
avoiding thus any mechanical constraint. In this condition,
the signal generated by the eye coil corresponded to gaze
orientation with respect to the field coils. Eye position
in orbit was obtained by subtracting head from gaze position signals. In case of table horizontal oscillation, the
position of gaze with respect to the room was computed as
the sum of the eye coil and table position signals.

3. RESULTS

Data obtained from the obliquus capitis cranialis will be
illustrated. The relations between muscle discharge and the
different parameters (eye and head position) are complex,
both in spontaneous or evoked gaze shifts.
Fig.1 shows an example of spontaneous exploratory behavior
in the light. Several observations can be made. (a) Eccentric positions of the head correspond to tonic discharges
of the muscles. This is particularly clear, in the example
shown, for the left obliquus (arrow 1). (b) Rapid changes
of head position are accompanied by phasic discharges (arrow 2).(c) Phasic discharges accompany most of the eye saccades. These saccades are most often in the same direction
as the ongoing head movement (arrows 3). (d) In some cases,

---

1 Research Associate N.F.S.R. Belgium

Roucoux, A. and Crommelinck, M. (eds.): Physiological and Pathological Aspects of Eye Movements.
© 1982, Dr W. Junk Publishers, The Hague, Boston, London. ISBN-13: 978-94-009-8002-0

the eye compensates for the head movement (arrow 4) and is driven in the direction opposite to the head: in this case, neck muscle activity is dissociated from eye position, but correlates well with head position. On fig.2 is represented a sample of visual scanning behavior. A piece of food was moved horizontally from left to right and vice-versa in front of the animal. The "pursuit" movement is characterized by: (a) a rather smooth alternating head movement, the velocity of which is modulated in synchrony with eye saccades; (b) series of eye saccades interspersed with compensatory movements.

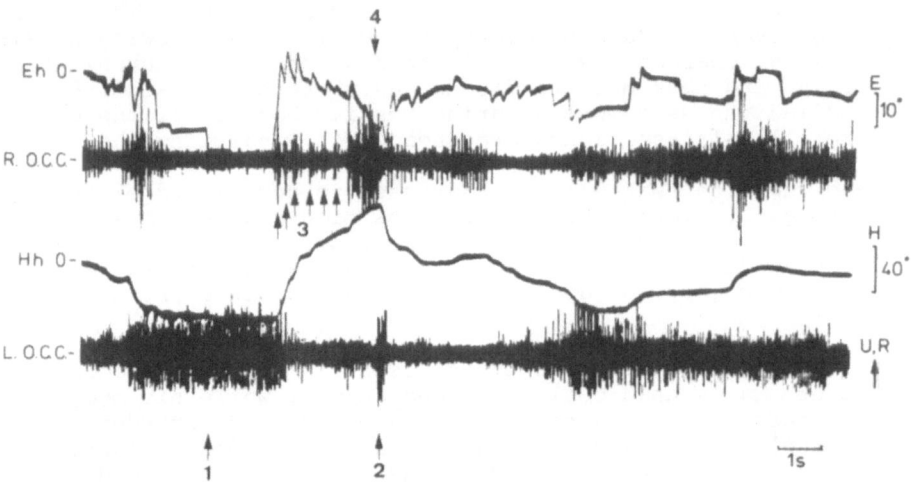

Fig.1. *Activity of right (R.O.C.C.) and left (L.O.C.C.) obliquus capitis cranialis muscles during spontaneous visual exploratory behavior of a head free alert cat. Eh: horizontal eye movements; Hh: horizontal head movements; R:right. Amplification of the eye position signal is 3 times higher than head's signal. Arrows point at particular events described in text.*

Gaze is characterized by a series of successive short fixations. The difference between the integrated activity of right and left obliquus muscles has been computed and represented on the third trace (R.O.C.C.-L.O.C.C.). The horizontal line (0) corresponds to an equal activity in both muscles, an upward deviation indicates a pre-eminence of the right muscle; the total amplitude is arbitrary. The muscle activity, besides showing a relationship with head position, is modulated by phasic elements: eye saccades and corresponding accelerations of the head. Gaze shifts are thus characterized by EMG bursts. During fixation periods, muscle activity decreases, often together with the eye compensatory movement. The consequence of the alternation of phasic discharges — linked to saccades — and decreases of activity — linked to gaze fixations — is that the muscle activity trace shows a "phase lead" of about 45 deg with respect to head position, the "periodic" movement of which occurs at a frequency of about 0.4 Hz.

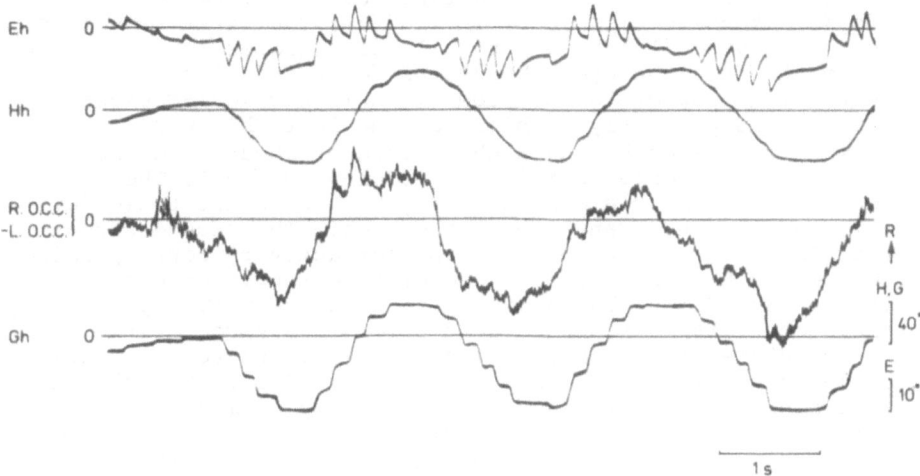

Fig.2. *Difference of rectified and integrated EMG's of right and left obliquus muscles (R.O.C.C.-L.O.C.C.) during visual scanning. Horizontal lines indicate zero horizontal position of eye (Eh), head (Hh) and gaze (Gh) and the EMG baseline.*

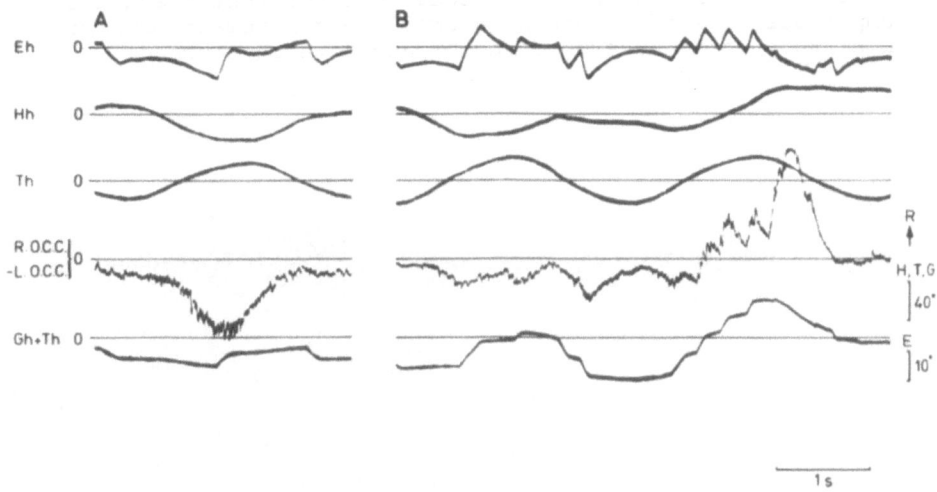

Fig. 3. *Difference of rectified and integrated EMG's of right and left obliquus muscles (R.O.C.C.-L.O.C.C.) of a head free alert cat during body horizontal oscillation. A: example of vestibulo-collic compensation. B: abolition of vestibulo-collic reflex by active visual exploration. Th: table horizontal position; Gh + Th: horizontal gaze position with respect to the room.*

During vestibular and optokinetic stimulation, induced by
horizontal body rotation in a textured visual background,
two situations could occur. In fig. 3A, the first situation
is illustrated. The head partially compensates for the table
movement while the eye compensates for residual head movements with respect to the room. In this particular example,
gaze is not perfectly stabilized. The left obliquus muscle
shows a discharge having a phase lead of about 30 degrees
(frequency of table oscillation is about 0.3 Hz). The absence of a right muscle discharge may be due to the tonic deviation of both head and eye to the right. The second situation is shown in fig.3B. The muscular activity corresponding
to the V.C.R., as described above, is strongly attenuated
in the first illustrated cycle and completely disappears in
the second. It is replaced by a strong discharge of the
right muscle corresponding to an anti-compensatory deviation
of the head. Moreover, this discharge is clearly modulated
in synchrony with eye saccades. Gaze displacement is anticompensatory and looks very similar to the active scanning
behavior shown in fig.2. This sequence ends up with a drift
of gaze, maybe caused by a mechanical limitation of head
movement. Situation A was observed when the animal's level
of alertness was rather low. On the other hand, situation B
prevailed when the cat was fully alert and visually explored
its environment.
Electrical stimulation of the Superior Colliculus (S.C.) was
also applied in the head free situation. An example is shown
in fig.4. The microelectrode was positioned very rostrally
in the S.C. and the evoked saccade was horizontal and had an
amplitude of a few degrees. A small head movement of similar
amplitude was also evoked, accompanying each saccade.

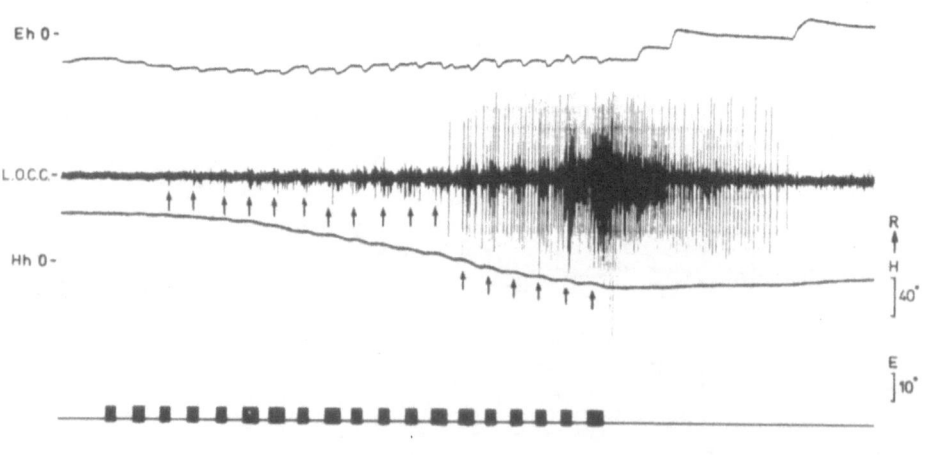

Fig.4. *EMG of left obliquus muscle together with horizontal
eye and head movements evoked by microstimulation of the
right Superior Colliculus anterior zone. Bottom trace indicates periods of stimulation. Arrows indicate muscle discharges synchronous to evoked eye saccades.*

As illustrated, repeated stimulation yields a total head displacement of 60 degrees. The left obliquus exhibits small phasic discharges (arrows) evoked by each stimulus, the amplitude of which progressively increases with head deviation. When the head attains its mid-position, a large motor unit is recruited and also discharges phasically. Other units are further recruited for more eccentric eye positions. Moreover, a tonic activity also appears at these eccentricities. At the end of the stimulation period, the head remains almost stationary and muscle activity decreases, to cease when the eye crosses its mid-position.

4. DISCUSSION

The relationship between neck muscles activity and eye and head movements cannot be simply described. Our preliminary analysis of the data shows that obliquus EMG activity appears to be first of all linked to phasic events: changes of head position but also eye saccades. Most of the time, as already underlined by Bizzi et al (1972) and also by Fuller (1981), head movements during visual scanning are "modulated" by eye saccades. Neck EMG clearly reflects this modulation and even sometimes magnifies it. It thus seems that the rather tight linkage of eye and head movements observed in head fixed condition subsists when the head actually moves. However, there are instances when this linkage fades away. This may occur during spontaneous head movements or passive body rotations. For instance, during table oscillations in the light, the V.C.R. either is present, sometimes with a gain close to 1 - the phase of muscle discharge is similar to that shown by Peterson et al (1980) —, or, when the animal seems to be "visually attentive", the V.C.R. is almost completely overshadowed by anti-compensatory movements, synchronized with eye saccades. The choice, again, seems to be between a "stabilizing" behavior or an "orienting" behavior. These data obtained with head free tend to support the hypothesis put forward in the preceding paper (Roucoux et al, this volume): the eye position signal may be sent or not to head motor centres.

S.C. stimulation experiments show results similar to those obtained with head fixed. Retinotopic saccades evoked in the anterior zone of cat's S.C. are accompanied by small head movements (Roucoux et al, 1980). These head movements shortly follow bursts of activity in the obliquus muscle. These bursts are modulated by initial eye position. This fact was interpreted in the preceding paper as a possible mechanism of change of coordinates from a retinotopic to a craniotopic system. However, with head free, all evoked head movements are similar in amplitude; but, as each eye saccade is followed by a compensatory drift back of about the same amplitude, the resulting displacement of the eye is negligible. Consequently, it is very difficult, in head free conditions, to demonstrate an influence of eye position on neck muscle activity. Our stimulation data presently do not bring any argument in favor or against the hypothesis of a change of coordinates in the head motor command.

The posterior zone of S.C. where saccade organization is different (craniotopic) has also been explored. Data are presently analyzed and will be reported later.

5. REFERENCES

Bizzi E, Kalil RE, Morasso P and Tagliasco V (1972) Central
 programming and peripheral feedback during eye-head coordination in monkeys, Bibl. Ophthal., 82, 220-232.

Fuller JH (1981) Eye and head movements during vestibular
 stimulation in the alert rabbit, Brain Research, 205, 363-
 381.

Peterson BW, Bilotto G, Fuller JH, Goldberg J and Leeman B
 (1981) Interaction of vestibular and neck reflexes in the
 control of gaze. In Fuchs A and Becker W, eds. Progress in
 Oculomotor Research, Developments in Neuroscience, vol.12,
 pp. 335-342, New York, Elsevier North-Holland Biomedical
 Press.

Roucoux A, Guitton D and Crommelinck M (1980) Stimulation of
 the Superior Colliculus in the alert cat. II. Eye and head
 movements evoked when the head is unrestrained, Exp.Brain
 Research, 39, 75-85.

BRAIN STEM NEURONS MEDIATING HORIZONTAL EYE POSITION
SIGNALS TO DORSAL NECK MUSCLES OF THE ALERT CAT

A. BERTHOZ, P.P. VIDAL, J. CORVISIER
Laboratoire de Physiologie Neurosensorielle du CNRS,
Paris, France

I. INTRODUCTION
It is well known that neck muscles are important not
only to allow volontary head movements but also to
stabilize the head in space and provide an adequate
setting of postural reflexes (Magnus, 1924; Rademaker, 1931). In the last ten years a number of studies have been devoted to the basic synaptic organisation of pathways controlling neck muscles. In the
cat most studies focused on the vestibular control
of neck muscles (Berthoz and Anderson, 1971; Ezure
and Sasaki, 1978; Peterson, see review in this volume) using the decerebrate preparation in which vestibular reflexes are free from cortical inhibition.
These studies lead to privilege the role of compensatory vestibular mechanisms (neck muscles pulling the
head in a direction opposite to head displacement).
By contrast a number of studies in the alert monkey
(Bizzi et al, 1971; Lestienne et al, 1981), rabbit
(Fuller, 1980 and 1981; Collewijn, 1977), and cat
(Roucoux et al, 1980; Guitton et al, 1980), stressed
the tight synergy between eye and head displacement
during volontary or evoked coordinated eye-head orienting movements. It therefore appears that neck muscles are controlled by distinct mechanisms which come
into play depending upon the strategy and purpose of
the movement.
The detailed neuronal organization subserving the
synergistic action of eye and head muscles is however
not known. Bender (1955), after several authors, hypothesized the presence, in the brain stem, of an "eye
centering system" whose operation required a close
cooperation between eye and head motor mechanisms.
The neuronal network for this system was supposed to
be around the abducens nucleus, in the area also
known as the "parabducens area" (see review in Baker
and Mc Crea, 1979).
More recently Bizzi et al (1972) hypothesized that a
parallel gaze signal was sent to eye and neck muscles
by a central generator leaving to peripheral sensory
feedback the role of adjusting reflexly the respective
positions of eye and head.
The recent finding of Vidal et al (1982) who showed
that in dorsal neck muscles of the cat the EMG is
tightly linked with the horizontal component of eye
position, suggests that eye position signals are carried to neck motoneurons by descending pathways. We
were therefore encouraged to search for neurons in the
brain stem mediating this effect and have recorded

Roucoux, A. and Crommelinck, M. (eds.): Physiological and Pathological Aspects of Eye Movements.
© 1982, *Dr W. Junk Publishers, The Hague, Boston, London.* ISBN-13: 978-94-009-8002-0

from reticular neurons in the periabducens area which
are candidates to project to neck muscles. In the present paper, we shall report new results concerning
reticular neurons and abducens motoneurons, and review, for the sake of comparison, some previous results concerning second order vestibular neurons (from
Berthoz et al, 1981).

2. METHODS
2.1. Preparation, stimulation and recording conditions
Experiments were performed on adult alert cats. Eye
movements were recorded with the search coil technique
with coils implanted chronically on the eye ball.
Identification of abducens motoneurons and abducens
nucleus field potential profiles were obtained by
antidromic stimulation of the VIth nerve with chronically implanted bipolar stimulating electrodes placed
near the nerve as it exits from the brain stem.
An opening of about 5mm in diameter was made in the
occipital bone and a funnel shaped chamber was formed
with dental cement. This chamber allowed penetration
of the brainstem through the cerebellum with glass
microelectrodes (1 to 1.5 µ tip) filled with NaCl.
Electromyographic (EMG) bipolar electrodes made of
stainless steel wire were implanted chronically in
various neck muscles (Splenius, Longissimus capitis,
Obliquus capitis cranialis and caudalis).
The head of the cat was fixed on the stereotaxic frame which was itself attached to a turntable. The head
of the animal was placed at a 25° nose down position.
The animal was completely alert and gently restrained with a cloth and elastic bandage.
Vestibular nystagmus could be induced by sinusoidal
rotation of the turntable in total darkness. Optokinetic stimulation could be added by rotation in the
light.
2.2. Data processing
Mid-position of the eye in the orbit was calculated
by averaging the results of two independent measurements:
a) the oculomotor range over a recording session of
about one hour was displayed on a memory oscilloscope
and mid-position was defined as the mean of extreme
horizontal eye movements.
b) the computer calculated mean value of the same
sample.
EMG was integrated with an analog integrator (5 msec
time constant). The integrated signal was sampled by
the computer for further processing. Instantaneous
firing rate of neuronal activity was calculated by
the computer with a time resolution of 10 µ sec.
Reticular neurons whose activity is reported here
were identified by their location with respect to the
antidromic field potential of the VIth nucleus. This
electrophysiological method has the advantage to allow numerous recording sessions in a single animal

and clearly establishes when a neuron is outside of
the boundaries of the VIth nucleus. (The field potential profile extends approximately 300 to 500 µ outside of the actual histological boundary of the abducens nucleus).

3. RESULTS
Whe shall report here only typical examples of the
results obtained. Full reports of the results will be
published elsewhere (Berthoz et al, 1982; Vidal et
al, in preparation). The behavior of respectively
abducens motoneurons, second order vestibular neurons, and dorsal neck motoneurons will be considered
in the following sections.

3.1. Relationship between neck muscle activity and
abducens motoneurons.
We have recorded simultaneously the vertical and horizontal components of eye movements, the extracellular activity of abducens motoneurones and neck
muscles EMG. Fig.1 illustrates a typical example of
recording. The firing of the motoneuron parallels
the firing of the ipsilateral longissimus muscle. It
is however interesting to note that in the EMG trace
of this record the large motor unit which overrides
the right EMG is not representative of the whole
pool of motoneurones. It fires when the eye is more
eccentric in the orbit than when the EMG actually
appears. The fact that motor units were recruited
at different eccentricities in the orbit was already
shown by Vidal et al (1982).
In order to define more precisely the relationship
between these neurons and eye movement we have plotted firing rate versus eye position. Fig.2A shows
another example of the records from the same neuron
as in fig.1. On fig.2B the rate-position curve for
the motoneurons is plotted (threshold with respect
to horizontal component of eye position: 5.9 degrees
to the right, slope 4.8 spikes per second per degree).
We were able to simultaneously record the activity
of two isolated motor units belonging to antagonistic
muscles. We have calculated the relationship between
their firing rate and horizontal eye position (fig.2C)
The noteworthy fact is that their firing rate is
proportional to the horizontal component of eye position in a range extending to about 15 degrees. Above
this value recruitement of other motor units preclu-
ded calculation of the firing rate. The threshold
with respect to horizontal eye position is .8 degrees
to the right and 1 degree to the left, the rate-position slopes are 3.9 and 3.7 spikes per second per
degree. They are therefore arranged in a push-pull
fashion with respect to the mid-position of the eye
in the orbit.
These data provide two results: first, the firing
frequency of at least some individual motor units

388

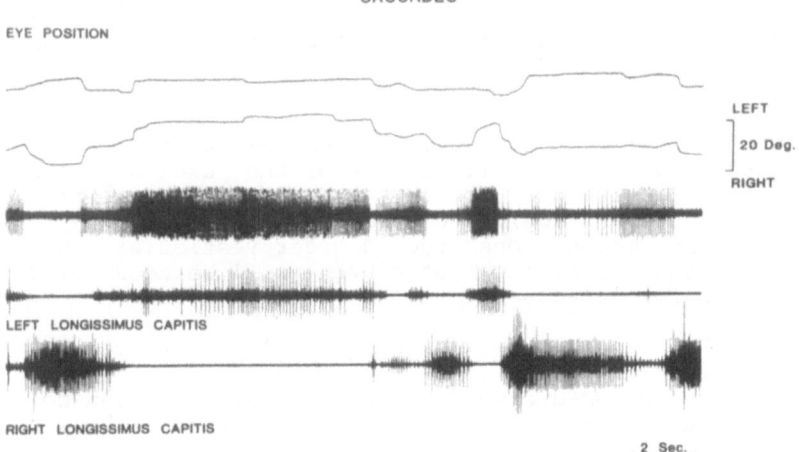

SACCADES

EYE POSITION

LEFT

20 Deg.

RIGHT

LEFT LONGISSIMUS CAPITIS

RIGHT LONGISSIMUS CAPITIS

2 Sec.

Fig.1. *Simultaneous recording of eye movement, dorsal neck muscle activity and firing of an abducens moto- neuron in the alert cat. From top to bottom: -Vertical and horizontal components of eye angular displacement.-Extracellular recording from an abdu- cens motoneuron.-EMG of left and right longissimus capitis muscles.*

in neck muscles is linearly related with ipsilateral horizontal angular eye position up to eccentricities of about 15 degrees with a threshold which is around mid-position in the orbit; second, they show that comparison of latencies of firing between abducens and neck motoneurons has no meaning because neck mo- toneurons firing is determined mainly by an <u>eye posi- tion threshold.</u>

3.2. <u>Are second order vestibular neurons candidates to carry eye position signals to neck muscles?</u>

Second order vestibular neurons which terminate in the abducens nucleus also give collaterals to the spinal cord (Yoshida et al, 1980; Mc Crea et al, 1981; Berthoz et al, 1981). Is has been shown that all type I neurons of this kind code the horizontal component of eye position during spontaneous fixation saccades. All the recorded neurons terminating in the contrala- teral abducens nucleus, in addition to collaterals branching in the periabducens area, prepositus hypo- glossi and contralateral vestibular nuclei, <u>send long collaterals to the spinal cord.</u> They therefore are good candidates to mediate eye position signals to neck motoneurons. Fig. 3 shows an example of such neuron (from Berthoz et al, 1981). During rotation in darkness it behaves like a typical type I vestibu-

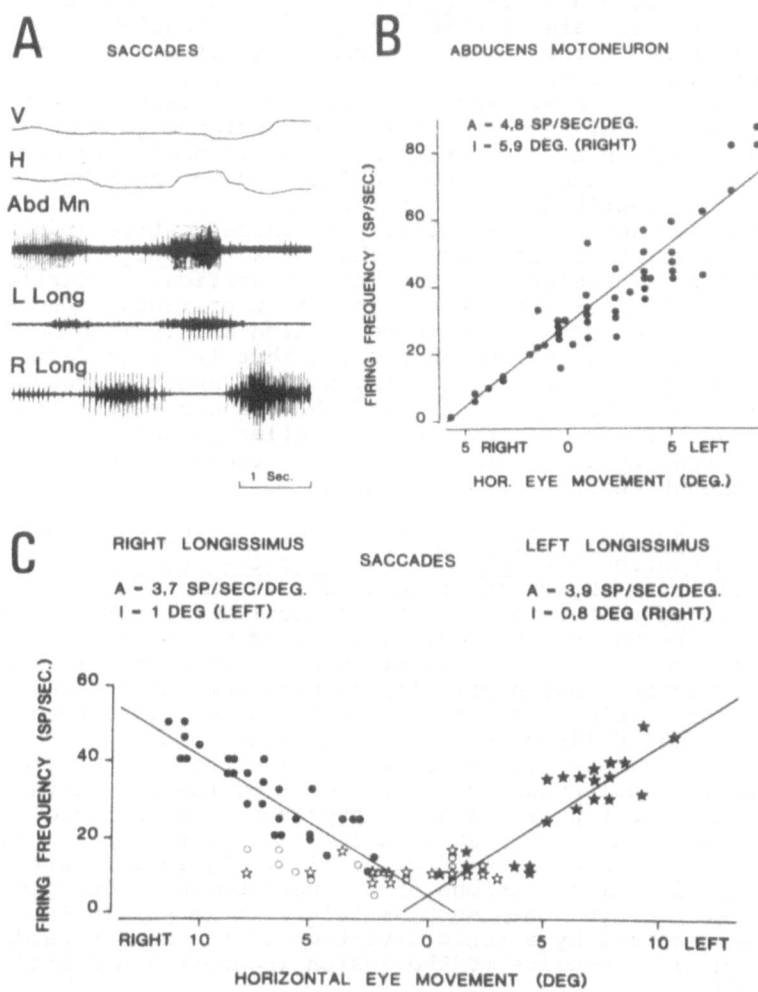

Fig.2. *Firing characteristics of an abducens motoneuron and two motor units of left and right longissimus
capitis muscles recorded simultaneously in an alert
cat.*
A- same records as in fig.1
*B- rate position curve for the abducens motoneuron. A
is the slope in spikes per second per degree and I,
the intercept of the regression line with the abscissa.
C- rate position curve for two isolated motor units
belonging respectively to the left (stars) and right
(dots) muscles. Unfilled stars and dots indicate firing
frequencies measured at the threshold when the motor
unit stops firing during the same fixation.*

lar neuron. Notice the large amplitude of the modulation in phase with <u>head velocity</u> (fig.3B and C).
The firing rate of this neuron can be modulated in
addition by the horizontal component of eye position
(fig.3A) and to a lesser degree by eye velocity.
Several arguments speak against the suggestion that
this type of neuron is the best candidate to provide
the horizontal eye position signal to neck motoneurons. (Although they are well suited to contribute
to the vestibulo-collic reflex).
The eye position sensitivity of these vestibular neurons is small compared to their head velocity sensitivity. Therefore if they had a significant synaptic
input to neck motoneurons in our experimental condition, the neck EMG would be related mainly with head
velocity, however we have shown that it is in fact
roughly related to the eye position. Another argument
is that Peterson et al (1980) have shown that the
phase of the vestibulo-collic reflex is not modified
by transection of the medial longitudial fasciculus
through which their axons descend.

3.3. Are reticular neurons in the periabducens area and pontine reticular formation better candidates?

All these objections focused our attention to another
area of the brain stem: the reticular formation below
and around the abducens nucleus. Peterson et al (1978)
had shown that subpopulations of neurons in this area
terminate monosynaptically on neck motoneurons and
particularly the dorsal part of nucleus gigantocel-
lularis. Cells of origin of the medial (and part of
lateral) reticulo-spinal tracts located in this area
receive polysynaptic activation from the labyrinth
and exhibit phase lagging responses similar to neck
muscles during galvanic vestibular stimulation in the
decerebrate cat (Peterson et al, 1975, 1980). Furthermore localized lesions of the periabducens zone give
specific syndromes such as lateral gaze paralysis
accompanied by a tonic deviation of the head towards
the side opposite to the lesion (Bennett and Savill,
1889).
These facts prompted our study of reticular neurons
in this area. We searched particularly for neurons
having a tight coupling of their firing discharge
with dorsal neck EMG in the alert head fixed cat.
Fig.4 illustrates a typical example of recordings
concerning a cell located below the abducens nucleus
at a depth of about 2mm. Traces show the vertical and
horizontal components of eye position, firing rate
of the neuron and EMG of left and right obliquus capitis muscles. The discharge rate of the neuron is
clearly related to the ipsilateral obliquus capitis
muscle EMG. Its firing frequency also follows horizontal eye position.
In order to analyze more quantitatively the behavior
of the neurons, instantaneous firing rate and inte-

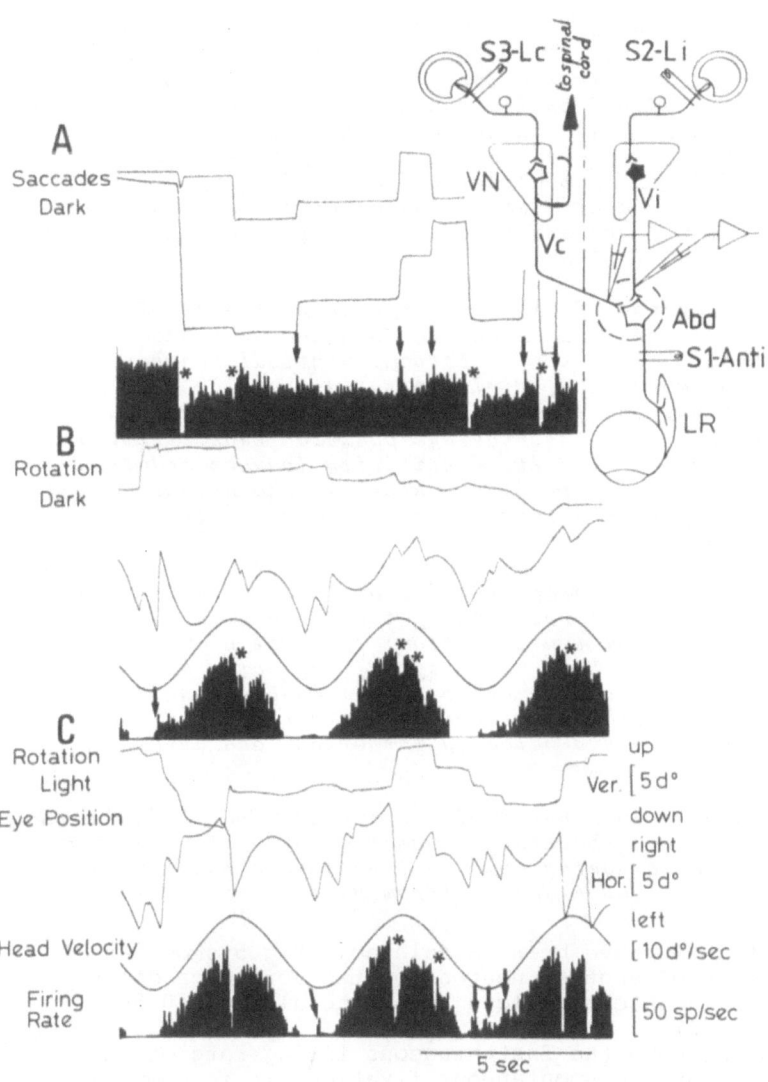

A
Saccades
Dark

B
Rotation
Dark

C
Rotation
Light

Eye Position

Head Velocity

Firing
Rate

S3-Lc   to spinal cord   S2-Li

VN   Vi

Vc

Abd

S1-Anti

LR

up
Ver. [5 d°
down

right
Hor. [5 d°
left
[10 d°/sec
[50 sp/sec

5 sec

Fig.3. *Intra-axonal recording of second order ves-*
tibular neurons in the alert cat.
Schema of the experimental paradigm. Stimulation and
recording sites. Stimulating electrodes (S2, S3)
are implanted in the ipsi (Li) and contralateral (Lc)
labyrinth for identification of second order vestibu-
lar nucleus (VN) neurons by orthodromic stimulation.
The intracellular recording site of the axons of
ipsi (Vi) or contralateral (Vc) projecting vestibular
neurons is identified in the abducens nucleus with
the help of the antidromic stimulation of the abdu-
cens nerve (S1-Anti).

A. Comparison of the discharge characteristics of a
second order Vc axon during spontaneous saccades and
nystagmus. From top to bottom: vertical and horizon-
tal eye movements, firing rate averaged over 50 mse-
cond bins. The figure shows a series of fixations in
darkness. Note that the eye position sensitivity and
saccadic eye velocity sensitivity (pauses and tran-
sient increases shown by asterisks and arrows during
off- and on direction saccades) occur in the absence
of visual input.

B. Discharge characteristics of the same neuron du-
ring sinusoidal rotation of the table at 0.2 Hz in
darkness. From top to bottom: vertical and horizontal
eye position, head velocity, firing rate. Note that
superimposed on the clear type I modulation in phase
with head velocity, there is a clear eye position
and saccadic eye velocity (asterisks and arrows)
sensitivity.

C. Same as in B but during sinusoidal rotation in the
illuminated laboratory (summation of vestibular and
optokinetic nystagmus). Calibrations shown here are
also valid for A and B. (From Berthoz et al, 1981).

grated EMG have been calculated. Fig.5 shows an
example of another neuron located ventro-caudally
to the abducens nucleus at a laterality of 0.8mm
(fig. 5B).
Fig.5A shows the instantaneous firing rate of the
neuron during spontaneous fixation. It is compared
with the integrated EMG of the ipsilateral longissimus capitis muscle. This neurons has a phasic discharge during saccades directed towards the ipsilateral side and a tonic component related to eye position. The instantaneous firing rate is clearly
correlated with ipsilateral neck EMG. This close
similarity between the two patterns of firing is
even more evident in fig.4C during vestibular nystag-

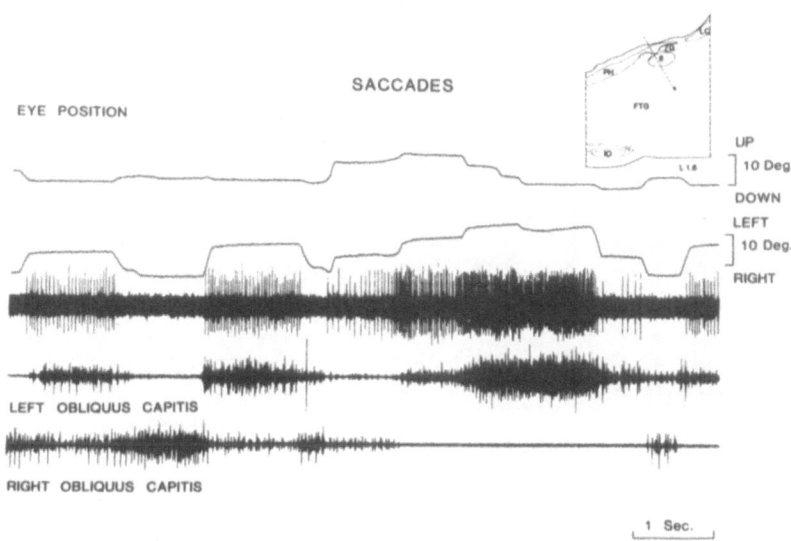

Fig.4. *Recording from a reticular neuron whose firing rate is related to neck EMG and horizontal eye position. The insert indicates the location of the neuron in the left brainstem. The dashed line indicates the electrode tract through the VIth nucleus. From top to bottom:*
- vertical and horizontal components of eye angular position
- extracellular recording of the reticular neuron
- EMG of respectively left and right obliquus capitis muscles.

mus. Mid-position of the eye in the orbit is indicated by the dashed line. Both the firing rate of the neuron and longissimus capitis EMG vary together with horizontal eye position. In our study we have encountered two extreme types of cells. The first type was mainly "tonic" (see classification in Robinson, 1981), it has a discharge rate related to the horizontal component of eye position, an absence of burst of discharge during rapid eye movements. These neurons sometimes paused during contralateral eye movements, and had a negative eye velocity sensitivity during contralateral eye movements. A second type was "burst-tonic". The discharge rate was modulated in relation with the horizontal component of eye position, with in addition, bursts during ipsilateral rapid eye movements but no pause during contralateral eye movements. These two groups of cells have been found in the reticular formation in an area roughly located at a depth of 1.3 to 3.3 mm beneath the abducens nucleus and anteroposterior coordinates (according

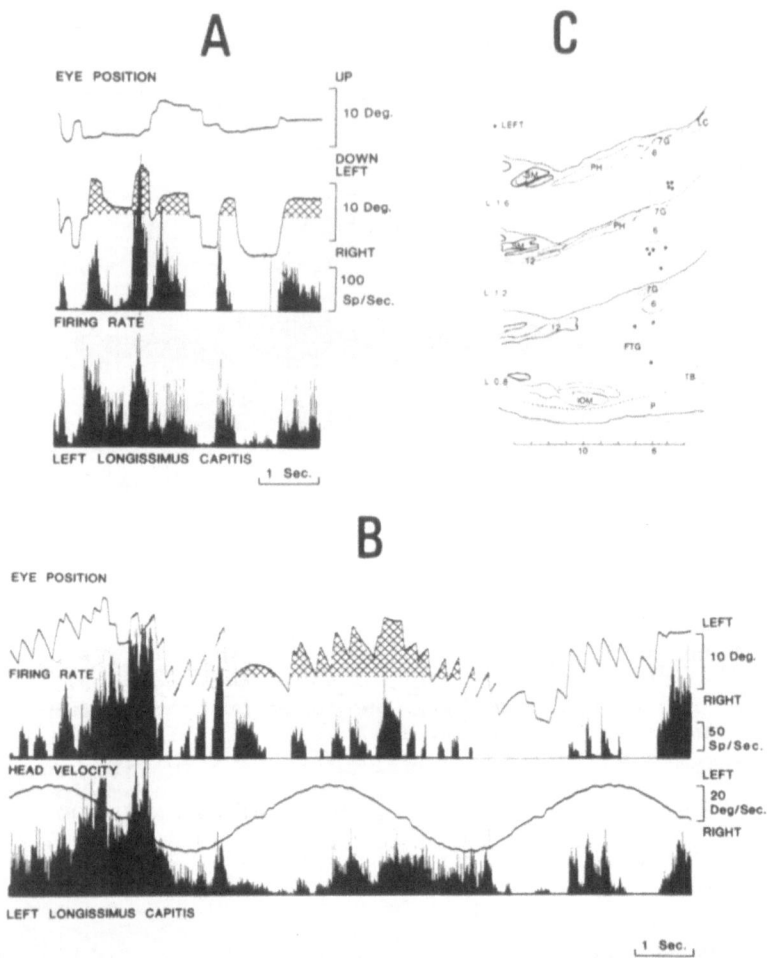

Fig.5. *Recording of a reticular cell, in the alert cat, whose discharge rate is related to EMG of ipsilateral longissimus capitis and to horizontal eye position.*
A- *Behavior of the neuron during spontaneous saccades and fixations.* From top to bottom: -Vertical and horizontal components of eye position. Instantaneous firing rate of the cell. Integrated EMG of the ipsilateral (left longissimus capitis). B- *Behavior of the neuron during vestibular nystagmus.* From top to bottom: -Horizontal eye position. Instantaneous firing rate of the neuron. Head velocity (turntable velocity). Integrated EMG of longissimus capitis muscle. C- *Diagram showing the location of the recorded cells in the left brainstem.* 6:abducens nucleus; 7G: genou of facial nerve; 12: hypoglossal nucleus, laterality: 0.8-1.2-1.6mm from the midline. Cross-hatched areas indicate moments when the eye occupies a position to the left of its mid-

line (corresponding to the straight bottom edge of those areas), in A, spontaneously and in B, during one oscillation cycle.

to the atlas of Berman) which vary from 5.3 to 7.2mm (fig. 5C). However we have only explored a small area around the abducens nucleus and they may be distributed more widely in the reticular formation.
A close examination of the records has revealed that in many occasions the neck EMG cannot be fully accounted for by the firing rate pattern of each individual neuron, but it seems that combining the firing profile of "burst tonic" and "tonic" neurons is sufficient to account for the EMG. We therefore suggest that neck EMG is the result of an addition of reticulo-spinal inputs with different dynamic properties.
It is interesting to compare the firing profile of the reticular neuron shown on fig.5B with the one of the second order vestibular neuron shown on fig. 3B and C. The former is clearly related to neck EMG and horizontal eye position whether the latter is mainly modulated by head velocity.

4. DISCUSSION
We conclude from the present study that cells, located around the abducens nucleus in the area described previously by Peterson (1980) as containing cells of origin of the medial reticulo-spinal tract and projecting to ipsilateral neck muscles, could be candidates to mediate the horizontal eye position signals found in dorsal neck muscles of the alert cat. It is obvious that, because of the absence of antidromic stimulation from the spinal cord, the neurons recorded here are only putative reticulo-spinal cells. It was however checked on every occasion that they are not mediating proprioceptive input from the neck to the reticular formation. The striking similarity between the firing pattern and neck EMG suggests that they are indeed premotor cells, although a reflection of interneuronal activity within the spinal cord cannot be excluded at this stage. A striking aspect of their firing characteristics which distinguishes them clearly from abducens motoneurons and prepositus neurons is the fact that they have a threshold around <u>mid-position of the eye in the orbit.</u> Is is therefore clear that they all fire only for ipsilateral eye position in the orbit (or ipsilateral beating field of nystagmus). The main question is: where does these signals originate from? Until now the identification of a tonic eye position generator is lacking and only the prepositus nucleus has been proposed as a possible candidate. It could be suggested that a common gaze generator modulates both abducens motoneurons and reticulo-spinal cells (in addition it may influence other structures such as the vestibular nuclei). Converging influences on reticular cells subsequently modify the original gaze command and induces a signal which is adapted for neck

motor control during a eye-head coordinated movement.
Another intriguing problem is the fact that neck
motoneuron discharge is in phase with eye position.
Because the vestibulo-spinal neurons whose firing
rate is coding mainly head velocity during head rotation do terminate on neck motoneurons it can be hypothesized either that their synaptic input is weak
(which is obviously wrong because compensatory vestibulo-collic reflexes do exist), or that some switching mechanisms occur. It may be that during an intentional strategy of synergistic eye-head movement,
descending (cortical?) influences inhibit the vestibulo-collic reflex. If this does not happen at vestibular nuclei level, it then could occur at spinal
cord level in the same way as many other reflexes
are blocked during voluntary movements. Different
descending tracts would therefore be involved in
different strategies ("compensatory" for the vestibulo-spinal tract, versus "eye-head coupling" for the
reticulo-spinal tract). These speculations are evi-
dently only working hypothesis which will have to be
confirmed by future experiments.

5. REFERENCE
Baker R and Mc Crea R (1979) The parabducens nucleus.
    In Asanuma H and Wilson VJ, ed. Integration in the
    nervous system, pp. 97-122, Tokyo-New York, Igaku-
    Shoin.
Bender MB (1955) The eye centering system, Arch. Neu-
    rol. and Psych., 73, 685-699.
Bennett AH and Savill T (1889) A case of permanent
    conjugate deviation of the eyes and head, the result
    of a lesion limited to the sixth nucleus; with re-
    marks on associated lateral movements of the eye
    balls and rotation of the head and neck, Brain 12,
    102-116.
Berthoz A and Anderson JH (1971) Frequency analysis
    of vestibular influence on extensor motoneurons.
    II. Relationship between neck and fore-limb exten-
    sors, Brain Res., 34, 376-380.
Berthoz A, Vidal PP and Corvisier J (1982) Are reti-
    cular neurons in the periabducens area mediating
    horizontal eye position signals to dorsal neck
    muscles of the cat? Soc. Neurosci. Abstr.(in press).
Berthoz A, Yoshida K and Vidal PP (1981) Horizontal
    eye movement signals in second-order vestibular nu-
    clei neurons in the cat. In Cohen B, ed. Vestibular
    and oculomotor physiology, vol. 374, pp. 144-156,
    Annals of the N.Y. Academy of Sciences.
Bizzi E, Kalil RE and Tagliasco V (1971) Eye-head
    coordination in monkeys: evidence for centrally pat-
    terned organization, Science, 173, 452-454.
Collewijn H (1977) Eye and head movements in freely
    moving rabbits, J. Physiol., 266, 471-498.
Ezure K and Sasaki S (1978) Frequency-response analy-
    sis of vestibular-induced neck reflex in cat.
    I. Characteristics of neural transmission from ho-

rizontal semicircular canal to neck motoneurons,
J. Neurophysiol., 41, 445-458.

Fuller JH (1980) Linkage of eye and head movements in
the alert rabbit, Brain Res., 194, 219-222.

Fuller JH (1981) Eye and head movements during vestibular stimulation in the alert rabbit, Brain Res.,
205, 363-381.

Guitton D, Crommelinck M and Roucoux A (1980) Stimulation of the superior colliculus in the alert cat.
I. Eye movements and neck EMG activity evoked when
the head is restrained, Exp. Brain Res., 39, 63-73.

Lestienne F, Whittington DA and Bizzi E (1981) Single
cell recording from the pontine reticular formation
in monkeys: behavior of preoculomotor neurons during
eye-head coordination. In Fuchs A and Becker W, eds.
Progress in Oculomotor Research, Developments in
Neuroscience, vol.12, pp. 325-333, Elsevier
North-Holland Biomedical Press.

Magnus R (1924) Köperstellung, Springer Ed. Berlin,
740pp.

Mc Crea RA, Yoshida K, Berthoz A and Baker R (1980)
Eye movement related activity and morphology of second order vestibular neurons terminating in the cat
abducens nucleus, Exp.Brain Res., 40, 468-473.

Mc Crea RA, Yoshida K, Evinger C and Berthoz A (1980)
The location, axonal arborization, and termination
sites of eye-movement-related secondary vestibular
neurons demonstrated by intra-axonal HRP injection
in the alert cat. In Fuchs A and Becker W, eds. Progress in Oculomotor Research, Developments in Neuroscience, vol.12, pp. 379-386, Elsevier North-Holland
Biomedical Press.

Peterson BW, Fillion M, Felpel LP and Abzug C (1975)
Responses of medial reticular neurons to stimulation
of the vestibular nerve, Exp. Brain Res., 22, 335-
350.

Peterson BW, Pitts NG, Fukushima K and Mackel R (1978)
Reticulo-spinal excitation and inhibition of neck
motoneurons , Exp. Brain Res., 32, 471-489.

Peterson BW, Fukushima K, Hirai N, Schor RH and
Wilson VJ (1980) Response of vestibulospinal and reticulospinal neurons to sinusoidal vestibular stimulation, J. Neurophysiol., 43, 1236-1250.

Rademaker GGT (1931) Das stehen, Springer Verlag,
59, 286-292.

Robinson DA (1981) The use of control systems analysis
in the neurophysiology of eye movements. In Cowan WM,
Hall ZW and Kandel ER, eds. Ann. Rev. Neurosc.,4,
pp. 463-503.

Roucoux A, Guitton D and Crommelinck M (1980) Stimulation of the superior colliculus in the alert cat.
II. Eye and head movements evoked when the head is
unrestrained, Exp. Brain Res., 39, 75-85.

Vidal PP, Roucoux A and Berthoz A (1982) Horizontal
eye position-related activity in neck muscles of the
alert cat, Exp. Brain Res., 46, 448-453.

Yoshida K, Berthoz A, Vidal PP and Mc Crea R (1981)
Eye movement related activity of identified second
order vestibular neurons in the cat. In Fuchs A
and Becker W, eds. Progress in Oculomotor Research,
Developments in Neuroscience, vol. 12,pp. 371-378,
Elsevier North-Holland Biomedical Press.

BEHAVIOR OF PONTINE CELLS DURING EYE-HEAD COORDINATION:
EVIDENCE OF GAZE SHIFT CODING BY PREOCULOMOTOR BURSTERS

F. LESTIENNE*, D. WHITTINGTON, E. BIZZI (Department of
Psychology. M.I.T., Cambridge, MA 02139 USA)

1. INTRODUCTION
The Pontine Reticular Formation (PRF)is known to be a preoculomotor area responsible for generating appropriate control signal to the extraocular musculature (Bender and
Shanzer, 1964, Büttner-Ennever and Henn, 1976; Cohen and
Henn, 1972; Eckmiller et al, 1980; Graybiel, 1977; Keller,
1974, 1977; Luschei and Fuchs, 1972; Sheibel and Sheibel,
1958; Sparks and Travis, 1971). In the Paramedian Pontine
Reticular Formation (PPRF) there are preoculomotor cells firing in relation to the pulse-step output and each phase of
the pulse step; i.e. burst units related to the pulse and
tonic units related to the steady position of the eye
(Keller, 1974; Luschei and Fuchs, 1972).
The PRF structure is also known to receive projections from
neck musculature and vestibular system (Brodal, 1974; Ladpli
and Brodal, 1963; Peterson et al, 1979; Pompeiano and Swett,
1963). Furthermore the PRF contains neurons with projection
to the neck muscles (Peterson et al, 1975).
If this PRF region has been studied extensively, however
most of the findings have been derived from experiments in
which the head was held fixed. In normal behavioral situation, head movements accompany changes in gaze fixation. The
interaction between eye movement and head movement has been
deduced from a series of studies (Bizzi et al, 1971, 1972;
Bizzi, 1974; Dichgans et al, 1973; Lanman, 1978; Morasso et
al, 1973). These findings have shown that coordinated eye
and head movements are linked through the vestibular system.
Indeed it was discovered that this coordination was accomplished by the simple strategy of using vestibular signal
generated by the moving head to diminish size of the saccade
and generate compensatory eye movement to maintain fixation
of the target during head turning (Dichgans et al, 1973;
Morasso et al, 1973). When the head is restrained, the total
gaze shift was accomplished by the eye saccade. Under such
conditions, it is not possible to separate cell activation
related to total gaze shift or size of saccadic eye movement.
In order to study some aspects of the PRF neural substrate
underlying eye-head coordination, single-unit recordings

* Present address: Lab. Physiologie Neurosensorielle. CNRS.
F. 75236 PARIS CEDEX 06.

Roucoux, A. and Crommelinck, M. (eds.): Physiological and Pathological Aspects of Eye Movements.
© *1982, Dr W. Junk Publishers, The Hague, Boston, London.* ISBN-13: 978-94-009-8002-0

combined with behavioral approaches were performed on alert
and unrestrained monkeys (Lestienne et al, 1981, 1982,
Whittington, 1980, Whittington et al, 1980).
The present paper is directed to analyse the effects of head
movement on the activity of two categories of preoculomotor
neurons, i.e.: burst unit and tonic unit.

2. METHODS

To record the activity of the PRF structures, four adult female monkeys (Macaca Mulatta) were trained to fixate, foveal-
ly, visual target. The target sequence consisted of a lumi-
nous spot of randomized (.4-1.5 sec) duration followed by the
superimposition of a horizontal or vertical hairline. The
monkeys received a reward of water for barpressing only during the presentation of the vertical hairline. The hairlines
required foveal fixation to be discriminated. When the hairline targets were presented at various positions in the monkey's periphery, they made coordinated eye-head movements to
direct their gaze to the targets. The size and direction of
the gaze shift were controlled by the experimenter's choice
of target position. The target could be presented at each of
nine target displays, spaced at 10° intervals from 40° left
of the midsagittal plane to 40° right of the midsagittal plane. The animal's head could also be restrained, forcing it to
make gaze shifts utilizing saccades only. This procedure also allowed accurate calibration of eye position, since the
monkeys had to be foveating to perform the discrimination.
After the monkeys became proficient at the visual discrimination task, they were anesthetized with Nembutal, and silver-
silver chloride electrodes were implanted for recording extraocular potentials of horizontal and vertical eye movements.
Screws were implanted in the monkey's skull for attachment
to a head movement recording apparatus. EMG electrodes were
placed in the splenii capitis muscles of the neck. A stainless steel recording well fixed to the skull, straddling the
midline above the cerebellum. The well was inclined posteriorly at about 17° and stereotaxically positioned to permit an
obliquely driven micro-electrode to reach the brainstem in
the area of the VI nucleus.
Approprialy designed teflon microelectrodes allowed to record
the activity of single brainstem neurons when the monkey is
free to move his head (Lestienne et al, 1981). The location
of the electrode tracks and the location of small electrolytic lesions placed at the tip of specific tracks were determined histologically.
During the experimental sessions, the monkeys sat in a primate chair with their torso restrained and their head attached by way of the skull screws to a head holder which limited head movement to rotation about the vertical axis. Head
movements were monitored from a potentiometer mechanically
coupled to the head holder.
The search procedure used was to make an electrode penetration with the monkey in apparatus and to examine each cell

encountered to see if it were related to eye movement or
head movement. Because during natural head movements both
neck proprioceptors and vestibular receptors are stimulated,
we devised a way to assess separately the contribution of these two modalities. To this end, we performed two maneuvers.
One procedure involved rotating the monkey about its vertical
axis with the head fixed with respect to the chair. In this
way only vestibular receptors were stimulated. In contrast,
the stimulation of neck afferents was obtained by maintaining
the monkey's head fixed with respect to the ground, while rotating the body.
During the recording sessions the variables were stored on a
FM recorder. The data were later digitized, displayed and analysed on a PDP 11/10 computer using appropriate analysis programs. Movement data were digitized in 10 msec. bins and spike data were digitized in 1 msec. bins. The use of trained
monkeys allowed averaging of a number of virtually identical
movements to known targets and the production of raster displays.

3. RESULTS AND DISCUSSION

The recordings comprising these experiments were made from
the Pontine Reticular Formation (PRF) within a 4mm radius of
the midpoint of a line connecting the VI nuclei. In these penetrations, a variety of cells were encountered; cells related to movements of the arm, head, torso, mouth, tongue,
and eyes, as well as many cells the activity of which was not
correlated with any variable being monitored or controlled.
Of the more than 500 cells encountered, 75 were head related,
while 141 were eye movement related cells which were well isolated and held for sufficient time to allow careful analysis.
The eye related cells to be presented in the present paper
feel into two classes; i.e.: tonic and burst.

3.1. Tonic Cells
By far the rarest of eye related cells in this study, this
group contains only eleven cells. Despite this, their behavior is quite uniform and of the four classes, this is the
most homogeneous. Tonic cells fire in relation to eye position in the orbit, and this seems to be a complete description of their activity. They are oblivious to the exertions
of the neck musculature and subject to vestibular influences
only insofar as those signals provide the command signal for
an eye movement. As observed by Robinson(1971, 1974), the
pattern of behavior for these cells when the head is restrained and fixations are made by saccades alone is one in which
the spike frequency increases and decreases in steps corresponding to the stepwise changes in fixation resulting from
saccadic movements. Figure 1 shows another aspect of these
cells' behavior not seen before. Here the head is free to move and the eye movement is no longer source of steps but
rather a more complex pattern typical of coordinated action
of the eye and head. The two recordings are for movements to

the left (1-A) and to the right (1-B), respectively, and
show averages of several movements (6 and 5, respectively).
The variables displayed are head position, eye position, and
the curve of instantaneous frequency of cell firing. The eye
movement consists of a saccadic portion smoothly blending
into a compensatory phase which serves to keep the gaze on
target during the head movement. Note that the curve of instantaneous frequency (dotted line) is a virtually perfect
fit, and that this is true for movements in both directions.

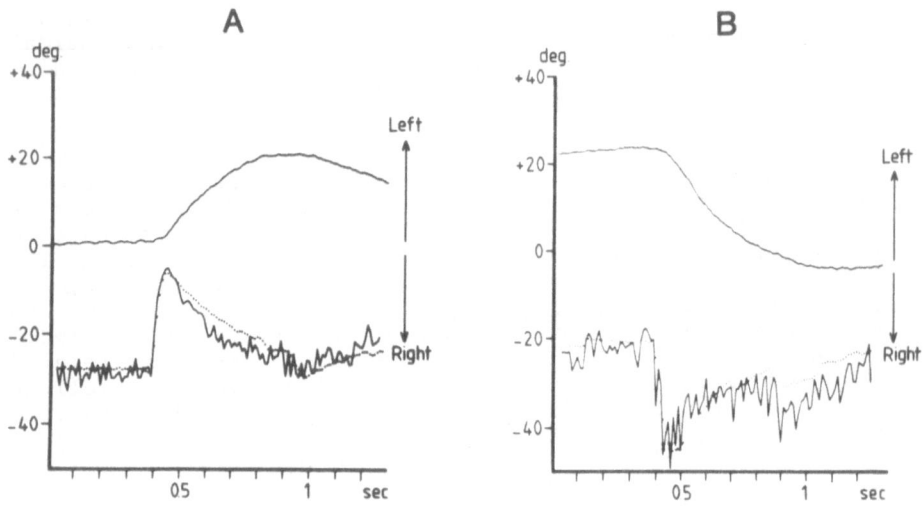

FIGURE 1. *Tonic cell firing for six coordinated eye-head movements to the left (A) and five coordinated eye-head movements to the right (B).*
*Upper solid line is averaged head position. Dotted line ave-
raged eye position. Remaining solid line is the inverted trace of the average of the reciprocal of interspike interval.*

Although the correlation between eye position and cell activity is quite good, another test was undertaken to make certain that neck activity, either afferent or efferent, was
not relevant to these cells' behavior. To test this, eye movements were recorded during neck stimulation when the monkey's body was being rotated back and forth while the head
was restrained. During this procedure there are, of course,
afferent signals from the neck and strenuous muscle contrac-
tions as the monkey resists the rotation.

Table 1 shows that the neck activity produces no significant difference in cell firing leading to the conclusion that these cells act independently of neck afference or efference.

Condition									
	a	b	r	a	b	r	a	b	r
(A)	11.1	18	.96	9.5	6	.90	17	1	.81
(B)	10.5	20	.83	8.5	4.5	.94	18.5	1.5	.84
	Unit 1			Unit 2			Unit 3		

TABLE 1. Slopes (a: spikes per degrees) and intercepts (b: degrees) of lines of best fit relating firing frequency versus eye position. r: correlation coefficients for the respective regression lines. The three units whose on-direction was leftward has been recorded during two experimental conditions: (A) head fixed while body is being rotated, (B) head fixed. Reconstruction of the penetrations shows that the majority of tonic cells were found within the VI nucleus, with the remainder scattered in an aera extending caudally and laterally to the VI nucleus (Whittington, 1980).

In conclusion our results have clearly demonstrated a tight correlation between tonic activity of these cells and the position of the eye within the orbit regardless of the position of the head or its movement. These results were not unexpected, since the activity of these neurons has been shown to correspond to the tonic firing rate of oculomotor neurons when the head was restrained (Henn and Cohen, 1976; Keller, 1974; Luschei and Fuchs, 1972) and to reflect the eye position during vestibularly induced eye movements (Robinson, 1971). Our results reinforce the hypothesis that the tonic cells have just two inputs: the eye command signals and the vestibular feedback signals.

3.2. Burst Cells
One of the first things one notices about burst cells is that there is a much greater diversity to them than their categorization by latency to eye movement would suggest. Most (45/52) of the bursting cells recorded in these experiments had latencies in the range of 5 to 10 ms, putting them in the category of short lead bursters. However, within this grouping there are at least three subclasses of bursters: (1) a class where firing rate is reasonably constant during the burst; (2) a class which fires fairly constantly at onset and then has sporadic spikes in the last half of the saccade; and (3) a class which fires intensely at onset and tapers off. Figure 2 shows the diversity of the class of short lead bursters.

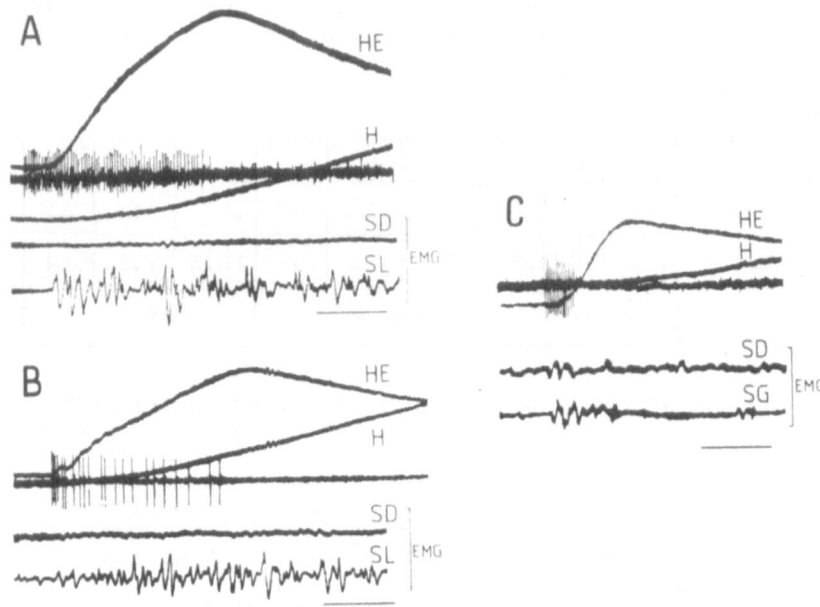

FIGURE 2. *Behavior of short lead burst cell.*
Unit activity recorded from three different short lead burst
units, one characterized by a constant intraburst discharge
(A), one by variable intraburst discharge (B) and one by
short burst at onset (C). H: head movement, HE: horizontal
eye movement, SD and SL: EMG activity of the right and left
splenii capitis, respectively.

Of these three types, the only group which shows a tight,
linear relation between the number of spikes in a burst and
saccade size is the constant rate group (Fig. 2A). Recently
Whittington et al (1980), Lestienne et al (1981, 1982) have
shown that these constant rate cells fall into two distinct
groups. One group shows a strong correlation between the
size of an associated saccade and the number of spikes in the
burst (fig. 3B), as might be expected from fixed experiments
by Luschei and Fuchs (1972). A second group, however was
one in which the number of spikes correlates with the size
of the shift of gaze, whether that shift was accomplished
entirely by eye movement, or made by a coordinated eye and
head movement (fig. 3A).

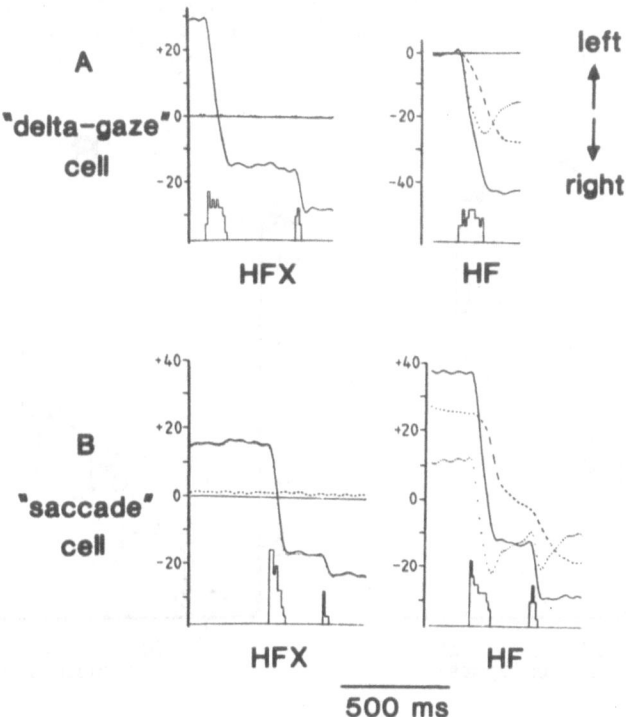

FIGURE 3. *Behavior of short lead burst unit (adapted from Lestienne et al, 1981, 1982).*
Response of cell whose discharges are related to (A) the total gaze shift including head movement contribution ("Delta-gaze" cell) and (B) the size of the saccadic eye movement ("Saccadic" cell). The three tracings are head movement (dashed line), horizontal eye movement (dotted line) and total gaze shift (solid line). At the bottom are spike histograms (cumulated discharges on bins of 10 msec). In A- Head fixed (HFX): size of the first saccade, 44°, number of spikes, 46. Head free (HF): size of the saccade, 24°, size of the total gaze shift, 41°, number of spikes, 47. In B- (HFX): size of the first saccade, 32°, number of spikes, 42. (HF): size of the first saccade, 36°, size of the total gaze shift, 50°, number of spikes, 41.

These two groups of cells, called "saccade" (S) cells for the class corresponding to the saccade size and "delta-gaze" (G) cells for the class corresponding to the size of the shift in gaze, are indistinguishable when the head does not

move during a shift in gaze. This is because the size of the
shift in gaze and the size of the sa<u>ccade</u> are identical under
these conditions. Figure 4 demonstrates the procedure used
to describe the behavior of the S and G cells (Lestienne et
al, 1981).

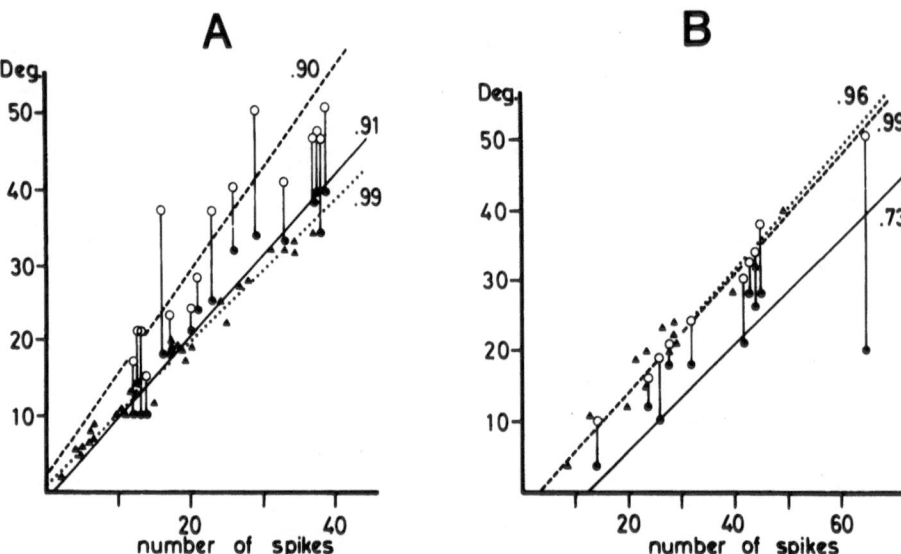

FIGURE 4. *Scatter plot of "Saccade" burster (A) and "Delta-
gaze" burster (B) (adapted from Lestienne et al, 1981).
The three types of symbols are: saccades head fixed (triangles and dotted regression line), saccades head free (filled
circles and solid regression line) connected to the respective head free gaze shifts (open circles and dashed regression
line) by a vertical solid line. This vertical line indicates
the amplitude of head contribution during eye-head movements.
In A notice coïncidence of head free saccade and head fixed
saccades, in B notice coïncidence of head fixed saccades and
head free gaze shifts.*

In this figure, the solid triangles show the relation between
the number of spikes in a burst and the size of the corresponding saccade when the head is restrained. Superimposed is
a plot relating the number of spikes in a burst to the size
of both the corresponding saccade and gaze shift when the
head is free to move. In this case, the points representing
saccade size (filled circles) are connected to their respective gaze shift size (open circles) by a vertical solid line.
Notice that the saccade size is always smaller than the gaze
shift and that the length of the line connecting them is
equal to the attendant head movement. Figure 4B clearly sup-

ports the claim that this is a G cell related to the size of
the shift in gaze, not the size of the saccade. In contrast,
consider Figure 4A which shows an S burster. Here, it is
saccade gaze, not gaze shift, that correlates with cell firing.
Figure 5 illustrates an other way of distinguishing between
S and G cells on the basis of averaging a number of identical movements to the same target. In order to induce series
of identical movements, we employed a paradigm in which the
target appears at regular intervals at a fixed location. Under these experimental conditions the head begins to move
well before ($\sim$ 200 msec) the saccade of the eye is initiated
(Bizzi et al, 1972). The saccadic movement is preceded and
followed by a compensatory eye movement (fig. 5A). Each set
of traces represents, for the same burst cell, the averaged
recordings of ten head free (5A) and ten head fixed (5B and
5C) responses to the presentation of visual targets. The
location of these targets was predictable.

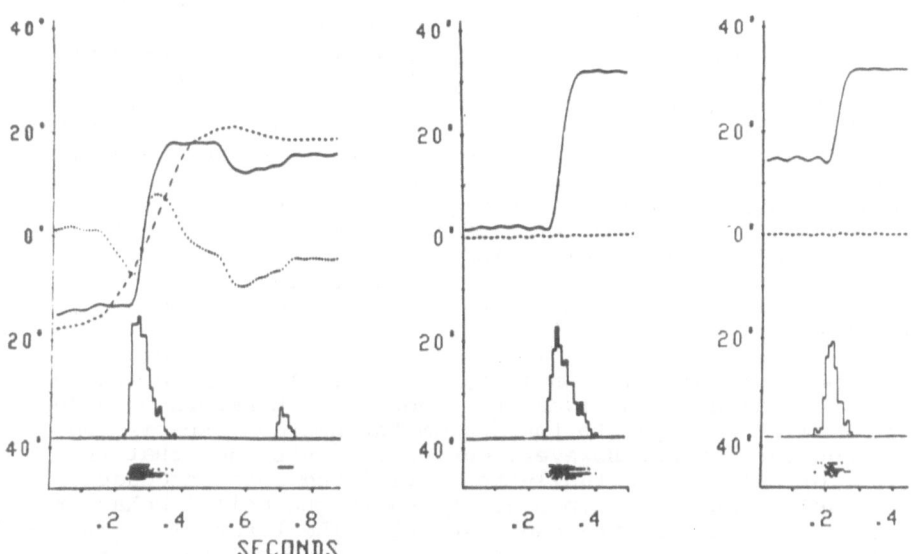

FIGURE 5. *Behavior of a "Delta-gaze" burster.*
For each of the three sets of traces the location of the
targets was predictable. The traces represent the averaged
recording of:
a) ten eye-head coordinations, the size of saccadic eye mo-
vement (dotted line), total shift in gaze (solid line) and
head movement (dashed line) are 30°, 20° and 40° respective-
ly.

b) ten 30° saccadic eye movements with head fixed
c) ten 20° saccadic eye movements with head fixed
The spike histogram (cumulated discharges in bins of 10 msec)
are shown at the bottom of each set of traces. The number of
spikes for each histogram are, from the left to the right,
120, 112 and 72 respectively.

What emerges from these recordings is a clear impression that
this cell is firing in relation to the size of the gaze shift
rather the size of the saccade. Indeed the averaged gaze shift
in A and B is equal (30°) and the cumulative histogram of
spikes is fairly the same (120 and 112 respectively). In contrast, concerning the size of the averaged saccadic eye movements, the results show that the cumulative histogram of
spikes in A and C is clearly different (120 and 72 respectively) although the averaged size of eye movements is equal
(20°).
We attempted to distinguish between the "G" and "S" cells on
the basis of latency to eye movement on the assumption that
the "G" cells were earlier in the processing chain than the
saccade cells, but the latencies were not significantly different. The role of other inputs, particularly neck afference
and efference, was also considered, and, as in the case of
the tonic cells, no effect of either could be detected in
the cell's behavior.
On the basis of histological examination, the majority of "S"
and "G" burst units were grouped into two different areas;
dorsal and ventral to the VI nucleus.Although "G" and "S"
cells occured in overlapping regions, a cluster of "G" cells
was identified by an electrolytic lesion. This region lies
ventral-caudal to the VI nucleus within about 2mm of the
midline (Whittington, 1980; Lestienne et al, 1981).
In conclusion previous neurophysiological (Cohen and Henn,
1972; Eckmiller et al, 1980; Keller, 1977; Luschei and Fuchs,
1972; Sparks and Travis, 1971) and anatomical studies
(Büttner-Ennever and Henn,1976; Graybiel, 1977) have led to
the acceptance of the idea that short-lead bursters provide
the excitatory input to the oculomotor neurons, specifying
saccade parameters. However, our experiments show that this
class of cells can actually be partitioned into "saccade" (S)
and "delta-gaze" (G) types according to the cells' behavior
during coordinated eye-head movements. The first class included cells whose firing activity was closely related to the
size of the saccadic eye movements, while in the second class
of bursters, the firing was correlated with the total gaze
shifts, including the head-movement contribution. This distinct behavior of "S" and "G" burst units raises the question
of the location of these neurons in the preoculomotor control
schema during coordinated eye and head movements. By assuming
an independant head control system which impinges upon the
preoculomotor control system only by vestibular feedback
(Bizzi et al, 1971; Dichgans et al, 1973; Morasso et al,
1973) we have tentatively characterized the "G" burster cells

as being upstream in preoculomotor processing at a level where the total shift in gaze is specified. Following this schema, the "S" burster cells are conceived to be further downstream toward the oculomotor plant at a point where the contribution of the head has been substracted out of the total gaze shift, presumably via the vestibulo-ocular reflex.

4. ACKNOWLEDGEMENTS
Research supported by NS 09343, NGR 22-009-798, EY 02621 and DGRST 80-7-0248.

5. REFERENCES
Bender MR and Shanzer S (1964) Oculomotor pathways defined by electrical stimulation and lesions in the brainstem of monkey. In The Oculomotor System, ed. by MB Bender, pp.81-140, Harper and Row, New York.
Bizzi E, Kalil RE and Tagliasco V (1971) Eye-head coordination in monkeys: evidence for centrally patterned organization, Science, 173, 452-454.
Bizzi E (1974) The coordination of eye-head movement, Sci. Am., 231, n°4, 100-106.
Brodal A (1974) Anatomy of vestibular nuclei and their connections. In Handbook of Sensory Physiology, vol.VIII, Vestibular System, Part I, Basic Mechanisms, ed. by HH Kornhuber, pp. 239-352, Springer-Verlag, New York.
Büttner-Ennever JA and Henn V (1976) An autoradiographic study of the pathways from the pontine reticular formation involved in horizontal eye movements, Brain Res., 108,155-164.
Cohen B and Henn V (1972) Unit activity in the pontine reticular formation associated with eye movements, Brain Res., 46, 403-410.
Dichgans J, Bizzi E, Morasso P and Tagliasco V (1973) Mechanisms underlying recovery of eye-head coordination following bilateral labyrinthectomy in monkeys, Exp. Brain Res., 18, 548-562.
Eckmiller R, Blair S and Westheimer G (1980) Fine structure of saccade bursts in macaque pontine neurons, Brain Res., 181, 460-464.
Graybiel AM (1977) Direct and indirect preoculomotor pathways of the brainstem: an autoradiographic study of the pontine reticular formation in the cat, J. Comp. Neurol., 175, 37-78.
Henn V and Cohen B (1976) Coding of information about rapid eye movement in the pontine reticular formation of alert monkeys, Brain Res., 108, 307-325.
Keller EL (1974) Participation of medial pontine reticular formation in eye movement generation in monkey, J. Neurophysiol., 37, 316-332.
Keller EL (1977) Control of saccadic eye movements by midline brainstem neurons. In Control of Gaze by Brainstem Neurons, ed. by R Baker and A Berthoz, pp. 327-336, Elsevier/North-Holland Biomedical Press, Amsterdam.

Ladpli R and Brodal A (1963) Experimental studies of the com-
misural and reticular formation projections from the vestibular nuclei in cat, Brain Res., 8, 65-96.

Lanman J, Bizzi E and Allum J (1978) The coordination of eye
and head movement during smooth pursuit, Brain Res., 153,
39-53.

Lestienne F, Whittington D and Bizzi E (1981) Single cell recording from the brain stem in monkey: behavior of preoculomotor neurons during eye-head coordination. In Progress in
oculomotor research, ed. by A Fuchs and W Becker, pp. 325-
333, Elsevier, New York.

Lestienne F, Whittington D and Bizzi E (1982) Activity of
brain stem neurons during eye-head coordination in alert monkey: behavior of eye-related neurons. In Spatially Oriented
Behavior, ed. by A Hein and M Jeannerod, in press, Springer-
Verlag, New York.

Luschei ES and Fuchs AF (1972) Activity of brainstem neurons
during eye movements of alert monkeys, J. Neurophysiol.,
35, 445-461.

Morasso P, Bizzi E and Dichgans J (1973) Adjustments of saccade characteristics during head movements, Exp. Brain Res.,
16, 492-500.

Peterson BW, Filion M, Felpel LP and Abzug C (1975) Responses
of medial reticular neurons to stimulation of the vestibular
nerve, Exp. Brain Res., 22, 335-350.

Peterson BW, Maunz RA, Pitts NG and Mackel RG (1975) Patterns
of projection and branching of reticulospinal neurons,
Exp. Brain Res., 23, 333-351.

Pompeiano O and Swett JE (1963) Actions of graded cutaneous
and muscular afferent volleys on brainstem units in the decerebrate cerebellectomized cat, Arch. Ital. Biol., 101,
584-613.

Robinson DA (1971) Models of oculomotor neural organization.
In The Control of Eye Movements, ed. by P Bach-y-Rita and
CC Collins, pp. 519-538, Academic, New York.

Robinson DA (1975) Oculomotor control signals. In Basic Mechanisms of Ocular Mobility and their Clinical Implications,
ed. by G Lennerstrand and P Bach-y-Rita, pp. 337-374,
Pergamon, Oxford.

Sheibel ME and Sheibel AB (1958) Structural substrates for
integrative patterns in the brainstem reticular core. In
Reticular Formation of the Brain, ed. by HH Jaspers,
LD Proctor, RS Knighton, WC Noshay and RT Costello,
pp. 31-35, Little Brown, Boston, Mass.

Sparks DL and Travis RP (1971) Firing patterns of reticular
formation neurons during horizontal eye movements, Brain
Res., 33, 477-481.

Whittington D (1980) The role of preoculomotor brainstem
neurons in coordinated eye-head movements, PhD Thesis, MIT.

Whittington D, Lestienne F and Bizzi E (1980) Preoculomotor
brainstem neurons recorded during eye-head coordination,
Soc. Neurosci. Abstr., vol. 6, p. 476.

COORDINATED EYE-HEAD MOVEMENTS IN THE CAT

R.M. DOUGLAS, D. GUITTON, and M. VOLLE. (Montreal Neurological Institute and Aviation Medical Research Unit, McGill University, Montreal, Quebec, Canada)

1. INTRODUCTION

Coordinated movements of the eyes and head were first studied systematically in the monkey by Bizzi et al. 1971; Morasso et al. 1973; and Dichgans et al. 1973. In these classic studies they showed that an animal, orienting to a randomly appearing visual target, encodes the same saccadic eye movement signal in both the head fixed and head free conditions. In the head free condition the vestibularly induced compensatory eye movement produced by the head movement is added linearly to the saccade signal. Since the compensatory eye movement is in the opposite direction to the saccade, saccade velocity and amplitude for a given target eccentricity are reduced. The elegance of this system is that an eye movement can be programmed independently of the head movement, and that a high degree of accuracy is achieved because the vestibulo-ocular reflex (VOR) enables the gaze to reach and stay on-target irrespective of what the head does. This strategy will be called the saccade attenuation (SA) strategy.

Blakemore, Donaghy (1980) have reported that the SA strategy is used by the cat. However two peculiarities of the cat with respect to the monkey suggest that the problem may be more complex. (1) The cat has an oculomotor range (OMR) of only 25° (e.g. Guitton et al. 1980) which is considerably less than that of the monkey, and yet Collewijn (1977) and Roucoux et al. (1981) have reported gaze shifts greater than 25°. If the SA strategy is valid in the cat, then such large gaze shifts require that, in the head free condition, the animal programs saccades larger than those it can make with its head fixed. (2) Haddad, Robinson (1977), and Blakemore, Donaghy (1980) have observed in the cat that a saccade of a given amplitude with head free is faster than one of equivalent amplitude with head fixed. The opposite is true in monkey (Morasso et al. 1973).

These points, suggest that the cat may be using a strategy that is different than that of the monkey. This possibility is reinforced by studies of the eye and head movements evoked by collicular stimulation in the alert cat (Guitton et al. 1980; Roucoux et al. 1980). These results have suggested that for gaze movements beyond the OMR, a vector addition (VA) strategy is used in which the eye and head trajectories are preprogrammed and proceed independently of each other. One feature of this hypothesis is that the VOR must be disabled during the saccade, a not so unlikely proposition since the VOR does pause during quick phases of vestibular nystagmus. The object of the present experiments was to describe in more detail the characteristics of coordinated eye and head movements made by alert cats. Special attention was paid to the possibility that the VA strategy may be used.

2. METHODS

Spontaneous active eye and head movements were studied in 5 adult cats which were kept in a high state of arousal by occasionally giving them food. The food was kept hidden behind a screen and brought around randomly to one side or the other, towards the cats, thus eliciting a wide range of head

Roucoux, A. and Crommelinck, M. (eds.): Physiological and Pathological Aspects of Eye Movements.
© *1982, Dr W. Junk Publishers, The Hague, Boston, London.* ISBN-13: 978-94-009-8002-0

412

amplitudes as the cats eagerly looked around for the food. Gaze (position of the visual axis with respect to the world) and head position were measured with the magnetic search coil method. The data were sampled, linearized and stored on-line on a computer, and eye position with respect to the head was computed by subtracting the head signal from the gaze. All displacements in which the rapid head movement began from a standstill or a maximum velocity of 10°/sec were analyzed. In our test conditions these constituted a large fraction of all the movements, with almost 200 being obtained in each 8 minute session. The data shown in each figure are from one session in one cat, but in every case, very similar data were obtained on other days in the same cat, and in the other 4 animals.

3. RESULTS

3.1 Horizontal gaze shifts within oculomotor range (<25°)

Fig. 1a shows an example of coordinated eye and head movements associated with relatively small gaze amplitudes in one cat. Gaze shifts occurred intermittently whenever there was a saccade, and any head movement between gaze saccades was cancelled by the VOR, thus giving a flat gaze trace. Saccades essentially never occurred without an accompanying head movement. Typically they occurred whenever the head showed a characteristic increase in velocity but a few occurred afterwards

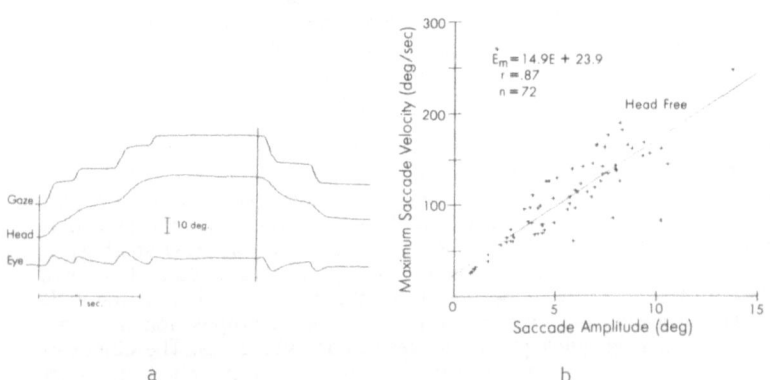

a   b

FIGURE 1. a) Example of coordinated eye-head movements made by a cat. Note that each gaze shift is accomplished with an eye saccade and a rapid head movement, and that the gaze is flat between saccades. The vertical bars mark the start of two movements, and in each case the saccade starts later than the head. b) Maximum velocity-amplitude relationship for horizontal saccades during active head movements. Only those saccades associated with gaze shifts < 25° have been included in this figure. Characteristics of linear regression line given in upper left in this and subsequent figures. E, amplitude of eye movement relative to the head. $\dot{E}_m$, maximum eye-re-head velocity.

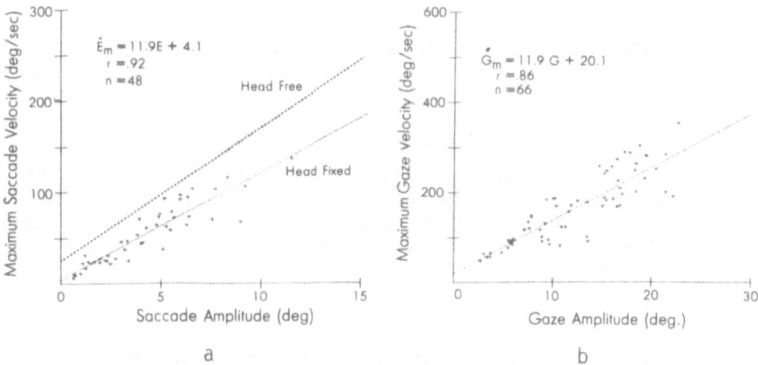

FIGURE 2. a) Maximum velocity-amplitude relationship for horizontal saccades when the head was held fixed. Dashed line taken from figures 1b. Note the higher velocities in the free head condition. b) Maximum velocity-amplitude relationship for horizontal gaze saccades in the head free condition. All gaze amplitudes greater than 25° have been excluded from the graph. G, gaze amplitude, $\dot{G}_m$, maximum gaze velocity.

while the head continued to move (eg 4th saccade from left in Fig. 1a). These latter movements may be vestibular quick phases, and were not analyzed here. In spite of the fact that the movements appear quite similar to those of the monkey, a more quantitative examination of the data showed that the pattern of coordination had two important differences. First, most of the saccades started after the head movement began. Second, saccades with head free were faster than those with head fixed. Fig. 1b shows the relationship between the maximum velocity reached during each saccade, and the saccade amplitude in a cat free to move its head. Only horizontal gaze shifts less than 25° are included. As is already well known for man, monkey and cat (for cat see Evinger, Fuchs, 1976; Guitton, Mandl, 1980), large amplitude saccades reach higher peak velocities. However in agreement with Haddad, Robinson (1977) and Blakemore, Donaghy (1980) and unlike the monkey, for a given saccade amplitude, a higher velocity on the average was obtained when the head was actively moved (Fig. 1b) than when the head was stationary (Fig. 2a). This was true over a wide range of saccade amplitudes for all cats. It could be argued that the SA strategy still is being used but that the cat programs very large saccades, and that the VOR reduces them to the size actually observed. The different amplitude-velocity relationships of Fig. 1b and 2a could then be explained by noting that the saccade maintains its maximum velocity for only a short portion of its time course and that the average velocity is considerably lower. As the head velocity is relatively constant throughout the saccade, the level of the compensatory VOR signal would constitute a larger percentage of the average velocity than of the peak velocity. Thus the amplitude, which is the product of the average velocity and saccade duration would be reduced proportionally more than the maximum velocity. This could produce the lower peak velocity versus amplitude relationship seen in the head fixed case.

Thus the SA hypothesis can account qualitatively for the observed data, and further, would predict that the velocity-amplitude relationship for the total gaze movement should be identical to that seen for saccades with head fixed. As can be seen from Fig. 2, there is a suggestion that this is true but the scatter in the data prohibits a firm conclusion.

A further interesting feature of Fig. 1a is that the duration of the saccadic gaze movement is greater than that of the movement of the eye with respect to the head (called here the eye movement). A considerable amount of the gaze shift takes place between the time the saccade velocity reaches zero and when the slow phase velocity attains unity gain. This observation is best explained by the SA strategy: a gaze movement is coded and the VOR associated with the fast head movement (see below) eventually overcomes and reverses the eye movement. In contrast, a more abrupt switch from saccade to full gain slow phase VOR, and thus equal durations, might be expected from the VA hypothesis.

3.2 Horizontal gaze shifts greater than the oculomotor range ($>25°$)

In agreement with Collewijn (1977) and Roucoux et al. (1981) all of our cats could produce large (up to 50°) single gaze and head shifts of amplitude greater than their oculomotor range. Beyond 25° the gaze velocity saturated (not shown in Fig. 2b). A characteristic feature of these displacements was that the velocity-time plots for the gaze and eye movements frequently were flat and did not exhibit the usual "bell-shaped" profile, seen in the small gaze shifts.

The large gaze shifts, like the small ones, had durations that exceeded those of the eye itself. The difference in duration was frequently very large. This observation is again more compatible with the SA strategy and suggests that the cat can program saccades larger than those it can make with its head fixed.

3.3 Head movements

Head movements were stereotyped. The accuracy of the head displacement is shown by the fact that its amplitude was equal to the total gaze shift (Fig. 3a). In man Barnes (1979) showed that the head movements are generally smaller than the target eccentricity. Moreover, in cat, this accuracy was accomplished despite the fact that the animals moved their heads extremely quickly, with peak velocities near those attained by saccades. Indeed the "saccade-like" nature of these head movements was reflected in a strong amplitude-velocity relationship.

A further interesting observation is that the eye saccade amplitude was a constant proportion of the head (or gaze) amplitude. Fig. 4 shows that the ratio was about 0.3 over the full saccade amplitude range, even for small gaze shifts which lay within the cats oculomotor range, and which theoretically could have been accomplished with only a saccade and no head movement.

3.4 Braked head movements

While all of the above results attest to the highly organized manner in which cats orient, none constitute conclusive evidence for either the SA or VA

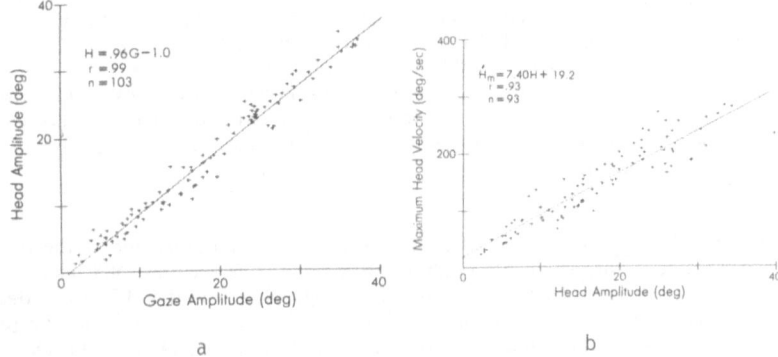

FIGURE 3. a) Final head amplitude versus gaze amplitude at end of eye saccade for horizontal movements. The graph shows that head amplitude equals gaze amplitude. H, head amplitude. b) Maximum velocity versus amplitude for horizontal head movements. The rather stereotyped nature of the head movements is reflected in the high correlation between maximum velocity reached by the head, and the final amplitude. $\dot{H}_m$, maximum head velocity.

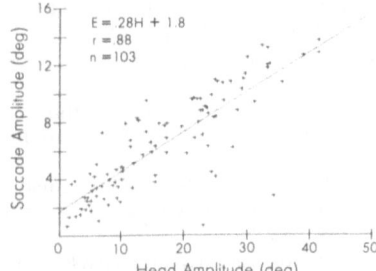

FIGURE 4 Relationship between the amplitudes of the horizontal components of the head movements and saccades. Oblique movements included. Larger saccades occur during larger head movements. A saccade amplitude is about 1/3 the head amplitude. The correlation improves if only horizontal movements are analyzed.

strategies. Current experiments are examining this issue further. In these, the cat's head is attached to an apparatus which permits braking a movement just prior to its initiation. The VOR addition hypothesis would predict that gaze still reaches the target. We find this to be true for gaze shifts less than 15 degrees. But in the two trained cats examined so far we have never observed saccades larger than 15° even when the head is blocked just before an intended movement of 30-40° in amplitude.

4. DISCUSSION

4.1 <u>Gaze shifts within OMR.</u> The tendency for gaze saccades, made with the head either fixed or free, to have similar characteristics suggests that

the cat uses the SA strategy within its OMR. A similar result was obtained by Roucoux et al (1981). This is supported by our braking experiments and corroborates the results of Blakemore, Donaghy (1980). Nevertheless, contrary to these authors' findings, our cats almost always generated saccades that began after the head movement and which were preceded by a short duration vestibularly induced compensatory rotation. This difference could be due to restrictions imposed by the head holder in the experiments of Blakemore, Donaghy (1980).

4.2 Gaze shifts beyond the OMR. If the SA strategy holds, and if the cat orients, say, to a target of 50° eccentricity, it must program a 50° saccade whose amplitude is reduced by about 70% (Fig. 4) to yield a 15° saccade. Both the programming of a saccade so far outside the OMR, and the large saccade attenuation are indeed surprising. Thus perhaps, beyond the OMR the cat uses the VA strategy. This would be compatible with the observation that the head movements were stereotyped in trajectory and equal to gaze amplitude. Our preliminary braking experiments also suggest the VA strategy. But if a different strategy were being used one might expect a discontinuity in the relation between saccade amplitude and head amplitude and none was found (Fig. 4b). A further complication for the VA strategy is that the gaze and eye saccades never terminated simultaneously.

REFERENCES

Barnes GR (1979) Vestibulo-ocular function during coordinated head and eye movements to acquire visual targets, J. Physiol. 287, 127-147.

Bizzi E, Kalil RE and Tagliasco V (1971) Eye-head coordination in monkeys: evidence for centrally patterned organization, Science, 173, 452-454

Blakemore C and Donaghy M (1980) Coordination of head and eyes in the gaze changing behaviour of cats, J. Physiol. 300, 317-335.

Collewijn H (1977) Gaze in freely moving subjects, In Baker and Berthoz A, eds. Control of gaze by brain stem neurons, 13-22. Amsterdam, Elsevier/North Holland.

Dichgans J, Bizzi E, Morasso P and Tagliasco V (1973) Mechanisms underlying recovery of eye-head coordination following bilateral labyrinthectomy in monkeys, Exp Brain Res. 18, 548-562.

Evinger, C and Fuchs AF (1976) Saccadic, smooth pursuit, and optokinetic eye movements of the trained cat, J. Physiol. 285, 209-229.

Guitton D and Mandl G (1980) A comparison between saccades and quick phases of vestibular nystagmus in the cat, Vision Res. 20, 865-874.

Guitton D, Crommelinck M and Roucoux A (1980) Stimulation of the superior colliculus in the alert cat. I. Eye movements and neck EMG activity evoked when the head in restrained. Exp. Brain Res. 39, 63-73.

Haddad GM and Robinson DA (1977) Cancellation of the vestibulo-ocular reflex during active and passive head movements in the normal cat, Soc. Neuroscience Abstr. 3, 155.

Morasso P, Bizzi E and Dichgans J (1973) Adjustment of saccade characteristics during head movements, Exp. Brain Res. 16, 492-500.

Roucoux A, Guitton D, and Crommelinck M (1980) Stimulation of the superior colliculus in the alert cat. II. Eye and head movements evoked when the head is unrestrained, Exp Brain Res. 39, 75-85.

Roucoux A, Crommelinck M, Guerit JM and Meulders M (1981) Two modes of eye-head coordination and the role of the vestibulo-ocular reflex in these two strategies, In Fuchs A and Becker W, eds. Functional Basis of Ocular Motility Disorders, 309-315. Amsterdam, Elsevier/North -Holland.

DYNAMICS OF COMPENSATORY VESTIBULAR REFLEXES IN THE GRASSFROG, RANA TEMPORARIA

N. DIERINGER, W. PRECHT
Institut für Hirnforschung, Universität Zürich

During locomotion, maintenance of clear vision and postural stability is a common problem for many animals.
As the body moves, passive head oscillations are reduced
by the action of compensatory vestibulo-collic and opto-
kinetic-collic reflexes, which cooperatively tend to
stabilize the position of the head in space. The slip
of retinal images is further reduced by the action of
these reflexes on the extraocular motor system i.e. the
vestibulo-ocular and the optokinetic-ocular reflexes.
In a natural situation (head free to move in response
to rotation of the whole body) all these reflexes are
active conjointly and simultaneously and 'stability' of
gaze results from their combined effects through the
collico-motor and the oculo-motor systems.

The properties of these reflexes can be expected
to be adjusted to the natural movement repertoire they
have to assist. Thus, it is not surprising to find many
species differences in the properties and in the central
organization of these reflexes. The motor repertoire of
amphibians is distinct enough from that of mammals, to
expect differences in the central organization of their
reflexes. If so, a comparison of the properties of these
differently organized networks might be helpful in understanding how and in which context these modifications
have come about.

COMPENSATORY HEAD AND EYE MOVEMENTS

Horizontal collic reflexes were studied in intact, unrestrained frogs with a magnetic search coil technique
(Dieringer, Precht, 1982). Stimuli consisted of sinusoidal oscillations of the body in the dark (vestibular)
or in the light in front of an earth-fixed visual surround (combined) or of a striped pattern, generated by
a shadow projector, oscillating around the animal (optokinetic). Eye movements evoked by similar stimuli
were recorded in animals with their head fixed.

Evoked head movements consisted of slow phases
that were rarely interrupted by quick phases and exhibited several marked non-linearities. Movements evoked
by rotation of the animal in the dark (VCR) showed a
frequency-dependent threshold above which the gain increased with stimulus amplitude to reach a frequency-
dependent plateau at which the system behaved approximately linear. Values measured in these linear ranges

Roucoux, A. and Crommelinck, M. (eds.): Physiological and Pathological Aspects of Eye Movements.
© *1982, Dr W. Junk Publishers, The Hague, Boston, London.* ISBN-13: 978-94-009-8002-0

418

are shown in Fig.1 (squares). The gain of optokinetically evoked head movements (OCR) was variable for small
amplitudes of sinusoidal stimulation, reached a frequency-
dependent plateau and decreased with a further increase
in stimulus amplitude. The gain and the phase values of
the OCR are shown in Fig.1 by circles.
These values are explained by a velocity-dependent gain

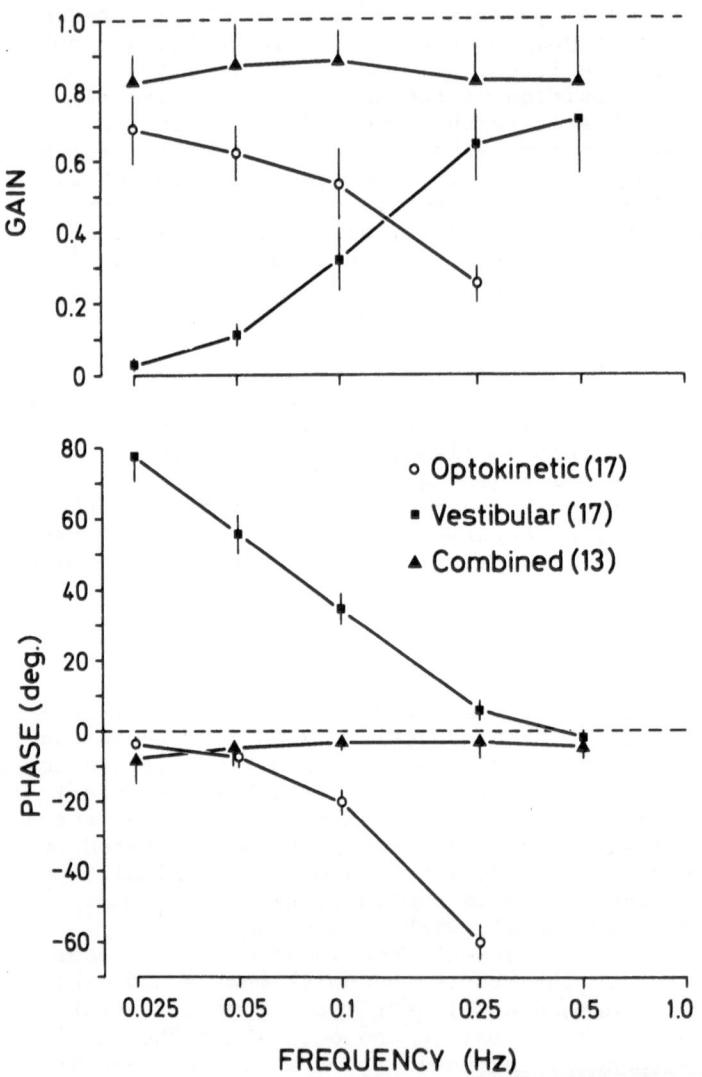

FIGURE 1. Bode plot showing gain and phase values of
collic responses evoked by optokinetic, vestibular and
combined stimulation. Data points represent means of
mean values from (N) animals. Phase values of responses
evoked by rotation of the animal were subtracted from 180°.

and a reaction time of the OCR of about 600 msec. This delayed onset was also observed in responses evoked by combined stimulation, provided peak acceleration was low (Fig.2).

In the light, head movements compensated in the linear range for about 80 to 90% of the imposed gaze shift with a small phase lag (0-10°) over the frequency range tested (Fig.1, triangles). Comparison of data observed during combined stimulation with those calculated from the values obtained for the VCR and the OCR suggest a vectorial addition of vestibularly and optokinetically evoked responses in the case of combined stimulation.

Eye movements in the absence of intended head movements were not observed. Evoked eye movements were limited in amplitude to ±4-6°. Quick phases were very rarely observed during sinusoidal stimulation. Instead the eyes saturated at an eccentric position as in Fig.2. In contrast to the VCR, vestibularly evoked eye movements (VOR) exhibited neither a threshold nor an amplitude-dependent gain below saturation. The mean phase values from 5 animals are shown in Fig. 3. Optokinetically evoked eye movements (OOR) as well as responses evoked by combined stimulation strongly depended on stimulus velocity and no linear range was found. The reaction time of the OOR was shorter (about 200 msec, Fig.2) and the phase lag at 0.25 Hz was less (about 20°) than that of the OCR.

These compensatory eye movements, even though severely restricted in amplitude, are large and fast enough when added to head movements to enable a frog, to stabilize his gaze over a wide range exclusively by means of slow phases. The two motor systems controlling movements of eye and head are matched in such a way that the non-linearities of the one (ocular) can compensate for the non-linearities of the other (collic).

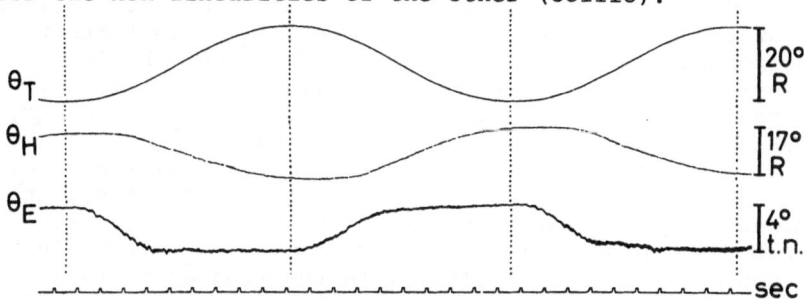

FIGURE 2. Comparison of collic and ocular responses to rotation of the animal in the light. Turning points of the table rotation (θ_T; 0.05 Hz) are indicated by dotted lines. θ_H and θ_E: Position of head and eye. Eye movements were recorded with the head fixed. R indicates a movement direction to the right and t.n. a temporo-nasal movement direction for the left eye.

RESPONSES IN VESTIBULAR NEURONS

In curarized frogs, primary afferent horizontal canal neurons were studied by Blanks and Precht (1976) and central vestibular neurons by Richter (1974) and Dieringer and Precht (unpubl.data). In comparison to similar studies in monkey and cat (see Goldberg,Fernández,1975;Precht, 1979;Baker et al.,1981) several differences were observed in the frog besides a 5 to 10 times lower resting rate:

1. Mean acceleration gain was several times higher in frog peripheral neurons (1.58 spikes/sec per degree/sec^2) but lower and similar in central vestibular neurons to that in cat and monkey (ca. 1 spike/sec per degree/sec^2).

2. Crossed inhibition between central vestibular neurons of synergistic canal pairs is missing in frog (Ozawa et al., 1974; Dieringer, Precht, 1979) as in lamprey (Rovainen, 1976) and toadfish (Korn et al.,1977).

3. Mean phase lag (re. head acceleration) is little smaller in frog primary afferents (Fig.3) than in cat or monkey, corresponding to a shorter cupular time constant of 3 sec (ca.4 in cat and 6 in monkey). Central vestibular neurons in the frog have a mean phase lag only little larger than that in primary afferents (Fig.3).

4. No central vestibular neurons were so far found in the frog that were reliably modulated by optokinetic stimuli.

Some of these differences might be causally related. Thus, according to the presence or absence of a functional commissural inhibition, the sensitivity from first- to second order vestibular neurons is either increased as in mammals (Shimazu,Precht,1966; but see Baker et al.,1981) or decreased as in the frog. This correlation is further corroborated by results obtained after hemilabyrinthectomy: in the cat (Markham et al.,1977) sensitivity of type I neurons on the intact side was strongly reduced, but not changed in the frog (unpubl.data).
        The time constants of central vestibular neurons in cat and monkey vary with the state of alertness. In decerebrate or drowsy animals the time constants are short due to a poorly functioning velocity integrating network (Raphan et al.,1977). In the frog as in rabbit (Collewjin et al.,1980) the estimated time constants of VOR (Fig.3) and of VCR (Fig.1) from frequency analyses are close to the cupular time constants (ca.3 sec), indicating that in both animals a velocity integrator is not charged during sinusoidal stimulation. Lack of positive behavioral evidence, together with point 4 leave serious doubts whether a frog has a functioning velocity integrator at all (Dieringer et al.,1982).

RESPONSES IN MOTONEURONS

Direct vestibulo-ocular projections are,as far as studied,
similarly organized as in cat or rabbit (see Precht,1979),
including inhibitory vestibulo-ocular connections.Neck
motoneurons also receive monosynaptic connections from
central vestibular neurons (Maeda et al.,1977). Is there
in the frog in parallel also an indirect pathway, partially integrating the vestibular velocity signal into a
position signal, as in the monkey (Skavensky,Robinson,
1973) and cat (Shinoda,Yoshida, 1974)?
We recorded the electromyographic (EMG) activity of several neck muscles involved in horizontal head movements
in frogs free to move their head or with their head fixed
and multi-unit activity from the abducens nerve of curarized frogs.

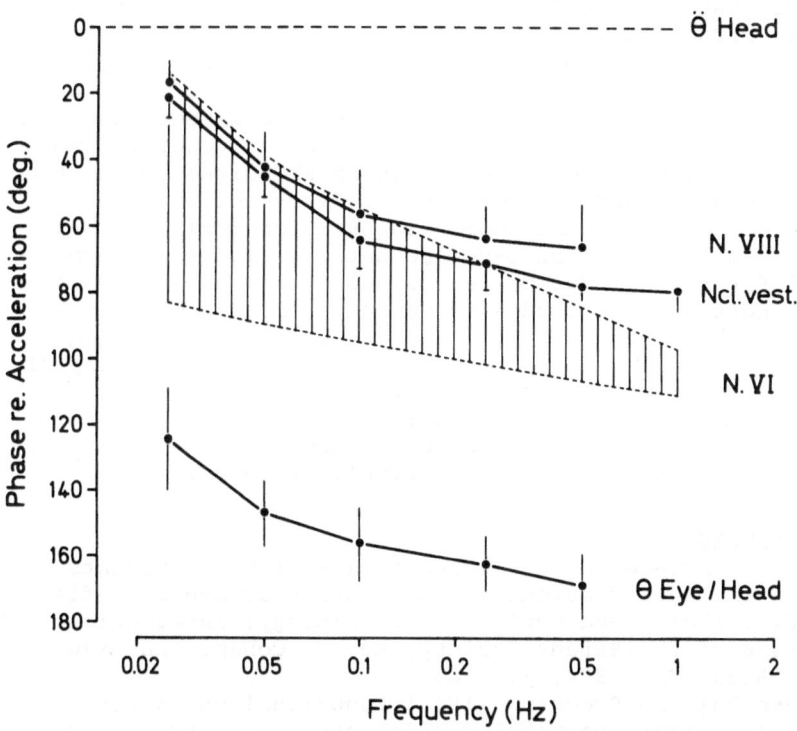

FIGURE 3. Bode diagram summarizing the phase shifts with
respect to head acceleration (θHead) in the VOR of the
frog. Mean values for primary vestibular afferents(N.VIII)
are from Blanks,Precht,1976. The dashed area outlines
phase values of abducens motoneurons recorded from the
VIth nerve. Neuronal data are from curarized preparations.
θ Eye/Head represents phase values of eye movements recorded in animals with their head fixed.

Most of these experiments gave very similar results:
The EMG activity in neck muscles and the spike activity
in most abducens nerve recordings showed amplitude-independent phase lags (determined by computer analysis) almost congruent with those of central vestibular neurons
between 0.025 and 0.5 Hz. In some abducens nerve recordings (30%), however, the phase lag was amplitude-dependent. At lower amplitudes consistently only spikes of
small size and with a larger phase lag were activated.
Increasingly larger stimulus amplitudes recruited in addition larger spikes and the phase lag decreased to reach
values overlapping with those obtained in other abducens
nerve, EMG or vestibular nucleus recordings. The range of
phase lags recorded in the abducens nerve is outlined in
Fig.3 by the dashed area.
It is tempting to interpretate these data in terms of the
two motor systems of the frog ("twitch" and "small nerve"
motor systems, see Simpson, 1976) innervating fast and
slow extraocular and skeletal muscle fibers:
The "small nerve" motor system has a lower reflex threshold, generates spikes that are small when recorded extracellularly (and are more difficult to detect) and slow
muscle fibers receiving this input do not generate action
potentials that are picked up as an EMG signal. Thus, the
EMG signals recorded might only reflect activity in the
"twitch" motor system, which in turn was activated only
by the direct vestibulo-collic pathway. The same might
hold for those abducens recordings, where the phase lag
was short and amplitude-independent. Then, however, the
larger phase lags observed in some abducens recordings
for small amplitudes, might be attributed to activity of
the "small nerve" motor system. The phase differences between these abducens and vestibular neurons suggest, that
in the frog as well an indirect pathway exists, that partially integrates central vestibular signals.

REFERENCES
Baker R, Evinger C and McCrea RA (1981) Some thoughts
about the three neurons in the vestibular ocular reflex.
In: Vestibular and Oculomotor Physiology: International
Meeting of the Bárány Society. Ed. B. Cohen. Ann. New
York Acad. Sci. 374, 171-188.
Blanks RHI and Precht W (1976) Functional characteriza-
tion of primary vestibular afferents in the frog. Exp.
Brain Res. 25, 369-390.
Collewijn H, Winterson BJ and van der Sten J (1980) Post-
rotatory nystagmus and optokinetic after-nystagmus in the
rabbit linear rather than exponential decay. Exp. Brain
Res. 40, 330-338.
Dieringer N and Precht W (1979) Mechanisms of compensa-
tion for vestibular deficits in the frog. Exp. Brain
Res. 36, 311-341.

Dieringer N and Precht W (1982) Compensatory head and
eye movements in the frog and their contribution to
stabilization of gaze. Exp. Brain Res. In press.
Dieringer N, Precht W and Cochran SL (1982) Is there a
velocity storage in the frog brain stem? Neurosci. Lett.
Suppl. In press.
Goldberg JM and Fernández C (1975) Vestibular Mechanisms.
Ann. Rev. Physiol. 37, 129-162.
Korn H, Sotelo C and Bennett MVL (1977) The lateral vestibular nucleus of the toadfish Opsanus Tau. N.Sci.2,851-884.
Maeda M, Magherini PC and Precht W (1977) Functional organization of vestibular and visual inputs to neck and fore-
limb motoneurons in the frog. J.Neurophysiol.40,225-243.
Markham CH, Yagi T and Curthoys IS (1977) The contribution
of the contralateral labyrinth to second order vestibular
neuronal activity in the cat. Brain Res. 138, 99-109.
Ozawa S, Precht W and Shimazu H (1974) Crossed effects on
central vestibular neurons in the horizontal canal system
of the frog. Exp. Brain Res. 19, 394-405.
Precht W (1979) Vestibular mechanisms. Ann. Rev. Neurosci. 2, 265-289.
Raphan T, Matsuo V and Cohen B (1979) Velocity storage in
the vestibulo-ocular reflex arc (VOR). Exp. Brain Res.
35, 229-248.
Richter A (1974) Antworten der Vestibulariskernneurone
des Frosches bei natürlicher Labyrinthreizung. Doct.
Thesis, Univ. Frankfurt.
Rovainen CM (1976) Vestibulo-ocular reflexes in the adult
sea lamprey. J. Comp. Physiol. 112, 159-164.
Shimazu H and Precht W (1966) Inhibition of central vestibular neurons from the contralateral labyrinth and its
mediating pathway. J. Neurophysiol. 29, 467-492.
Shinoda Y and Yoshida K (1974) Dynamic characteristics
of responses to horizontal head angular acceleration in
vestibuloocular pathway in the cat. J. Neurophysiol. 37,
653-673
Simpson JI (1976) Functional synaptology of the spinal
cord. In: Frog Neurobiology. Eds. R. Llinás and W. Precht.
Springer-Verlag Berlin, Heidelberg, New York.
Skavensky AA and Robinson DA (1973) Role of abducens
neurons in vestibuloocular reflex. J. Neurophysiol. 36,
724-738.

This work is supported by grants from the Swiss National Science Foundation (3.505.79 and 3.616.80) and
from the Dr.Eric Slack-Gyr Foundation.

"VISUO-SPINAL ATAXIA" CAUSED BY DISORDERS OF EYE MOVEMENTS [+]

Th. Brandt, J. Esser, W. Büchele, S. Krafczyk

(Neurological Clinic with Clinical Neurophysiology, Alfried Krupp Hospital, Essen, Federal Republic of Germany)

The characteristics of central and peripheral disorders of ocular motility constitute valuable diagnostic signs for the clinician. For the patient, however, they result in a variety of distressing symptoms such as oscillopsia, diplopia, blurred vision, spatial disorientation or ocular vertigo including postural imbalance. Ocular vertigo (Adler, 1941) arises from an intersensory mismatch when visual information is at variance with vestibular and somatosensory inputs. The perceptual and postural consequences of ocular motor disorders are often neglected and it is the purpose of the present paper to deal especially with those of the ocular vertigo symptoms which can be regarded as visuo-spinal in origin.

The sudden onset of an <u>extraocular muscle paresis</u> as well as <u>acquired ocular oscillations</u> often induce ocular vertigo, particularly associated with voluntary eye or head movements. This also affects locomotion and postural balance since vision is a major cue for postural stabilization. In order to maintain postural stability in the upright position, afferent (vestibular; somato-sensory; visual) signals must be generated as an input for compensation of natural fore-aft and lateral body sways.

<u>Postural imbalance</u> with ocular motor disorders can be attributed to an acute sensory deficiency of visual localization of objects in egocentric coordinates; this is calculated from both the position of the target on the retina and the awareness of eye position in the head. Visually guided motor performance requires accurate information about gaze direction and body position relative to the surround. An extraocular muscle paresis as well as acquired ocular oscillations, however, cause a dissociation of subjective visual and somatosensory straight ahead (Brandt, Büchele, 1979) because the involuntary deviation from the "expected eye position" (due to the efference copy signal) is not compensated by adaequate afferent extraretinal information (fig. 1, $\alpha \neq \alpha'$). Thus, the mismatch between the expected and actual eye position is responsible for the direction specific distortion of locomotion and reaching movements as well as increased body sway amplitudes which can be measured by posturography (fig. 2, 3, 4). Increased body sway can be interpreted as a visuo-spinal imbalance

[+] supported by Deutsche Forschungsgemeinschaft (DFG)

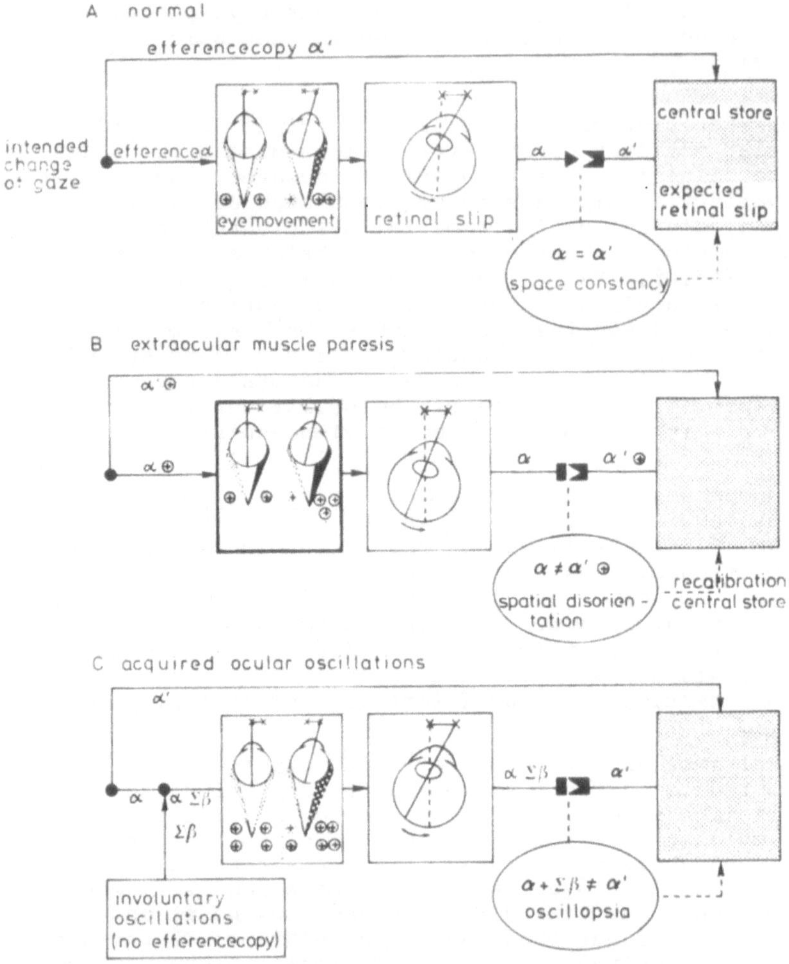

FIGURE 1. Pathomechanisms of ocular vertigo: A) In
normals the voluntary impulse to perform a change of gaze
releases the efference α to the eye muscles as well as an
appropriate efference copy signal α' to a central store.
This store contains the memory for the expected retinal
slip due to the particular intended eye movement as
calibrated prior to disease onset. Space constancy is
maintained if the comparison of the actual with the
expected retinal slip is $\alpha = \alpha'$. B) With an acute extraocular muscle paresis spatial disorientation occurs
because the expected slip α' $\oplus$ - as dependent on the
greater effort which is required for the movement -
exeeds the actual slip α, $\alpha \neq \alpha'$ $\oplus$. Eye movement
exercises, however, promote a rearrangement of the central
store with subsequent diminution of the mismatch.
C) Acquired ocular oscillations are not associated with an
efference copy and therefore cause oscillopsia, $\alpha \Sigma \beta \neq \alpha'$.

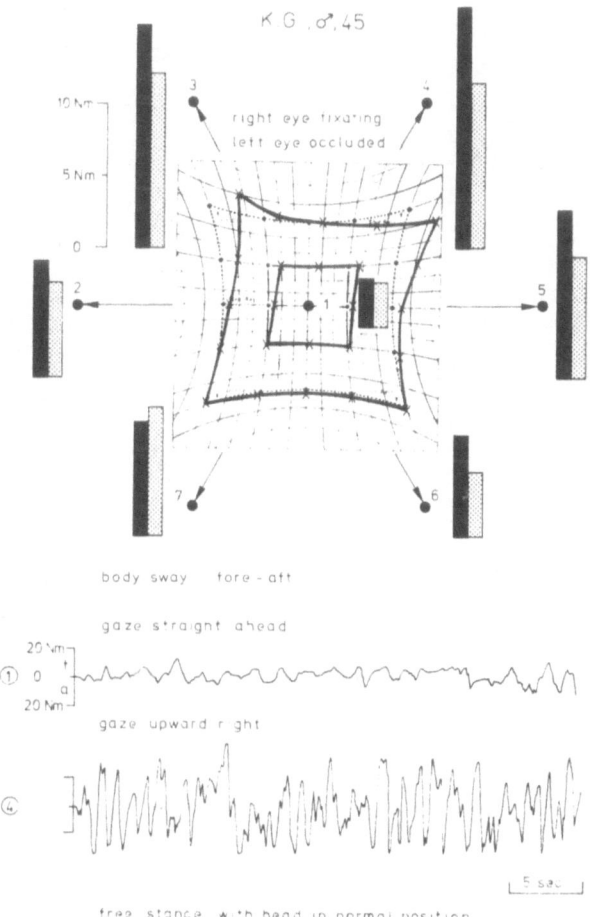

FIGURE 2. Posturography of the fore-aft (black columns)
and lateral (shaded columns) body sway with free upright
stance in a patient suffering from an acquired paresis of
the rectus superior and an overaction of the obliquus
inferior, as indicated by the investigation with the
Hess-Lees screen (top). Root mean square values RMS
(Nm = Newton meters) of body sway are minimal in the
primary position of gaze (1) and increase significantly
when the gaze is directed 45° towards the optimal range
of action of the affected extraocular muscles (3; 4).
Original recordings of the fore-aft sway with gaze
conditions 1 and 4 are depicted at the bottom.

428

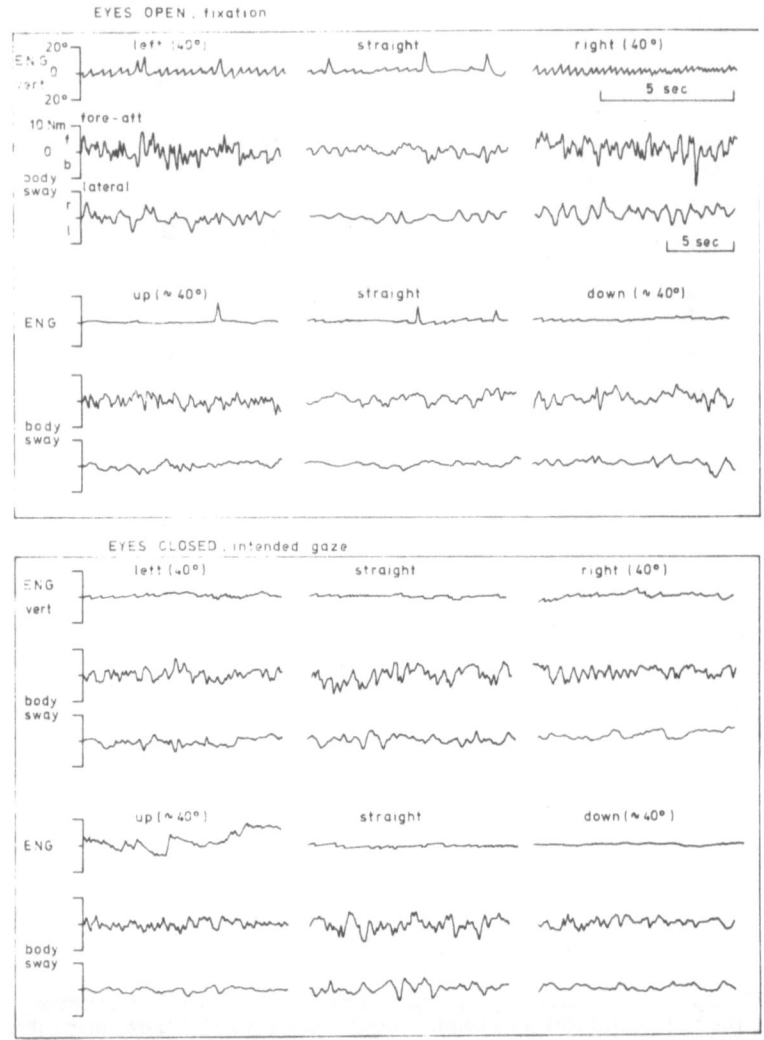

FIGURE 3. Simultaneous recordings in a patient with down-beat nystagmus of vertical electronystagmography, and fore-aft and lateral body sway during standing with the head straight. With the eyes open and fixation of a stationary target the nystagmus amplitude is dependent on the lateral direction of gaze as is postural imbalance (top). Intended change of gaze with eyes closed, however, has no comparable effect on nystagmus amplitude or body sway (bottom).

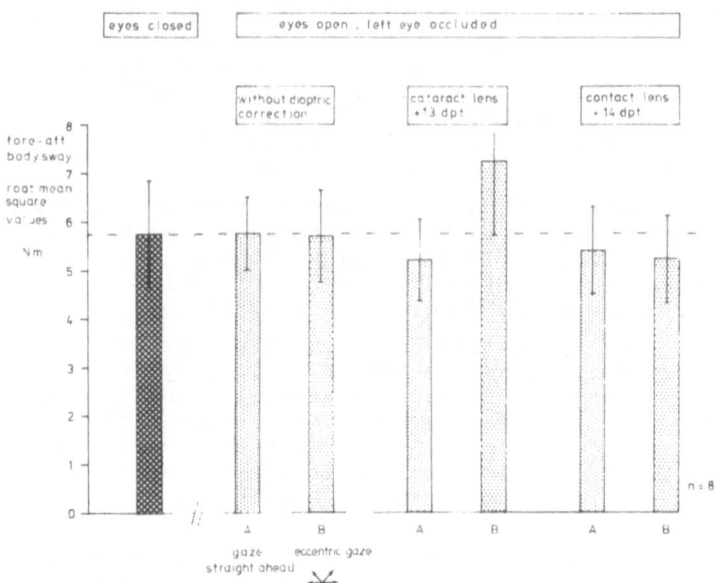

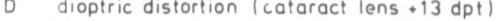

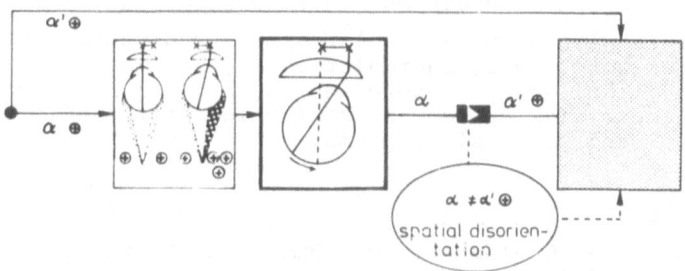

D   dioptric distortion (cataract lens +13 dpt)

FIGURE 4. Gaze dependent postural imbalance with upright
stance (RMS values of fore-aft sway in Newton meters) in
a patient with aphakia due to cataract surgery, wearing a
cataract lense for the first time (top). Spatial
disorientation and subsequent postural imbalance with
eccentric gaze can be attributed to the strong prismatic
distortion when looking through the peripheral parts of
the lense (bottom).

consequent to the disparate retinal slip as compared to
the expected pattern calibrated prior to the disease
onset. The disturbance of spatial localization and
oscillopsia is not restriced to the fovea but involves
the entire visual field and therefore affects the two
modes of visual processing, "focal" and "ambient",
respectively. The ambient mode relies on afferent
information from the peripheral field and subserves
spatial orientation and postural balance.

Postural imbalance with acute extraocular muscle paresis
is particularly apparent when voluntary head movements
are performed (Brandt, 1982) or with intended gaze
towards the direction of optimal range of action of the
paretic muscle (fig. 2; Esser et al., 1981).

Involuntary ocular oscillations such as acquired pendular
nystagmus, spasmus nutans, superior oblique myokymia or
downbeat nystagmus, are not associated with an appropriate
efference copy and therefore cause oscillopsia and visual
ataxia even without precipitating voluntary head and eye
movements. The increased sway amplitudes increase with the
gaze dependent increased nystagmus amplitude, as does the
oscillopsia (fig. 3).

Finally, as mentioned by Adler in 1941, "individuals who
wear strong lenses for the first time, particularly
cataract lenses, also suffer from the strong prismatic
effect produced from looking through the peripheral parts
of the lense" and exhibit an increased body sway (fig.4).

In patients with acquired ocular motility disturbances
as well as with acute abnormalities in the dioptric
apparatus, head and eye exercises may promote sensory
rearrangement with subsequent diminution of the described
perceptual and postural symptoms.

REFERENCES

Adler FH (1941) Ocular vertigo. Am. Acad. Ophthal.
Otolaryng., 27-31.
Brandt Th (1982) The relationship between retinal image
slip, oscillopsia, and postural imbalance. In Lennerstrand
G, Lee DS and Keller El, eds. Functional Basis of Ocular
Motility Disorders, Oxford, Pergamon (in press).
Brandt Th, Büchele W (1979) Ocular myasthenia: Visual
disturbance of posture and gait. Agressologie 2o,
195-196.
Esser J, Krafczyk S, Brandt Th (1981) Posturographie der
visuellen Standataxie bei infranukleären Okulomotorik-
störungen. Arbeitstagung, Deutsche Gesellschaft für
Neurologie, München

EYE-HEAD-HAND COORDINATION

C. PRABLANC and B. BIGUER, Lab. de Neuropsychologie
Expérimentale, Inserm unité 94, 69500 Bron, FRANCE

1. INTRODUCTION

The execution of such a simple task as pointing with the finger
at a small visual target within the prehension space involves a
series of sensory and sensorimotor processes in order to trigger
the activation of the appropriate muscles and their synergistic
control. Contrary to a situation of avoidance reaction where
detection is the prime triggering stimulus, localization of the
target with respect to the subject's body is here the initial
source of the motor response. This spatial encoding needs
knowledge of the head position with respect to the trunk, eye
position with respect to the head, and finally retinal position of
the target. An inaccurate response of a pointing may have two
sources of variation, one in the spatial encoding of the target,
the other one in the arm-forearm motor program. In a normal
situation the vision of both the hand movement (called
reafference) and of the target will allow for a correction of the
motor program if it were to be inaccurate. We will focus in this
study mainly on the spatial encoding aspects, discarding the role
of error correction based on the vision of both the hand and the
target. This will be achieved either by never seeing the hand (no
reafference condition) or by cutting the target off before the
visible hand moves and thus preventing any error detection on the
retina. As strategies are determinant in the ordering of a complex
sequence, the instructions given to the subjects all throughout
the different experimental conditions will be the same as to the
final goal : to realize the best compromise between velocity and
accuracy of the hand pointing.

2. PROCEDURES

2.1. <u>Materials and methods</u> The first experimental set up is
schematically shown on figure 1. Targets presentation was
performed through a matrix of light emitting diodes. The subject
could see binocularly the virtual image of the target through a
semi-reflecting mirror. The space between surfaces Q and R could
either be illuminated, allowing the subject to see his whole arm,
or be made completely dark. Eye movements were recorded
binocularly with an EOG technique. A logic pulse could be used to
cut off the target at the onset of the goal directed saccade,
preventing retinal feedback. Hand position was recorded by a
thimble attached to the subject's forefinger, which indicated its
coordinates on the surface R. Targets were presented as step
stimuli along horizontal or sagittal directions at 8 positions ;
they always stepped from the center C' to a peripheral random
target. When pointing under peripheral vision the subject
continuously fixated a target 2 mm ahead of the center. The
interstimulus interval and the sequence of positions were
randomized in order to avoid anticipation adjustments responsible
for latency variations (Requin, 1978 ; Becker, 1972).
The second experimental apparatus was similar to the first one,
with a polar (angular) stimulation and arm recording instead of a
cartesian one. Additional signals made it possible to record

Roucoux, A. and Crommelinck, M. (eds.): Physiological and Pathological Aspects of Eye Movements.
© *1982, Dr W. Junk Publishers, The Hague, Boston, London.* ISBN-13: 978-94-009-8002-0

432

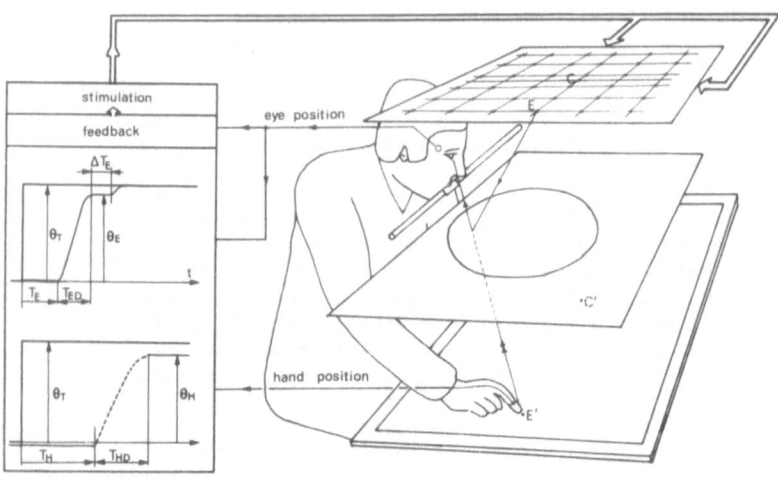

Fig. 1. Experimental apparatus showing on surface P the matrix of targets. The subject with his head fixed, sees the target on surface R through a semi-reflecting mirror. He can point starting from C' to an E' target either when seeing both the target and his hand (reafference) or with his hand unseen (no reafference). Horizontal eye movements are recorded by an electrooculographic technique, and hand position by a thimble attached to the finger ; and transmitting its coordinates. Eye velocity can be used to trigger a feedback stimulation : for instance the onset of a saccade can cut off the target. T_E, T_{ED},θ_E and T_H, T_{HD}, θ_H are respectively for eye and hand the latency, duration of movement, and position of the response. (from Prablanc et al 1979).

Fig. 2. Saccadic eye movements in response to (a) continuous target ; (b) with time presentation = 200 ms LC : central fixation point LP : 20° nasal target. T_1 is the latency of the main saccade with respect to the onset of LP. T_2 is the delay between the end of the main saccade and the beginning of the corrective saccade. The main features in situation b was the absence of the corrective saccade and the persistent residual retinal error $(\Delta\alpha)$ at the end of the main saccade (from Prablanc and Jeannerod, 1975,pp 465-471)

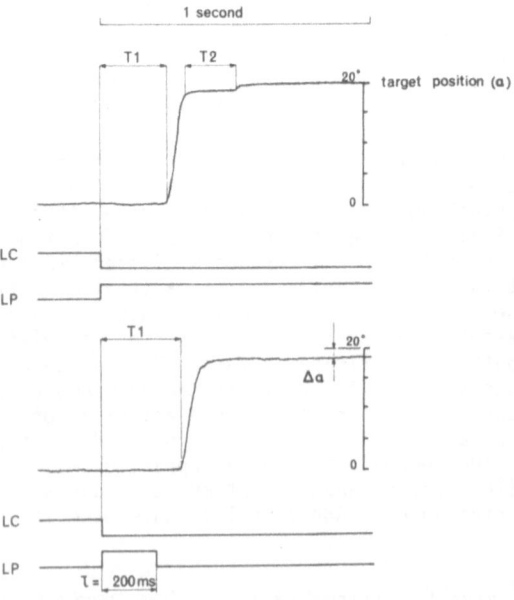

simultaneously eye-head-hand positions and neck and biceps electromyographic activities (emgs). Head movement was recorded with an helmet attached to a potentiometer and emgs with surface electrodes (right splenius capitis for the neck and biceps brachialis for the arm).

Three experiments were performed : Exp. 1 investigated mainly the role of the extraretinal signal of the saccade on the accuracy of the pointing. It was performed under continuous vision of the whole hand-arm, but at the onset of the goal directed saccade the target was turned off. Exp. II was a study of the sequence of the overall response (eye-head and hand positions) and of the corresponding control signals (neck and biceps emgs). Exp. III investigated only the role of the head orientation response on the accuracy of the hand pointing.

2.2. Does the saccade efference copy play a role in the arm response ?

When a subject is asked to point the most quickly and accurately as possible at a peripheral target, his head beeing restrained and without further instruction regarding eye movement, one observe within 200 msec a goal directed saccade followed by the onset of hand movement 80-100 msec later. It is important to know whether this delayed hand response is the result of a serial processing in which the efference copy of the saccade could be used for the encoding of the hand motor program or whether it is a motor processing parallel to the oculomotor response.

Goal directed saccades corresponding to retinal stimulus beyond 10 degrees of eccentricity are known to be composed of two clustered saccades : a first hypometric saccade of 90 % of the extent of the retinal eccentricity, followed by a small corrective saccade, 150 msec later, bringing the fovea onto the stimulus (Bartz, 1962 ; Becker, Fuchs, 1969 ; Becker, 1972 ; Prablanc, Jeannerod, 1975 ; Hallett, 1978 ; Deubel et al, 1982). There are two types of corrective saccades 1) when the error of the primary saccade is large (> 15 %) secondary saccades occur, which are triggered by extraretinal signals, their latency is usually very short (≤ 100 msec) but they are not fully corrective ; 2) when the error is smaller than 10 % corrective saccade generally need a retinal feedback to be triggered, and the line of gaze remain in an uncorrected error if no retinal feedback is available (Fig. 2). In the further study we will take into account only those single saccadic responses to a brief target.

As regards hand pointing accuracy we will see whether the oculomotor efference copy of the initial saccade can be the relevant triggering signal for the encoding of the arm motor program. In that case there should be a correlation between the hypometry of the saccade and the sign of hand pointing error. In order to discriminate whether the hand pointing error relied upon peripheral retinal uncertainly or oculomotor inaccuracy, two sessions were performed with visual reafferences from the arm : in the first session, pointings at the targets were done under peripheral vision (P.V.) while continously fixating a central point ; in such a condition, visual reafferences from the arm and vision of the target are useless in correcting any motor program error. In the second session restricted vision (R.V.) the onset of the goal directed saccade turned the target off, preventing any comparison between the arm reafferences and the position of the target.

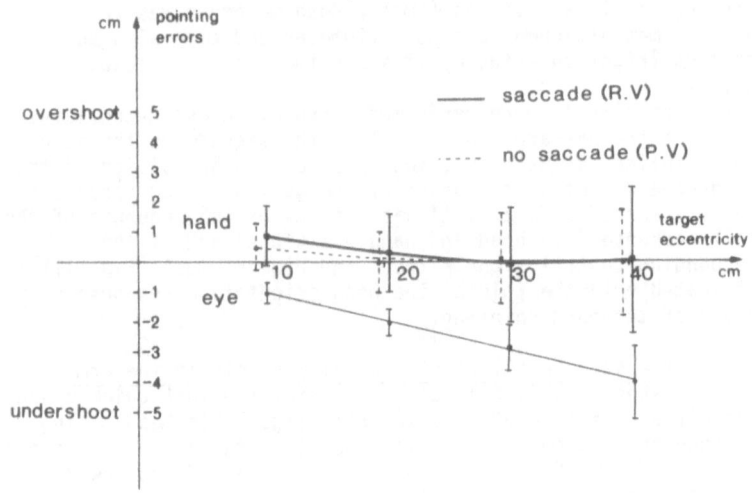

Fig. 3. Hand pointing errors in the two different conditions described in the text : restricted vision (R.V.) and peripheral vision (P.V.). Note that in both conditions, the distribution of errors is practically surimposed. In addition, in the restricted vision condition, the hypometry of saccades does not seem to be reflected upon the hand pointing.

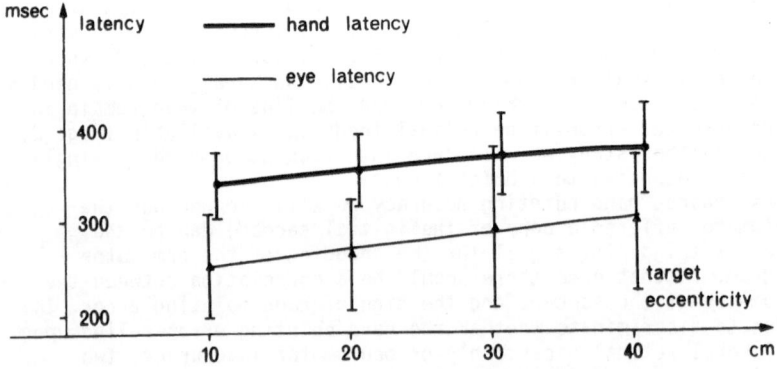

Fig. 4. Mean latency of the eye and hand movement with respect to target eccentricity. Across the different eccentricities the onset of hand movement followed that of the eye by 80-100 msec. In this experiment, the head was kept fixed.

Results

Errors of hand pointing and of the initial saccade toward the target versus eccentricity on the right side ipsilateral to the arm are represented on figure 3.

In peripheral vision the mean hand pointings slightly overshoot the target for small eccentricities, then become centered around the target for larger ones. Their variance increases as eccentricity, reflecting the corresponding decay of visual acuity on the peripheral retina.

In restricted vision where the initial saccade turns the target off, a quite linear relationship between stimulus eccentricity and saccadic initial error is observed, while the hand pointing errors distribution is practically superimposed on the one under peripheral vision, the only difference beeing a higher variance. Thus the hypometry of saccades does not seem to be reflected upon the hand pointing. In addition, within a constant target eccentricity, a correlation analysis between hand error versus eye error revealed to be nonsignificant ($r = 0.05$), making very unlikely the saccade efference copy as a quantitative signal to compute the arm motor program. If not used for the computation of the arm motor program, the efference copy could be used as a triggering signal for the arm movement initiation ; and indeed figure 4 shows that eye and arm latencies follow the same parallel course versus target eccentricity with a nearly constant difference of about 85 msec, as it has also been observed in an oculo-manual tracking task on a display (Angel et al. 1970). However the degree of coupling between eye and arm latency, within a constant target eccentricity, appear much looser ($r = 0.45$).

Contrary to fast movements performed without spatial goal, where arm movement duration is found to be almost independent from its extent, duration was found here to be highly dependent upon target eccentricity ($F = 33.4$, $p < 0.001$). In the R.V. condition this increased duration with eccentricity cannot be explained by a processing of arm visual reafferences and target position, the target beeing turned off at the onset of the saccade i.e. about 85 msec before the onset of arm movement ; thus if this additional time rely upon a feedback processing, it may be more likely upon kinaesthesis.

2.3. Initiation of the eye-head-hand responses and of their emg signals. When a subject has to point quickly and accurately, he makes a saccade followed by a head orientation and then by an arm movement. The eye-head sequence in a visual orientation is well documented (Bizzi, 1971 ; Warabi, 1977 ; Barnes, 1979 ; Zangemeister, Stark, 1981) it consists of a saccade followed 40 msec later by the head movement associated with a compensatory eye movement equal and opposite to the head displacement, through the vestibulo-ocular reflex (VOR).

In order to study the overt sequence of eye-head and arm movement in our pointing task, an experiment was conducted with a simultaneous recording of eye, head, arm positions and neck and biceps emgs (biceps was chosen as the muscle signalling onset of arm movement each pointing beginning by a lift from the surface).

Subjects participated on two sessions with and without visual reafferences from the arm with the same procedures as in the previous experiment. They were not given any instruction regarding the sequence of responses.

Results

The typical sequence is represented on figure 5 : a saccade is first triggered 220 msec after the target onset followed by the head movement 40 msec later, and then by an arm movement 100 msec later. Head movement produces compensatory eye movements which stabilize gaze in space, but as the initial saccade is hypometric a corrective saccade is triggered, superimposed on the compensatory eye movements, bringing the gaze onto the target. Emg signals from neck and biceps appear to be close to the saccade onset which itself is known to follow the extraocular muscle emg 10 msec later (Breinin, Kugelberg, 1955 ; Fuchs, Luschei, 1970 ; Henn, Cohen, 1973). If the two different conditions (reafference or no reafference) have no effect on the eye latency, the arm latency is slightly longer without reafferences (t = 15 msec). The mean latencies of eye movements, neck emg and biceps emg versus target eccentricity are represented on figure 6. Saccade latency is slightly but significantly increasing with eccentricity as observed previously by several authors (Bartz, 1962 ; White et al, Prablanc, Jeannerod, 1974 ; Biguer et al, 1982). Biceps and neck emgs have a decreasing latency from 10 to 20 degrees, but are then consistently increasing with eccentricity (F = 3.62, p < 0.02). A correlation analysis performed within each of the 20, 30 and 40 degrees targets shows a significant but loose link between emgs and eye movement latency, as can be seen on table I. A possible explanation for this loose but significant correlation between latencies and for a non unity regression slope is that there is a first common stage corresponding to the visual process of target detection and localization, followed by parallel decisions of the different motor programs having independent variations.

TABLE I. Relationships between eye and neck-biceps emg latencies.
T_E : eye movement latency
T_N : neck emg latency
T_B : biceps emg latency

CONDITION		Correlation Coefficient	Regression Slope
REAFFERENCE	$T_N = f \ (T_E)$	0.34	0.47
	$T_B = f \ (T_E)$	0.41	0.47
NO REAFFERENCE	$T_N = f \ (T_E)$	0.39	0.50
	$T_B = f \ (T_E)$	0.39	0.47

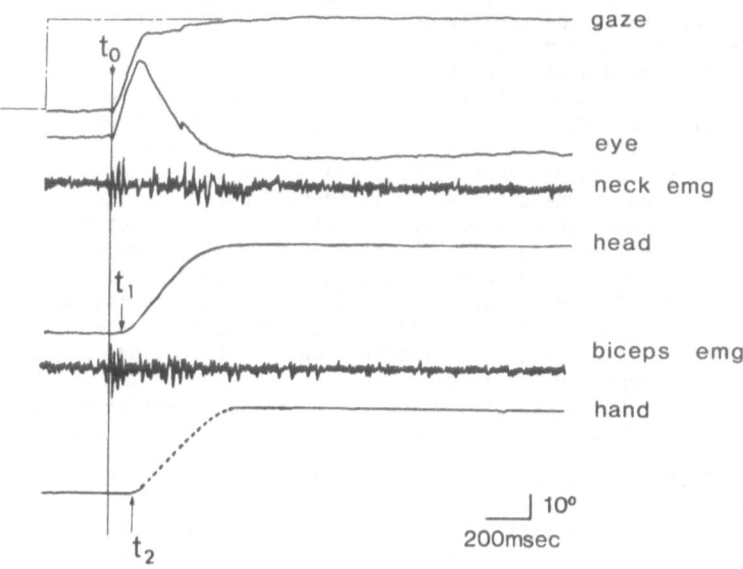

Fig. 5. A typical example of eye, head and hand movements toward a single visual target within the extrapersonal space. While overt movements are sequential (t_0, t_1 t_2), the biceps and neck emg latencies are practically synchronized with the gaze latency. On the bottom curve, dotted lines indicate that hand trajectory is lost.

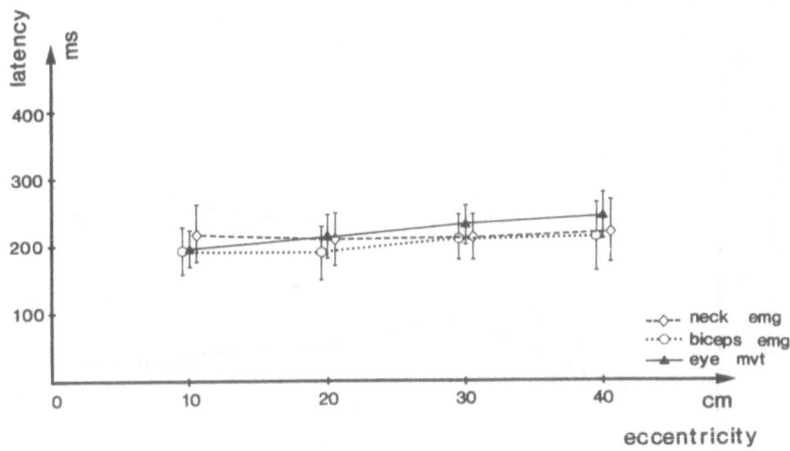

Fig. 6. Mean latencies and standard deviations for neck and biceps emg and eye movement. Data for this figure are averaged from five subjects. They have been obtained in the condition without visual reafferences from the hand movement.

438

2.4. Influence of head orientation on hand pointing accuracy The
mechanism of eye-head orientation toward a peripheral stimulus has
been shown to be practically independent from neck proprioceptive
information, the final goal i.e. gaze orientation beeing reached
with the same dynamics, whatever the situation, providing
vestibular system is intact (Bizzi, 1979). However if from a motor
point of view neck afferences are not crucial, spatial encoding of
visual information rely heavily on those signals, which importance
has been stressed by Cohen (1961), who showed that after dorsal
roots section, monkeys had an impaired goal directed reaching,
though they were able to maintain fixation on the object to
reach. In addition the role of active head mobilization in
updating afferent information has been suggested by Paillard
(1971) and Paillard, Beaubaton (1976). However in a pointing task,
when visual reafferences from the arm are present and eye
movements allowed, a clear difference between head fixed or head
free conditions can hardly been observed ; indeed if the localization were to be inaccurate on the basis of a poor extra-retinal
signal related to a too extreme position of the eyeball within the
orbit, an inaccurate arm motor program would be corrected all
throughout the movement by the visual reafferences of the arm
dynamic error.

In order to estimate the role of head orientation response
toward the target on hand pointing accuracy, two sessions were
performed both without visual arm reafferences, one with the head
restrained in a straight position, the other with the head freely
moving.
Results

The absolute hand pointing errors versus eccentricity are
represented on figure 7. For 10 cm, as the head does not naturally
move, errors are not different, up to 20 cm errors increase in
both conditions though slower for the head free condition, then
for 30 and 40 cm, "head free" errors decrease down to the same
magnitude as for small eccentricities and become significantly
smaller than "head fixed" errors (t = 3.09 ; p < 0.01).

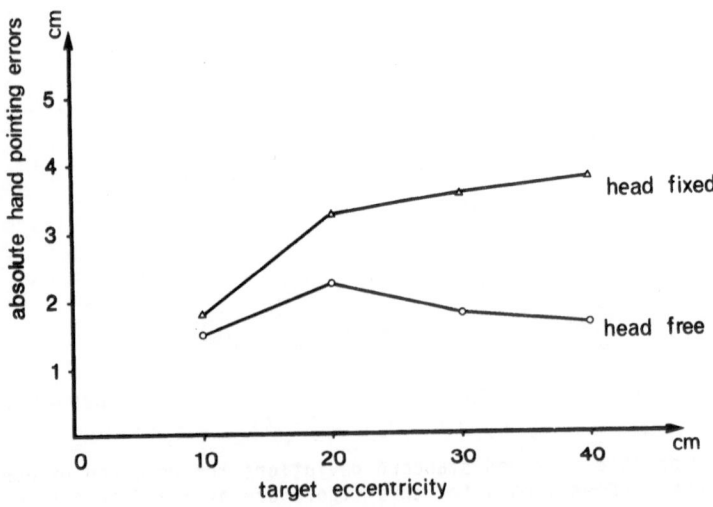

Fig. 7.

3. DISCUSSION

The different experiments of optimals eye-head-hand coordination in a pointing task indicate a clustering of control signals systematically observed with or without visual reafferences from the arm, and which occur within a time interval of about 50 msec, although movements of the different systems appear sequential, reflecting only their own inertial properties. However, these control signals are unlikely to be issued from an oculomotor efference copy generator because they do not show a sharp covariation. This is also supported by the absence of correlation between the eye position signal issued from the saccade and the hand pointing accuracy under fixed head condition. Their latencies from the onset of the target probably share a common process of detection and localization on the peripheral retina ; the second part of the latencies have more or less independent variations, the less sensitive to various conditions beeing the eye latency as also shown by Zangmeister, Stark (1982), the hand latency beeing sensitive to the presence or absence of its visual reafferences (Prablanc et al 1979 ; Herman et al 1981), and head latency has been shown to depend also on conditions under which head movement is elicited (Bizzi et al 1972 ; Barnes, 1979).

The improvement of arm pointing accuracy when head is free has some indirect but important implications. The sequence of activation of the different motor programs stays within a 50-70 msec average timing, with either fixed or free head. In the same arm pointing task, Biguer (1981) has shown that arm and head movements had approximately the same durations ranging from 300 to 550 msec for targets from 10 to 40 cm. If, as observed, an adjustment of the arm motor program has occured when the head is free, it cannot be through reafferences from the final head positions. The dynamic reafferent neck informations and the corresponding recentering of the eyeball within the orbit which could improve the accuracy of the extraretinal signal, can be considered as possible mechanisms for spatial information sharpening and for motor program adjustments in the absence of visual arm reafferences. However this hypothesis neads further investigations of the distribution of extra-retinal and head position signal errors.

Acknowledgements. We would like to thank all our subjects for their patience and collaboration. We are grateful to J.F. Echallier and C. Urquizar for their computing and electronic assistance and to M. Althabe and S. Bello for making up this paper.

REFERENCES

Angel RW, Alston W and Garland H (1970) Functional relations between the manual and oculomotor control systems, Exp. Neurol. 27, 248-257.

Barnes GR (1979) Vestibulo-ocular function during coordinated head and eye movements to acquire visual targets, J. Physiol., 287, 127-147.

Bartz AE (1962) Eye movement latency, duration and response time as a function of angular displacement, J. Exp. Psychol., 64, 318-324.

Becker W (1972) The control of eye movements in the saccadic system, Bibliotheca Ophthal., 82, 233-243.

Becker W and Fuchs AF (1969) Further properties of the human saccadic system : eye movements and correction saccades with and without visual fixation points, Vision Res., 9, 1247-1258.

Biguer B (1981) Coordination visuomotrice : séquence d'activation et contrôle des mouvements visuellement guidés. Thèse de Doctorat 3è cycle de Neurobiologie, Université Claude Bernard, Lyon.

Biguer B, Jeannerod M and Prablanc C (1982) The coordination of eye, head and arm movements during reaching at a single visual target, Exp. Brain Res., 46, 301-304.

Bizzi E, Kalil RE, Tagliasco V (1971) Eye-head coordination in monkeys : evidence for centrally patterned organization, Science, 173, 452-454.

Bizzi E, Kalil RE and Morasso P (1972) Two modes of active eye-head coordination in monkeys, Brain Res., 40, 45-48.

Breinin G and Kugelberg E (1955) Electromyography of the human extraocular muscles, Arch. Ophthalmol., 54, 200-210.

Cohen LA (1961) Role of the eye and neck proprioceptive mechanisms in body orientation and motor coordination, J. Neurophysiol., 24, 1-11.

Deubel H, Wolf W and Hauske G (1982) Corrective saccades : effect of shifting the saccade goal, Vision Res., 22, 353-364.

Fuchs AF and Luschei E (1970) Firing patterns of abducens neurons of alert monkeys in relationship to horizontal eye movements, J. Neurophysiol., 33, 382-392.

Hallett PE (1978) Primary and secondary saccades to goals defined by instructions, Vision Res., 18, 1279-1296.

Henn V and Cohen B (1973) Quantitative analysis of activity in eye muscle motoneurons during saccadic eye movements and positions of fixation, J. Neurophysiol., 36, 115-124.

Herman R, Herman R and Maulucci R (1981) Visually triggered eye-arm movements in man, Exp. Brain Res., 42, 392-398.

Paillard J and Beaubaton D (1978) De la coordination visuomotrice à l'organisation de la saisie manuelle. In Hecaen H and Jeannerod M, ed. Du contrôle moteur à l'organisation du geste, pp 225-260. Masson, Paris.

Paillard J (1971) Les déterminants moteurs de l'organisation spatiale, Cahiers de Psychol., 14, 261-316.

Prablanc C, Echallier JF, Komilis E and Jeannerod M (1979) Optimal response of eye and hand motor systems in pointing at a visual target I Spatio temporal characteristics of eye and hand movements and their relationships when varying the amount ov visual information, Biol. Cybernetics, 35, 113-124.

Prablanc C and Jeannerod M (1974) Latence et précision de saccades en fonction de l'intensité, de la durée et de la position rétinienne d'un stimulus, Rev. E.E.G. Neurophysiol., 3, 484-488.

Prablanc C and Jeannerod M (1975) Corrective saccades : dependence
on retinal reafferent signals, Vision Res., 15, 465-469.
Requin J (1978) Spéficité des ajustements préparatoires à
l'exécution du programme moteur. In Hecaen H and Jeannerod M, ed.
Du contrôle moteur à l'organisation du geste, pp 84-129. Masson,
Paris.
Warabi T (1977) The reaction time of eye-head coordination in man,
Neurosc. Let., 6, 47-51.
White CT, Eason C and Barlett NR (1962) Latency and duration of
eye movements in the horizontal plane, J. Opt. Soc. Am., 52, 210-
213.
Zangemeister WH, Meinberg O, Stark L and Hoyt WF (1982) Eye-head
coordination in homonymous hemianopia, J. Neurol. 226, 243-254.
Zangemeister WH and Stark L (1981) Active head rotation and eye-
head coordination, Ann. New-York Sci., 374, 540-559.

LIST OF PARTICIPANTS

AL ANSARI Amir, Laboratoire de Neurophysiologie, Univer-
    sité Catholique de Louvain, UCL 5449, Avenue Hippo-
    crate, 54, B-1200 Bruxelles, Belgium - tel. 02-
    7623400 ext. 5447.

BAKER Robert, Dept. of Physiology, New York University,
    Medical Center, 550 First Avenue, New York, N.Y.
    10016, USA - tel. 212-340-5402.

BARMACK Neal H., Physiology Section, The Biological
    Sciences Group, The University of Connecticut,
    Storrs, CT 06268, USA - tel. 203-486-4562.

BARNES Graham, Behavioural Sciences Div., R.A.F. Insti-
    tute of Aviation Medicine, Farnborough, Hants, U.K.
    - tel. 0252 24461 X-4406.

BECKER Wolfgang, Sektion Neurophysiologie, Universität
    Ulm, Ob. Eselberg, D-7900 Ulm, Germany - tel. 0731-
    1762335.

BEHRENS Frank, Institut of Physiology, Freie Universität
    Berlin, Arnimallee 22, D-1000 Berlin 33, FRG.

BERTHOZ Alain, Centre National de la Recherche Scienti-
    fique, Laboratoire de Physiologie Neurosensorielle,
    15, rue de l'Ecole de Médecine, F-75270 Paris Cedex
    06, France - tel. 3292177/3296154.

BITTENCOURT Paulo R.M., Depto de Clinica Medica (Neuro-
    logia) Hospital de Clinicas da U.F.P., Rua General
    Carneiro, Curitiba-PR-80000, Brazil - tel. 41-242-
    2426.

BÖHMER Andreas, Kantonspital Zürich, Neurologische Klinik
    Rämistrasse 100, CH-8091 Zürich, Switzerland.

BOUR L.J., Laboratory of Medical Physics and Biophysics,
    Geert Grooteplein N 21, NL-6526 EZ Nijmegen, The
    Netherlands - tel. 080-514237/514945.

BRANDT Thomas, Neurological Clinic with Clinical Neuro-
    physiology, Alfried Krupp Hospital, D-4300 Essen,
    FRG - 0201-4342527.

BÜCHELE Wolfgang, Neurological Clinic with Clinical Neu-
    rophysiology, Alfried Krupp Hospital, D-4300 Essen,
    FRG. - tel. 0201-4342527.

BUIZZA Angelo, Ist. Informatica e Sistemistica, Univers.
di Pavia, Strada Nuova 106/C, I-27100 Pavia, Italy -
tel. 39-382-29142.

BÜTTNER Ulrich, Dept. of Neurology, Univ. of Düsseldorf,
Moorenstr. 5, D-4000 Düsseldorf, FRG - tel. 211-
3118460.

BÜTTNER-ENNEVER Jean, Curieweg 27, D-4000 Düsseldorf - 13
FRG - tel. 0211-750425.

CAZIN Lionel, Université de Rouen, Laboratoire de Physiologie Animale, 10, Bd de Broglie, F-76130 Mont Saint
Aignan, France - tel. 35-982850.

CHAMBERS Brian R., MRC Neuro-otology Unit, National Hospital, Queen Sq., London WC1, U.K. - tel. 8373611
ext. 254.

CLEMENT G., Laboratoire de Physiologie Neurosensorielle,
15 rue de l'Ecole de Médecine, F-75270 Paris Cedex
06, France - tel. 3292177/3296154.

COHEN Bernard, Department of Neurology, Annenberg 21-24,
Mount Sinaï School of Medicine, 1 Gustave L. Levy
Place, New York, USA 10029 - tel. 212-650-7068.

COLLEWIJN Han, Faculteit der Geneeskunde, Dept. Physiology I, Erasmus Universiteit, Postbus 1738, NL -
Rotterdam 3000 DR, The Netherlands - tel. 010-
639111.

COMPAGNIONI Laura, Via Vanni n°2, 91100 Viterbo, Italy -
tel. 0761-220245.

CROMMELINCK Marc, Laboratoire de Neurophysiologie, Facul-
té de Médecine, UCL 5449, Université Catholique de
Louvain, 54, avenue Hippocrate, B-1200 Bruxelles,
Belgium - tel. 02-7623400 ext. 5447.

CULEE Christine, Laboratoire de Neurophysiologie, Facul-
té de Médecine, UCL 5449, Université Cahtolique de
Louvain, 54, avenue Hippocrate, B-1200 Bruxelles,
Belgium - tel. 02-7623400 ext. 5447.

DAUNICHT Wolfgang J., Dept. Biocybernetics, Inst. Phys.
Biol., University of Dusseldorf, D-4000 Dusseldorf,
FRG - tel. 0211-311-4538.

DEMANEZ Jean-Pierre, Hôpital de Bavière, Service ORL,
Boulevard de la Constitution, 66, B-4020 Liège,
Belgium.

DIERINGER Norbert, Institut für Hirnforschung der Universität Zürich, A. Forelstrasse, 1, CH-8029 Zürich,
Switzerland - tel. 01-533000.

DUYSSENS Jacques, Laboratorium voor Neuro en Psychofysiologie, Campus Gasthuisberg, Herestraat,
B-3000 Leuven, Belgium.

ECKMILLER Rolf, Ph. D., Div. of Biocybernetics, Dept.
of Biophysics, University of Düsseldorf, D-4000
Düsseldorf, FRG - tel. 0211-311-4540.

ESSER Joachim, Neurological Clinic with Clinical Neurophysiology, Alfried Krupp Hospital, Alfried Krupp
Str. 21, D-4300 Essen, FRG.

GIOANNI Henri, Laboratoire de Psychophysiologie Sensorielle, 9, quai St-Bernard, Bât. B., 3ème ét.,
F-75005 Paris, France - tel. 1-3362525 ext. 3233,
3400.

GRESTY Michael, M.R.C. National Hospital, Queen Square,
London WC1, U.K. - tel. 837-3611 ext. 254.

GRÜSSER Otto-Joachim, Dept. Physiology, Freie Universität, Arnimallee 22, D-1000 Berlin 33, FRG - tel.
030-8382543.

GUITTON Daniel, Montréal Neurological Institute, 3801
University St., Montréal H3A 2B4, Canada - tel. 514-
284-4711.

HENN Volker, Dept. of Neurology, University Hospital, CH-
8091 Zürich, Switzerland - tel. 01-2553285.

HEPP Klaus, Institut für Theoretische Physik, E.T.H., CH-
8093 Zürich, Switzerland - tel. 1-3772580.

HIGHSTEIN Stephen M., Dept. Neuroscience, Kennedy Center,
Albert Einstein College of Medicine, 1410 Pelham
PKY. S., Bronx, N.Y., 10461, USA - tel. 212-430-
2958.

HOFFMANN Klaus-Peter, Abt. Neurobiologie (Bio IV) Universität Ulm Postfach 4066, D-7900 Ulm, FRG - tel.
1763228 (a.c.0731).

INCHINGOLO Paolo, Dept. of Elettrotecnica, Elettronica e
Informatica, University of Trieste, v. Valerio 10,
I-34100 Trieste, Italy - tel. 39-40-574044.

JUDGE Stuart J., University Laboratory of Physiology,
Parks Road, Oxford OX1 3PT, U.K. - tel. 0865-57451.

JURGENS Reinhart, Sektion Neurophysiologie, Universität
Ulm, Oberer Eselberg, D-7900 Ulm, FRG - tel. 0049-
0731-1762335.

KITSOS Thomas, St Andreas Hospital-University, Clinic,
Patras, Greece - tel. 222812

446

KOENIG Eberhard, Neurologische Klinik, Liebermeister-
    strasse 18-20, D-7400 Tubingen, FRG - tel. 07071-
    292064/292046.

KOMMERELL Guntram, Klinikum der Albert-Ludwigs-Universi-
    tät, Universitäts-Augenklinik, Killianstrasse 5,
    D-7800 Freiburg i.Br., FRG - tel. 0761-2704002.

KRAFCZYK Siegbert, Neurological Clinic with Clinical
    Neurophysiology, Alfried Krupp Hospital, Alfried
    Krupp Str. 21, D-4300 Essen, FRG - tel. 0201-434-1.

LESTIENNE Francis, Laboratoire de Physiologie Neurosenso-
    rielle, CNRS, 15, rue de l'Ecole de Médecine, F-
    75270 Paris Cedex 06, France - tel. 1-3296154.

MAGNIN Michel, INSERM Unité 94, 16, avenue du Doyen
    Lépine, F-69500 Bron, France - tél. 7-8546578.

MAIOLI Claudio, I.F.C.N.-C.N.R., Via Mario Bianco, 9,
    I-20131 Milano, Italy - tel. 02-2840227.

MARKNER Christine, Abt. Vergleiehende Neurobiologie,
    Oberer Eselberg, Universität Ulm, D-7900 Ulm, FRG -
    tel. 0731-176-3228.

MERGNER Thomas, Sekt. Neurophysiologie, Universität Ulm,
    Oberer Eselberg, D-7900 Ulm, FRG - tel. 0731-176-
    2332.

MEULDERS Michel, Laboratoire de Neurophysiologie, UCL
    5449, Faculté de Médecine, Université Catholique de
    Louvain, Avenue Hippocrate, 54, B-1200 Bruxelles,
    Belgium - tel. 02-7623400 ext. 5449.

MIRA Eugenio, Otolaryngological Clinic, University of Pa-
    via, I-27100 Pavia, Italy - tel. 39-382-21072.

NAPPO Agostino, Via Vanni n°2, I-91100 Viterbo, Italy -
    tel. 0761-220245.

OTTES Fenno P., Lab. for Medical Physics & Biophysics,
    University of Nijmegen, Geert Grooteplein Noord 21,
    NL-6525 EZ Nijmegen, The Netherlands - tel. 80-514237

PAUSE Max, Institute of Physiology, Freie Universität
    Berlin, Arnimallee 22, D-1000 Berlin 33, FRG.

PETERSON Barry W., Dept. of Physiology, Northwestern
    University Medical School, 303 East Chicago Ave,
    Chicago IL 60611, USA - tel. 312-649-6216.

PIERROT-DESEILLIGNY Charles, Hôpital de la Salpêtrière,
    Bd de l'Hôpital, F-75013 Paris, France - tel. 584-
    14-12.

PRABLANC Claude, Unité 94, Laboratoire de Neuropsychologie Expérimentale INSERM, 16, Avenue Doyen Lépine, F-69500 Bron, France - tel. 7-8546578.

PRECHT Wolfgang, Brain Research Institute, University of Zürich, August Forelstr. 1, CH-8029 Zürich, Switzerland - tel. 533000.

REBER Annie, Université de Rouen, Laboratoire de Physiologie Animale, 10 bd. de Broglie, F-76130 Mont Saint Aignan, France - tel. 35- 982850.

REISINE Harvey, Neurology Dept. University Hospital Zürich, CH-8091 Zürich, Switzerland - tel. 255-3591.

REULEN Jos P.J., Dept. of Medical Physics, Vrije Universiteit, van der Boechorstst. 7, NL-1081 Amsterdam, The Netherlands - tel. 020-5482753.

REY J., Laboratoire de Psychophysiologie sensorielle, 9, quai St-Bernard, Bât.B, 3me ét., F-75005 Paris, France - tel. 1-3362525 ext. 3233/3400

ROBINSON David A., Depts. of Ophthalmology and Biomedical Engineering, The Johns Hopkins Univ., Baltimore, Maryland, USA - tel. 301-955-3587.

RON Samuel, Occupational Health and Rehabilitation Inst. at Loewenstein Hospital, Raanana 43100, Israël - tel. 052-91103.

ROUCOUX André, Laboratoire de Neurophysiologie, UCL 5449, Faculté de Médecine, Université Catholique de Louvain, Avenue Hippocrate, 54, B-1200 Bruxelles, Belgium - tel. 02-7623400 ext. 5447.

ROUCOUX-HANUS Marguerite, Laboratoire de Neurophysiologie, UCL 5449, Faculté de Médecine, Université Catholique de Louvain, Avenue Hippocrate, 54, B-1200 Bruxelles, Belgium - tel. 02-7623400 ext. 5447.

SCHMID Roberto, Istituto di Informatica e Sistemistica, Universita di Pavia, Strada Nuova 106/C, I-27100 Pavia, Italy - tel. 39-382-29142.

TAMMINGA Ernst Peter, Dept. of Physiology, Erasmus University, P.O. Box 1738, NL-3000 DR Rotterdam, The Netherlands - tel. 10-635770.

GISBERGEN Jan, Laboratory of Medical Physics and Biophysics, Geert Grooteplein N 21, NL-6525 EZ Nijmegen, The Netherlands - tel. 080-513326/514237.

VERAART Claude, Laboratoire de Neurophysiologie, UCL 5449, Faculté de Médecine, Université Catholique de Louvain, Avenue Hippocrate, 54, B-1200 Bruxelles, Belgium - tel. 02-7623400 ext. 5446.

VIDAL Pierre-Paul, Laboratoire de Physiologie Neuro-
    sensorielle CNRS, 15 rue de l'Ecole de Médecine,
    F-75006, Paris, France - tel. 3292177/3296154.

VILLALOBOS Julio, Laboratoire de Psychophysiologie
    Sensorielle, 9, quai St-Bernard, Bât. B, 3ème ét.,
    F-75005 Paris, France - tel. 1-3362525 ext. 3233/
    3400.

VIVIANI Paolo, Istituto di Fisiologia dei, Centri Nervo-
    si - CNR, 9, Via Mario Bianco, I-20131 Milano,
    Italy - tel. 39-2-2849220.

WAESPE Walter, Neurologische Klinik, Universität Zürich,
    Rämistr. 100, CH-8091 Zürich, Switzerland - tel. 01-
    2551111.

ZAMBARBIERI Daniela, Istituto di Informatico e Sistemis-
    tica, Universita di Pavia, Strada Nuova 106/C,
    I-27100 Pavia, Italy - tel. 39-382-29142.

ZEE David S., Depts of Neurology and Ophthalmology, The
    Johns Hopkins University, Baltimore, Maryland, USA
    - tel. 301-955-3319.

ZICOT-HOUTERS Laure, Rue Collard Trouillet, 51, B-4100
    Seraing, Belgium.

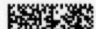